Core Curriculum *for* OCCUPATIONAL & ENVIRONMENTAL HEALTH NURSING

American Association of
Occupational Health Nurses, Inc.

THIRD EDITION

Edited by

MARY K. SALAZAR, EdD, RN, COHN-S, FAAN, FAAOHN

Professor
Department of Psychosocial and Community Health
University of Washington School of Nursing
Seattle, Washington

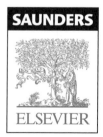

SAUNDERS

ELSEVIER

BP45

SAUNDERS
ELSEVIER

11830 Westline Industrial Drive
St. Louis, Missouri 63146

Core Curriculum for Occupational & Environmental Health Nursing   ISBN-13: 978-1-4160-2374-6
Copyright © 2006, Mosby Inc.   ISBN-10: 1-4160-2374-7

NOTICE

Nursing is an ever-changing field. Standard safety precautions must be followed, but as new research and clinical experience broaden our knowledge, changes in treatment and drug therapy may become necessary or appropriate. Readers are advised to check the most current product information provided by the manufacturer of each drug to be administered to verify the recommended dose, the method and duration of administration, and contraindications. It is the responsibility of the licensed prescriber, relying on experience and knowledge of the patient, to determine dosages and the best treatment for each individual patient. Neither the publisher nor the author assumes any liability for any injury and/or damage to persons or property arising from this publication.

Previous editions copyrighted 1997, 2001

ISBN-13: 978-1-4160-2374-6
ISBN-10: 1-4160-2374-7

Acquisitions Editor: Linda Thomas
Developmental Editor: Barbara Watts
Publishing Services Manager: Jeff Patterson
Project Manager: Jeanne Genz
Designer: Teresa McBryan

Working together to grow
libraries in developing countries
www.elsevier.com | www.bookaid.org | www.sabre.org

ELSEVIER   BOOK AID International   Sabre Foundation

Printed in the United States of America

Last digit is the print number: 9 8 7 6 5 4 3 2 1

12/19/06

CONTRIBUTORS

Jacqueline Agnew, PhD, MPH, COHN-S, FAAN
Professor & Director, Education and Research Center in Occupational Health and Safety
Johns Hopkins Bloomberg School of Hygiene and Public Health
Baltimore, Maryland

Mary C. Amann, RN, MS, COHN-S/CM, FAAOHN
Consultant, Occupational Health and Safety Information Management
Winter Park, Colorado

Randal D. Beaton, PhD, EMT
Research Professor
Department of Psychosocial and Community Health
School of Nursing
Adjunct Research Professor, Department of Health Services
School of Public Health and Community Medicine
Faculty, Northwest Center for Public Health Practice
University of Washington
Seattle, Washington

Anna M. Bruck, MN, RN, COHN-S
Lecturer, School of Nursing
Occupational Health Nurse, Employee Health Clinic
University of Washington
Seattle, Washington

Barbara Burgel, MS, RN, COHN-S, FAAN
Clinical Professor and Adult Nurse Practitioner
Occupational and Environmental Health Nursing Program
University of California, San Francisco
School of Nursing
San Francisco, California

Kay N. Campbell, EdD, RN-C, COHN-S
US Manager, Employee Health Services and Resilience
GlaxoSmithKline
Research Triangle Park, North Carolina

Eleanor McCarthy Chamberlin, RN, COHN-S, CCM
Occupational Health Nurse Consultant
Indialantic, Florida

Frances Childre, MS, RNC, ANP, COHN-S
National Manager—Health Services
Comprehensive Health Services, Inc.
Vienna, Virginia

Catherine Connon, PhD, RN
Lecturer
Department of Psychosocial and Community Health
University of Washington School of Nursing
Seattle, Washington

Deborah V. DiBenedetto, MBA, BSN, RN, COHN-S/CM, ABDA, FAAOHN
Manager Health and Productivity, The Kellogg Company
President, DVD Associates, LLC
Past-President, AAOHN
Battle Creek, Michigan

Mary E. Dirksen, MN, RN, COHN-S
Medical Field Volunteer
Doctors Without Borders / Médecins Sans Frontières
New York, NY
Employee Health Nurse / Infection Control Consultant
Harborview Medical Center
Seattle, Washington

Michelle Kom Gochnour, MN, RN, COHN-S
Occupational Health Nurse Consultant
Occupational Health Services
Children's Hospital and Regional
    Medical Center
Clinical Facility
Department of Psychosocial and
    Community Health
School of Nursing
University of Washington
Seattle, Washington

Marilyn L. Hau MS, RN-C, COHN-S, OHST, ASP, CHMM
Director of Environmental Health and
    Safety
University of Illinois at Chicago
Chicago Illinois

Diane Knoblauch, JD, MSN, RN
Attorney
Knoblauch Law Offices
Toledo, Ohio

Elizabeth Lawhorn, MSN, RN, COHN-S, CCM
U.S. Production Clinical Coordinator
ExxonMobil Corporation
Medicine and Occupational Health—
    Americas
Houston, Texas

Jane A. Lipscomb, Ph.D., RN, FAAN
Professor
University of Maryland
School of Nursing
Baltimore, Maryland

Sally L. Lusk, PhD, RN, FAAN, FAAOHN
Professor Emerita
University of Michigan School of Nursing
Ann Arbor, Michigan

Mary Miller, MN, RN
Occupational Health Nurse
Washington State Department of Labor
    and Industries
Olympia, Washington

Karin D. Myerson, BSN, RN, COHN-S
Director, Occupational Health
Washington Hospital Center
Washington, DC

Jane Parker-Conrad, PhD, RN, FAAOHN
Occupational Health Consultant
Knoxville, Tennessee

Jean Randolph, RN, COHN-S/CM, MPA
Occupational Health Manager
Children's Healthcare of Atlanta
Atlanta, Georgia

Delbert M. Raymond III, PhD, RN
Assistant Professor
Wayne State University College of
    Nursing
Detroit, Michigan

Lori K. Rieth, RN, MS, COHN-S/CM
Health and Disability Management
    Consulting
L. Reith & Associates
Grays Lake, Illinois

Bonnie Rogers, DrPH, COHN-S, LNCC, FAAN
Associate Professor
Director, North Carolina Occupational
    Safety and Health Education and
    Research Center
Director, Occupational Health Nursing
    Program
School of Public Health
University of North Carolina at Chapel
    Hill
Chapel Hill, North Carolina

Mary K. Salazar, EdD, RN, COHN-S, FAAN, FAAOHN
Professor
Department of Psychosocial and
    Community Health
University of Washington School of
    Nursing
Seattle, Washington

Barbara Sattler, RN, DrPH, FAAN
Associate Professor
Director, Environmental Health
  Education Center
University of Maryland School of Nursing
Baltimore, Maryland

Denise L. Souza, MSN, RN, ARNP,
COHN-S
Manager/Administrator, Occupational
  Health
Weyerhaeuser
Federal Way, Washington

Patricia B. Strasser, PhD, RN, COHN-
S/CM
Owner
Partners in BusinessHealth Solutions, Inc.
Toledo, Ohio

Weldonna Toth, MS, PhD, RN
Clinical Informaticist
CongniTech Corp
Salt Lake City, Utah

Joy E. Wachs, PhD, APRN, BC,
FAAOHN
Professor, Family/Community
  Nursing
East Tennessee State University
Mountain City, Tennessee

Mary Lou Wassel, MEd, RN, COHN-
S/CM, ARM
Senior Loss Control Representative
Companion Property & Casualty
  Group
Yorktown, Virginia

FOREWORD

The American Association of Occupational Health Nurses (AAOHN) proudly presents the third edition of its Core Curriculum for Occupational and Environmental Health Nursing. This widely used reference continues to provide a comprehensive framework for occupational and environmental health nursing practice. It includes newly updated material throughout, plus a chapter on disaster planning and management, a topic of ongoing emphasis since the horrific events of September 11, 2001. All of this reflects the dynamic and evolving role that occupational and environmental health nurses assume in promoting the health of workers and preventing injuries and illnesses.

Changes in the work force, workplace, and health care affect the delivery of occupational health services. Of continued importance will be the control of health-care costs within the context of integrated worker health, safety, and productivity management programs. While many chronic conditions are preventable through lifestyle choices, more can be done through coordinated programs that incorporate health promotion and health protection. Occupational and environmental health nurses must be aware of work-force and workplace trends to design and provide health care programs and services that are appropriate and strategic, many of which are described throughout the text.

The Core Curriculum, in conjunction with the Code of Ethics, Standards of Practice, and Competencies, as established by AAOHN, the professional association for occupational and environmental health nurses, provides the basis for scope of practice, knowledge, skills, and the ethical and legal framework in the specialty area. This resource will prove invaluable to practicing occupational health professionals with varying backgrounds or levels of preparation, those considering a career in occupational safety and health, and others wanting a refresher of major concepts and principles. We hope you will find this latest edition of the AAOHN Core Curriculum for Occupational and Environmental Health Nursing a valuable resource.

Susan A. Randolph,
President
AAOHN

PREFACE

In 1997, the American Association of Occupational Health Nurses released the first edition of the core curriculum for occupational and environmental health nursing. This text, which is designed to serve as a comprehensive resource and practical guide for occupational and environmental health nurses, is divided into three major sections. The first section, called "Foundations of Occupational and Environmental Health Nursing Practice," provides the theoretical and conceptual overview of this specialty area including the traditions, the basic concepts and the sciences that serve as the underpinnings of occupational health and safety practice, education and research. Topics in this section include leadership and management, business and economic trends, and ethical and legal issues that shape and influence our specialty. The second section, "Strategies and Approaches to Occupational and Environmental Health Nursing Practice," provides an in-depth guide to the practical aspects of our specialty. It begins with an overview of the strategic processes that are essential to the development of a comprehensive health and safety program; it then describes specific programs and services such as direct care, disability case management and health promotion. The section concludes with several examples of specific programs that are often offered in occupational settings. The final section, "Advancing Professionalism in Occupational and Environmental Health Nursing," highlights issues and activities that facilitate the development of knowledge and that contribute to occupational and environmental health nurses' professional growth and development.

While the important core elements presented in the initial text have been retained in the two subsequent editions (including this one), the information in the last two editions has been designed to broaden and deepen the occupational and environmental health nurses' knowledge and understanding of this complex area of practice. The content for these later editions were influenced by social, economic and political changes that have affected the nature of our practice. They also include content related to changes in health care delivery that have the potential to affect workers. A major change in the second edition was the increased emphasis on environmental health, which was consistent with changes that were occurring within professional practice and reflected in other documents developed by AAOHN. The word "environment" was added to the title, and a chapter focusing on environmental health was added. Other additions to the second edition included new chapters focusing on psychosocial factors in the occupational setting, case management and information management systems.

Although it has been merely five years since the publication of the second edition, the roles and functions of occupational and environmental health nurses continues to evolve and develop as a result of internal and external influences. An increasing number of workers are telecommuting; American workers are getting older and more ethnically and culturally diverse; and the characteristics of the work environment are being affected by modern day information and communication systems. As science and technology advance, as the globalization of the workplace increases, and as new societal threats emerge, the hazards faced by workers are also affected. These many changes in the work life of American workers are reflected in this third edition. Some examples of new and expanded content include recently passed regulations such as HIPPA (Health Insurance

Portability and Accountability Act) and CLIA (Clinical Laboratory Improvement Amendments) (Chapter 3); innovative models of leadership and management (Chapter 7), advanced safety measures such as comprehensive containment approaches (Chapter 10), and valuable updates on specific worksite programs (i.e., hearing loss prevention, drug and alcohol testing, international travel) (Chapter 16). A major contribution to this third edition is the inclusion of one additional chapter focusing on disaster management. This was partially inspired by the events of September 11, 2001, but it is also reflective of the increased importance of the occupational and environmental health nurses' role in the event of any disaster, natural or man-made. As in previous editions, the appendices that supplement this text were carefully selected to complement the content that is included in these 18 chapters. The appendices include a glossary, a list of useful occupational health and safety resources, and relevant websites.

It is important to remind ourselves why we do what we do. We are members of an extraordinarily successful group of professionals whose primary role is to protect workers and worker populations from work-related injury and illnesses—and, without a doubt, we are making strides towards the achievement of this goal. It is notable, for example, that since the passage of the Occupational Safety and Health Act in 1970, occupational injury and illness rates have decreased by 40 percent and workplace fatalities by more than 60 percent. In fact, recorded occupational fatalities in recent years have been at an all time low. Nevertheless, we cannot rest on our laurels. A core premise of occupational health and safety is that *all* workplace injuries and illnesses are preventable; thus despite our achievements, much work remains to be done to assure the protection of our nation's workers.

It is an exciting time to be an occupational and environmental health nurse. Nurses in our specialty are assuming innovative roles and increasing responsibilities as they strive to respond to a changing and more complex work environment. The complexity of providing effective occupational health services is compounded by a constantly changing social, economic and political climate, by many challenges related to health care delivery, and by rapid and multiple technological changes. Indeed, the prevention of injury and disease is the most critical role for occupational health and safety professionals, and occupational and environmental health nurses are in a key position to make that happen! It is hoped that this text will inform you so that you can be effective in your efforts to achieve this end, that the information contained herein will assist you as you become leaders and managers in your organizations, and, importantly, that you will be inspired to carry the banner in multiple forums on behalf of the health and safety of workers everywhere.

Mary K. Salazar
Managing Editor

ACKNOWLEDGMENTS

The completion of this third edition of the *Core Curriculum for Occupational and Environmental Health Nursing* is a result of the dedication and hard work of numerous individuals. I am especially grateful to the chapter authors for the excellence of their work and the timeliness of their contributions. Thanks to each and every one of you for your patience and perseverance in meeting what seemed to be an impossible timeline. Your dedication and commitment to occupational and environmental health nursing is inspiring! I am honored to have had this opportunity to work with you on this important endeavor.

Thanks, too, to the many others who worked behind the scenes to assure the high quality of this publication. These include American Association of Occupational Health Nurses' staff members, Marcia Noble, MN, RN, former Director of Professional Practice, Dean M. Burgess, MSN, RN, COHN-S, Directors of Professional Affairs and Ann Cox, MN, RN, CAE, Executive Director; the Elsevier staff, especially Linda Thomas, Managing Editor, Barbara Watts, Developmental Editor and Jeanne Genz, Project Manager; Mary Love, Senior Secretary in the University of Washington School of Nursing, who assisted with the preparation of some of the figures; and Brenda James, who assisted with the review of the reference lists.

I also want to acknowledge the support and encouragement from friends and family, especially Jerry, Mike, Gretchen, Brenda, Darren, Carolyn, Kaitlyn, Brittany and Alyssa; also thanks to Sheila and John and Gene and Marilu. You are all wonderful!

Lastly but importantly, I want to thank the members of the American Association of Occupational Health Nurses for their dedication and commitment to the health and safety of our nation's workers.

CONTENTS

SECTION ONE

Foundations of Occupational and Environmental Health Nursing Practice

1. *Occupational and Environmental Health Nursing: An Overview,* 3
   MARY E. DIRKSEN

   Introduction to Occupational Health and Safety, 3
   Historical Perspective on Work and Occupational Health, 4
   Evolution of Occupational Health and Safety, 7
   Brief History of Workers' Compensation, 13
   The Occupational Safety and Health Act, 14
   National Health Goals: Healthy People and Healthy Communities, 15
   Occupational Health in the International Community, 15
   The Workplace: Occupational Hazards and Their Impact on Workers, 17
   Work-Related Injury and Illness, 19
   Assessment and Prevention of Occupational and Environmental
       Injury and Illness, 23
   History and Evolution of Occupational and Environmental
       Health Nursing, 24
   The Practice of Occupational and Environmental Health
       Nursing, 25
   Future Opportunities and Challenges, 31

2. *Workers and Worker Populations,* 35
   SALLY L. LUSK, DELBERT M. RAYMOND III, CATHERINE CONNON, AND MARY MILLER

   Demographic and Social Trends, 35
   Technologic Trends, 38
   Females in the Workforce, 40
   Minorities in the Workforce, 41
   Age of Workers, 42
   Children in the Workforce, 44
   Contingent and Other Alternative Workers, 48
   Workers in Labor Unions, 50
   Disabled Workers, 51
   Agricultural Workers, 53
   Construction Workers, 56
   Health Care Workers, 58
   International (Expatriate) Workers, 63

3. *Legal and Ethical Issues,* 71
DIANE KNOBLAUCH AND PATRICIA B. STRASSER

Sources of Law, 71
Basic Legal Concepts Relevant to Occupational and
  Environmental Health Nursing Practice, 72
Legal Responsibilities of the Occupational and Environmental
  Health Nurse, 73
Occupational Safety and Health Act (Public Law 91-596), 73
Americans with Disabilities Act (ADA) of 1990, 77
Family and Medical Leave Act (FMLA) of 1993 (29CFR825.118), 79
The Department of Transportation, 81
Clinical Laboratory Improvement Amendments (CLIA), 82
Documentation, 83
Recordkeeping, 84
Access to Employee Medical and Exposure Records, 88
HIPAA (Health Insurance Portability and Accountability
  Act, 1996), 90
Overview of Workers' Compensation, 93
Overview of Workers' Compensation Benefits, 94
Professional Position on Ethics, 95
Ethics: Definitions and Principles, 95
Ethical Conflicts, 96

4. *Economic, Political, and Business Forces,* 101
DEBORAH V. DIBENEDETTO

Introduction to Economics, 101
Economic State of the Nation, 103
The Impact of Economics on the Individual, 104
Changes in the National Economy, 105
Factors Affecting National and Global Competitiveness, 105
International Trade Status of the Nation, 106
The Global Marketplace, 107
Implications for the Occupational and Environmental
  Health Nurse, 108
Business Trends, 108
Major Business Issues, 109
Implications for Occupational and Environmental Health Nursing, 112
Health Care Reform and Managed Health Care, 113
Overview of Managed Care, 113
Quality Controls in Managed Care, 114
Judging Standards of Care, 115
Defining and Evaluating Quality Outcomes, 115
Implications for Occupational and Environmental Health Nursing, 116

5. *Scientific Foundations of Occupational and Environmental Health Nursing Practice,   119*
JACQUELINE AGNEW

Nursing Science,   119
Nursing Science in the Context of Public Health,   119
Evolution of Occupational and Environmental Health
    Nursing Practice,   121
Epidemiology,   123
Overview of Epidemiologic Terms and Principles,   123
Measures of Association,   124
Sources of Epidemiologic Data,   124
Comparisons of Rates,   125
Types of Rates,   125
Inferential Statistics,   126
Overview of Study Designs,   126
Bias and Confounding in Epidemiologic Studies,   127
Screening,   129
Toxicology,   130
Overview of Toxicologic Terms and Principles,   130
Major Exposure Routes,   131
The Dose-Response Relationship,   132
Nature of Effects,   132
The Fate of Toxins in the Body,   133
Endogenous and Exogenous Host Factors,   133
Examples of Exposures and Their Effects,   134
Industrial Hygiene,   141
Overview of Industrial Hygiene,   141
Sources of Information to Facilitate Hazard Recognition,   141
Sampling Methods,   142
Airborne Contaminants,   143
Control Strategies for Occupational Exposures,   143
Ergonomics,   143
Overview of Ergonomic Terms and Principles,   143
Work-Related Musculoskeletal Disorders,   144
High-Risk Jobs,   145
Evaluating Risk Factors,   145
Ergonomic Improvements,   146
Injury Epidemiology,   147
Occupational Injury Epidemiology,   147
Countermeasures,   147
Implications for Occupational and Environmental Health
    Nurses,   148
Social and Behavioral Sciences,   149

Effects of Social Conditions and Behavior on Health,   149
Health Promotion and Risk Reduction,   150

6. *Environmental Health,   153*
BARBARA SATTLER AND JANE LIPSCOMB

Introduction,   153
Environmental Health Assessment,   155
Children and Environmental Health,   158
Environmental Justice and Advocacy,   160
Risk Assessment, Risk Management, and Risk Communication,   161
Federal Agencies,   165
Public Health Infrastructure,   168
Accessing Information and the "Right to Know,"   169
Environmental Health Risks Across Settings,   172
Environmental Health Risks in the Home,   172
Environmental Risks in Schools,   174
Environmental Risks in the Community,   175
Industrial Pollutants,   179
Nurses' Roles in Environmental Health,   179
General Environmental Health Competency for Nurses,   179
The Institute of Medicine's Recommendations on Nursing
    Practice, Education, Research, and Advocacy,   180

7. *Principles of Leadership and Management,   183*
JOY E. WACHS AND FRANCES CHILDRE

Leadership,   183
Vision,   184
Relationship,   185
Strategic Planning,   186
Management Theories: Historical Perspective,   187
The Management Process,   189
Phase 1 of Task Cycle®: *Making Goals Clear and Important,   190*
Phase 2 of Task Cycle®: *Planning and Problem-Solving,   191*
Phase 3 of Task Cycle®: *Facilitating the Work of Others,   194*
Phase 4 of Task Cycle®: *Obtaining and Providing Feedback,   200*
Phase 5 of Task Cycle®: *Monitoring and Adjusting the Process,   205*
Phase 6 of Task Cycle®: *Reinforcing Performance,   207*
Power: Concern for Influencing People,   208
The Image of the Occupational and Environmental Health Nurse,   209
Customer Service,   209

8. *Information Management in the Occupational Health Setting,   215*
MARY C. AMANN AND DONNI TOTH

Introduction to Nursing Informatics,   215

Tools Available to the Occupational and Environmental
Health Nurse,   216
Selecting and Implementing Information Management Systems,   217
The Internet,   224
Intranets,   227
Security,   227
Office Management Programs,   229
Implications for Occupational and Environmental Health Nursing,   230

SECTION TWO

Strategies and Approaches to Occupational and Environmental Health Nursing Practice

9. *Developing, Implementing, and Evaluating Comprehensive Occupational Health and Safety Programs,*   237
KARIN D. MYERSON AND JANE PARKER-CONRAD

Assessment,   237
Program Planning,   239
Program Implementation,   241
Program Evaluation,   242
Methods of Evaluation,   248
Cost-Effective and Cost-Benefit Programs and Services,   249
Other Health and Safety Program Considerations,   251

10. *Prevention of Occupational Injuries and Illnesses,*   255
MARILYN L. HAU

Recognition and Identification,   255
First Steps in a Prevention Program,   255
Methods of Identifying Hazards,   256
Hazard Evaluation and Analysis,   264
Purpose of Hazard Evaluation and Analysis,   265
Industry Standards,   265
Risk Analysis,   267
Exposure Monitoring,   268
Worker Populations Analysis,   271
Prevention and Control,   274
Prevention and Control Approaches That Focus on Engineering
Controls,   274
Prevention and Control Approaches That Focus on Administrative
Controls,   279
Prevention and Control Approaches That Focus on Personal Protective
Equipment,   285
Prevention and Control program That Focus on Comprehensive
Containment Approaches,   290

11. *Direct Care in the Occupational Setting, 295*
BARBARA BURGEL

Direct Care Professional Practice Concepts,   295
Overview of Direct Care,   296
Health History,   300
The Physical Examination,   302
Clinical Decision Making,   307
Practice Guidelines,   309
Application of Levels of Prevention to Direct Care Activities,   310
Evaluating Outcomes,   323

12. *Disability Case Management, 331*
MARY LOU WASSEL, JEAN RANDOLPH, AND LORI K. RIETH

Case Management,   331
Important Case Management Terms,   331
Historical Perspective,   333
Case Management Services: Practice Settings and Providers,   337
Team Roles and Responsibilities,   338
Steps in Program Development,   340
Return to Work (RTW),   345
Integrated Disability Management Programs,   359
Federal Acts,   360
Delivery Models,   360

13. *Disaster Planning and Management, 365*
MARILYN L. HAU

Disaster Characteristics,   365
Disaster Planning and Preparedness,   369
Disaster Response,   377
Disaster Recovery,   385
Natural Hazard-Specific Considerations (FEMA, 2004),   386
Technologic Hazard-Specific Considerations,   387
Conflict-Related Hazard-Specific Considerations,   389
Terrorism,   390
Template Emergency Preparedness/Disaster Management Plan,   397
Appendices to Include in a Written Plan,   405

14. *Health Promotion and Adult Education, 409*
KAY N. CAMPBELL

Overview of Health Promotion,   409
National Health Promotion Objectives,   413
Health Models,   413
Behavior Change Theories and Models,   416
Levels of Prevention,   420
Framework for a Health Promotion Program,   420
Lifestyle and Health Promotion,   424

Employee Assistance Programs (EAPs),   431
Introduction to Adult Education,   433
Philosophies of Adult Education,   434
Motivating Adults to Learn,   436
Teaching Methods and Techniques,   437
Effective Presentations,   437

15. *Managing Psychosocial Factors in the Occupational Setting,*   451
MARY K. SALAZAR AND RANDAL D. BEATON

Overview of Psychosocial Factors,   451
Psychosocial Hazards,   453
Occupational Stress,   460
Effects of Stress on Workers,   461
Effects of Stress on Organizations,   462
Occupational Stress Models,   462
An Ecologic Approach to Occupational Stress,   464
Managing Psychosocial Factors in the Occupational Setting,   465
Evaluating Interventions That Promote Psychosocial Health
    in the Occupational Setting,   468

16. *Examples of Occupational Health and Safety Programs,*   473
MICHELLE KOM GOCHNOUR, ANNIE BRUCK, AND DENISE SOUZA

Hearing-loss Prevention Programs and Services,   473
Noise-Induced Hearing Loss,   473
Purposes of a Hearing-loss Prevention Program,   474
Roles and Responsibilities Related to Hearing-loss Prevention
    Programs,   475
Assessment and Control of Noise Exposure,   476
Worker Training and Education,   477
Hearing Protection Devices,   479
Audiometric Testing,   480
Monitoring and Evaluating a Hearing-loss Protection Program,   482
Ergonomics Programs,   483
Overview of Ergonomics,   483
Work-Related Musculoskeletal Disorders,   484
Ergonomic Regulation and Guidelines,   485
Purposes of Ergonomics Programs and Services,   486
Ergonomics Programs and Services,   486
Training and Education,   491
Management of Work-Related Musculoskeletal Disorders (WMSD) as
    Part of a Comprehensive Ergonomics Program,   492
Documentation and Recordkeeping,   492
Program Evaluation,   493
Hazard Communication Programs and Services, 494
Hazardous Chemical Exposure,   494
Purposes of a Hazard Communications Program,   494
Management Roles and Responsibilities,   494

Description of the Programs and Services,   495
Elements of the HazCom Program,   496
Material Safety Data Sheets (MSDSs), 497
Trade Secrets,   498
Container Labeling and Warning Requirements,   498
Recordkeeping,   498
Evaluation,   498
Drug and Alcohol Programs and Services,   499
Mandated Drug and Alcohol Programs,   499
Establishing a Drug-Free Workplace,   500
Purposes of a Drug and Alcohol Testing Program,   502
Program Components,   502
Methods and Procedures of a Drug and Alcohol Testing Program,   503
Employee Assistance Programs,   505
Training and Education,   505
Consequences of Drug and Alcohol Abuse and Return to Duty,   506
International Travel Health and Safety Program,   506
International Business and the International Work Force,   506
Roles and Responsibilities Related to International Travel Programs,   507
Health and Safety Education for Travel,   508
Control of Prevalent Communicable Diseases,   511
Post-Travel Evaluation for Long-Term Travelers,   512

SECTION THREE

Advancing Professionalism in Occupational and Environmental Health Nursing

17.   *Research,   519*
BONNIE ROGERS

Professional Mandates for Research,   519
Research Roles of Occupational and Environmental Health Nurses
    by Education Level,   519
Purposes of Research,   520
Ethics in Research,   520
Research Development,   521
Research Dissemination,   526
Research Utilization,   526
Research Priorities,   527
Evaluating Research,   528
Funding Research,   529

18. *Professional Issues: Advancing the Specialty,*   *533*
ELEANOR MCCARTHY CHAMBERLIN AND ELIZABETH LAWHORN

Professional Associations,   533
Professional Credentialing in Nursing,   534
Competency in Occupational and Environmental Health Nursing,   537
Strategies for Advancing the Discipline and Practice,   538
Role Expansion,   540
Partnerships in Occupational and Environmental Health,   542

APPENDIXES

I. *Occupational and Environmental Health and Safety Resources,*   *545*
II. *Glossary,*   *551*
III. *Acronyms,*   *557*
IV. *Websites,*   *562*
V. *Occupational Safety and Health Administration Act of 1970,*   *565*
VI. *Competencies in Occupational and Environmental Health Nursing,*   *567*
VII. *Standards of Occupational and Environmental Health Nursing,*   *568*
VIII. *American Association of Occupational Health Nurses' Code of Ethics,*   *570*
IX. *Legislation Related to Occupational Health and Safety,*   *571*

INDEX,   575

SECTION ONE

Foundations of Occupational and Environmental Health Nursing Practice

~

CHAPTER

1

Occupational and Environmental Health Nursing: An Overview

Mary E. Dirksen

The primary focus of occupational and environmental health nursing practice is preventing work-related illnesses and injuries and promoting health and safety among workers, worker populations, and communities. Achieving these goals requires a clear understanding of the basic terminology used in this specialty and knowledge of the principles that underpin occupational and environmental health nursing practice, education, and research. This chapter presents an overview of the traditions and concepts inherent to the field, and a historical perspective of the development of the profession and practice.

I Introduction to Occupational Health and Safety

A The mission of occupational health and safety is "to assure so far as possible every working man and woman in the nation safe and healthful working conditions" (United States Congress, Occupational Safety and Health Act, 1970; see Appendix V).

B The primary objectives of occupational health and safety practice include the following:

1. Preventing work-related illnesses and injuries through a systematic process of assessment, data collection, planning, intervention, and evaluation
2. Evaluating and treating work-related injury or illness
3. Promoting health and safety behaviors among workers and worker populations
4. Implementing hazard prevention and abatement interventions that promote safe and healthy work environments while remaining consistent with organizational goals
5. Advocating organizational attention to environmental concerns on behalf of workers, their families, and the broader community

C The goals and objectives of occupational health and safety practice are achieved through the collaboration of multiple professional disciplines, which may include the following, depending on the needs of the work setting and the scope of the organization's occupational health program:

1. *Occupational and environmental health nurses* focus on promoting, protecting, restoring, and maintaining workers' health within the context of a safe and healthful work environment.

3

2. *Occupational physicians* focus on preventing, detecting, and treating work-related diseases and injuries.

3. *Industrial hygienists* identify, evaluate, and control toxic exposures and hazards in the work environment.

4. *Safety engineers* and other safety professionals focus on preventing occupational injuries and maintaining or creating safe workplaces and safe work practices.

5. Other professionals provide specific expertise as required by the occupational health and safety program and service needs of the organization; these could include *epidemiologists, toxicologists, industrial engineers, ergonomists, health educators, occupational and physical therapists,* and *vocational rehabilitation specialists.*

D **The workplace is characterized by multidimensional and complex environments that affect worker health and safety. These environments include the following (Figure 1-1):**

1. Social: the meaning of work, the social milieu of the worker (including the worker's baseline health status) and the structure of work

2. Cultural: beliefs, attitudes, and values related to work

3. Political: the prevalent ideology in a society; the distribution of power and level of governmental support for worker health and safety

4. Economic: the levels of unemployment, competition, and wage regulation, and the overall health of the local economy

5. Organizational: corporate mission, philosophy, and values; financial and structural viability of the organization; job security issues; and production structure and requirements

E **Occupational health and safety should be considered an integral part of all health programs and services.**

1. Most Americans are directly or indirectly affected by hazards in the workplace.

2. Occupational health and safety programs and services affect not only the worker, but also the worker's family, significant others, community, and the larger society.

F **Occupational and environmental health sciences are in an early stage of development; much remains to be learned about the effect of the work environment on the health and safety of workers.**

II Historical Perspective on Work and Occupational Health

The concept and value of work is fundamental to every nation, race, culture, and time.

A **The earliest reference to occupational health was made by Hippocrates.**

1. Hippocrates recognized clusters of specific diseases that were more prevalent in craftsmen by 400 BC (Hunter, 1978).

2. Pliny the Elder (23-79 AD) observed ancient miners wearing protective breathing devices to avoid inhaling toxic dusts and vapors.

B **Much work in the Middle Ages (roughly 500-1500 AD) occurred in homes and small shops.**

1. Profitable work consisted primarily of crafts and arts using various metals, chemicals, and minerals, the use of which was accompanied by observed adverse health effects.

2. Most manufacturing was conducted in rural homes, although some occurred in guild shops in towns.

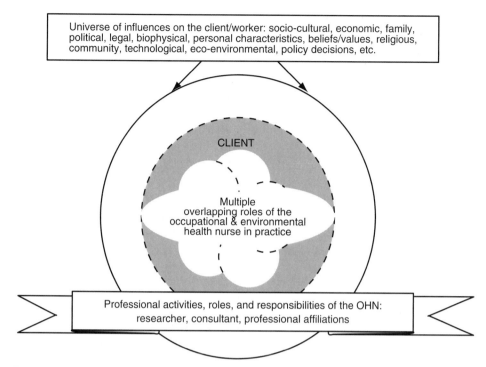

FIGURE 1-1 *A model for occupational and environmental health nursing.*

This model illustrates the interconnectedness and fluidity of the elements constituting and affected by the practice of occupational and environmental health nursing. The clients, whether individual workers, aggregates of workers, or an organization's administration, are influenced by the universe of work-related and external variables, all of which affect the individual, collective, or organizational state of health and safety. The roles and responsibilities of the occupational and environmental health nurse overlap. All interactions between the occupational health nurse and the client are bound together and guided by the professional responsibilities and activities engaged in by the occupational and environmental health nurse. The junction at which the occupational health nurse and the client meet, each bringing their individual and collective experience to the interaction (as illustrated by the broken lines), represents the common ground where health and safety goals are mutually determined and realized. (Source: Dirksen, et al., 1994)

3. Increased competition resulted in increased production and escalating work hazards.

C Some notable commentaries on occupational health and safety were presented in the pre-industrial age.
  1. Georgius Agricola (1494-1555 AD) described the ailments of miners, such as joint, lung, and eye problems.
  2. Paracelsus (1493-1541 AD):
     a. Identified acute and chronic health effects in craftsmen exposed to metal smelting fumes
     b. Articulated the principle paradigm of toxicology, the dose/response ratio, when he wrote: "All substances are poisons; there is none which is not. Only the dose differentiates a poison from a remedy."
  3. Bernardino Ramazzini (1633-1714 AD), considered the "father of occupational medicine:"

    a. Published *De Morbis Artifactum Diatriba (The Diseases of Workmen)* in 1713, describing more than 100 different trade occupations, their associated hazards, and various methods of protection for tradespeople, including protective clothing, adequate ventilation, and proper working posture

    b. Noted that workers "who hoped for a subsistence . . . are too often repaid with the most dangerous diseases" (Ramazzini, 1993, p. 39)

    c. Encouraged physicians to inquire into their patients' occupations as part of their assessments

D **A major shift in working conditions occurred during the industrial revolution (mid-18th to mid-19th century).**

1. Ordinary citizens' lifestyles in European and American societies were transformed by the shift from agrarian or home-based hand manufacturing to urban-based industrial processes.

2. Power-driven machinery introduced dramatic changes in production and work process.

    a. Mass factory production began in England in 1718 with the first mechanized silk-textile mill.

    b. Machine-driven jobs became specialized and work became monotonous.

3. The economic and social impact of work-related injury, illness, and death became evident with the high rates of factory workers affected.

E **American workers' health and safety were profoundly affected by the industrial revolution.**

1. American economic focus shifted from agriculture to industry.

    a. Millions flocked to urban industrial centers for the promise of cash wages and an improved lifestyle.

    b. Company-owned housing districts became overcrowded, unsanitary centers of poverty and communicable disease.

    c. The abundant labor supply gave rise to massive exploitation of women, children, and non–English speaking immigrants; child labor, indentured servitude, and slavery were routine.

2. Trends toward division of labor, ownership of the means of production, and capitalism emerged.

    a. Accidents and workplace deaths were considered inevitable and acceptable consequences of progress.

    b. The industrial ethic of the time placed profit and property rights above human rights.

3. Working conditions were abysmal; machines were largely without protective devices and accidental-death rates were high.

F **During the industrial and postindustrial eras, responsibility for work-related injuries and illnesses was placed on the worker rather than on the hazards that caused injury and illness.**

1. Company-based industrial medicine programs and services focused on pre-employment physical examinations.

2. Primary causes of accidents were identified as lack of English language skills, inexperience, and worker carelessness.

3. Prevention strategies were aimed at altering worker behaviors rather than controlling or preventing workplace hazard sources.

4. The economic and social conditions prevalent in the early 20th century led to a rise in the number of industrial nurses.

5. Alice Hamilton (1869-1970), considered the "matriarch of American occupational health":
   a. Was the first American physician to devote her life's work to industrial health
   b. Studied and documented the adverse human effects associated with occupational exposure to industrial toxins such as lead, arsenic, carbon monoxide, and solvents
   c. Published *Industrial Poisons in the United States* (1925) and *Exploring the Dangerous Trades* (1943)
   d. Served as editor of *The Journal of Industrial Hygiene*

III Evolution of Occupational Health and Safety

A Government agencies and legislation focusing on workplace health and safety emerged during the industrial revolution (Appendix VII)

1. Formal workplace regulation began in the textile manufacturing sector in England; between 1802 and 1891, eight Factory Acts were passed, aimed at improving conditions for laborers, including:
   a. Limiting working hours to 12 hours daily, which at the time was an improvement
   b. Raising the minimal age limit for working children from 10 years to 11 years
   c. Prohibiting the employment of pregnant women within 1 month of delivery
   d. Requiring that workplace injuries or deaths be reported to a surgeon, who was required to investigate the cause and report the result to the factory inspector
   e. Requiring protective fencing for machinery
2. In the United States, Massachusetts created the first factory inspection department in 1867.
3. State and federal reporting requirements for industrial accidents began in the late 1800s.
4. The concerns of workers and occupational health and safety professionals have historically and often been misperceived as opposing those of the business sector; hence passage of state and federal legislation aimed at improving the conditions of workers and workplaces is often won only after overwhelming evidence and an intensive lobbying effort or after a disastrous industrial accident. Box 1-1 presents federal agencies and legislation governing workers and workplaces.

B Organized labor has been involved in occupational health and safety in various capacities. (Box 1-2, pp.10-12, presents a chronology of significant events in the labor movement.)

1. As workers began to assert their demands for workplace health and safety reforms, tensions between labor and management increased.
2. Among the few early strategies effective in improving workplace conditions were labor strikes and lawsuits brought by injured workers against employers.
3. Although union membership has been steadily decreasing from a high of 20% in 1983, the influence of these organizations reaches far beyond their unionized workplaces.
4. In 2003, 12.9% of U.S. workforce consisted of union members (US Department of Labor [USDL], Bureau of Labor Statistics [BLS], 2004a).

BOX 1-1

State and federal agencies and legislation affecting occupational and environmental health in the United States

1867	The first factory inspection department was created in Massachusetts
1869	The Bureau of Labor Statistics was established Pennsylvania passed legislation requiring two exits from all mines
1877	Employer Liability Law was passed Massachusetts passed the first law requiring safeguards for hazardous machinery
1884	The Federal Bureau of Labor, reorganized as the United States Department of Labor (USDL) in 1913, was created to "foster, promote and develop the welfare of wage earners in the United States" (from William B. Wilson, first USDL secretary, 1913-1921).
1907	The U.S. Department of Interior created the Bureau of Mines to investigate accidents, examine health hazards, and make recommendations for improvements
1911	Wisconsin passed the first effective worker's compensation law
1912	The U.S. Public Health Service (USPHS) was established to scientifically investigate and analyze the effects of toxins on individual workers
1913	The U.S. Department of Labor was established The National Council of Industrial Safety was organized, and renamed two years later as the National Safety Council to collect and document occupational injury and illness data
1916	The Office of Worker's Compensation Programs (OWCP) was established for federal employees
1933	The New Deal, introduced by President Franklin D. Roosevelt, included occupational health reform statutes, and encouraged a renewed advocacy for workplace health and safety—efforts that had waned in the anti-labor sentiment following World War I
1934	The Division of Labor Standards was established to collaborate with other organizations to develop safety codes and standards, disseminate information about chemical hazards to workers, and improve the efficacy of factory inspection processes
1935	The Social Security Act was signed into law
1935	The National Labor Relations Act of 1935 (Wagner Act) was enacted to govern relations between workers and management which had, before that time, been confrontational, litigious, and sometimes violent
1938	The Fair Labor Standards Act (FLSA) established the first minimum wage at 25 cents/hour, which was well below what most covered workers already earned; additionally, FLSA initiated the 8-hour workday
1963	The Equal Pay Act banned wage discrimination based on gender
1964	The Civil Rights Act banned institutional forms of racial discrimination
1968	The standard 8-hour workday was federally legislated

Sources: Houghton Mifflin, US DOL

BOX 1-1

State and federal agencies and legislation affecting occupational and environmental health in the United States—cont'd

1970 The Occupational Safety and Health Act (OSH Act) was signed into law and established the Occupational Safety and Health Administration (OSHA) as an agency within the USDL and

The OSH Act established the National Institute for Occupational Safety and Health (NIOSH) as an institute within the USPHS; it is currently positioned within the Centers for Disease Control and Prevention (CDC)

1977 The Federal Mine Safety Act was passed

1986 The Superfund Amendments and Reauthorization Act (SARA) was passed

The Community Right-to-Know Act was passed, requiring that the public be made aware of any potentially hazardous materials used by local industries

1990 The Amended Clean Air Act of 1970 was passed

1993 The Family and Medical Leave Act required covered employers to provide up to 12 weeks unpaid leave and continued medical benefits to eligible employees during any 12-month period

1997 Tuberculosis standard was proposed and defeated

2000 After a 10-year effort by OSHA and state OSH Administrations, a federal ergonomic standard was released; it was overturned the following year by the president and congress

---

5. Labor unions represent and pursue the collective interests of workers in matters of health and safety, often in collaboration with occupational health and safety professionals.
   a. Unionized workers are more likely to be informed about the presence of health and safety hazards than are nonunion workers in the same jobs.
   b. Successful campaigns conducted by labor unions include, but are not limited to, the following:
      1) The 8-hour work day, which was federally legislated in 1968
      2) Overtime compensation
      3) Employer-paid health insurance for industrial workers
      4) Regulations aimed at protecting farm and field workers against the dangers of pesticide exposure, including lengthening re-entry periods beyond state and federal standards, requiring testing of farm workers on a regular basis to monitor exposure levels, and restricting the use of dangerous pesticides
      5) Occupational Safety and Health Administration's (OSHA) Cotton Dust Standard of 1978
      6) OSHA's Occupational Tuberculosis Standard, which was proposed in 1997, after years of lobbying mainly by the health care and social services sectors; OSHA withdrew its proposed standard after intense opposition by business and employer groups

> ## BOX 1-2
> *A chronology of the organized labor movement in the United States*
>
> | | |
> |---|---|
> | 1600s | Agriculture was the major U.S. industry |
> | 1739 | Boston shipyard workers formed the first political organization, called the "Caucus" |
> | 1750 | Trade associations developed among carpenters, tailors, and iron-workers |
> | 1780s | American and European economies shifted to a merchant/capitalist system |
> | 1786 | Philadelphia printers conducted the first successful strike for higher wages |
> | 1791 | Philadelphia carpenters waged the first strike in the building trades, demanding a 10-hour workday |
> | 1836 | The 10-hour workday was initiated after a general labor strike in Philadelphia the previous year |
> | 1866 | The National Labor Union was established following an economic depression |
> | 1867 | Factory inspection was introduced in Massachusetts |
> | 1868 | The first barrier safeguard patent was awarded |
> | 1869 | The Noble and Holy Knights of Labor, one of the earliest labor unions, which admitted into membership both skilled and unskilled workers of both sexes, was formed and began agitating for workplace safety laws |
> | 1869 | The Colored National Labor Union was formed |
> | 1876 | The Socialist Labor Party established its headquarters in Newark, New Jersey; the party was renamed in 1877 as the Workingmen's Party of America |
> | 1882 | The first Labor Day Parade was organized in New York City |
> | 1886 | The American Federation of Labor (AFL) was founded |
> | 1890 | The United Mine Workers Union was founded in Ohio |
> | 1892 | The first recorded workplace safety program was established in an Illinois steel plant, in response to a flywheel explosion |
> | 1900 | International Ladies Garment Workers Union was founded, primarily to organize workers at Triangle Shirtwaist Factory |
> | 1903 | The Women's Trade Union League was formed at the AFL convention |
> | 1905 | Industrial Workers of the World (IWW or Wobblies) was founded; it aimed to organize all unions into a labor solidarity in preparation to topple capitalism. IWW is now remembered for organizing women, blacks, new immigrants, and unskilled and migratory laborers, all of whom the AFL had shunned |
> | 1909 | "Uprising of the 20,000"—female shirtwaist makers in New York City strike against sweatshop conditions |
> | 1911 | Triangle Shirtwaist Factory fire in New York City killed 146 workers, trapped by the lack of fire escapes and locked exit doors |
> | 1919 | 20% of American workers walked out in a great strike wave, including national clothing, coal, and steel workers |
> | 1925 | The nation's first African-American union, the Brotherhood of Sleeping Car Porters, was founded; although receiving support from the AFL, the union was opposed by the Pullman Company, and the brotherhood did not receive an international charter until 1936 |

BOX 1-2

*A chronology of the organized labor movement
in the United States—cont'd*

1933	The New Deal was introduced to congress by President Roosevelt to stimulate the economy after the Great Depression had increased unemployment by 12 million in three years; millions found employment in federally sponsored works programs
1935	The National Labor Relations Act of 1935 (Wagner Act) legalized union practices such as collective bargaining and the closed shops, and outlawed certain anti-union practices such as blacklisting
1935	United Auto Workers (UAW) was founded, now representing Automobile, Aerospace and Agricultural Implement Workers of America
1937	The Committee for Industrial Organizations (CIO), at that time a constituency of the AFL, organized strikes in all major industries
1938	The Congress of Industrial Organizations (CIO) was formed as an independent federation
1943	The CIO formed the first political action committee to get out the vote for President Roosevelt
1946	The Full Employment Act was signed to increase national employment
1947	The Labor-Management Relations Act (Taft-Hartley Act), ostensibly enacted to govern relations between workers and management, in fact restricted union behavior and the activities of union members in order to allow commerce to develop
1955	The AFL and the CIO unified
1962	Federal employees gained the right to organize and bargain collectively
1962	National Farm Workers Association (NFWA) was formed by Caesar Chavez
1963	March on Washington for Jobs and Justice occurred
1966	NFWA and the Agricultural Workers Organizing Committee merged to form the United Farm Workers (UFW) and became an affiliate of the AFL-CIO
1969	End of Kennedy/Johnson era aided development of depressed areas, urban renewal, and anti-discrimination initiatives
1960s-1970s	Rise in debate began over environmental protection vis-à-vis jobs Affirmative Action and Equal Opportunity Acts were signed
1972	The Coalition of Black Trade Unionists was formed
1973	The Labor Council for Latin American Advancement was founded
1974	The Coalition of Labor Union Women was founded
1980s	Major industries were deregulated.
1992	The Asian Pacific American Labor Alliance was created within the AFL-CIO
	By the end of the Reagan/Bush era, less than 18% of workers were affiliated with a labor union, compared with half the labor force, directly following World War II
1990s	Technology began to surpass ethical guidelines. For example, inherited conditions may one day bar a choice of occupation; the use of random drug testing in non–safety-sensitive occupations raises ethical and privacy questions

(Continued)

BOX 1-2

A chronology of the organized labor movement in the United States—cont'd

1997	Pride At Work, a national coalition of lesbian, gay, bisexual and transgender workers and their supporters, becomes an AFL-CIO constituency group
1997	An estimated 30,000 to 50,000 working-family activists marched in Seattle to tell the World Trade Organization and its allies, "If the global economy doesn't work for working families, it doesn't work."
1999	5,000 North Carolina textile workers gained a union contract after a 25-year struggle

Sources: http://www.aflcio.org/http://www.afscme.org/, http://www.spartacus.schoolnet.co.uk/USATv.htm

---

    7) A new enforcement policy regarding respiratory protection, which became effective in 2004

    8) Defeat of legislation that would have given the president the ability to "Fast-Track" trade legislation without assured protection of workers' rights and the environment in 1997

C **Public pressure and social activism have had an important influence on workplace health and safety over the years.**

    1. Increasing societal intolerance of the exploitation and abuse of women and children in the mid-19th century led to factory reform and inspection legislation, which included provisions for limited working hours and a minimum age for child employment.

    2. Workplace disasters are often dramatic in terms of mortality, and have provided the impetus for both general and specific changes in workplace safety regulations.

      a. After the 1911 Triangle Shirtwaist Factory fire killed 146 workers who were trapped by the lack of fire escapes and management's practice of locking all exits to keep workers from leaving the job for breaks, the New York legislature yielded to public pressure to improve industrial working conditions, calling for tougher municipal building codes and more stringent factory inspections in New York and elsewhere.

      b. Public outrage contributed to the Coal Mine Health and Safety Act of 1969, after a mining accident killed 78 miners in West Virginia the previous year.

    3. Advances in occupational health regulation have often occurred in concert with major environmental protection laws.

      a. Social activism in the 1960s raised awareness of the link between environmental and occupational health concerns and work processes.

      b. After publication of *Silent Spring* (Carson, 1963), public attention was directed at the human health and environmental consequences of certain pesticides, leading to production and usage bans of some products.

      c. Increased societal awareness of the hazards of chemical exposure has resulted in the development of comprehensive protective interventions aimed at both the workplace in general and the management of manufacturing by-products and waste.

d. Environmental impact studies, aimed at protecting both the local ecology and the population, are now required in many jurisdictions before establishing new industrial enterprises.

4. The efforts of organized labor have both assisted and been influenced by the concerns for social justice and equality.

a. The 1941 March on Washington, led by A. Philip Randolph, president of the Brotherhood of Sleeping Car Porters, led to the creation of the Fair Employment Practices Committee.

b. The civil rights movement in the 1960s raised public awareness of the effects of racism, which drew national attention to the struggles of farm workers in California and eventually nationwide.

5. In the 1970s, a growing wellness/health promotion movement encouraged employers to implement workplace wellness programs and services.

a. The goal of these wellness programs and services was to reduce costs by enhancing awareness of self-care, decreasing absenteeism, improving worker morale, and increasing productivity.

b. Critics of the movement maintained that these programs and services shifted blame from the work environment to the individual worker, repeating a trend from earlier years.

c. Concerns were also raised about potential discrimination against populations at risk (e.g., smokers, obese workers, hypertensives).

IV Brief History of Workers' Compensation[1]

A **Before the passage of workers' compensation laws, injured workers and the survivors of workers killed on the job could be compensated for their loss or medical costs only through litigation.**

B **Employers were historically protected from loss claims under three common legal defenses:**

1. The *assumption-of-risk* defense assumed that workers were aware of occupational hazards and accepted the risk inherent to their jobs.

2. The *fellow servant rule* assumed that if a co-worker contributed to an accident or injury, that co-worker should be responsible for compensating the injured worker.

3. The concept of *contributory negligence* held that the employer was not liable if the employee contributed in any way to the injury; this defense strategy argued that physical harm would not have come to the worker had he or she been paying attention to the task, overriding the importance of a lack of protective devices.

C **Workers' compensation legislation was intended to protect business from lengthy litigation and prevent injured workers from becoming wards of the state.**

1. Workers' compensation laws were first enacted in Germany in 1884, and were widespread in Europe by the late 1890s.

2. In the United States, the first workers' compensation law was passed in Wisconsin in 1911.

---

[1]See Chapter 3 for a more detailed discussion of this content.

   a. Between 1911 and 1921, 25 states enacted workers' compensation laws.
   b. All 50 states and the District of Columbia now have workers' compensation laws; the last statute was enacted in Mississippi in 1948.
3. Each jurisdiction has administrative control over its own system, but there are several elements required of all statutes.
   a. Negligence or assumption of fault is not material to a claim, although it must be clear that the injury or illness occurred as a result of work-related processes.
   b. Benefits are made available by employers' payment of premiums to the established administrative system.
   c. Workers forfeit their right to sue their employer in exchange for prompt and reasonable compensation.
4. Employers lose their immunity from litigation if any of the following conditions are present:
   a. An injury is caused by an employer's intentional act.
   b. The employer is not in compliance with the state workers' compensation regulations.
   c. Punitive action is taken against the employee in retaliation for filing a claim or otherwise pursuing workers' compensation benefits.

V The Occupational Safety and Health Act[1]

A **Passage of the Occupational Safety and Health Act of 1970 (Appendix V) underscored two major points:**
1. Many occupational hazards are controllable, and their resulting work-related injuries and illnesses are preventable.
2. Primary responsibility for providing safe and healthful working environments rests with the employer.

B **Individual states may manage their own occupational health and safety programs and services with federal approval of the state plan, which is contingent upon a demonstrated ability to provide the essential elements required by the federal plan; 26 states currently manage their own OSHA-approved state plans. (See Box 3-1 for list of states.)**

C **The OSH Act of 1970 established three separate bodies with distinct functions:**
1. The Occupational Safety and Health Administration (OSHA), positioned within the United States Department of Labor (USDL), promulgates, administers, and enforces workplace health and safety standards, and establishes reporting and recordkeeping procedures to monitor the number and type of job-related injuries and illnesses.
2. The National Institute for Occupational Safety and Health (NIOSH) located in the U.S. Department of Health and Human Services (DHHS) as part of the Centers for Disease Control and Prevention (CDC), conducts occupational health and safety research, provides education, and makes health and safety recommendations to OSHA and the nation's employers.
3. The Occupational Safety and Health Review Commission, a separate entity independent from OSHA, primarily arbitrates disputes between employers and OSHA regarding citations and proposed fines.

---

[1]See Chapter 3 for a more detailed discussion of this content.

VI National Health Goals: Healthy People and Healthy Communities

A *Healthy People 2010* (DHHS, 2000) outlines a comprehensive, nationwide health-promotion and disease-prevention agenda in 28 public-health focus areas, including occupational health and safety and environmental health.

B *Healthy People 2010* is designed to achieve two overarching goals:
1. Increase quality and years of healthy life
2. Eliminate health disparities

C The underlying premise of *Healthy People 2010* is that "the health of the individual is almost inseparable from the health of the larger community."

D *Healthy People 2010* builds on initiatives and objectives pursued over the past two decades, aiming for measurable and achievable public health objectives. Interim evaluations in the occupational and environmental health and safety focus area have and will continue to result in the following:
1. New objectives to address emerging work-related concerns
2. Revision, replacement, or elimination of objectives that cannot be tracked reliably or have low relative value for monitoring improved outcomes in worker health and safety.

E The *Healthy People 2010* goal for Chapter 20, Occupational Safety and Health, is to "promote the health and safety of people at work through prevention and early intervention" (US DHHS, 2000). Specific objectives related to occupational health and safety are summarized in Box 1-3.

F The *Healthy People 2010* goal for Chapter 8, Environmental Health, is to "promote health for all through a healthy environment" (US DHHS, 2000). Specific objectives related to environmental health are summarized in Box 1-3.

G *Healthy Communities 2000: Model Standards* (American Public Health Association, 1991) was developed to help implement national health objectives for community populations, including working populations, by providing a "framework for incremental improvement in community health status through preventive health service programming."

VII Occupational Health in the International Community

A Occupational health and safety programs and services in developing countries face many societal, cultural, and political challenges, including the following:
1. Poor general working conditions
2. Substandard wages
3. Lack of political commitment; corruption at many levels
4. Lack of awareness among the working population of both their hazardous occupational exposures and their rights as workers to safe working conditions
5. Inadequate workers' compensation, or no worker's compensation at all
6. Inadequate health and safety legislation; non-enforcement of existing laws
7. Exploitation of the labor force, including child labor
8. Lack of regulation related to environmental pollution and degradation
9. Inadequate supply of occupational health and safety expertise
10. Hazardous industries, operations, equipment, machinery, and products often imported from developed countries where they may be banned

---

BOX 1-3

Healthy People 2010—summary of topics addressed in objectives

Chapter 20: Occupational Safety and Health

Work-related injury deaths
Work-related injuries
Overexertion or repetitive motion
Pneumoconiosis deaths
Work-related homicides
Work-related assaults
Elevated blood lead levels from work exposure
Occupational skin diseases or disorders
Worksite stress reduction programs
Needlestick injuries
Work-related, noise-induced hearing loss

Chapter 8: Environmental Health

Outdoor air quality
Water quality
Toxins and waste
Healthy homes and healthy communities
Infrastructure and surveillance
Global environmental health

Source: www.healthypeople.gov/Document/HTML/Volume2/20OccHS.htm.

B **International organizations committed to occupational health and safety include the following:**

1. The World Health Organization (WHO), which was established in 1948 to promote international cooperation to improve health conditions.
   a. The purpose of WHO is "to promote the attainment of the highest level of health by all people in the world" (WHO, 1994).
   b. Following the 1994 Declaration on Occupational Health for All, WHO developed a global strategy on occupational health (WHO, 1995).
   c. In 1990, WHO created a global network of Occupational Health Collaborating Centers.
2. The International Labor Organization (ILO), which was established in 1919 to protect the life and health of working men and women and to control occupational hazards. Its services include the following:
   a. Policy and advisory guidance through its International Program for the Improvement of Working Conditions and Environment
   b. Provision of information through its International Occupational Safety and Health Information Center in Geneva, Switzerland (known as CIS in the European Union)
3. The European Commission, which has developed directives aimed at harmonizing national occupational health and safety laws in European Union members.
4. The International Commission on Occupational Health (ICOH), an international scientific society established in 1906, which is recognized by the United Nations as a nongovernmental organization.
   a. The purpose of ICOH is to foster the scientific progress, knowledge, and development of occupational health in the international community.
   b. ICOH has a close working relationship with WHO, ILO, and other United Nations agencies.

    c. Since 1969, ICOH's Scientific Committee on Occupational Health Nursing has produced nine reports for occupational health nurses internationally.

C **The trend towards globalization of trade, while economically beneficial, is introducing a host of occupational hazards to developing countries, where 75% of the global workforce lives and where the technical and social infrastructure is lacking to protect workers from these hazards (World Health Organization [WHO], 1999a).**

D **The International Labour Organization (ILO) estimates that the overall economic losses resulting from work-related diseases and injuries are approximately 4% of the world's gross national product (WHO, 1999b).**

VIII The Workplace: Occupational Hazards and Their Impact on Workers

The range of workplace hazards with actual or potential effects on worker health and safety is as broad and varied as work itself. The nature of occupational hazards changes with the evolution of work processes but can be broadly categorized as physical, chemical, biological, mechanical, and/or psychosocial.

A *Physical hazards* **are agents or forces inherent to the nature of a work environment or process that may cause tissue damage or other physical harm.**

1. Environmental noise contamination is the single most prevalent occupational hazard; its hazard potential is generally underestimated.
   a. Each year, more than 30 million workers are exposed to continuous or impulse noise at levels sufficient to cause measurable hearing loss (National Institute for Occupational Safety and Health [NIOSH], 2001).
   b. Environmental noise contamination can elicit physiologic and psychologic stress reactions resulting in neuro-endocrine stimulation capable of adversely affecting multiple body systems (Lusk, Ronis, Kazanis, Eakin, Hong & Raymond, 2003; Lusk, Hagerty, Gillespie & Caruso, 2002; Penney, Earl, 2004; Suter, 1993).
2. Thermal stress experienced by working in conditions of excessive heat or cold can lead to multiple pathologies, including cardiovascular and metabolic disturbances, central and peripheral neurologic alterations, and mental status changes, resulting in impaired judgment and performance and increased risk of accidents.
3. Sustained or repeated body contact with vibrating surfaces has been associated with neurologic, neurovascular, and musculoskeletal changes and visual and gastrointestinal disorders.
4. Other examples of physical hazards include ionizing radiation (isotopes, X-rays, radium), non-ionizing radiation (welding flash, ultraviolet rays, microwaves, sunburn), electric and magnetic fields, hyperbaric environments, and lasers.

B **Chemical hazards occur in various forms and have varying effects on workers.**

1. The American National Standards Institute classifies chemicals as dusts/particulates, fumes, mists, vapors, and gases.
2. Chemical formulations include solutions, metals, solvents, aerosols, pharmaceutics, oils, synthetic textiles, pesticides, and explosives.
3. Commercial products are often formulated with various additives and stabilizers, which may themselves be toxic.

4. An estimated 32 million workers are annually exposed to one or more chemical hazards that may cause, contribute to, or exacerbate serious adverse health effects.
5. NIOSH has identified 13,000 toxic substances and 2000 carcinogens that pose threats to human health in the workplace.
6. Regulation of safe exposure limits for chemical substances requires clear scientific evidence of pathologic effects; the burden of proof lies with OHSA, which relies on evidence from NIOSH and other research entities.
7. Primary routes of chemical exposure are inhalation, transdermal absorption, and ingestion; deleterious effects range from local reactions to systemic or end-organ damage.
   a. Acute effects—usually linked to a single high-dose incident with an identifiable offending substance
   b. Chronic effects—evolve insidiously, presenting multiple challenges in establishing causal relationships to exposures
   c. Allergic reactions—not consistent with the usual population dose-response curve

C **Biologic hazards found in the work environment include viruses, bacteria, fungi, molds, and parasites.**
1. Exposure to biologic agents can be direct or indirect, and occurs through one of three routes of transmission: airborne, droplet, or contact.
2. Many occupations are at risk of exposure to biohazards.
   a. The occupational risk of exposure to infectious agents among employees in health care and related fields is well documented.
   b. Workers who have contact with animals or animal products may be at risk for zoonotic diseases.
   c. Workers whose jobs involve contact with soil are at risk for parasitic diseases and bacterial or fungal infections.
3. Prevention and control methods include immunization, isolation of the agent, engineering control measures (e.g., effective ventilation mechanics), personal protective gear, and hand washing.
4. Challenges to prevention and control include the following:
   a. Emerging infectious agents (CDC, 1998b)—more than 30 new infectious processes have been detected in the past two decades, including Lyme disease, Legionnaire's disease, human immunodeficiency virus/acquired immunodeficiency syndrome, necrotizing fasciitis, avian influenza, hantavirus, and Ebola fever
   b. The potential that terrorists may release biohazards in the workplace (Chapter 13)
   c. Drug resistance and organism mutation because of overuse of antibiotics and lapses in treatment regimens

D **Mechanical hazards are elements of the workplace that lead to stress or injury through an incompatibility between the design of the workplace or work processes and human physiology.**
1. Mechanical hazards might also be termed *biomechanical,* because they represent not only an interface between equipment and humans, but also the physiologic mechanics required to perform work duties.
2. The effect of this incompatibility is most often exacted on the musculoskeletal and peripheral nervous systems, but other body systems may be affected as well.

3. The identification, analysis, and abatement of biomechanical hazards are often a function of *applied ergonomics*.[2]
4. Effects of biomechanical stresses can be temporary or result in permanent disability.
   a. Acute effects include musculoskeletal injuries resulting from overexertion, slips, falls, or other accidents; muscular strain or fatigue resulting from forceful exertion or awkward positioning; and visual fatigue.
   b. Chronic effects include Raynaud's syndrome resulting from the use of vibrating power tools; cumulative trauma injuries stemming from repeated or sustained motions resulting in neurologic and musculoskeletal disorders; and chronic back pain resulting from improper lifting or awkward, abrupt movements.
   c. Biomechanical injuries may impair mobility, strength, tactile capabilities, or motor control; recovery is often long-term and may be incomplete.
5. Prevention and control of biomechanical pathologies is best achieved through engineering designs that focus on manipulating the elements of the work facilities and processes to accommodate the characteristics, capabilities, and expectations of the worker.

E **Psychosocial hazards have become an internationally recognized problem of epidemic proportions.**
1. The ILO reports that more than 50% of workers in industrialized countries complain of job-related stress and its adverse consequences (WHO, 1999b).
2. Psychosocial hazards are often difficult to identify and even more difficult to quantify because of their intangible and insidious nature and the variable responses among individuals.
3. Workplace psychosocial distress stem from multiple sources internal and external to the organization (Chapter 15).
4. Psychosocial stress hazards that occur in the workplace may have the following characteristics:
   a. They may be manifested physically, psychologically, or behaviorally, with outcomes detrimental to the individual, co-workers, and general workplace morale and productivity.
   b. They may have economic implications to the organization, including lost productivity, costs related to medical benefits, temporary help, and employee turnover, and losses related to the impact of stressed employees on customer relations.
   c. They may be symptomatic of widespread organizational problems rather than isolated incidents, indicating a need for systemic solutions.

IX Work-Related Injury and Illness

A **OSHA definitions distinguish the differences between occupational injuries and illnesses.**
1. An *occupational injury* is any injury, such as a cut, fracture, sprain, amputation, etc., that results from a single instantaneous exposure or incident in the work environment.
2. An *occupational illness* is any abnormal condition or disorder, other than one resulting from an occupational injury, caused by exposure to environmental

---

[2]Chapter 16 presents an example of an ergonomics program.

factors associated with employment, including acute or chronic illnesses that may be caused by inhalation, absorption, ingestion, or direct contact.

B **There are some challenges in accurately defining the extent of occupational and environmental injury and illness.**

1. Statistical data on occupational injury and illness rates are dependent upon thorough and accurate incident reporting.
   a. Statistical accuracy can be compromised when the differentiation between illnesses or injuries is not clear (e.g., chronic disorders such as back pain, multiple chemical sensitivity, or cumulative trauma disorders may result from single or repeated injurious events).
   b. There is no national reporting system for occupation-related chronic disease or death; while occupational health and safety professionals are acutely aware of the importance of reporting the work-relatedness of an injury or illness, reports on occupationally related morbidity and mortality from general practice nurses and physicians depend on the diligence and awareness of the health care practitioner of the importance of such reporting.
2. Underreporting of work-related incidents is a well-recognized phenomenon, and occurs on several levels:
   a. Governmental surveillance criteria do not require gathering data on certain categories of workers.
   b. Employees may not report nonacute incidents or those not requiring medical attention, or may not recognize the work-relatedness of a disorder.
   c. The organizational culture may discourage reporting incidents or filing workers' compensation claims through incentive measures and other tactics.
   d. Death certificates may lack information about work-relatedness; only 67% to 90% of all occupational fatalities resulting from injury can be identified through the death certificate (CDC, 1998a).
3. Work-related illnesses are more difficult to quantify than injuries and are more likely to be underreported.
   a. Diseases related to occupational exposures are indistinguishable from those caused by non–work-related sources.
   b. The onset of illness resulting from occupational exposure is often subtle, occurring years after the exposure.
   c. Health care providers may not recognize the relationship of a worker's presenting symptoms to past or present occupations or may find the determination of relative causation of work-related hazards to a disorder difficult because of genetic or behavioral variables that have the potential to affect the disorder.

C **Occupational injuries pose a major threat to American workers.**

1. More than 4.1 million recordable nonfatal workplace injuries were reported in 2002 (USDL, BLS, 2004b).
   a. The most common nonfatal work injuries involving days away from work have consistently been related to overexertion and contact with objects or equipment, e.g., being struck by objects or being caught in, under, or between objects (National Safety Council [NSC], 2004).
   b. Nonfatal workplace injuries resulting in temporary or permanent disability are estimated at 3.7 million annually (NSC, 2003).
2. Injury rates tend to be higher in mid-sized organizations, with 50-249 employees, than in either smaller or larger organizations (USDL, BLS, 2003).

3. Workplace fatalities resulting from accidents and injuries have declined from 21 per 100,000 full-time workers in 1912, when surveillance began, to an estimated 4.2 per 100,000 in all private industry in 2003 (www.bls.gov/iif/home).
   a. In 2003, 5559 work-related injury deaths, of which 560 were homicides, were reported, averaging approximately 15 per day (USDL, BLS, 2002).
   b. The three most hazardous industries in terms of fatalities have long been mining, agriculture, and construction, with rates reported at 23.5, 22.7, and 12.2 per 100,000 full time workers, respectively; however, agricultural mortality rate has been estimated by other sources at more than 50 per 100,000 (NIOSH, 2004).
4. Underlying or root causes of workplace accidents stem from the human-hazard interface, and injuries are often the result of deficiencies in adhering to safety precautions, either at the organizational/administrative level or by the individual worker.

D Occupational illnesses, though fewer in number, are also a serious concern.
1. Work-related illness morbidity and mortality figures are more difficult to quantify and more likely to be underreported than are injuries.
2. Occupational illnesses are categorized by the Bureau of Labor Statistics as skin diseases or disorders, respiratory conditions, poisonings and all other illnesses.
3. The manufacturing sector accounts for nearly 45% of all reported occupational illnesses in private industry (USDL, BLS, 2003).
4. Despite the elimination of repeated trauma or repetitive motion disorders as a separate occupational illness category in 2002, and the relocation of this category to "all other illnesses," the evidence shows the continued impact of these disorders:
   a. The median number of days away from work related to repetitive motion disorders is 19 days (USDL, BLS, 2002).
   b. More than 35% of repetitive motion disorders require more than 31 days away from work (USDL, BLS, 2002).
   c. In 1999, repetitive motion disorders accounted for 65% of all occupational illnesses (NIOSH, 2001b).
   d. The costs associated with work-related musculoskeletal disorders, of which one third is attributable to repetitive motion or overexertion, is estimated to range from $13 billion to $54 billion annually (NIOSH, 2001b).
   e. The incidence of repeated trauma disorders more than tripled between 1987 and 1994.
5. Skin disorders are the second most prevalent work-related illness, and the most common non–trauma-related illness (USDL, BLS, 2003).
   a. Skin disorders represent over 15% of all reported occupational disease (USDL, BLS, 2003).
   b. In the workplace, skin is an important route of exposure to chemicals and other contaminants, some of which can cause systemic disorders as well as local skin reactions.
   c. There is no occupation or industry without potential exposure to the diverse agents that cause allergic and irritant dermatitis. Manufacturing has the greatest number of cases, but the highest rate for new case diagnosis is in agriculture, forestry, and fishing.

    d. The estimated total costs, including lost workdays and loss of productivity associated with occupational skin disease may reach $1 billion annually.

  6. The prevalence of occupation-related chronic respiratory disease is difficult to determine; however, NIOSH estimates that up to 30% of 10 million cases of asthma in the general population may be attributable to workplace exposure (www.2a.cdc.gov/nora/NaddinfoAsthma.html).

    a. More than 20 million U.S. workers are exposed to substances that can cause airway diseases.

    b. The estimated annual cost related to occupational asthma is approximately $400 million.

  7. Hazardous occupational exposures are considered substantial contributors to many other disease processes, affecting nearly every body system.

  8. New disorders have emerged with evolving technologies and work processes that present new challenges to occupational health and safety professionals, including sick-building syndrome, multiple-chemical sensitivity, cumulative trauma disorders, and the effects of new uses for existing chemicals.

E **There are multiple economic impacts of occupational and environmental injury and illness.**

  1. The direct costs of occupational injuries and illnesses are estimated at $45.8 billion, and include wage and productivity losses, medical costs, and administrative expenses such as time spent investigating incidents and writing accident reports.

  2. Indirect costs are estimated at $229 billion, and include but are not limited to overtime payment, hiring temporary workers, recruiting and training new workers, and remediation of faulty safety equipment.

  3. More than 20 million productive days are lost annually due to workplace injuries and illness reported in all private sector industries combined.

    a. In 2002, 1.4 million cases of nonfatal injuries and illnesses required days away from work beyond the day of the incident; the occupations with the greatest number of such injuries and illnesses were truck drivers, nurse aids, orderlies, and attendants (USDL, BLS, 2004b).

    b. Consistently over the past decade, the number of injury and illness cases requiring 30 or more days away from work is higher than any category of lesser time loss, indicating the severity of these cases.

  4. Economic estimates of loss do not include the impact on communities and families, such as pain and suffering, lowered workplace morale because of the loss of a co-worker, the strain of taking care of a disabled family member, or the loss of the injured employee's contributions to community activities.

F **Sources of information and data on occupational injury and illness include the following:**

  1. U.S. Department of Labor, Bureau of Labor Statistics (www.bls.gov)

  2. National Safety Council (www.nsc.org)

  3. Workers' compensation records

  4. State and federal occupational health and safety administrations (www.osha.gov)

  5. National Institute for Occupational Safety and Health (www.cdc.gov/niosh)

  6. International Labor Organization (www.ilo.org)

X Assessment and Prevention of Occupational and Environmental Injury and Illness

A Theoretically, all occupational and environmental injuries and illnesses are preventable.

1. Prevention measures include modifying hazardous workplace conditions, preventing contact between the hazard and the worker, and educating and training workers regarding safe work practices.
2. The efficacy of prevention strategies depends on the accurate assessment of the following:
   a. Hazardous workplace conditions
   b. Actual or potential risk of employee exposure, previous similar exposures, and preexisting health conditions that may impact the severity of the exposure
3. The prevention of workplace injury and illness cannot be effectively achieved without genuine corporate commitment.

B Hazards in the workplace can be assessed by the following approaches:[3]

1. Actual or potential hazards are identified through site surveys, record audits, accident investigations, chemical inventory analyses, or other methods.
2. Exposure monitoring quantitatively assesses exposures to known, suspected, or reasonably predicted hazards such as chemicals, noise, or atmospheric conditions.
3. Process safety analysis focuses on assessing the hazards inherent to specific work processes such as ergonomic analysis or production line safety.
4. Population analysis takes an epidemiologic approach to identifying work-related hazards.

C Assessment of occupational and environmental illness involves multiple strategies.

1. There are no specialized diagnostic procedures to identify the work-relatedness of a disorder, making the occupational and environmental exposure history the crucial tool to accurate diagnosis and appropriate treatment recommendations.
2. The key components of the occupational and environmental exposure history include the following (Levy & Wegman, 2000):
   a. Descriptions of all jobs held
   b. Environmental (work/home/school/community) exposures, and protective mechanisms and interventions in use
   c. Temporal relationship between symptoms and work schedule or between symptoms and exposure
   d. Epidemiology of similar symptoms or illnesses among peers
   e. Incidental exposures—descriptions of nonemployment activities
3. The accurate determination of the work-relatedness of an illness provides benefits to the following:
   a. The individual worker who receives an accurate diagnosis, relevant treatment recommendations, and meaningful prevention measures to reduce or eliminate the source of the exposure
   b. The population of workers, who, through an investigative assessment of the hazard, benefit from the implementation of prevention strategies

---

[3]Chapter 10 presents a more detailed discussion.

aimed at groups of workers in work environments similar to the affected employee

c. The organization, which avoids the costs of unnecessary diagnostic procedures, medications, or referrals

XI History and Evolution of Occupational and Environmental Health Nursing

The evolution of industrial nursing paralleled the growth of industry.

A **Industrial nursing, with its roots in 19th-century Great Britain, emerged as a new specialty field during the era of rapid industrialization (McGrath, 1946; American Association of Industrial Nurses, 1976).**

1. The philosophy of care of industrial nursing was based on the concepts and principles of public health nursing.
2. Early industrial nurses were public health nurses employed by mining and manufacturing companies and department stores to:
   a. Provide primary and community health services to employees and their families
   b. Focus on preventing and treating communicable diseases
3. Earliest recorded industrial nurses included the following:
   a. Phillippa Flowerday was hired in 1878 by the J.J. Coleman Mustard Company in England to provide home care to workers and their families.
   b. Betty Moulder, generally considered the first American occupational health nurse, was reportedly hired by a group of coal mining companies to care for miners and their families in the late 1880s.
   c. Ada Mayo Stewart was hired in 1895 by the Vermont Marble Company; in 1896, she became the superintendent of the company-built hospital in Proctor.

B **As the profession developed into the early 20th century, the focus remained on public and community health services.**

1. In 1909, the Milwaukee Visiting Nurse Association placed a nurse in a plant to offer public health services in order to demonstrate the economic value of the service.
2. For the most part, industrial nurses remained visiting nurses until workers' compensation laws were instituted, at which time first-aid stations were opened in plants.
3. In 1916, Florence Wright, in an address to the National Safety Council, described the valuable work done by the industrial nurse as follows:
   a. Promotes pleasant industrial relations
   b. Reduces time lost through accident and illness
   c. Minimizes the results of accidents by providing first aid and subsequent care under the direction of the surgeon
   d. Searches out the causes of illness and accidents through cooperation with employers and outside agencies in the community and the home
   e. Makes possible the healthy, happy, thrifty home life in the families of those visited, preventing waste of life and health and increasing the efficiency of each member
4. In 1916, Ella Phillips Crandall described the roles of occupational health nurses as follows:
   a. First aid and dispensary service
   b. Hospital duty

    c. Making rounds in industrial plants to inspect conditions and observe employees

    d. Consultation, chiefly for women

    e. Teaching health and hygiene classes

    f. Making home visits to provide nursing and social services, including domestic education in food economics, cookery, and budgeting

    g. Keeping records of occupational diseases and injuries, and of the relationship of employment to disease and mortality

C Occupational health nursing organizations have defined the profession, guided its development, and established its professional foundations (Box 1-4).

XII The Practice of Occupational and Environmental Health Nursing

A Occupational and environmental health nursing is a unique, complex, and multidimensional practice (See Figure 1-1).

1. Occupational and environmental health nurses are professionally accountable to workers, employers, communities, and their profession and are responsible for their own professional development.

2. Multiple work-related and external variables influence the health of workers and workplaces and the outcomes of the occupational and environmental health and safety program.

B Occupational and environmental health nursing is the specialty practice that provides for and delivers health and safety programs and services to workers, worker populations, and community groups (AAOHN, 2004a).

1. The practice focuses on promotion and restoration of health, prevention of illness and injury, and protection from work related and environmental hazards.

2. The research-based foundation of occupational and environmental health nursing derives its theoretic, conceptual, and factual framework from a multidisciplinary scientific base, which includes, but is not limited to nursing, medical, public health and social/behavioral sciences, and business and management theories.

3. The basis for the scope of practice, knowledge, skill, and the legal and ethical framework in occupational and environmental health nursing is provided by AAOHN Standards of Practice (AAOHN, 2004a, Appendix VII), the AAOHN Code of Ethics (AAOHN, 2004b, Appendix VI), core competencies (AAOHN, 2003; Appendix VIII), and the Core Curriculum for Occupational and Environmental Health Nursing.

4. Standards of occupational and environmental health nursing are developed by the profession to define and advance practice and to provide a framework for evaluation. AAOHN has identified 11 professional practice standards that describe the accountability of the practitioner, reflect the values and priorities of the profession, and describe a competent level of performance regarding the nursing process and professional roles of the occupational and environmental health nurse (AAOHN, 2004a) (Appendix VII).

5. The AAOHN has delineated nine categories of competency in occupational and environmental health nursing. Three levels of achievement are identified within each category—competence, proficiency, and expertise—with the competent levels considered core for practice in the specialty (AAOHN, 2003) (Appendix VIII).

BOX 1-4

Historical development of occupational and environmental health nursing organizations

1913 The first industrial nurse registry was opened in Boston for the purpose of supplying emergency room nurses to factories

1915 The Boston Industrial Nurses' Club was formed, the forerunner of the New England Association of Industrial Nurses

1916 The Factory Nurses' Conference was formed, admitting only graduate, state-registered nurses who belonged to the American Nurses' Association

1917 Boston University's College of Business Administration offered the first industrial nurse educational course

1922 The Factory Nurses' Conference changed its name to the American Association of Industrial Nurses (AAIN) to more closely identify with the industrial physicians' group

1933 The AAIN merged with the New England Association of Industrial Nurses

1938 The first annual joint conference of the industrial nurses' associations of New England, New Jersey, New York, and Philadelphia met in New York City

1942 On April 19, at the Philadelphia conference, the AAIN became a national organization, created by 300 nurses from 16 states; Catherine R. Dempsey was its first president

1943 The first annual meeting of the new AAIN was held in New York City, describing its objectives as:
- To develop sound standards of education and practice in industrial nursing
- To cooperate with physicians, management, safety professionals, and other allied groups in conserving the health of industrial workers
- To promote mutual understanding of the goals of occupational health and safety programs and services among these groups
- To interpret the objectives and ideals of industrial nurses to the professional and lay world
- To bring industrial nursing participation into the plans for advancing industrial and community health

1944 AAIN prepared an "Outline of Basic College Courses for Industrial Nurses" and distributed it to colleges and universities in the United States
Industrial Nursing became the official publication of AAIN

1949 Publishing of *Industrial Nursing* was halted because of increased publishing costs; a newsletter was substituted

1953 *Nurses Journal* was re-established, winning several awards in the years that followed

1964 AAIN copyrighted its publication as the *American Association of Industrial Nurses Journal, The Journal of Occupational Health Nursing*

BOX 1-4

Historical development of occupational and environmental health nursing organizations—cont'd

1966	A committee consisting of members from AAIN, the American Industrial Hygiene Association, the Industrial Medical Association, and the American Academy of Occupational Medicine was established to study the formation of an American Board of Certification for Occupational Health Nurses
1969	The name of the journal became *Occupational Health Nursing*, the official journal of the American Association of Industrial Nurses
1971	The American Board for Occupational Health Nurses was established as a separate organization whose purpose was certification of occupational health nurses
1977	To better reflect the expanded activities of its members in health promotion and disease prevention, and the variety of settings in which they practice, AAIN, Inc. changed its name to the American Association of Occupational Health Nurses, Inc. (AAOHN)
1983	The official headquarters of AAOHN moved from New York City to Atlanta, Georgia
1986	The journal became known as the *AAOHN Journal*, the official journal of the American Association of Occupational Health Nurses
1988	Occupational health nursing celebrated its centennial year
1992	AAOHN celebrated its 50th anniversary with 12,500 members
1996	AAOHN was awarded a cooperative agreement by the Agency for Toxic Substances and Disease Registry (ATSDR) to develop and provide environmental health information to AAOHN members, other nursing professionals, and community groups
1997	The first edition of the core curriculum was published; it was entitled *AAOHN Core Curriculum for Occupational Health Nursing*
1998	The importance of environmental health concerns to occupational health nurses was reflected through the addition of the term "occupational *and environmental*" to AAOHN's mission statement, by-laws, standards of practice, and other AAOHN publications
2001	The second edition of the core curriculum, entitled *Core Curriculum for Occupational and Environmental Health Nursing* was published
2005	The *Core Curriculum for Occupational and Environmental Health Nursing*, 3rd edition, was published

E Functional roles and primary responsibilities of the occupational and environmental health nurse are determined by a number of factors, including the nature of the work and its associated hazards, the number of employees, the organizational structure, and the organization's administrative and financial support for the program.

1. The practice of the occupational and environmental health nurse and the breadth and depth of an organization's health and safety program vary in accordance with the needs and resources of the work setting.
2. Functional roles and primary responsibilities of the occupational and environmental health nurse have been delineated by a job analysis study conducted by the American Board of Occupational Health Nurses as part of its content validation process for certification examination (Salazar, Kemerer, Amann and Fabrey, 2002).
   a. Clinician—Primary responsibilities aimed at preventing work-related and non–work-related health problems and restoring and maintaining health; duties may include hazard assessment and surveillance, and investigation of illness and injury events
   b. Case manager—Coordinates health and rehabilitation services for an individual worker from the onset of an injury or illness to an optimal return to work status or a satisfactory alternative; may include case management for nonoccupational maladies
   c. Occupational health services coordinator—Functions as the single occupational health nurse for a business or organization
   d. Health promotion specialist—Develops and manages a comprehensive, multilevel, broad-range health promotion program that supports organizational business objectives
   e. Manager/administrator—Directs, administers, and evaluates an occupational and environmental health and safety service and its policies, ensuring legal, regulatory, and ethical compliance while maintaining consistency with organizational goals and objectives
   f. Nurse practitioner—Uses additional specialized preparation meeting state requirements for advanced practice nursing to critically evaluate the health status of workers through health histories, physical assessments, and diagnostic tests
   g. Corporate director—Responsible for the total occupational and environmental health and safety program at the policy-making level
   h. Consultant—Serves as an advisor for developing, selecting, implementing, and evaluating occupational and environmental health and safety services
   i. Educator—Assumes programmatic and administrative responsibilities for curricula and/or clinical experiences in occupational and environmental health nursing
   j. Researcher—Identifies occupational and environmental health problems, develops researchable questions with consideration for research priorities, assesses study feasibility, and initiates and conducts research studies using all elements of the research process
3. Many occupational and environmental health nurses work in more than one of these roles simultaneously; for example, a nurse whose primary role is as a clinician may also serve as a health promotion specialist, educator, and case manager.
4. Additional responsibilities required for a successful occupational health and safety program include the following:
   a. Development of professional rapport with employees and employers
   b. Development of collegial and cooperative relationships with members of the interdisciplinary health and safety team
   c. Establishing a liaison with community referral agencies and resources
   d. Establishing a network of professional resources

    e. Maintenance and enhancement of professional competence in occupational and environmental health and related subspecialties through continuing education and other professional development activities

5. Emergency preparedness and disaster planning have long been recognized as within the realm of responsibility for occupational and environmental health nurses (AAOHN, 2004c); the events of September 11, 2001 have highlighted the importance of this occupational and environmental health nursing role.

6. Broader environmental issues are increasingly being recognized as within the domain of occupational health practice, partly because of the following:

    a. Recognition of the link between environmental conditions and human disease

    b. Greater understanding of the impact of industry and its byproducts on the environment

    c. The occupational health nurse's unique, integrated body of scientific knowledge that can be drawn upon to advocate for practices that impact workers, the community, and environmental health (See Chapter 6.)

F **Occupational and environmental health nurses who have pursued additional specialized education or training have expanded their roles to various nontraditional areas, including:**

1. Risk management

    a. Responsibilities include anticipating and controlling potential causes of human and financial loss related to occupational health and safety incidents.

    b. Risk managers help manage insurance coverage for workers' compensation and other health- and disability-related insurance products.

2. Safety officer

    a. Functional activities may include some tasks usually performed by industrial hygienists or other safety professionals.

    b. A primary responsibility is maintaining organizational regulatory compliance.

3. Counseling services for work-related or non–work-related concerns, many of which may adversely impact the employee's work effort

    a. The occupational health nurse counselor addresses the worker's psychosocial needs, wellness/health promotion concerns, and other health or work-related concerns.

    b. The occupational health nurse counselor may assume primary responsibility for managing the employee assistance program (EAP); in workplaces where this service is outsourced, the occupational health nurse may be the first contact for referral to the EAP.

4. Occupational and environmental health nurses are increasingly called upon to manage benefit programs and advise management regarding the development of integrated benefit plans.

5. An increasing number of occupational and environmental health nurses are self-employed, working as independent contractors in many of these roles.

G **Research is fundamental to the practice of occupational and environmental health nurses, both in guiding practice decisions and in building the body of knowledge in the field (Chapter 17).**

1. The AAOHN has identified a set of research priorities, which are periodically reviewed and updated to reflect the evolving nature of the work environment and its related hazards, and emphasizes the expanding role of the occupational and environmental health nurse.
2. NIOSH has developed the National Occupational Research Agenda (NORA) to guide the broader research goals in the field of occupational and environmental health (NIOSH, 1996).

H **Practice settings for occupational and environmental health nurses are as diverse as the many types of businesses in existence, and include:**
1. Industrial, business, or corporate settings
   a. Organizations with more than 250 employees are most likely to employ occupational and environmental health nurses.
   b. Firms with relatively high occupational injury and illness rates are more likely to employ occupational health nurses.
   c. The most common employer-based sites include manufacturers, service providers, and the transportation, communication, and utility industries.
   d. At the organizational administrative level, the occupational and environmental health nurse may be focused primarily on policy development and program oversight.
2. Insurers and third-party administrators (TPAs)
   a. Occupational and environmental health nurses monitor and manage the work-related injury and illness of patients for whom insurers and TPAs provide workers' compensation insurance coverage.
   b. Insurers and TPAs provide occupational health and safety consultation to their clients, including:
      1) Employee and supervisor training
      2) Program and regulatory compliance audits
      3) Health screening and surveillance
      4) Management support
      5) Case management protocol development
      6) Injury and illness trend analysis
3. Government and regulatory agencies
   a. Government agencies employ occupational health nurses as consultants, analysts, program developers, and compliance officers; they also provide occupational health services for government employees.
   b. Governmental and regulatory agencies focus their services and activities on populations rather than individual clients.
   c. Agencies may be federal (e.g., US PHS, OSHA, NIOSH), state (e.g., state health and safety administrations, state health departments), or local (e.g., city or county health departments).
4. Utilization review and case management firms
   a. Occupational and environmental health nurses may work directly with employees and employers, through insurers and third party administrators, or in managed care settings.
   b. Health care services and return-to-work interventions are monitored and managed by occupational and environmental health nurses individually with the employee or as an oversight service for the organization.
   c. The ultimate objectives are to provide cost-effective, quality health care and to facilitate the employee's return to an optimally expected level of work.

d. A utilization review and case management firm may exist in a range of organizations, from an independent nurse practice to a large multimillion-dollar firm.

5. Consulting firms
   a. Consulting services provided to client employers encompass evaluation and audit activities, training, trend analysis, program and system development, and management support.
   b. Consulting firms may be:
      1) Independent occupational and environmental health and safety consulting firms
      2) Finance-oriented consulting firms, such as insurance or accounting firms
      3) An independent practice owned and managed by one or more occupational health nurses
6. Research or academic organizations
   a. Occupational and environmental health nurses may serve as the lead or coinvestigator of research focusing on occupational health and safety problems.
   b. Occupational and environmental health training and education programs are delivered by occupational and environmental health nursing educators.

XIII Future Opportunities and Challenges

A **Globally, workplaces and workforces are changing as a result of demographic, social, and technologic changes.**

1. Changes in the United States that affect workers and the workplace include the following:
   a. The demographics of the country, and consequently the workforce, are changing.
      1) By 2010, an estimated 40% of the U.S. workforce will be aged 45 years or older. Older workers are at increased risk for fatal work injuries, require more time to return to work following an injury or illness, and are less likely to receive training as their jobs change (US DHHS PHS, 2004).
      2) The increasing population of newly immigrated workers faces particular challenges in the work environment, including unfamiliarity with laws and labor standards in the U.S.
   b. Managed care is replacing "free choice" as the predominant system for the delivery of health care in this country; employers have a major role in the provision of health care packages for employees.
   c. The information, technology, and service industries are expanding; the manufacturing industry is shrinking as a result of company closures, global economics, and increased automation.
   d. In the United States, health care and computer related occupations will account for 15 of the 20 fastest growing occupations over the coming decade (USDL, BLS, 2004c).
   e. Increasingly, businesses are choosing such cost-cutting measures as hiring part-time and temporary workers, using subcontractors for specialized work, and outsourcing selected services or entire divisions abroad.
   f. Technology is affecting communication patterns and the nature of work for many Americans.

g. Because many workers are telecommuting, occupational hazards in the home setting pose an additional hazard for some workers.

2. Immigration and the development of multinational corporations have increased the likelihood that occupational and environmental health nurses will be working with an ethnically and racially diverse workforce.

a. Culturally based norms, beliefs, and behaviors affect work ethics, practices, and health-related values.

b. Multilingual workforces are increasingly common, creating communication challenges.

3. These and other trends affecting occupational health and safety are discussed in detail in Chapter 2.

B **Implications for occupational and environmental health nurses are as follows:**

1. Health and safety services provided must be adjusted to accommodate a changing workforce and its changing needs.

2. Occupational and environmental health nurses have a professional responsibility to keep abreast of changes in the field by reading professional literature and participating in continuing education and other forms of professional development.

3. Increasing opportunities exist for global and international practice, teaching, and research.

4. Occupational and environmental health nurses should participate in an effort to ensure that industries exported to developing countries incorporate adequate occupational and environmental safeguards.

5. Continual expansion of the occupational and environmental health nurses' functional roles, especially those relating to direct clinical interventions and management/administrative responsibilities, is creating additional opportunities to affect the health and safety of working populations.

REFERENCES

American Association of Industrial Nurses. (1976). *The nurse in industry*. New York: AAIN.

American Association of Occupational Health Nurses, Inc. (AAOHN). (1997). *Guidelines for developing job descriptions in occupational and environmental health nursing*. Atlanta, GA: AAOHN.

American Association of Occupational Health Nurses, Inc. (AAOHN). (1998). Research priorities in occupational and environmental health nursing. Retrieved from http://www.aaohn.org/practice/priorities. Accessed 30 October 2004.

American Association of Occupational Health Nurses, Inc. (AAOHN). (2003). Competencies in Occupational and Environmental Health Nursing. *AAOHN Journal, 51* (7), 290-302.

American Association of Occupational Health Nurses, Inc. (AAOHN). (2004a). *Standards of occupational and environmental health nursing*. Atlanta, GA: AAOHN Publications.

American Association of Occupational Health Nurses, Inc. (AAOHN). (2004b). *AAOHN code of ethics and interpretative statements*. Atlanta, GA: AAOHN Publications.

American Association of Occupational Health Nurses, Inc. (AAOHN). (2004c). Position Statement: The occupational health nurse's role in all-hazard preparedness. Retrieved from http://www.aaohn.org/practice/positions. Accessed 30 October 2004.

American Public Health Association (APHA). (1991). *Healthy communities 2000: Model standards* (3rd ed.). Washington, DC: APHA.

Carson, R. (1963). *Silent spring*. Boston: Houghton Mifflin.

Centers for Disease Control and Prevention (CDC). (1998a). Fatal occupational injuries—United States, 1980-1994. *MMWR Morbidity and Mortality Weekly*, 47, (15), 297-302.

Centers for Disease Control and Prevention (CDC). (1998b). Preventing emerging infectious diseases: A strategy for the 21st century overview of the updated CDC plan. *MMWR Morbidity and Mortality Weekly, 47 (RR15)*, 1-14.

Hunter, D. (1978). *The diseases of occupations* (6th ed.). London: Hodder & Stroughton.

Levy, B.S. & Wegman, D.H. (2000). Occupational health: An overview. In B.S. Levy & D.H. Wegman (Eds.), *Occupational health: Recognizing and preventing work-related disease and injury* (4th ed.) (pp.3-26). Boston: Little, Brown and Company.

Lusk, S.L., Gillespie, B., Ziemba, R.A., Caruso, C.C., & Hagerty, B.M. (1996). *Noise effects on cardiovascular and stress related diseases*. (Final Report to The United Auto Workers/General Motors National Joint Committee on Health and Safety and its Occupational Health Advisory Board).

McGrath, D.J. (1946). *Nursing in commerce and industry*. New York: The Commonwealth Fund.

Moll van Charante, A.W., & Mulder, P.G. (1990). Perceptual acuity and the risk of industrial accident. *American Journal of Epidemiology, 131 (4)*, 652-663.

National Institute for Occupational Safety and Health (NIOSH). (1996). *National occupational research agenda (NORA)*. U.S. Department of Health and Human Services, Public Health Service, Centers for Disease Control and Prevention (Publication No. 96-115). Cincinnati, OH: NIOSH. Retrieved from http://www.2acdc.gov/NORA. Accessed 31 October 2004.

National Institute for Occupational Safety and Health (NIOSH). (2001a).Work-related hearing loss. DHHS (NIOSH) Publication No. 2001-103. Retrieved from http://www.cdc.gov/niosh/topics/noise/a bouthlp/docs/worker-hearingloss_factSheet.pdf. Accessed 22 December 2004.

National Institute for Occupational Safety and Health (NIOSH). (2001b). National occupational research agenda for musculoskeletal disorders: research topics for the next decade – a report by the NORA musculoskeletal disorders team.

DHHS (NIOSH) Publication No. 2001-117. Retrieved from http://www.cdc.gov/niosh/pdfs/2001-117. Accessed 30 November 2004.

National Institute for Occupational Safety and Health (NIOSH). (2004). High-risk industries and occupations. Worker Health Chartbook, 2004. Retrieved from http://www. 2acdc.gov/niosh-chartbook/ch4. Accessed 31 October 2004.

National Safety Council (NSC). (2003). Report on injuries in America, 2002. In *Injury facts, 2003 edition*. Itasca, IL: NSC. Retrieved from http://www.nsc.org/library. Accessed 31 October 2004.

Ramazzini, B. (1993). *The diseases of workmen* (Translated from the Latin *De morbis artificium diatriba of 1713*, by Wilmer Care Wright). Thunder Bay, Ontario: OH&S Press.

Salazar, M.K., Kemerer, S., Amann, M.C., & Fabrey, L.J. (2002). Defining the roles and functions of occupational and environmental health nurses: results of a national job analysis. *American Association of Occupational Health Nurses Journal, 50* (1), 16-25

Suter, A.H. (1993). *Hearing conservation manual: Council for Accreditation in Occupational Hearing Conservation* (3rd ed.). Milwaukee, WI: Council for Accreditation in Occupational hearing Conservation.

U.S. Department of Health and Human Services (DHHS). (2000). *Healthy People 2010* (Conference Edition, in two volumes). Washington, DC: U.S. Government Printing Office. Retrieved from http://www.healthpeople.gov/Document/HTML/Volume2. Accessed 11 October 2004).

US Department of Health and Human Services – Public Health Service (US DHHS PHS). (2004). Progress review: occupational safety and health. retrieved from http://www.healthpeople.gov/data/ 2010prog/focus20. Accessed 31 October 2004.

US Department of Labor (USDL), Bureau of Labor Statistics (BLS). (2002). Injury, illness and fatalities: non-fatal cases involving days away from work: selected characteristics. Retrieved from http://www.bls.gov/iif. Accessed 7 November 2004.

US Department of Labor (USDL), Bureau of Labor Statistics (BLS). (2003). Workplace injuries and illnesses in 2002. Press Release USDL 03-913. Retrieved from http://www.bls.gov/iif/home. htm. Accessed 7 November 2004.

US Department of Labor (USDL), Bureau of Labor Statistics (BLS). (2004a). Union membership declines again in 2003. Retrieved from http://www.bls.gov/opub/ted/2004/jan/wk3/art03.htm. Accessed 23 November 2004.

US Department of Labor (USDL), Bureau of Labor Statistics (BLS). (2004b). Lost-worktime injuries and illnesses: characteristics and resulting days away from work, 2002. Press Release USDL 04-460. Retrieved from http://www. bls.gov/iif/home.htm. Accessed 7 November 2004.

US Department of Labor (USDL), Bureau of Labor Statistics (BLS, 2004c). Tomorrow's jobs. Retrieved from http://www.bls.gov/home. Accessed 11 October 2004.

World Health Organization (WHO). (1994). *Declaration on occupational health for all*. Geneva, Switzerland: WHO.

World Health Organization. (1995). *Global strategy on occupational health for all—the way to health at work*. Geneva, Switzerland: WHO.

World Health Organization (WHO). (1999a). *Occupational health: ethically correct, economically sound* (Fact Sheet No. 84, revised June 1999). Geneva, Switzerland: WHO.

World Health Organization (WHO). (1999b). *The burden of occupational illness: UN agencies sound the alarm* (Press Release PR-99-31). Geneva, Switzerland: WHO.

CHAPTER

2

Workers and Worker Populations

SALLY L. LUSK, DELBERT M. RAYMOND III,
CATHERINE CONNON, AND MARY MILLER

Workers and workplaces are affected by changes and trends that occur in the larger society. It is essential that occupational and environmental health nurses be knowledgeable about these trends and their potential effects on the workforce. This chapter provides an overview of current demographic, social, and technologic trends and describes some of the many worker populations that characterize the modern workplace.

I Demographic and Social Trends

A Supportive and explanatory data

1. Workforce changes reflect changes in the general population.
   a. Assuming no change in immigration laws and fertility rates, the U.S. population will increase by nearly 24% between 2000 and 2025 (U.S. Census Bureau, 2004).
   b. Between 2000 and 2010, the size of the labor force is expected to increase by 17 million, a growth rate of about 1.1% per year, roughly the same as for the 1990s (Fullerton & Toossi, 2001).
   c. The workforce will experience an increase in the proportion of female workers, an increase in the average age of workers, and continued, though variable, growth of all ethnic groups.
   d. The Hispanic labor force will expand faster than the rest of the labor force (Karoly & Panis, 2004).
2. Despite predictions of shorter work days and more vacation time, the number of working hours among Americans has increased relentlessly in recent years (Womens Wall Street, 2005).
   a. Compared with 1969, the average American now works 163 more hours per year.
      1) About 25% of workers spend 49 or more hours on the job each week; and 11% work 60 hours or more.
      2) Overall, salaried workers, especially managers and professional employees, work longer hours than hourly workers.
   b. Americans have less leisure time than many European countries; for example, Swedish workers get 5 to 8 weeks' vacation per year; German, French and English workers average 6 weeks per year (Salary.com, 2004).

c. Flextime and job sharing are work options increasingly important to workers to handle competing demands of work and family (Schaffner & Van Horn, 2003).

3. Virtual offices, or offices without walls, are increasingly used as telecommuting options to reduce office costs and commuting time (Dent, 2000; National Institute of Occupational Safety and Health [NIOSH], 2002).

a. Telework/telecommuters were approximately 10% of the workforce population in 2000, with potential for dramatic increases (VanHorn & Storen, 2003).

b. In 2001, half of those who usually worked at home (defined as at least one day per week) were wage and salary workers who took work home from the job on an unpaid basis; another 17% had a formal arrangement with their employer to be paid for the work they did at home; the remaining 30% were self-employed (U. S. Department of Labor [USDL], Bureau of Labor Statistics [BLS] 2002, March).

c. The trend towards "a seamless work-life paradigm" may affect the health and safety of home workers (NIOSH, 2002).

1) Because of less commuting and a less stressful environment, working at home may result in fewer occupational injuries and illnesses.

2) On the other hand, lack of safety oversight, the introduction of workplace hazards into the home, and isolation from peers may increase stress and the potential for injury occurrence.

d. By 2006, nearly one half of all U.S. workers will be employed in industries that produce or intensively use information technology, products, and services (USDL, 1999).

4. Health care benefits provided at work sites are undergoing rapid changes.

a. Changes in business and political environments have led to drastic reductions in employer-provided health care insurance (Schaffner &Van Horn, 2003).

b. Workers are increasingly being required to pay more out-of-pocket expenses and may have a reduced choice of providers (American Health Consultants, 2003).

5. The National Institute for Occupational Safety and Health (NIOSH, 2002) has identified stress at work as a leading occupational health and safety problem.

a. The organization of work is a major contributor to workplace stress; work organization refers to the following (NIOSH, 2002; 1996):

1) Scheduling of work (work-rest schedules, number of hours of work, shift work)

2) Job design (complexity of tasks, skill and effort required, degree of worker control)

3) Interpersonal aspects of work (relationships with supervisors and co-workers)

4) Career concerns (job security and growth opportunities)

5) Management style (participatory versus autocratic)

6) Organizational characteristics (climate, culture, communications)

b. Layoffs and corporate downsizing are occurring with greater frequency (Klein, 2003; NIOSH, 1996).

c. Longer hours, compressed work weeks, shift work, reduced job security, and part-time and temporary work are realities of the modern workplace (NIOSH, 1996).

      d. See Chapter 15 for more information about stress and the organization of work.

6. Violence in the workplace is a serious concern for American workers; workplace violence includes any action that threatens or causes harm to workers or to the work environment.

      a. Workplace violence may result in lost work time and wages, reduced productivity, medical costs, worker compensation payments, legal and security expenses (Federal Bureau of Investigation [FBI], 2002).

      b. "By impacting society as a whole, [workplace violence] damages trust, harms the community, and threatens the sense of security every worker has a right to feel while on the job" (FBI, 2002).

      c. Although there are warning signs for workplace violence, most workers fail to recognize these signs in potential offenders (e.g., mood change, negative behavior, verbal threats); in fact, an AAOHN survey found that less than 4% of respondents were able to recognize these "red flag" behaviors (AAOHN, 2003).

      d. Workplaces that have violence prevention and education programs are much more likely to identify and prevent dangerous situations before they occur (AAOHN, 2003; FBI, 2002).

      e. Chapters 13 and 15 have more detailed information about workplace violence.

7. Terrorism is an increasing concern worldwide (see Chapter 13).

      a. Terrorism is defined by Title 22 of the United States Code, Section 2656f(d):

         1) The term *terrorism* means premeditated, politically motivated violence perpetrated against noncombatant targets by subnational groups or clandestine agents, usually intended to influence an audience.

         2) The term *international terrorism* means terrorism involving citizens or the territory of more than one country.

         3) The term *terrorist group* means any group practicing, or having significant subgroups that practice, international terrorism.

      b. According to the Emergency Response and Research Institute, in 2001, 6318 civilians, security personnel, and terrorists were killed and 4160 were wounded in international terrorist attacks (Emergency Response and Research Institute, 2002); a large percentage of these were workers.

B **Implications for occupational and environmental health nurses**

1. Occupational and environmental health nurses will need to take into account the changing population and workforce when designing and implementing work-site programs and services.

2. Changes in health care benefits may influence the type of services available to workers from their primary providers; this then may influence the choice of services provided at work sites.

3. Workers may need assistance in handling conflicting demands.

4. Occupational and environmental health nurses may have less opportunity for face-to-face communication with workers; thus they will have to develop less-personal methods of communication with off-site workers.

5. Occupational and environmental health nurses need to be alert to the potentially dangerous effects of fatigue on work-site health and safety.

6. Programs and services are needed to help employers identify and prevent potentially dangerous or explosive personal reactions because of stress or mental illness (Bennett, Cook, & Pelletier, 2003).

7. Appropriate violence prevention and control measures should be developed for the work setting.
8. A comprehensive plan for dealing with terrorism-related events should be in place in every work site to protect employees, customers, the community, and the business (Figure 2-1 provides security recommendations for businesses; also see Chapter 13).

II Technologic Trends

A Explanatory and supportive data

1. The service sector is the most rapidly growing job sector in the United States; between 2002 and 2012, it is anticipated that (USDL, ASP, 2004; NIOSH, 2004a):
   a. Service sector jobs will account for 96% of the new wage and salary jobs generated; manufacturing's share of total jobs will decline.
   b. Computer technology and health care will have the most growth during this period.
2. Demand for skilled work is increasing and educational requirements for jobs are shifting.
   a. Six out of ten workers were unskilled in the 1950s; currently, six out of ten workers are skilled (Schaffner & Van Horn, 2003).
   b. Occupations requiring an associate degree or higher education accounted for 25% of all jobs in 1998; an associate degree or higher education will be required for 40% of the job growth from 1998-2008.
   c. All but 1 of the 50 highest paying occupations requires at least a bachelors' degree (USDL, BLS, 2004, June).
   d. The pay gap between those with education and those without has more than doubled since the mid-1980s (Moe, 2003).
3. Equipment using increasingly high technology will be used in all work settings.
   a. Advances in technology have increased the speed of production and the subsequent demands on workers.
   b. The increasing use of computers at home *and* work has caused higher incidences of cumulative trauma disorders (also called repetitive strain injuries or overuse syndrome).
   c. Automation (robots, robotic systems, and automated machinery) eliminates certain types of jobs, so fewer workers are responsible for complex systems (Levy & Wegman, 2000).

B Implications for occupational and environmental health nurses

1. Because service sector jobs require more interaction with people, they are more likely to involve stress, confrontation, and violence.
2. Occupational stress related to job ambiguity, role uncertainty, and job insecurity may become increasingly apparent as technologic changes are implemented.
3. New technologies will present new hazards that will need to be considered in occupational disease surveillance and prevention; the additive effect of home and recreational use of the technologies will also need to evaluated.

HOMELAND SECURITY ADVISORY SYSTEM RECOMMENDATIONS

Businesses

Risk of Attack	Recommended Actions
SEVERE (Red)	• **Complete recommended actions at lower levels** • Listen to radio/TV for current information/instructions • Be alert to suspicious activity and report it to proper authorities immediately • Work with local community leaders, emergency management, government agencies, community organizations, and utilities to meet immediate needs of the community • Determine need to close business based on circumstances and in accordance with written emergency plan • Be prepared to work with a dispersed or smaller work force • Ensure mental health counselors available for employees
HIGH (Orange)	• **Complete recommended actions at lower levels** • Be alert to suspicious activity and report it to proper authorities • Review emergency plans to include continuity of operations and media materials on hand • Determine need to restrict access to business or provide private security firm support/reinforcement • Contact vendors/suppliers to confirm their emergency response plan procedures • If a need is announced, contact nearest blood collection agency and offer to organize a blood drive
ELEVATED (Yellow)	• **Complete recommended actions at lower levels** • Be alert to suspicious activity and report it to proper authorities • Contact private security firm for security risk assessment and to determine availability of support/reinforcement • Contact voluntary organizations you support to determine how you can provide assistance in case of emergency
GUARDED (Blue)	• **Complete recommended actions at lower levels** • Be alert to suspicious activity and report it to proper authorities • Dialogue with community leaders, emergency management, government agencies, community organizations and utilities about disaster preparedness • Ensure emergency communication plan updated to include purchase of needed equipment. • Ask the local Red Cross chapter to provide a "Terrorism: Preparing for the Unexpected" presentation at your workplace for employees
LOW (Green)	• Use Red Cross *Emergency Management Guide for Business and Industry* to develop written emergency plans to address all hazards. Include an emergency communication plan to notify employees of activities; designate an off-site 'report to' location in case of evacuation. • Develop continuity of operations plan to include designating alternate work facility/location for business • Arrange for staff to take a Red Cross CPR/AED and first aid course • Obtain copies of *Terrorism: Preparing for the Unexpected* and *Preparing Your Business for the Unthinkable* brochures from your local Red Cross chapter for distribution to all employees/management as appropriate.

Your LOCAL AMERICAN RED CROSS CHAPTER has materials available to assist you in developing preparedness capabilities.

ARC 1466 (Rev. 8-2002)

FIGURE 2-1 *Recommended actions for business based on risk of attack.©American National Red Cross, Aug, 2002. All Rights Reserved. Reprinted with permission.*

III Females in the Workforce

An increasing proportion of workers is female.

A Supportive and explanatory data

1. Demographics
   a. In 2003, 60% of females age 16 and older were in the labor force, up from 51% in 1977; since 2000 the labor force participation of females age 16 to 24 has declined (NIOSH, 2004a) and the growth in participation has slowed substantially (USDL, 2003, October).
   b. The proportion of female workers is expected to increase to 48% by 2010 (NIOSH, 2004a).
   c. White, African American, and Asian females participated at essentially the same rate (56%); Hispanic females had the lowest rate of participation in the labor force in 2002 (53%) (USDL, BLS, 2004, February).
   d. The participation rate of women with children has declined since 1999 but is still affected by the age of their children as follows (USDL, BLS, 2004, February):
      1) Mothers with children age 6 to 17: 75% participation
      2) Mothers with children under age 6: 59% participation
      3) Mothers with children under age 3: 56% participation
   e. Since 1975, the labor force participation rate of mothers with children under age 18 has grown from 47% to 72%; by 2002, two-thirds of all mothers in married-couple families were employed (USDL, Women's Bureau [WB], 2004, February).
   f. Females between the ages of 55 and 64 have steadily increased their labor force participation rates from 42.0% in 1985 to 49.2% in 1995 and to 56.6% in 2003 (USDL,WB, 2004).
   g. In 1970, wives' earnings accounted for almost 27% (median) of their families' incomes; by 2001, the proportion had grown to 34% (USDL,WB 2004).
2. Social factors
   a. Females are disproportionately represented in the lower-paying service sector occupations; job segregation by gender continues.
   b. Females have greater responsibilities for care of dependents, both children and the elderly; more females are single custodial parents than males; 72% of caregivers of the elderly are female (USDL, WB, 1998, May).
   c. To meet family and work responsibilities, females may neglect behaviors that promote and maintain their own health (American Association of University Women Educational Foundation, 2003).
3. Work-related factors
   a. Females are often shorter, lighter, and not as physically strong as males; as a result, they may be more at risk for certain types of injuries.
   b. Higher rates of work-related musculoskeletal disorders have been reported in females as compared with males; risk factors may include differences in stature and physiology and the nature of jobs performed by females.
   c. Lung cancer rates are increasing faster in females than in males.
   d. Work-site exposures that present reproductive hazards are a serious consideration for female workers. (Note: Reproductive hazards are also a serious consideration for male workers.)
   e. Sources of work-related stress for females often reflect conflicts between meeting work demands and family and self-care needs (Speilberger, Vagg, & Wasala, 2003).

B **Implications for occupational and environmental health nurses**
1. Work-site programs and services should address the specific needs and problems of females. These programs and services may include education, support groups, referral to community resources, and other strategies that promote health and safety.
   a. Programs and services related to prenatal care, female's health, and menopause concerns should be increased.
   b. Programs related to early detection of breast, uterine, and ovarian cancer should be offered.
   c. Support for caregiver roles assumed outside of work may be required.
   d. Work-site day care for children and dependent adults may be needed.
   e. Females should be targeted for smoking cessation programs and services in view of their increasing smoking rates.
2. Work-site adjustments will need to be made to accommodate biologic characteristics of female workers.
   a. Work stations should be adjusted to accommodate females' stature.
   b. Ergonomic programs and services should be targeted to females to prevent work-related musculoskeletal disorders.
   c. Surveillance for potential reproductive hazards should be conducted.
   d. Personal protective equipment that fits females should be provided.
   e. Because job stress can result from a variety of working conditions, attention should be directed toward the following (Swanson, 2000):
      1) Eliminating sex discrimination and harassment
      2) Developing coping skills
      3) Promoting participation in decision making
      4) Expanding opportunities for advancement
      5) Providing family support programs and services

IV Minorities in the Workforce

An increasing proportion of the population consists of minority groups. Minority populations in the United States are defined as American Indian and Alaska Native (AI/AN), Asian American, African-American (black), Hispanic or Latino, and Native Hawaiian and Other Pacific Islanders (NHOPI) (U.S. Department of Health and Human Services [US DHHS], 2004).

A **Supportive and explanatory data**
1. Demographic and social factors
   a. Because of immigration and the growth of resident minority populations, the United States is becoming increasingly a multiracial, multiethnic society.
   b. By 2010, Hispanics will replace African-Americans as the largest minority group (US Census Bureau, March, 2004).
   c. By 2040, minorities will increase to almost one-half of the population (US Census Bureau, March, 2004).
   d. Minority status has been found to contribute to health disparities, even when controlling for insurance status and access to primary care physicians (Cohen, 2003).
   e. Leading causes of death differ by minority group; for example, hypertension is more common among African-Americans, diabetes among Native Americans, and chronic liver disease among Hispanics.
2. Employment factors

a. In 2000, 12.6% of the U.S. labor force was foreign born (USDL, BLS, 2001).

b. Minorities tend to work disproportionately in high-risk occupations; thus they suffer a disproportionate burden of morbidity and mortality (USDL, BLS, 2001).

c. Nonwhite workers experience higher unemployment rates than white workers (USDL, BLS, 2001).

d. Hispanic and African-American workers have a lower median household income than white workers (Schaffner & Van Horn, 2003).

e. Changes in labor-force composition include continued growth in females' participation, a decline in males', and continued growth by all racial groups (white, black, Hispanic, Asian, and other) (USDL, BLS, 2001).

B **Implications for occupational and environmental health nurses**

1. Because of the increasing number of minority workers, occupational and environmental health nurses will need to have greater knowledge of and make greater use of multicultural approaches.

2. Occupational and environmental health nurses will need increased knowledge of diseases that are common in certain minorities.

3. For workers with fewer educational opportunities, remedial programs offered at the work site will present avenues to attain new skills and knowledge.

4. To ensure participation, work-site health and safety programs and services will need to consider the special needs of workers who are non–English-speaking or who have low literacy levels.

V Age of Workers

The average age of the workforce is increasing.

A **Supportive and explanatory data**

1. Demographic and social factors

a. The U.S. population is growing older; the median age of Americans is projected to climb from 35.5 in 2000 to 40.7 by the year 2050 (Karoly & Panis, 2004).

b. In 2003, there were 21.2 million workers age 55 and older, which was 15.4% of total employment (USDL,WB, 2004, September).

c. More elderly workers are returning to or remaining in the workforce.

d. People are living longer. In 1965 the typical male worker would spend 13 years in retirement, today that has increased to 18 years (Committee for Economic Development, 2003).

e. The number of elderly per working adult is increasing. It is expected that the number of people 65 years of age per 100 working-age Americans will nearly double from 18.6 in 2000 to 34.9 by 2050 (Karoly & Panis, 2004).

f. Savings for retirement for middle-aged workers who suffer a reduction in salary or disruption of employment will be seriously affected.

2. Employment and work-related factors

a. U.S. law has changed; there is no longer a mandatory retirement age for workers in nearly all job categories.

b. The middle-aged and older worker is more likely to have responsibilities for a dependent elderly parent or spouse.

c. Often retirees would like to work, but they confront many barriers (i.e., physical, social, and emotional); additionally they may experience reductions in pension plan payments (Committee for Economic Development, 2003).

d. By 2010, middle age and older age groups will outnumber younger workers (NIOSH, 2004a)

e. Retired workers represent an important worker pool (Committee for Economic Development, 2003).

f. Workers over 55 are 30% less likely to be injured on the job, but when injured, take two weeks longer on average to recover (Tetrick & Quick, 2003).

B **Implications for occupational and environmental health nurses**

1. Occupational and environmental health nurses should consider the following strategies to address the special needs and problems of older workers:

   a. Programs and services to prevent and treat musculoskeletal disorders related to poor ergonomics

   b. Increased light at work sites to improve visibility, because light requirements increase with age

   c. Increased attention to measures to ensure adequate hearing ability

   d. Increased support for caregiver roles assumed outside of work

   e. Promotion of work-site or community day-care facilities for dependent adults

   f. More programs and services focusing on the illnesses more common in middle age, such as cardiovascular disease and cancer

   g. More programs and services to prepare workers for retirement

2. Interactions with older workers should allow for possible decreases in their ability to hear, process information, and handle new technology (Box 2-1).

BOX 2-1

Recommendations for training programs for older workers

Training Programs for Older Workers Should:

- Allow self-paced learning
- Use training materials with high-contrast colors and bold typeface
- Avoid posting training materials above eye level
- Speak clearly and distinctly during training sessions
- Use adult learning principles to train older adults in new skills
- Provide a friendly, supportive environment
- Eliminate jargon from the work site, or at least explain it from the start
- Use multiple training methodologies
- Use older workers to teach other older adults
- Build upon valuable life experiences
- Link learning with rewards
- Give older learners something in writing to help reinforce learning

Source: Fyock, 1990.

3. Disease prevention programs and services may become increasingly important to employers as a means of decreasing health care costs, including the costs of supplemental health care insurance.

4. As corporations attempt to improve their profit picture by reducing employment of mid-level middle-aged workers, programs and services will be needed to assist workers with job and career transitions.

5. Occupational and environmental health nurses should ensure that wellness programs and services take into consideration the needs and interests of older workers.

6. Health promotion by mail has been successful in reducing health care costs of retirees and decreasing health-risk behaviors; this approach represents an opportunity for occupational and environmental health nurses to implement a cost-savings program (Lusk, 1995).

VI Children in the Workforce

A significant percentage of children (12 to 17 years of age) work some time each year.

A **Supportive and explanatory data**

1. Demographics

   a. The minimum age for youth employment in the United States is 14 years, except for certain agricultural jobs in which 12- and 13-year-olds are permitted to work; children working on family farms are exempt from regulations and typically work at a much younger age.

   b. The minimum age for hazardous job activities is 18 years of age in non-agricultural settings, but 16 years of age in agriculture.

   c. Children who work in exploitative situations like sweatshops, largely out of view of regulators or the public, account for a small fraction of those engaged in work in the United States (Castillo, Davis, & Wegman, 1999).

   d. In 2001, it was estimated that nearly 3.7 million 15- to 17-year-old youths were employed in the United States (US General Accounting Office [US GAO], 2002); these figures exclude many 14-year-olds and do not include various job activities, such as newspaper carriers and family businesses, including farming.

   e. It is estimated that at least 44% of 16- to 17-year-olds work some time during the year, and most teens work some time during their high school years.

   f. Most minors are employed in the retail trade, primarily restaurants and grocery stores; service industries; and agriculture (Mardis & Pratt, 2003; Runyan, 2000).

   g Approximately 4% of youth are employed illegally in violation of the laws restricting the hours of work or the prohibited hazardous occupations (U.S. GAO, 2002).

   h. Low-income and minority children are less likely to be employed and, when employed, work more hours and in more hazardous jobs than high-income youths (U.S. GAO, 2002).

2. Injury and illness data

   a. Although most adolescents work part-time, their injury rate has been found to be two times higher than for adults, based on the number of hours worked (NIOSH, 2004; Miller & Kaufman, 1998).

b. An average of 70 adolescents die from injuries at work each year, and nearly 230,000 suffer nonfatal injuries, a substantial number of which require treatment in hospital emergency departments (NIOSH, 2003).

c. More than half of work-related injuries occur in restaurants, the majority of which are fast-food establishments (Mardis & Pratt, 2003); other high-risk industries include retail stores, agriculture, construction, and manufacturing (Runyan & Zakocs, 2000).

d. Many nonfatal injuries involve working with knives, hot oil and cooking appliances, working on wet and greasy floors, and overexertion from heavy lifting; lacerations, strains and sprains, contusions, and burns are the most common injuries (NIOSH, 2003).

e. Adolescent Latino farmworkers are routinely involved with handling pesticides without proper training or use of personal protective equipment; in addition to the lack of age-appropriate materials, language issues and lack of knowledge about risk are barriers to adequate protection (McCauley, et al., 2002).

f. Overall, 40% of work-related fatalities among children occur in agriculture, primarily crop production and 50% of children who died while working in agriculture were under the age of 15 (U.S. GAO, 2002).

g. Retail trades had the second highest number of fatalities; the majority of deaths in retail are due to assaults and violent acts (NIOSH, 2003).

h. About 44% of occupational fatalities among minors involve motor vehicles (i.e., highway collisions, falls from moving vehicles); other common causes are being caught or compressed by equipment or being struck by a falling object (US GAO, 2002).

i. Boys are 8 times more likely to die in the workplace than girls (U. S. GAO, 2002).

3. Work-related factors

a. Federal and state child labor laws regulate youth employment and establish the permitted hours of work, prohibited work activities, and administrative requirements.

b. Use of a permit system for minors to work is required in 41 states, either for the employer to hire minors or for a minor to be employed; youths who work without a work permit are more likely to perform dangerous job tasks and less likely to receive appropriate health and safety training than those with permits (Delp, et al., 2002).

c. It is estimated that more than 75% of employers of young workers are unfamiliar with child labor laws (NIOSH, 2003).

d. Data suggest that a substantial percentage of occupational fatalities among youths are associated with violations of child labor regulations (NIOSH, 2003); nonetheless, in many instances youths are killed doing work currently allowed under the child labor regulations.

e. The Fair Labor Standards Act (FLSA) of 1938, the federal law regulating youth employment, has undergone few substantive changes since 1970 to reflect changes in the patterns of work for young people, the nature of work and associated hazards, and knowledge about the health and safety risks young workers face; state laws differ in their level of protection.

f. Little research has been done to evaluate children for acute, chronic, or latent effects from exposure to toxic chemicals, such as pesticides, or to physical hazards, such as noise; the long-term effects of injuries sustained during early work experiences is also unknown.

4. Social factors
   a. The failure to prevent work-related injuries and provide adequate protection to children in the workplace is a serious public health problem.
   b. The United States leads all other industrialized nations in the employment of youth (Wegman & Davis, 1999).
   c. Children who work have two jobs—education and employment—but typically their work is not connected to their educational needs and goals.
   d. Contributing factors for the increase in the number of children working include social pressure, high level of consumerism, acceptance of child employment, availability of low-skilled jobs, lower wages, growing poverty, relaxation in law enforcement, and increasing immigration.
   e. Teens are inexperienced workers and less likely to recognize hazards or to understand their legal rights on the job; teens may not feel capable of speaking up to an adult supervisor or refusing to do a task that is inappropriate or dangerous, especially if they desire to be treated more like adults than children.
   f. Biology and physiologic immaturity of adolescence puts youth at greater risk for disruption of organ system function as a result of chemical exposures; rapid changes occur in a number of organ systems during this developmental period including reproductive, respiratory, skeletal, immune, and central nervous system (Golub, 2000).
   g. The number of hours worked by teens may affect academic performance and lower educational attainment, diminish participation in peer and family activities, and increase the risk of substance abuse and other minor deviant behaviors (Carskadon, 2004; Dornbusch, 2004).
   h. Adolescents have a physiologic need for more sleep than adults; longer and later work hours may lead to sleep deprivation and thus to falling asleep in school, and increased levels of stress, anxiety, and depression (Carskadon, 1990; Kelman, 1999; Steinberg & Dornbusch, 1991; Steinberg & Cauffman, 1995).
   i. In addition to possible disability leading to lost work time, work-related injuries contribute to missed school time and other age-appropriate activities (Zierold, et al, 2004; Parker, et al., 1994).

B **Implications for occupational and environmental health nurses**
   1. Advocacy
   a. Reinforce that teens have the right to a safe and healthy work environment.
   b. Participate in partnerships with diverse members of the community to develop a comprehensive educational approach that addresses the health and safety needs of young workers; such programs and services should include parents, employers, educators, health care providers, teens, and others (NIOSH, 1999; Zakocs, et al., 1998; Occupational Safety and Health Reporter, 2002).
   c. Encourage educators, who play a role in approving work permits or authorization forms that allow teens to work, to use this opportunity to monitor the appropriateness of planned work activities and hours of work, and ensure that they do not interfere with the student's education; provide information to schools regarding available health and safety curricula for students (Miara, et al., 2003).

    d. Reinforce to employers that they are responsible for providing a safe and healthy work environment and must provide adequate (i.e., extra) supervision and training for young workers and assign only age-appropriate activities.

    e. Educate primary care and adolescent health care providers to inquire about their patients' work activities and provide appropriate anticipatory guidance; workers' compensation should be obtained for work-related injuries or exposures where appropriate.

    f. Promote job opportunities that provide both educational opportunities and a balanced schedule for youths to allow participation in family and peer activities.

    g. Encourage teens to be involved in the development and delivery of health and safety training programs and services; such programs and services increase acceptance among peers and enhance their own investment in protecting themselves and understanding their rights.

    h. Advocate that enforcement of existing regulations should be strengthened; existing child labor regulations should also be updated to reflect their appropriateness in the current work environment; agricultural regulations should be updated to be consistent with the nonagricultural restrictions for hazardous activities.

2. Education and outreach

    a. Occupational health and safety professionals and public health injury control experts should be educated regarding the risk of occupational injury for children and adolescents and develop cross-training programs and services regarding occupational hazards for youth and prevention strategies.

    b. Workplace health and safety training programs and services (e.g., hazard communication, injury and illness prevention, safe task performance) should be age appropriate; teen workers should be encouraged to ask questions and refuse to perform activities that they have not been trained to do or that are too dangerous.

    c. Front-line supervisors and adult co-workers who directly interact with young workers should receive extra training about the special needs of young workers; mentoring programs and services to buddy experienced workers with new ones should be established by employers.

    d. Education about occupational health and safety issues, including work-related rights and responsibilities, should be provided in all high schools; occupational health and safety curricula have been shown to be successful in secondary education (Reed, Westneat, & Kidd, 2003).

    e. Farm families should be involved in educational and prevention activities to increase awareness of the risk of injury in the home and farm work environment.

3. Research

    a. More research is needed to examine the association of factors, such as work experience, gender, work setting, and pace of work, with the occurrence of hazardous exposures and injuries among adolescents.

    b. More research is needed regarding the association between work intensity and injury, including the number of hours worked per day and per week; more understanding about working late night hours during adolescence is also needed.

c. Research leading to a better understanding of age-appropriate work activities in agricultural and nonagricultural settings is crucial.

d. Intervention research projects should be developed to evaluate the effectiveness of training programs and services, such as apprenticeship and other vocational education programs; integration of occupational health and safety curriculum in high schools; programs and services aimed at providing training to employers of youth about their special needs; and enforcement of federal and state child labor regulations.

e. More surveys of teens regarding their beliefs and attitudes about safety on the job should be undertaken; more information is needed to assess the effectiveness of interventions aimed at reaching youth and to identify relevant health communication and training techniques, including issues regarding literacy, language, and cultural differences.

f. Research of the long-term impacts of early work-related exposures and injuries should be done, including evaluation of disability outcomes and psychosocial responses, attitudes toward work and the risk of occupational hazards, biologic effects of toxic exposures, and changes in career options as a result of injury; in addition, the special needs of young workers with disabilities requires more attention.

VII Contingent and Other Alternative Workers

The use of contingent and alternative workers is markedly increasing. The Bureau of Labor Statistics (USDL, BLS, 1999) defines contingent work as any job in which an individual does not have an explicit or implicit contract for long-term employment.

A **Supportive and explanatory data**
1. Demographics
   a. In 2001, 8.6 million workers were identified as independent contractors, 2.1 million worked "on-call," 1.2 million worked for temporary agencies, 633,000 worked for contract firms, and 5.4 million held contingent jobs (USDL, BLS, 2001, May).
   b. Since the 1990s, the contingent workforce has grown two to four times as fast as overall employment (Benner, 2003).
   c. While often offering flexible work arrangements, contingent workers tend to have lower median weekly earnings than workers with traditional jobs (Schaffner & Van Horn, 2003).
   d. The model selected for using contingent workers is influenced by the following factors (Mayall, 1995):
      1) Volume, periodicity, and duration of work
      2) Skill required for the work
      3) Labor supply
      4) Cost of hiring, benefits, and job security
      5) Legislation and unions
   e. From 42% to 49% of contingent workers work part-time (USDL, BLS, 2001, May).
   f. All types of workers may be employed as temporary workers (e.g., doctors and nurses, bank officers, attorneys, and corporate executives) (Theodore & Peck, 2002).
   g. Contingent workers are over-represented in professions, with teachers accounting for more than 10% of all contingent workers (Polivka, 1996).

    h. The trend among large corporations is to outsource their occupational health services, with the following results:

        1) Occupational and environmental health nursing positions may be eliminated.

        2) Nurses with inadequate occupational health and safety preparation may deliver work-site services.

    i. Contingent workers, as compared with noncontingent workers are:

        1) More likely to be female, black, and in services, construction, or agriculture industries (USDL,BLS, 2001, May).

        2) More than twice as likely to be aged 16 to 24 than noncontingent workers and thus more likely to be enrolled in school and less likely to have health insurance and pension benefits through the employer (USDL, BLS, 2001, May).

    j. Over one-half (52%) of contingent workers would prefer a long-term job (USDL, BLS, 2001, May).

2. Work-related factors (Lenz, 1994)

    a. Alternative workers may be co-employed. *Co-employment* is the term used to describe ". . . a relationship between two or more employers in which each has actual or potential legal rights and duties with respect to the same employee or group of employees" (Lenz, 1994, p. 13).

    b. Co-employment influences civil rights, workers' compensation, labor relations and practices, workers' benefits, reasonable accommodation for the disabled, work-site safety, and job training.

        1) Liability is generally determined by the employer's relationship with or actions toward the worker.

        2) Workers' compensation and unemployment insurance laws related to co-employment vary by state in terms of single or joint responsibility.

        3) Generally, health and pension benefits, if any, are provided by the staffing agency (that is, the agency that provides workers for an employer); although few workers receive these benefits now, they may increase as work assignments become more long-term.

    c. The Americans with Disabilities Act (ADA) requires reasonable accommodation on the part of the staffing agency and the work-site employer, but it is not clear regarding specific responsibilities related to alternative workers, making cooperation essential.

    d. Under the ADA, staffing companies have the right to ask relevant health questions before considering a worker for a specific job assignment.

    e. Work-site employers, rather than staffing agencies, are required to maintain OSHA records of workers' illnesses and injuries and to provide work-site safety programs and services; however, staffing agencies are responsible for workers' compensation coverage.

    f. A greater use of staffing agencies is expected in the future.

    g. Temporary workers may be less willing to report illnesses or injuries because of fear that doing so may interfere with the possibility of being hired as a long-term employee (Morris, 1999).

    h. Use of temporary employees offers a business the opportunity to more carefully screen and evaluate potential employees (Theodore & Peck, 2002).

3. Health considerations
   a. Because contingent or alternative workers are less likely to have health insurance than noncontingent or nonalternative workers (USDL, BLS, 2001, May), obtaining health care may be difficult.
   b. The lack of job security may increase contingent and alternative workers' stress.
   c. Tensions may exist between contingent workers and regular workers in a given job site.
   d. The lack of an emotional and psychologic attachment to a place of employment may have a negative effect on a worker's health.

B **Implications for occupational and environmental health nurses**
   1. Occupational and environmental health nurses in some organizations will be providing services to an increasing number of temporary workers.
   2. Because alternative workers are less likely to have health insurance, they will be constrained in their follow-up of recommendations for preventive care and ongoing treatment of chronic problems.
   3. Occupational and environmental health nurses must be familiar with state and federal laws governing the obligations of work-site employers and staffing agencies regarding civil rights, disabilities, safety education, and job training.
   4. Occupational and environmental health nurses may be involved in negotiating arrangements between the staffing agency and the work-site employer regarding selection criteria, care of injured workers, disability adjustments, and safety education.
   5. Because the majority of temporary workers are female, all implications for female workers cited earlier apply to this group as well (Section III. B).
   6. Stress-reduction programs and services may be particularly important at work sites with large numbers of contingent workers.
   7. Alternative workers may need extra help in assessing jobs for hazards and direction regarding job training and job safety.
   8. As corporations outsource their health care services, more occupational and environmental health nurses may experience the challenges of being temporary workers; occupational and environmental health nurses may need to move into entrepreneurial roles to sell their services to industry.

VIII Workers in Labor Unions

A decreasing proportion of workers are represented by labor unions.

A **Supportive and explanatory data**
   1. In contrast with other developed countries, American unions have seen a decline in membership from a high of 35% of workers in the 1950s to less than 13% in 2003 (USDL, BLS, 2004a).
   2. Although an increase in the number of union workers was seen in 1999, a decrease of 369,000 occurred from 2002 to 2003. A total of 15.6 million workers were union members in 2003 (USDL, BLS, 2004a).
   3. The percentage of workers belonging to unions varies by type of employer, as illustrated by the following figures (USDL, BLS, 2004a):
      a. Government—37%
      b. Public utilities—26%
      c. Transportation—26%
      d. Construction—16%
      e. Manufacturing—14%
      f. Agriculture—2%

4. Union membership is highest among local government workers (service groups that include teachers, police officers, and firefighters) at 43% (USDL, BLS, 2004a).
5. The highest unionization rate across demographic groups is for employed African American men; a little more than 17% are members of unions (USDL, BLS, 2004a).
6. From 1983 to 1999, union membership has declined more among men (25% to 14%) than females (15% to 11%) (USDL, BLS, 2004a).
7. Factors contributing to the decline in union membership include the following (Ziegler, 1994):
   a. International competition
   b. More diversified and specialized production techniques
   c. Deregulation of industries
   d. Increased use of part-time and temporary workers
   e. Failure of unions to focus on recruitment
   f. Disenchantment with union leadership
   g. Lack of enforcement of labor laws

B **Implications for occupational and environmental health nurses**
   1. In work sites without union contracts, occupational and environmental health nurses may serve as the primary advocate for the promotion of occupational health and safety programs and services.
   2. In work sites without unions, occupational and environmental health nurses may have the primary responsibility for ensuring that workers are informed and knowledgeable about health and safety hazards in the workplace.
   3. Occupational and environmental health nurses need to involve worker representatives in program planning and implementation, whether they are from the union or other work-team structures.

IX Disabled Workers

An increased number of disabled workers require accommodation.

A **Supportive and explanatory data**
   1. Demographics and social factors
      a. In 2002, over 18 million persons (9.9% of the working-age population [ages 16 to 64]), had work disabilities (U.S. Census Bureau, 2003, table No. 557).
      b. In 2004, among persons aged 16 to 64 years, 7.2% of all work disabilities were severe (U.S. Census Bureau, 2004a).
      c. Work disability increases with age, as follows (U.S. Census Bureau, 2003, table No. 557):
         1) 3.6% of persons 16 to 24 years of age
         2) 5.9% of persons 25 to 34 years of age
         3) 8.7% of persons 35 to 44 years of age
         4) 12.8% of persons 45 to 54 years of age
         5) 22.0% of persons 55 to 64 years of age
      d. In 2002, more females had work disabilities than males (10.1% vs. 9.8%), and more African-Americans had work disabilities than Caucasians (15.3% vs. 9.3%) (U.S. Census Bureau, 2003, table No. 557).
      e. In 2002, the unemployment rate among persons with a work disability (aged 16 to 64) decreased with age, as follows (U.S. Census Bureau, 2003, table No. 613):

1) 29.8% for persons 16 to 24 years of age
2) 17.1% for persons 25 to 34 years of age
3) 15.1% for persons 35 to 44 years of age
4) 10.0% for persons 45 to 54 years of age
5) 8.0% for persons 55 to 64 years of age

  f. Educational level is inversely associated with work disability, as shown by the following figures for ages 16 to 64 (U.S. Census Bureau, 2004a):
1) 20.5% disability for those with less than high school education (8th grade or less)
2) 12.9% disability for those with high school education (9th through 12th grade)
3) 7.0% disability for those with some college education

  g. Among persons aged 16 to 64 with a work disability, those with a bachelor's degree or higher, were nearly twice as likely to be employed, compared with those with a high school diploma as their highest level of formal education (43.1% vs. 24.4%) (U.S. Census Bureau, 2004b).

2. Work-related factors
  a. From 1997 to 2001, the number of disabling injuries occurring on the job increased from 3.8 million to 3.9 million. The number of worker deaths on the job increased from 5,200 to 5,300 over the same period (U.S. Census Bureau, 2003, table No. 649).
  b. In 2001, deaths and disabling on-the-job injuries accounted for 85 million days of production time lost, representing a 6.25% increase over days of production time lost in 2000 (U.S. Census Bureau, 2003, table No. 650).
  c. In 2004, the unemployment rate for persons aged 16 to 64 with work disabilities was estimated at 15.2%, whereas the unemployment rate for persons of the same age group without work disabilities was less than half of that (5.8%) (U.S. Census Bureau, 2004b).
  d. By 2001, more disabling injuries occurred to persons employed in services, trade, manufacturing, and government than in other industry groups, whereas the industries of mining and quarrying, and agriculture had the highest death rates (31.8 per 100,000 workers, and 21.3 per 100,000 workers, respectively) (U.S. Census Bureau, 2003, table No. 649).
  e. Among persons with work disabilities aged 16 to 64 years, females were more likely to receive food stamps (20.3% vs. 12.9%), reside in public housing (8.2% vs. 5.1%), reside in subsidized housing (4.6% vs. 2.4%), and were less likely to be covered by Medicaid (62.2% vs. 70.3%) than were males (U.S. Census Bureau, 2003, table No. 557).
  f. Among persons with work disabilities aged 16 to 64 years, females had a higher unemployment rate compared to males (15.9% vs. 14.7%). However, among persons without work disabilities for that same age group, females had a lower unemployment rate than did males (5.3% vs. 6.4%) (U.S. Census Bureau, 2004b).

B **Implications for occupational and environmental health nurses**
1. Increased attention will need to be given in the workplace to specific needs of disabled workers.
2. Work-site adjustments will be needed to accommodate physical limitations of disabled or functionally impaired workers; these include:
  a. Modification of equipment
  b. Installation of mechanic aids
  c. Job restructuring

    d. Work-schedule modifications

    e. Additional training or conditioning

3. Job requirements, including job tasks, will need to be clearly defined.

4. Programs and services need to be directed at preventing work-related disabling conditions or functional impairments.

5. Comprehensive surveillance programs and services, including hazard and health surveillance, should be incorporated into existing health monitoring systems.

NOTE: Information about the Americans with Disabilities Act can be found in Chapter 3.

X Agricultural Workers

A Supportive and explanatory data

1. Characteristics of the population

    a. Agriculture ranks among the most hazardous industries.

    b. Farm workers are classified into three categories:

      1) Family members who work on their family's farm

      2) Hired farm workers who live locally and work in seasonal agricultural jobs (sometimes called seasonal farmworkers)

      3) Migrant farm workers who are hired farm workers who live outside of the area

    c. All three categories of farm workers often include children as workers.

    d. Migrant workers are subject to all hazards described for any farm worker, plus those associated with frequent moves, poor housing, poverty, social and cultural isolation, lack of health insurance, and work-related musculoskeletal disorders caused by the postures required for harvesting (Arcury, Quandt, Cavey, Elmore, and Russell, 2001).

    e. Hired local (seasonal) farm workers may experience the same problems as migrant workers except for the frequent moves.

    f. Migrant and seasonal farm workers have lower levels of education and wages and, often, only seasonal work with no benefits; these farm workers are among the lowest paid and least protected workers in the United States (National Center for Farmworker Health, 2001).

    g. All farm workers, including family members who work on their farms, are likely to be underinsured for health care.

2. Illnesses and injuries

    a. Including only farms employing 11 or more workers, agricultural production workers have one of the highest incidences (just below construction workers and health care workers) of occupational injuries and illnesses—6.5 cases per 100 full-time workers versus 5.3 for all private industry (USDL, BLS, 2003, December).

    b. In 2003, 150,000 agricultural work injuries and 730 farm-related deaths occurred (National Safety Council, 2003).

    c. Approximately one half of the injuries and deaths involved family farmers; one half involved seasonal farm workers or individuals working in other industries classified as agricultural (fishing, agricultural services, and forestry, excluding logging) (National Safety Council [NSC], 2003).

    d. Every day about 500 agricultural workers incur disabling injuries; about one half result in permanent impairment (NIOSH, 1996).

3. Causes of injury and illness
   a. Machinery and equipment are the most common cause of injury and death on the farm (OSHA, 2002). These include the following:
      1) Rollovers of tractors or harvesting equipment that cause crushing or amputation injuries; one half of deaths are caused by tractors
      2) Power take-off equipment (machinery with a long, powered, rotating shaft) that can twist the worker around the shaft, causing suffocation, scalping, and avulsion injuries
      3) Machinery running in enclosed spaces that can cause carbon monoxide poisoning
   b. Farm machinery may cause noise-induced hearing loss (NIHL).
      1) NIHL may occur at an earlier age and be more severe among farm workers (Thelin, et al., 1983; Wright, 1993).
      2) Approximately 25% of male farm workers in one study had a hearing loss affecting communication by age 30, and 50% by age 50 (Karlovich, et al., 1988).
      3) Hearing loss has been documented in high school students involved in farm work, suggesting that the hearing loss seen in adult farmers may begin in childhood (Broste, et al., 1989).
      4) Noise-induced hearing loss can be prevented through engineering changes to equipment to reduce the noise levels and by workers' use of hearing protection (Lusk, Ronis, & Kerr, 1995).
   c. Safety features in farm equipment
      1) New equipment may have built-in safety features; however, much of the machinery in use is older.
      2) Even new machines may be altered to circumvent safety features that are perceived as interfering with efficiency.
   d. Agricultural workers are exposed to a number of hazardous materials (Table 2-1).
   e. Exposure can be prevented through proper work practices and use of personal protective equipment.
4. The NIOSH Agricultural Initiative, developed in 1990, is a comprehensive research-based intervention program to reduce injury and disease among agricultural workers and their families.
   a. The Agricultural Initiative is designed to accomplish the following (Cordes and Rea, 1991):
      1) Assign nurses to rural areas to talk about prevention and distribute information about injury and illness prevention to farmers
      2) Assess incidence of injury and illness
      3) Provide cancer screening and assess cancer rates
      4) Evaluate farms for safety hazards and determine the incidence of illness among farm family members
      5) Award academic grants to establish new centers and support applied research; as of 2005, nine universities have established agricultural safety and health centers
   b. An Occupational Health Nurse in Agricultural Communities (OHNAC) program was initiated with 31 nurses in rural hospitals, clinics, and health departments in 10 states to provide surveillance of illnesses and injuries related to agricultural work (Connon, et al., 1993).

TABLE 2-1

Hazards to agricultural workers

Hazardous substance	Health effects
Anhydrous ammonia fertilizer	Contact can cause irritation, burns, or asphyxiation (Wright, 1993).
Insecticides and herbicides	Used to increase crop productivity, they can cause coma and death; they have been associated with increased incidence of cancer (Blair & Zahn, 1991; Wright, 1993).
Fungal spores and moldy grains	Cause "farmer's lung," a chronic debilitating condition (Wright, 1993).
Nitrogen oxides	Found in silos, these can cause chemical pneumonitis and pulmonary edema (Wright, 1993).
Methane gases	Gases formed in manure holding tanks and live stock confinement buildings can cause asphyxiation (Wright, 1993).
Extreme heat and cold	Because they work outside, agricultural workers may suffer heat exhaustion or frostbite. Because of their extensive exposure to the sun, they have higher rates of skin cancer and melanoma (Brown, 1991; Blair & Zahn, 1991).
Occupational infections	These infections, acquired from working with soil, animals, and animal wastes, affect thousands of farm workers each year, causing disability (Kligman, Peate, & Cordes, 1991).

B Implications for occupational and environmental health nurses

1. Agricultural workers generally do not receive services focused on their occupational health and safety needs.
2. There is an opportunity and need for collaboration between community health services and occupational and environmental health nurses to meet the needs of agricultural workers, including the following:
   a. Improved recordkeeping and a national monitoring and surveillance system for agricultural occupational illnesses and injuries
   b. Input regarding occupational health and safety illnesses and injuries into federally sponsored programs and services, such as migrant worker programs and services
   c. Improving farm families' understanding of and ability to appropriately respond to hazards that may result in their children's illness or injury
3. NIOSH's OHNAC program begins to address the needs of agricultural workers, but it is available to only a small proportion of agricultural workers.
4. Although the role of the occupational and environmental health nurse working in agriculture has been described (Randolph and Migliozzi, 1993), studies are needed to determine the effectiveness of interventions to prevent illness and injury related to agriculture.
5. Intervention programs and services may include improved engineering standards for equipment, advocacy for legislation related to agricultural health and safety, and education of agricultural workers (Cordes and Rea, 1991).

6. Nurses not trained in occupational and environmental health nursing nonetheless need information regarding agricultural hazards in order to assess and treat rural residents.

XI Construction Workers

A **Supportive and explanatory data**

1. Characteristics of population
   a. In 2002, 6.7 million wage and salary jobs and 1.6 million self-employed were in construction, making it one of the nation's largest industries (USDL, BLS, 2004b).
   b. The construction industry is divided into three major segments.
      1) *Construction of buildings contractors*, or *general contractors*, build residential, industrial, commercial, and other buildings (23.5%)
      2) *Heavy and civil engineering construction contractors* build sewers, roads, highways, bridges, tunnels, and other projects (13.8%)
      3) *Specialty trade contractors* are engaged in specialized activities such as carpentry, painting, plumbing, and electrical work (62.7%) (USDL.BLS, 2004b)
   c. In 2001, more than 80% of construction establishments had fewer than 10 employees (NIOSH, 2004). Few small establishments have formal health and safety programs and services.
   d. Construction workers are a diverse and mobile population that comprises numerous specialists and skilled and semiskilled workers on job sites that are varied and changeable (Lusk, Ronis & Hogan, 1997).
   e. Workers in the skilled and semiskilled trades tend to identify more with their trade than with the employer and are often self-supervised.
   f. A higher proportion of construction workers are without health insurance (27%) compared with the total for all industries (16%) (Center to Protect Workers' Rights, 2002).

2. Work characteristics
   a. A significant portion of construction work is done outdoors, and indoor activities occur in relatively small spaces.
   b. Job sites are temporary; workers may work on several different job sites in a single day.
   c. The variability of the job sites, job conditions, tools used, and patterns of employment inhibit the use of environmental and engineering controls to reduce hazards (Lusk, Ronis, & Hogan, 1997).

3. Injury and illness data
   a. In 2002, cases of work-related injury and illness were 7.1 per 100 full-time construction workers, which is significantly higher (40% higher) than the 5.3 rate for the entire private sector (Henshaw, 2004).
   b. Because injury rates are calculated with numbers of workers rather than hours worked as the denominator, the rates of construction worker fatalities may be underestimated because of part-time employment or overtime work.
   c. Although those establishments with fewer than 20 employees employed only 38.2% of the workforce, fatal occupational injuries among these smaller establishments accounted for more than 55.5% of fatal occupational injuries in 2001 (NIOSH, 2004a).

d. In the year 2000 while fatality rates declined for non-Hispanic workers, there was a 24% increase in fatal injuries in construction work among Hispanic workers (NIOSH, 2001).

e. Fatalities and injuries in the construction industry are often a result of falls, 4.3 per 100,000 full-time workers NIOSH, 2004a).

f. In 2002, construction fatalities were reduced by 9%, a drop from 1225 to 1121 (Henshaw, 2004).

g. Because of the large amount of time spent outdoors, construction workers are at increased risk from the effects of heat, cold, and sun exposure.

h. Construction workers have high rates of hearing loss, but typically have not received training programs to promote use of hearing protection (Lusk, et al., 1999).

i. Construction health hazards have been characterized as ranging "from A to Z" (Table 2-2).

j. Exposure to hazardous materials may spread to family members when construction workers carry home toxic substances on their clothing and tools.

TABLE 2-2

Examples of construction hazards A to Z

Hazardous substance	Sources of exposure
Asbestos	Pipe insulation, asbestos concrete building materials, roofing felts
Beryllium	Beryllium-copper alloys
Carbon monoxide	Gasoline-powered engines and power tools
Diesel emissions	Portable power tools, heavy equipment
Electromagnetic radiation	X-radiography, UV from welding
Formaldehyde	Plywood, particleboard, carpet
Gasoline	Operating and refueling equipment
Heat stress	Roofing, carpentry
Insect bites	Ticks or other insects
J-Band radio energy	Construction around radar sites
Ketones	Adhesives, glues, mastics
Lead	Fumes from hot work on painted structural elements
Metal fumes	Welding, cutting, and burning metal
Noise	Heavy equipment, portable power tools
Overexertion	Handling materials, lifting
Polynuclear aromatics	Combustion products
Q-switched lasers	Surveying, aligning sewer pipe
Repetitive trauma	Laying carpet, tying rebar
Styrene	Plastic materials
Tar	Roofing materials, coatings and linings for underground tanks and pipelines
Urethane paints	Decomposition products, including hydrogen cyanide
Vibration	Pneumatic tools
Welding fumes	Lead, copper, cadmium, iron, chrome, nickel
Xylene	Paints, glues, adhesives, mastics
Zinc	Fumes from cutting galvanized metals

Source: Rekus, 1994.

UV, Ultraviolet.

4. Standards for hearing-conservation programs and services are less stringent for construction than for manufacturers, even though construction workers are exposed to excessive noise in many of their job sites.
   a. No requirement exists for periodic noise monitoring, dosimetry, periodic audiometric testing, or worker education.
   b. In 2002, OSHA placed a notice on their docket for a standard for hearing conservation programs in construction, but as of 2005, it was downgraded from pre-rule to long term action stage (Laborers' Health and safety fund of North America (LHSFNA), 2005).
   c. "Many hazardous exposures result from inadequacies in access to information, measurement technology, and personal protective equipment" (Ringen, et al., 1995).

B **Implications for occupational and environmental health nurses**
1. Construction workers are underserved by occupational health and safety programs and services; therefore there is a need for new programs and services to reach this segment of the worker population.
2. Programs and services should focus on the major hazards of the construction industry—falls, machinery, chemicals, and noise.
3. Because construction workers work for multiple employers, there may be opportunities for entrepreneurial nurses to provide occupational health and safety services.
4. Ensuring health and safety in construction is complex, involving short-term work sites, changing hazards, and multiple crews working in close proximity (NIOSH, 1996b, July).
5. Because of the strong identification with the trade, trade union groups represent potential avenues for providing occupational health and safety services to construction workers.

XII Health Care Workers

A **Supportive and explanatory data**
1. Demographics and trends
   a. Health care and related services is one of the largest industries in the nation, employing about 11.3 million in 1998, of which more than two million were registered nurses and nearly a half million were self-employed (Kelenson and Tate, 2000; USDL, BLS, 2000).
   b. The health care industry employs a diverse population in a variety of occupational segments; it includes workers from all socioeconomic strata with varying levels of education, training, and English language skills, including the following:
      1) Professional specialties such as physicians, registered nurses, social workers, and therapists
      2) Service occupations such as nurse aides, medical assistants, dietary aides, janitors and housekeepers, and personal care and home health aides
      3) Technicians and support personnel such as health information and laboratory technicians, dental hygienists, clerical staff, and others
      4) Executive and administrative personnel
   c. More than 460,000 establishments make up the health industry, varying greatly in terms of size, staffing, and organization (USDL, BLS, 2000).

1) Hospitals constitute less than 2% of all private health service establishments, but employ nearly 40% of all workers in the industry; when government hospitals are included, the proportion rises to nearly half of all workers.

2) Nearly two thirds of hospital employees work in establishments with more than 1,000 workers.

3) More than half of all non-hospital health establishments employ fewer than five workers.

d. Much of the health care industry workforce is employed part-time; many of these workers are students, parents of young children, dual job holders, and older workers.

e. Health care professionals tend to be older than workers in other industries, particularly in specialties requiring higher levels of education and training; the percent of workers 55 and older in nursing and health-related fields will increase from 12 to 18 percent between 2000 and 2008 (USDL, WB, 2004).

f. Growth in the health care industry is expected to exceed that of other industries for at least another decade (USDL, BLS, 2000).

1) Between 1986 and 1996, nearly one out of every nine new jobs created by the economy was in the health care industry.

2) Between 1998 and 2008, approximately 14% of all new jobs will be in the health care industry, adding about 2.8 million new jobs.

3) Employment in the health care industry is projected to increase 26% through 2008, compared with an average of 15% for all industries; the greatest growth will be concentrated outside the inpatient hospital sector.

4) By 2008, 12 of the 30 fastest growing occupations will be in the health care industry.

g. The changing landscape of the health care industry and the evolving national demographics will continue to redistribute the workforce (Kelenson and Tate, 2000; USDL, BLS, 2000):

1) Advancing medical technology enables increasingly sophisticated treatments and procedures to be provided in ambulatory clinics, provider offices, residential care facilities, and private homes.

2) The aging of the general population will require more home care and personal care services and residential nursing facilities; these segments of the industry will increase by 58% to 80% between 1998 and 2008.

3) As advances in medical technology increase the survival rate of severely ill or traumatically injured patients, more extensive therapy and rehabilitation facilities will be required.

2. Work environment

a. The North American Industrial Classification System (NAICS) sector 62, *Health Care and Social Assistance,* categorizes nine work environments in the health care industry (US DHHS, Center for Medicare and Medicaid Services [CMS], 2005):

1) Offices of physicians

2) Offices and clinics of dentists

3) Offices and clinics of other health practitioners

4) Outpatient care centers

5) Medical and diagnostic laboratories

    6) Home health agencies
    7) Other ambulatory health care
    8) Hospitals
    9) Nursing and residential care facilities
  b. Two thirds of all private health establishments are physician or dentist offices.
  c. Many who are employed in the health care industry have little or no direct health care delivery functions, yet may be exposed to the same occupational hazards.
  d. Most segments of the health services industry are not heavily unionized; in 1998, 14.9% of hospital workers and 10.7% of workers in nursing and personal care facilities were covered by union contracts.
  e. Very few hospital-based facilities offer comprehensive health promotion programs and services for employees (Rogers, 2002).
  f. Personnel who provide home care are exposed to many of the hazards traditionally associated with acute-care settings in addition to those unique to residential environments (e.g., traffic accidents, falls inside and outside homes, and increased risk of overexertion injuries). Mechanical lifting devices are rarely available in patients' homes (USDL, BLS, 2000).
  g. In 2002, the incidence of nonfatal occupational injuries in health care workers was equal to that of construction workers (6.9 per 100 full-time equivalents), the highest for all worker groups; incidence rates for health care workers (HCWs) by employment setting, compared to the rate for all service industries at 4.3, were as follows (USDL, BLS, 2003, December):
    1) Nursing and personal care facilities—12.1
    2) Hospitals—8.9
    3) HCWs providing residential care—5.5
  h. Needlestick and other sharps injuries present a significant risk of blood-borne pathogen infection to direct caregivers and others working in the health care environment.
    1) OSHA has responded to this risk by issuing a revised Bloodborne Pathogen Compliance Directive (1999) emphasizing the importance of implementing safer medical technologies, such as needleless systems, among other administrative, engineering, and training requirements.
    2) Several states have introduced or passed legislation aimed at requiring health care establishments to evaluate and make available safer medical devices.
  i. HCWs and others in the industry who regularly don latex gloves are at increased risk for developing latex allergy; an estimated 6.2% to 30% of HCWs are allergic to latex (Lopes, Benatti, & Zollner, 2004).
  j. Workers in health care delivery environments are routinely exposed to biologic hazards at rates far exceeding the exposure to the general population, including the following general categories (Table 2-3 lists the most significant biologic hazards):
    1) Bloodborne pathogens
    2) Airborne pathogens
    3) Vaccine-preventable communicable diseases
  k. Workers in health care facilities are often exposed to chemical hazards, which may contribute to sensitization or allergy, such as the following:
    1) Anesthetic gases

TABLE 2-3

Selected biologic occupational hazards to health care workers

Biologic/infectious agent	Major sources of exposure
Hepatitis A, E	Feces
Hepatitis B (HBV), Hepatitis C	Blood and body fluids
Hepatitis D (found only in patients with HBV)	Blood and body fluids
Human immunodeficiency virus	Blood and body fluids
Cytomegalovirus	Blood and body fluids
Rubeola (hard measles, red measles, 10-day)	Respiratory secretions (direct contact, droplet)
Mumps	Saliva (droplet, direct contact)
Rubella (German measles, 3-day)	Respiratory secretions (direct/indirect contact, droplet, airborne); virus shed in urine and stool
Influenza	Respiratory secretions, airborne droplet
Varicella zoster virus:	Indirect contact with freshly soiled articles
• Chickenpox	Respiratory secretions (direct contact, airborne)
• Shingles	Secretions of lesions, saliva
Herpes simplex virus	Secretions of lesions, saliva
Tuberculosis (pulmonary)	Airborne droplet
Salmonella, Shigella, Campylobacter	Feces
Parvovirus B19	Airborne droplet
Adenovirus	Airborne droplet, possibly by contact
Respiratory syncytial virus	Respiratory secretions (direct/indirect, droplet)
Pertussis	Airborne droplet, respiratory secretions
Scabies	Direct skin contact with infected lesions
Methicillin resistant staph aureus	Contact with purulent lesion, airborne (rare)
Fungal infections: dermatitis, parenychia	Frequently moist skin; direct contact

Source: Chin, 2000; DiBenedetto, 1995; Sepkowitz, 1996.

      2) Chemotherapeutic and antineoplastic agents
      3) Disinfectants, detergents
      4) Sterilizing agents
      5) Solvents
      6) Latex proteins
      7) Tissue fixatives and reagents
  k. Workers in health industries are regularly exposed to multiple physical and environmental hazards (Box 2-2).
  l. Psychologic and emotional hazards in health care fields stem from the following sources and may result in the effects listed in Box 2-3.
      1) Dealing directly with human suffering
      2) Ethical dilemmas regarding client care decisions
      3) Work overloads, staff shortages, hectic work schedules
      4) Cyclic job insecurity
      5) Verbal and physical aggression
      6) Working rotating or nighttime shifts

B Implications for occupational and environmental health nurses
  1. Collaborative relationships between occupational health and safety professionals and administrative personnel can effectively facilitate the prevention, control, and abatement of occupational hazards, thereby reducing a number of risks.

BOX 2-2

Physical and environmental hazards in health care settings

- Needlesticks are the most commonly reported injury among HCWs.
- Over one half of all reported back injuries occur within the health care field.
- Radiation may be ionizing or nonionizing.
  - Ionizing radiation has cumulative detrimental effects to all living tissue, including fetal tissue.
  - Nonionizing radiation poses thermal and light hazards to skin and eyes.
- Workers in health care are at greater risk for violent incidents than in other industries.
- Noise levels in housekeeping, dietary, laboratories, engineering, laundry, some nursing units, and other departments are often recorded at 80 dBA or higher.
- Ergonomic hazards in health care include cluttered hallways, patient rooms crowded with equipment, wet floors, the need to maneuver multiple pieces of equipment, awkward patient transfers, and the fast pace of emergent situations.
- Verbal and physical aggression is increasing in health care work environments.
- Lasers, a type of electromagnetic radiation increasingly used in health care settings, pose a risk of tissue trauma, particularly to vulnerable tissue, such as the eye.

BOX 2-3

Adverse effects of psychologic stress in health care workers

- Higher incidence of depression than in the general population
- Higher incidence of chemical substance addiction than in the general population
- Career burnout
- Psychologic and physical effects of shift work:
  - Chronic fatigue
  - Alterations in mood and personality
  - Strained interpersonal relationships; decreased socialization
  - Disorders of sleeping, eating, and elimination
  - Decreased alertness; higher rates of accidents
  - Increased rates of infertility or decreased fertility and other adverse reproductive outcomes among workers who rotate shifts
- Anxiety-related disorders, including altered work performance, related to actual or potential exposures to biologic, chemical, or other occupational hazards

2. As occupational hazards become known (e.g., latex allergies) and new technologies emerge (e.g., safer needle systems), occupational and environmental health nurses have a responsibility to advocate for organizational policies that address these issues.

3. The wide variety of workers in health industries, with their varying educational levels and job tasks, requires that occupational health and safety services and information be customized to the audience.

4. Comprehensive employee health services need to be made available to all health care workers, including those who work off-site, those who provide home care services, night shift workers, and workers with no patient-care responsibilities.

5. There is a need for health establishments to offer more comprehensive health promotion programs and services to employees.

6. There may be increased opportunities for occupational and environmental health nurses to offer health and safety services to independent and alternative practitioners, as the public increases its demand for such professional services as acupuncture, naturopathy, hypnosis, chiropractic, and others.

7. As health establishments reorganize and merge, occupational and environmental health nurses will increasingly be responsible for the health and safety of employees in satellite and ambulatory clinics and associated service facilities, such as long term care facilities, that are affiliated with health care consortiums.

8. Health and safety services for home care workers need to be expanded to include assessments of the client's living environment; occupational and environmental health nurses may be able to advocate for temporary equipment to reduce the risk of injury.

9. Organizational policies and procedures to prevent, and a crisis plan to handle, violent incidents should be developed (USDL, OSHA, 1996).

10. Attention to the health and safety concerns of workers of childbearing age, particularly with respect to reproductive hazards, continues to be needed.

XIII International (Expatriate) Workers

A **Supportive and explanatory data**

1. Demographics and trends
   a. Because of the increase in globalization, the number of expatriates has dramatically increased in the last three decades; it is estimated that about 350,000 U.S. nationals work abroad each year (Baruch & Altman, 2002; Blonigen, 1998).
   b. Other factors that have contributed to the growth of international business are trade policy reforms that favor businesses, and economic and regulatory incentives.
   c. The employees of some large multinational companies log thousands of business trips each year; for example, the World Bank in Washington DC sends about 5,000 workers on more than 18,000 business trips each year.
   d. Ninety percent of U.S. expatriates are male; the percentage of female expatriates is increasing.

e. New capitalistic and developing nations enthusiastically recruit business enterprises and skilled labor from the United States and other developed nations.

2. The international workplace
   a. Approximately 80% of U.S. companies with expatriate workers provide pre-departure orientation regarding health issues; of these, only 42% offer orientation to all expatriate workers.
   b. Health systems abroad vary widely; some may not be able to offer the quality or quantity of services to which U.S. workers are accustomed.
   c. Some studies suggest that workers who travel seek health care more often than workers who do not travel; for example, traveling males are 80% more likely to seek health care than non-traveling males, and traveling females are 18% more likely than their non-traveling counterparts (Rose, 2001).
   d. Local business, cultural, and social norms abroad may differ significantly from those in the U.S. workplace; a lack of understanding of norms may lead to interpersonal conflict and workplace stress among expatriate workers.
   e. Economic and environmental regulatory incentives that help recruit multinational companies to foreign locations may also contribute to unsafe, unhealthy, and repressive working conditions for local workers (Baruch & Altman, 2002; Blonigen, 1998).
   f. Hazardous industries relocated in developing and newly industrialized countries are often without adequate worker health and safety precautions.
   g. Although international guidelines for selected toxicants exist, efforts to develop international uniform occupational exposure limits have been unsuccessful; political and social forces often influence scientific decisions about exposure limits (Levy & Rest, 1996).
   h. Terrorist activities such as kidnapping or hostage taking are an increasing concern for international travelers in this post-9/11 world; multinational companies and their workers are often the target of dissident groups wanting to make a political statement.

B **Implications for occupational and environmental health nurses**
1. The breadth and depth of pre-departure orientation related to the health issues of U.S. nationals planning to work abroad will need to be increased. (Chapter 16 presents an example of an international travel program).
2. U.S. nationals who are dispatched to work abroad need appropriate vaccinations against infectious agents endemic to the destination country.
3. Contingency plans for accessing local emergency services and for emergency evacuation should be developed.
4. Occupational health and safety programs and services need to be sensitive to regional management practices and cultural norms.
5. Occupational and environmental health nurses can be advocates for ethical practices related to child labor, females' health, and other workplace health and safety issues.
6. Occupational and environmental health nurses responsible for the health and safety of expatriate workers can gain valuable advice and insight from such international resources as the WHO, ILO, and International Safety Council.

REFERENCES

American Association of Occupational Health Nurses (2003). *Standards of occupational and environmental health nursing.* Atlanta, GA: AAOHN Publications.

American Association of University Women Educational Foundation (2003). *Women at work.* Washington, DC: AAUW Educational Foundation.

American Health Consultants (2003). Changing health care environment can make discharge planning a juggling act; Patients have more out-of-pocket expenses, changing benefits. *Hospital Case Management, 11*(4), 49-64.

American National Red Cross (2002, August) Homeland security advisory system recommendations: Businesses. American National Red Cross. Available at http://www.redcross.org/ services/ disaster/beprepared/hsas. html

American Public Health Association (APHA) (2002). Protection of Child and Adolescent Workers, Policy Statement 2001-9. *Am J Public Health 92*, 461-462.

Arcury, T.A., Quandt, S.A., Cravey, A.J., Elmore, R.C., & Russell, G.B. (2001). Farmworkers reports of pesticide safety and sanitation in the work environment. *American Journal of Industrial Medicine, 39*, 487-498.

Baruch, Y., & Altman, Y. (2002). Expatriation and repatriation in MNCs: A taxonomy. *Human Resource Management, 41*(2), 239-259.

Benner, C. (2003). Shock absorbers in the new economy. In Schaffner, H.A., & Van Horn, C.E., (Eds.), *A nation at work: The Heldrich guide to the American workforce* (pp. 221-225). New Brunswick, NJ: Rutgers University Press.

Bennett, J. B., Cook, R. F., & Pelletier, K .R. (2003). Toward an integrated framework for comprehensive organizational wellness: Concepts, practices and research in workplace health promotion. In Quick, J.C., & Tetrick, L.E. (Eds.), *Handbook of occupational health psychology* (pp. 69-96). Washington, DC: American Psychological Association.

Blair, A., & Zahn, S. H. (1991). Cancer among farmers. In D. H. Cordes & D. F. Rea (Eds.), *Occupational Medicine: Health Hazards of Farming. State of the Art Reviews, 6*(3) 335–354.

Blonigen, M. (1998). Managing global operations: focus on expatriates. *Decision Line,* Retrieved December 28, 2004 from http://www.decisionsciences.org/DecisionLine/Vol29/29_4/pom_29_4.pdf.

Broste, S. K., Hanson, D. A., Strand, R. L., & Stueland, D. T. (1989). Hearing loss among high school farm students. *American Journal of Public Health, 79*, 619-622.

Brown, W. D. (1991). Heat and cold in farm workers. In D. H. Cordes & D. F. Rea (Eds.), *Occupational Medicine: Health Hazards of Farming. State of the Art Reviews, 6*(3) 371–390. Philadelphia: Hanley & Belfus, Inc.

Carskadon, M. (1990). Patterns of sleep and sleepiness in adolescents. *Pediatrician, 17,* 5-12.

Carskadon, M. A. (2004). Factors influencing sleep patterns of adolescents. In M, A. Carskadon (Ed.), *Adolescent sleep patterns: Biological, social, and psychological influences.* Cambridge, UK: Cambridge University Press, pp. 4-26.

Castillo, D., Davis, L., & Wegman, D. (1999). Young workers. *Occupational medicine: State of the art reviews, 14*(3), 519-536.

Center to Protect Workers' Rights (CPWR). (2002). *The construction chart book* (3rd ed). Washington, DC: CPWR.

Chin, J. (Ed.). (2000). Control of communicable diseases manual (17th ed.). Washington DC: American Public Health Association.

Cohen, J. J., (2003). Disparities in health care: An overview. *Academic Emergency Medicine, 10,* 1155-1160.

Committee for Economic Development (2003). New opportunities for older workers. In H. A. .Schaffner & C. E. Van Horn (Eds.), *A nation at work: The Heldrich guide to the American workforce* (pp. 372-376). New Brunswick, NJ: Rutgers University Press.

Connon, C. L., Freund, E., & Ehlers, J. K. (1993). The occupational health nurse in agricultural communities program: Identifying and preventing agriculturally related illnesses and injuries. *AAOHN Journal, 41,* 422-428.

Cordes, D.H., & Rea, D.F. (1991). Farming: A hazardous occupation. In D.H. Cordes & D.F. Rea (Eds.), *Occupational medicine: Health hazards of farming. State of the art reviews, 6(3)* 327-334. Philadelphia: Hanley & Belfus, Inc.

Delp, L., Runyan, C. W., Brown, M., Bowling, J. M., & Jahan, S. A. (2002). Role of work permits in teen workers' experience. *American Journal of Industrial Medicine*, 41(6), 477-482.

Dent, H. S., Jr. (2000). The roaring 2000s. New York: Simon & Schuster.

DiBenedetto, D. V. (1995). Occupational hazards of the health care industry: Protecting health care workers. *AAOHN Journal*, 43 (3), 131–137.

Dornbusch S. M. (2004). Sleep and adolescence: A social psychologist's perspective. In: M. A. Carskadon (Ed.), *Adolescent sleep patterns: Biological, social, and psychological influences* (pp. 1-3). Cambridge, UK: Cambridge University Press.

Emergency Response and Research Institute (2002). *Summary of emergency response and research terrorism statistics: 2001 and 2002*. Available at http://www.emergency.com/.

Federal Bureau of Investigation (2002). Workplace violence: Issues in response. Quantico, VA: Critical Incident Response Group: National Center for Analysis of Violent Crime.

Fullerton, H., & Toossi, M. (2001, November). Labor force projections to 2010: Steady growth and changing composition. *Monthly Labor Review*, 124(11), 21-38.

Fyock, C. D. (1990). *America's work force is coming of age*. Lexington, MA: Lexington Books.

Golub, M. S. (2000). Adolescent health and the environment. *Environmental Health Perspectives*, 108(4):355-362.

Henshaw, J. L. (2004, February) Speech at the 14th Annual Construction Safety Conference Chicagoland Construction Safety Council Chicago, Illinois. Available at http://www.osha.gov/

Karlovich, R. S., Wiley, T. L., Tweed, T., & Jensen, D. V. (1988). Hearing sensitivity in farmers. *Public Health Reports*, 103(1), 61-71.

Karoly, L. A., & Panis, C. W. (2004). The 21st century at work; Forces shaping the future workforce and workplace in the United States. Santa Monica, CA: Rand Corporation.

Kelenson, J. W., & Tate, P. (2000). The 1998-2008 job outlook in brief. Occupational Outlook Quarterly, (Spring, 2000). Available at http://www.bls.gov.oco/.

Kelman, B. (1999). The sleep needs of adolescents. *Journal of School Nursing*, 15(3), 14-19.

Klein, N. (2003). The discarded factory: Degraded production in the age of the superbrand. In H. A. Schaffner & C. E. Van Horn (Eds.), A nation at work: The Heldrich guide to the American workforce (pp. 189-198). New Brunswick, NJ: Rutgers University Press.

Kligman, E. W., Peate, W. F., & Cordes, D. H. (1991). *Occupational infections in farm workers. In D. H. Cordes & D. F. Rea (Eds.), Occupational Medicine: Health Hazards of Farming. State of the Art Reviews*, 6(3), 429–446. Philadelphia: Hanley & Belfus, Inc.

Kraus, L. E., & Stoddard, S. (1991). Chartbook on work disability in the United States. An InfoUse report. Washington, DC: U.S. National Institute on Disability and Rehabilitation Research.

Laborers' Health & Safety Fund of North America (LHSFNA) (2005, February). Hearing conservation squelched at OSHA. *Lifelines online*. Washington, D. C.: LHSFNA. Available at http://www.lhsfna.org/

Levy, B. S., & Rest, K. M. (1996). Policies to protect and promote workers' health are necessary for sustainable human development. In G. Shahi, B. S. Levy, A. Binger, T. Kjellstrom, & R. Lawrence (Eds.), *International perspectives in environment, health and development: Toward a sustainable world* (pp. 486-496). New York: Springer.

Levy, B. S., & Wegman, D. H. (2000). *Occupational health: Recognizing and preventing work-related disease and injury*, (4th ed.). Boston: Little, Brown and Company.

Lopes, R. A., Benatti, M. C., & Zollner, R. L. (2004). A review of latex sensitivity related to the use of latex gloves in hospitals. *AORN Journal*, 80(1), 64-71.

Lusk, S. L., Hong, O. S., Ronis, D. L., Kerr, M. J., Eakin, B. L., & Early, M. R. (1999). Effectiveness of an intervention to increase construction workers' use of hearing protection. *Human Factors*, 41(3), 487-494.

Lusk, S. L., Ronis, D. L., & Hogan, M. M. (1997). Test of the health promotion model as a causal model of construction workers' use of heavy protection. *Research in Nursing and Health*, 20, 183-194.

Lusk, S. L., Ronis, D. L., & Kerr, M. J. (1995). Predictors of hearing protection use among workers: Implications for training programs. *Human Factors, 37*(3), 635-640.

Mardis, A. L., & Pratt, S. G. (2003). Nonfatal injuries to young workers in the retail trades and service industries in 1998. *Journal of Occupational and Environmental Medicine, 45*(3), 316-323.

McCauley, L. A., Sticker, D., Bryan, C., Lasarev, M. R., & Scherer, J. A. (2002). Pesticide knowledge and risk perception among adolescent Latino farmworkers. *Journal of Agricultural Safety and Health, 8*(4), 397-409.

Miara, C., Gallagher, S., Bush, D., & Dewey, R. (2003). Developing an effective tool for teaching teens about workplace safety. *American Journal of Health Education,* Supplement 34(5):S 30-34.

Moe, M. (2003). The knowledge web. In H. A. Schaffner & C. E. Van Horn (Eds), *A nation at work: The Heldrich guide to the American workforce* (pp. 329-336). New Brunswick, NJ: Rutgers University Press.

Morris, J. (1999). Injury experience of temporary workers in a manufacturing setting. Factors that increase vulnerability. *AAOHN Journal, 47*(10), 470-478.

National Center for Farmworker Health (2001). *Migrant health issues. Introduction.* Monograph series: Bethesda, MD: Migrant Health Branch.

National Institute for Occupational Safety and Health (NIOSH) Facts, (1996a, July). Agriculture safety and health. Available at http://www.cdc.gov/niosh/agfc.html.

National Institute for Occupational Safety and Health (NIOSH). (2003). *NIOSH Alert: Preventing deaths, injuries and illnesses of young workers.* (DHHS [NIOSH] Publication No. 2003-12b. Cincinnati, OH: U.S. Department of Health and Human Services.

National Institute for Occupational Safety and Health (NIOSH) (1999). *Promoting safe work for young workers: A community-based approach,* (DHHS [NIOSH] Publication No. 99-14. Cincinnati, OH: U.S. Department of Health and Human Services.

National Institute for Occupational Safety and Health (NIOSH) (2005). *Emergency preparedness for business.* NIOSH Health and Safety Topic. Retrieved March 1, 2005 from http://www.cdc.gov/niosh/topics/prepared

National Institute for Occupational Safety and Health (2001, December 19). *NIOSH adds Spanish-language web section with job health, safety information.* Retrieved February 1, 2002, from http://www.cdc.gov/niosh/spansite.html

National Institute for Occupational Safety and Health (NIOSH, 2004a). *Worker health chartbook.* NIOSH Publication No. 2004-146.

National Institute for Occupational Safety and Health (2002). Recommendations to the U.S. Department of Labor for Changes to Hazardous Orders, May 3, 2002. U.S. Department of Health and Human Services. Available from http://youthrules.dol.gov/niosh_recs_to_dol_050302.pdf, accessed September 16, 2004.

National Institute for Occupational Safety and Health (2004). Work-related Injury Statistics Query System. Available at http://www2.cdc.gov/risqs, accessed September 2, 2004.

National Safety Council (NSC). (2003). *Report on Injuries in America, 2002.* Itasca, IL: NSC.

Occupational Safety and Health Reporter (2002). *State focuses on fast-food industry to address teenager safety at work.* 32(5), pp.96-97.

Parker, D., Carl, W., French, L., & Martin, F. (1994). Characteristics of adolescent work injuries reported to the Minnesota Department of Labor and Industry. American Journal of Public Health, 84(4), 606-611.

Polivka, A. E. (1996, October). A profile of contingent workers. *Monthly Labor Review, 119*(10), 10-21.

Randolph, S. A., & Migliozzi, A. A. (1993). The role of the agricultural health nurse: Bringing together community and occupational health. *AAOHN Journal,* 41, 429-433.

Reed, D. B., Westneat, S. C., & Kidd, P. (2003). Observation study of students who completed a high school agricultural safety education program. *Journal of Agricultural Safety and Health, 9*(4), 275-283.

Rekus, J. F. (1994, May). Chronic risks in construction. *Occupational Health & Safety,* 103–104, 106–108, 129.

Ringen, K., Englund, A., Welch, L., Weeks, J. L., & Seegal, J. L. (1995). Perspectives of the future. In K. Ringen et al., (Eds.), *Occupational medicine: Construction safety and health. State of the art reviews, 10*(2), 445-451. Philadelphia: Hanley & Belfus, Inc.

Rogers, B. (2002). *Occupational health nursing: Concepts and practice* (2nd ed.). Philadelphia: W.B. Saunders.

Rose, S. R. (2001). 2001 international travel guide (12th ed.). Northhampton, MA: Travel Medicine, Inc.

Runyan, C. W., & Zakocs, R. C. (2000). Epidemiology and prevention of injuries among adolescent workers in the Untied States. Annual Review of Public Health, 21, 247-269.

Salary.com (2004). Whatever happened to leisure time? Retrieved on December 30, 2004 from http://www.salary.com/site-search/layoutscripts/sisl_display.asp?filename=&path=/destinationsearch/benefits/part_par64_body.html

Schaffner, H. A., & Van Horn, C. E., (2003). *A nation at work: The Heldrich guide to the American workforce.* New Brunswick, NJ: Rutgers University Press.

Sepkowitz, K. A. (1996). Occupationally-acquired infections in health care workers. Part 1. *Annals of Internal Medicine,* 125(10), 826–834.

Solomon, C. M. (1994). Global operations demand that HR rethink diversity. *Personnel Journal, 73*(7), 40-50.

Spielberger, C. D., Vagg, P. R., Wasala, C. F. (2003). Occupational stress: Job pressures and lack of support. In J. C. Quick & L. E. Tetrick (Eds.), *Handbook of occupational health psychology* (pp. 185-200). Washington, DC: American Psychological Association.

Steinberg, L., & Dornbusch, S. (1991). Negative correlates of part-time employment during adolescence: Replication and elaboration. *Developmental Psychology, 27,* 304-313.

Steinberg L, & Cauffman E. (1995). The impact of employment on adolescent development. In R..Vasta (Ed.), *Annals of child development (11)* (p. 136). Philadelphia, PA: Jessica Kingsley Publishers.

Swanson, N.G. (2000). Working women and stress. *Journal of the American Medical Women's Association, 55*(2), 76-79.

Tetrick, L. E., & Quick, J. C. (2003). Prevention at work: Public health in occupational settings. In J.C. Quick, & L.E. Tetrick (Eds.), *Handbook of occupational health psychology* (pp. 3-18). Washington, DC: American Psychological Association.

Thelin, J. W., Joseph, D. J., Davis, W. E., Baker, D. E., & Hosokawa, M. C. (1983).

High-frequency hearing loss in male farmers of Missouri. *Public Health Reports, 98*(3), 268-272.

Theodore, N., & Peck, J. (2002). The temporary staffing industry: Growth imperatives and limits to contingency. *Economic Geography, 78*(4); 463-494.

U.S. Census Bureau. (2003). *Statistical abstract of the United States: 2003.* (Tables 557, 613, 649, 650) (123rd ed.). Washington D.C.

U.S. Census Bureau. (2004a). Current population survey. Table 1. Selected characteristics of civilians 16 to 74 years old with a work disability, by educational attainment and sex: 2004, accessed on 2/28/2005. at http://www.census.gov/hhes/www/disability/cps/cps103.html

U.S. Census Bureau. (2004b). Current population survey. Table 2. Labor Force Status. Work Disability Status of Civilians 16 to 74 Years Old, by Educational Attainment and Sex: 2004, accessed on 2/28/2005 at http://www.census.gov/hhes/www/disability/cps/cps204.html.

U.S. Census Bureau (2004, April) International data base. Available at http://www.census.gov/ipc/www/idbnew.html..

U.S. Census Bureau (2004, March) U.S. Interim projections by age, sex, race, and Hispanic origin. Available at http://www.census.gov/ipc/www/usinterim-proj.

U.S. Department of Health and Human Services (DHHS). U.S. Public Health Service. (2000). *Healthy people 2010,* 2nd ed., Vol. I and II. S/N 017-001-00547-9. Washington, DC: U.S. Government Printing Office.

U.S. Department of Health and Human Services (DHHS), Center for Medicare and Medicaid Services. (2005).

U.S. Department of Health and Human Services (DHHS), Office of Minority Affairs. (2004). Racial and ethnic populations. Available at http://www.cdc.gov/omh/Populations/populations.htm

U.S. Department of Labor. (1999). *Futurework: Trends and challenges for work in the 21st century.* Available at http://www.dol.gov/dol/asp/public/futurework/report/main.htm.

U.S. Department of Labor (2003, October). Women at work: A Visual essay. Monthly Labor Review.

U.S. Department of Labor, Assistant Secretary for Policy (USDL ASP. (2004).*America's dynamic workforce.* Available at http://www.dol.gov/ asp/ media/reports/workforce/toc.htm.

U.S. Department of Labor, Bureau of Labor Statistics (USDL BLS). (2000). *Career guide to industries: Health services.* Available at http://www.bls.gov/ oco/cg

U.S. Department of Labor, Bureau of Labor Statistics (USDL BLS). (2001). *Report on the American workforce.* Available at http://www.bls.gov/opub/rtaw:htm

U.S. Department of Labor, Bureau of Labor Statistics (USDL BLS). (2001, May). *Employed contingent and noncontingent workers by selected characteristics, February 2001.* Available at http:// www.dol.gov/

U. S Department of Labor, Bureau of Labor Statistics (USDL BLS). (2002, March 1). *Work at home in 2001. USDL 02-107.* Available at http://www.bls.gov/cps/

U.S. Department of Labor, Bureau of Labor Statistics (USDL BLS) (2003, December). *Industry illness and injury data.* Available at http://www.bls.gov/ iif/oshwc/osh/os/ostb1236.pdf

U.S. Department of Labor, Bureau of Labor Statistics (USDL BLS). (2004a). *Union members summary/technical information.* (USDL 04-53). Available at http://www.bls.gov/cps/

U.S. Department of Labor, Bureau of Labor Statistics. (USDL, BLS), (2004b). *Career guide to industries, 2004-05 Edition, Construction.* Available at http:// www.bls.gov/oco/cg/cgs003.htm

U.S. Department of Labor, Bureau of Labor Statistics (USDL, BLS) (February 2004). *Women in the labor force: A Databook. USDL.report* 973

U.S. Department of Labor, Bureau of Labor Statistics (USDL BLS). (2004, June). *Tomorrow's jobs.* Available: http:// www.dol.gov

U.S. Department of Labor, Occupational Safety and Health Administration (USDL OSHA). (1996). *Guidelines for preventing workplace violence for health care and social service workers* (OSHA 348). Washington, DC: U.S. Government Printing Office.

U.S. Department of Labor, Women's Bureau (USDL WB). (2004, September). *Quick facts on older workers.* Available at http://www.dol.gov/wb

U.S. Department of Labor, Women's Bureau (USDL WB). (1998, May*). Work and elder care: facts for caregivers and their employers.* Available at http://dol.gov/ dol/wb/public/wbpugs/elderc.html

U.S. General Accounting Office (2002). *Child labor: Labor can strengthen its efforts to protect children who work.* Publication No. GAO-02-880. Washington, DC: U.S. General Accounting Office.

U.S. General Accounting Office (1990). *Child labor: Characteristics of working children.* Publication No. GAO/HRD-90-116. Washington, DC: General Accounting Office.

Van Horn, C.E., & Storen, D. (2003). Is telework coming of age? Evaluating the potential benefits of telework. In H. A. Schaffner & C. E. Van Horn (Eds), *A nation at work: The Heldrich guide to the American workforce* (pp. 280-288). New Brunswick, NJ: Rutgers University Press.

Wegman, D., & Davis, L. (1999). Protecting youth at work. *American Journal of Industrial Medicine, 36,* 579-583.

Wegman, D.H. (1999). Older workers. *Occupational Medicine State of the Art Review, 14*(3), 537-57.

Weller, N. F., Cooper, S. P., Tortolero, S. R., Kelder, S. H., & Hassan, S. (2003). Work-related injury among South Texas middle school students: prevalence and patterns. *Southern Medical Journal,* 96(12), 1213-1220.

Womens Wall Street (2005). Whatever happened to leisure time? Available at http://www.womenswallstreet.com/ Retrieved January 2, 2005.

Wright, K.A. (1993). Management of agricultural injuries and illness. *Nursing Clinics of North America, 28,* 253-266.

Zakocs R. C., Runyan, C. W., Schulman, M. D., Dunn, K. A., & Evensen, C. T. (1998). Improving safety for teens working in the retail trade sector: Opportunities and obstacles. *American Journal of Industrial Medicine, 34,* 342-350.

Ziegler, R. H. (1994). *American workers, American unions.* Baltimore: John Hopkins University Press (pp. 193-205).

Zierold, K. M., Garman, S., & Anderson, H. (2004). Summer work and injury among middle school students aged 10-14 years. *Occupational and Environmental Medicine,* 61, 518-522.

CHAPTER

3

Legal and Ethical Issues

DIANE KNOBLAUCH AND PATRICIA B. STRASSER

Legal and ethical issues often arise in the occupational setting. It is essential that occupational and environmental health nurses be familiar with state and federal regulations that affect workers in their work settings and that they clearly understand their professional responsibility with regard to those regulations. Furthermore, they must be prepared to respond effectively to the various ethical concerns that can arise in a competitive environment, which often breeds conflicting opinions and moral dilemmas. The information in this chapter provides a broad overview of government regulations and ethical principles that can serve as a guide to occupational and environmental health nursing practice.

I Sources of Law

A *Common law* **is the body of law formed by court decisions of individual disputes that establishes judicial precedent. These legal precedents are generally relied upon in deciding similar future cases in the same jurisdiction.**

1. Deference is accorded to decisions made by higher courts within the same jurisdiction; state courts have precedence over local courts, appellate courts over lower courts, and the Supreme Court over appellate courts.
2. Courts follow past precedents to promote the uniform and predictable application of common law rules based on changing societal values, norms, and cultures; however, courts can reinterpret prior decisions or the application of law to a subject matter in current, future, and past cases.

B *Statutes* **are laws created by state or federal legislatures.**

1. Statutes modify existing law or regulate new subject matter.
2. The legislature can delegate the responsibility for promulgating rules and regulations about a particular matter to an administrative agency.
3. Statutes may preempt rules and regulations of administrative agencies.
4. Statutes reflect societal norms and social order; thus laws are enacted or codified as a result of societal changes.

C *Federal law* **is based on the United States Constitution, which is the basis of all other laws; that is, state statutes must comply with and be at least as strict as federal law.**

D *State law* **regulates activities within the state's jurisdiction.**

1. *Civil law* addresses the rights and duties of persons within that state; an example is the Nurse Practice Act.
2. *Criminal law* is enacted to preserve public order.

3. *Administrative law* consists of rules and regulations established by administrative agencies within each state that give effect to the state laws; for example, the State Board of Nursing is an administrative agency that oversees, monitors, and enforces the Nurse Practice Act within the state.

II Basic Legal Concepts Relevant to Occupational and Environmental Health Nursing Practice

A *Tort* **refers to a private wrong against the person or property of another; examples include fraud, invasion of privacy, and defamation. These wrongs are compensated with money damages.**

B *Nursing negligence* **is the omission (failure to do something) or commission (doing something) that violates the standard of care of an occupational and environmental health nurse.**

1. *Standard of care* refers to what the average, reasonable, and prudent occupational and environmental health nurse would do in the same or similar circumstances; the "reasonable occupational health nurse standard."
2. *Duty* is the obligation that an occupational and environmental health nurse has to workers in a specific work setting to prevent foreseeable harm. For example, if workers are at risk of exposure to toxin *a*, the occupational and environmental health nurse has a *duty* to ensure that monitoring is conducted and appropriate action is taken to prevent adverse effects from toxin *a*.
   a. Breach of duty occurs when the occupational and environmental health nurse fails to provide care according to the "reasonable occupational health nurse standard."
   b. There are some circumstances in which exceptions have been identified to the duty of an occupational and environmental health nurse; for example, in an emergency if there is an unreasonable risk of harm to the occupational and environmental health nurse.
3. Examples of negligence include the following:
   a. Failure to assess and make proper nursing diagnosis
   b. Failure to observe and monitor
   c. Failure to take action
   d. Failure to communicate danger
   e. Delay in obtaining assistance
   f. Medication errors
   g. Failure to obtain informed consent

C *Informed consent* **means that a worker's decision about a treatment or action plan is made with a clear understanding, including material risks, benefits, and alternative treatments (i.e., complete notice).**

1. To give informed consent, the worker must be advised of the following:
   a. Nature and purpose of proposed treatment
   b. Diagnosis
   c. Material risks of proposed treatment
   d. Alternative treatments
   e. Consequences of lack of treatment
2. The purposes of informed consent include the following:
   a. Allows the worker to make a decision based upon all known information
   b. Ensures accountability of health professionals

3. In order to be valid, informed consent must have the following characteristics:
   a. Given freely and without coercion
   b. Given with full understanding
4. The person giving informed consent must be mentally, physically, and legally competent.

D *Malpractice* **is negligence that involves professional misconduct or unreasonable lack of skill.**
   1. State statutes will determine the civil action for misconduct by the occupational and environmental health nurse.
   2. *Malpractice* implies that a higher standard of care is owed to the client than the standard implied by simple negligence.
   3. Malpractice suits require expert testimony to help the jury understand the standard of care owed to a client by the reasonably prudent occupational and environmental health nurse.

E *Statute of limitation* **is the period of time within which a lawsuit must be filed after a tort occurs.**
   1. Typically, the statute of limitation for negligence is 2 years.
   2. The statute of limitation for malpractice is typically 1 year.

III Legal Responsibilities of the Occupational and Environmental Health Nurse

A **Occupational and environmental health nurses are responsible for maintaining a current knowledge of the laws affecting occupational health practice in the jurisdiction where they practice, including the following:**
   1. Changes in state administrative rules for the practice of nursing, for example, the State Board of Nursing
   2. Changes in state administrative rules that affect the practice of the occupational and environmental health nurse, for example, the State Board of Pharmacy, State Board of Medicine
   3. Changes in state and federal legislation (laws) that affect the practice of the occupational and environmental health nurse

B **Because of the dynamic and evolving nature of occupational and environmental health nursing practice, there may be inconsistencies between actual practice and legal guidelines of practice.**
   1. Laws, rules, and regulations that are enacted are dynamic; thus they may be challenged as professional practice evolves.
   2. The interpretation of laws, rules, and regulations may change as new cases are decided (common law) and legal precedents are established.

IV Occupational Safety and Health Act (Public Law 91-596)

A **The OSH Act was signed into law on December 29, 1970. The purpose of the OSH Act is to "Assure so far as possible every working man and woman in the Nation safe and healthful working conditions and to preserve our human resources." (Appendix V)**
   1. The OSH Act applies to employers and workers within the United States and any territory under U.S. jurisdiction.
   2. The OSH Act does not apply to self-employed persons, immediate members of family farms that do not employ outside workers, industries regulated by

other federal agencies, such as mining, nuclear, and air transportation, or state and local governments.

B **OSHA, a regulatory agency within the U.S. Department of Labor (USDL), was created as a result of the OSH Act.**

1. The Occupational Safety and Health Administration (OSHA) is responsible for enacting, administering, and enforcing standards to provide workplace health and safety and was the first attempt by Congress to provide a comprehensive program to protect the health and safety of American workers.
2. States may choose to administer their own occupational health and safety program, with the following provisions:
   a. OSHA approves the state program.
   b. The state's program applies to all workers and includes state, local and private sector workers.
   c. The state's statutes must be as strict as federal OSHA requirements; otherwise, OSHA statutes apply. However, states can be more restrictive; i.e., place a higher standard on workplace health and safety.
      (Box 3-1 provides a list of states that have established Occupational Safety and Health Administrations.)
3. General Duty Clause of the OSH Act: Employers are required to furnish all workers "employment and a place of employment which are free from recognized hazards that are causing or are likely to cause death or serious physical harm." The General Duty Clause can be invoked for hazards not covered by an OSHA standard as an important means of protecting workers, because setting standards is often a slow process.

C **OSHA has the responsibility to promulgate legally enforceable occupational health and safety standards in accordance with Section 6 of the OSH Act.**

1. Standards are developed to eliminate or reduce risks; compliance with standards must occur to the technologic and economic extent possible.

BOX 3-1

States and territories with Occupational Safety and Health Administrations

Alaska	Michigan	South Carolina
Arizona	Minnesota	Tennessee
California	Nevada	Utah
Connecticut*	New Jersey*	Vermont
Hawaii	New Mexico	Virginia
Indiana	New York*	Virgin Islands*
Iowa	North Carolina	Washington
Kentucky	Oregon	Wyoming
Maryland	Puerto Rico	

From www.OSHA.gov (2004 web site).

*Plans cover public sector employees only.

NOTE: Employers should contact their state agency to determine the current status of a state-regulated OSHA.

2. OSHA standards must be reasonably necessary or appropriate to provide safe or healthful employment and places of employment.

3. The development of standards is an interdisciplinary process involving individuals from the fields of health care, epidemiology, law, economics, and industrial hygiene; standards are written by OSHA employees and invited consultants.

4. OSHA standards are developed by a public rule-making process that includes the following features:
   a. Public notice: the proposed standard and date of public hearing, which are published in the Federal Register
   b. Public hearings: scheduled forums for public input
   c. Public comment: written or offered at public hearings

5. OSHA has enacted some standards, a complete list of which can be found at the OSHA web site (http://www.osha.gov/).

6. OSHA can implement emergency standards as proposed permanent standards effective for 6 months.

7. There are 23 standards that have medical surveillance provisions (Box 3-2).

8. OSHA part 1910 Occupational Safety and Health Standards sub-part Z is a series of tables, known as the *Z tables*, which list permissible exposure limits for substances for which specific standards are in place and for those for which a standard has not been generated.

D **OSHA is authorized to enforce established standards by performing inspections, with or without advance notice to the employer.**

1. Inspections may include a review of records, walk-through, and worker interviews.

2. OSHA has established a system of inspection priorities; inspections occur in the following order (OSHA, n.d.):
   a. Imminent danger situations; that is, when there is reasonable certainty that danger exists that can be expected to cause death or serious physical

---

BOX 3-2

OSHA standards requiring medical surveillance

Acrylonitrile	DBCP
Arsenic (Inorganic)	Ethylene Oxide
Asbestos (General Industry)	Formaldehyde
Asbestos (Construction and	HAZWOPER
Shipyards)	Hazardous Chemicals in Laboratories
Benzene	Lead
Bloodborne Pathogens	Methylenedianiline
1,3-Butadiene	Methylene Chloride
Cadmium	Noise
Carcinogens (Suspect)	Respiratory Protection
Coke Oven Emissions	Vinyl Chloride
Compressed Air Environments	
Cotton Dust	

DBCP, dibromochloropropane; *HAZWOPER*, Hazardous Waste Operations and Emergency Response Standard.

harm immediately or before the danger can be eliminated through normal enforcement procedures

b. Fatalities and catastrophes resulting in hospitalization of three or more workers; these situations must be reported to OSHA by the employer within 8 hours of the incident

c. Worker complaints of alleged violation of standards or of unsafe or unhealthful working conditions

d. Follow-up inspections to confirm abatement of previously identified violations

e. Planned inspections aimed at special high hazard industries, occupations, or substances

3. Workers or authorized worker representatives may request OSHA to perform an inspection.

a. If an inspection occurs, the employer has a right to see a copy of the complaint.

b. The worker's name will be withheld from the complaint if the worker requests.

c. While inspections can occur without advance notice, employers have a right to refuse entry without a court order.

4. OSHA may issue citations identifying violations and specifying the penalty associated with each violation.

E OSHA consults with business and industry about health and safety issues; these consultation services primarily target small businesses.

1. The OSHA consultation service is a voluntary program primarily focused on lending assistance to employers to make the workplace free of or safe from recognized hazards.

2. Generally, this service is not punitive; employers who use it are not subject to fines, providing that efforts are being made to correct deficiencies.

3. Employers can request an OSHA consultation to accomplish the following:
   a. Identify and correct hazards
   b. Provide technical assistance related to work site hazards
   c. Provide education and training to health and safety personnel

4. Although the consultation service is funded by OSHA, the services are delivered by state governments using well-trained professional staff.

5. OSHA produces a variety of publications designed to provide a basic understanding of occupational health and safety issues and to help with compliance issues.

6. OSHA provides basic to advanced occupational health and safety classes through the OSHA Training Institute.

F OSHA's Voluntary Protection Program (VPP) was adopted in 1982 (AAOHN, 2004a).

1. VPP was initiated as a cooperative effort among industry management, labor, and OSHA to recognize excellence in employer-provided programs and services that go beyond basic regulatory compliance.

2. VPP requirements include the following:
   a. A comprehensive written program demonstrating management commitment and planning
   b. A thorough work site analysis
   c. Hazard prevention and control systems
   d. Safety and health training

e. Active worker involvement

f. A lost workday case rate of below 50% of the national average for the specific industry (based on a review of 3 years of OSHA 300 logs)

g. Periodic program evaluation with annual report submission

h. Worker commitment

3. Participating employers are eligible for VPP awards. Award levels are as follows:

   a. Star: exemplary work sites with comprehensive, successful safety and health management systems

   b. Merit: effective stepping-stone to "Star." Merit sites have good safety and health management systems, but these systems need some improvement to be judged excellent

   c. Star Demonstration: designed for work sites with Star quality safety and health protection to test alternatives to current Star requirements

4. Complete information about OSHA's VPP can be found at http://www.osha.gov/oshprogs/vpp/.

G **In 1988, OSHA instituted measures to ensure nursing representation in policy making.**

1. In 1988, the first occupational and environmental health nurse was hired by OSHA.

2. In 1988, an Occupational Health Nurse Intern Program was introduced; this program is available to nurses in graduate school who are specializing in occupational health.

3. In 1993, the Office of Occupational Health Nursing was formally recognized and established.

H **NIOSH, an institute within the Centers for Disease Control and Prevention (CDC), U.S. Department of Health and Human Services (US DHHS), was also created by the OSH Act.**

1. NIOSH conducts or funds occupational health and safety research to establish safe levels of toxic materials; this research is the basis for OSHA standards.

2. NIOSH also provides training and education to occupational health and safety professionals, including graduate programs for occupational health nurses.

I **The Occupational Safety and Health Review Commission (OSHRC) is an independent regulatory commission authorized by the OSH Act (http://www.oshrc.gov/).**

1. OSHRC members are appointed by the President with Senate approval.

2. OSHRC is responsible for handling appeals filed by employers who have received OSHA citations.

   a. Employers must file a Notice of Contest within 15 days of receiving an OSHA citation.

   b. OSHRC assigns the appeal to an administrative appeal judge.

   c. Appeal of an OSHRC decision is made to a U.S. Court of Appeals.

V Americans with Disabilities Act (ADA) of 1990

A **The ADA is wide-ranging legislation intended to make American society more accessible to people with disabilities (http://www.eeoc.gov/policy.ada).**

1. Disability is defined as:
   a. A physical or mental impairment that substantially limits one or more major life activities
   b. A record of such an impairment
   c. Being regarded as having such an impairment
2. Title I of the ADA applies to employers (including public and private employers, employment agencies, and labor unions) with more than 15 employees.
3. Businesses must protect the rights of "qualified individuals with disabilities" in all aspects of employment, including the application process, hiring, firing, compensation and benefits, and training.

B **A qualified person with a disability is one who can perform the essential functions of the job with or without "reasonable accommodation"**
   1. Reasonable accommodation is any modification or adjustment to a job or the work environment that will enable a qualified applicant or worker with a disability to participate in the application process or perform essential job functions.
   2. Reasonable accommodation may include the following:
      a. Making existing facilities used by workers readily accessible to and usable by persons with disabilities
      b. Restructuring the job, modifying work schedules, or reassigning the worker to a vacant position
      c. Acquiring or modifying equipment or devices; modifying examinations, training materials, or policies; or providing qualified readers or interpreters
   3. Considerations related to providing reasonable accommodation include the following (AAOHN, 1994):
      a. Decisions should be made by a multidisciplinary team that includes health and safety professionals, human resources staff, and management.
      b. The affected worker should be consulted regarding accommodations.
      c. Community resources and national agencies can provide information that can assist with the process of accommodation.
      d. The "reasonableness" of accommodation is based on cost and impact on the business.

C **The ADA affects employment inquiries and medical examinations in the following ways (Equal Employment Opportunity Commission [EEOC], 2000):**
   1. Employers may not ask job applicants about the existence, nature, or severity of a disability; however, they may ask about the applicant's ability to perform specific job functions.
   2. A medical examination may be performed after a conditional offer of employment has been made, if examinations are required for all entering workers in similar jobs; the post-offer examination does not have to be job related.
   3. If an individual is not hired because of the post-offer examination:
      a. The reason for not hiring must be job-related and consistent with business need.
      b. The employer must show that no reasonable accommodation was available or that accommodation would impose an undue hardship.

4. Post-offer examinations may disqualify a person if it is determined the individual poses a "direct threat" in the workplace (i.e., a significant risk of substantial harm to the health and safety of the individual or others).

5. After a person is employed, any medical examination or medical inquiry must be job-related and consistent with business necessity.

6. Results of medical examinations must be maintained in a confidential manner in medical files that are separate from other worker information and available under limited conditions.

D The EEOC enforces and regulates Title I of the ADA.

VI Family and Medical Leave Act (FMLA) of 1993 (29CFR825.118)

A FMLA entitles eligible workers to take up to 12 weeks of unpaid, job-protected leave in a 12-month period for the following reasons: (http://www.dol.gov/dol/esa/regs/statutes/whd/fmla).

1. The birth and care of the worker's newborn child
2. Adoption or foster placement of a child with the worker
3. The care of a parent, spouse, or child with a serious health condition
4. The worker's inability to work because of a serious health condition

B To be eligible for leave under the FMLA, the following conditions must be satisfied:

1. The worker must work for a covered employer in a covered location (at least 50 workers employed within 75 miles).
2. The worker must have worked for the employer for a total of 12 months and worked at least 1,250 hours during the 12 months immediately before the leave.

C Under some circumstances, workers may take FMLA leave on an intermittent basis (e.g., in blocks of time or by reducing a normal work schedule).

D For the complete definition of a *serious health condition* refer to Box 3-3.

E Rights and responsibilities under FMLA include the following:

1. The worker has the right to return to the same or equivalent position with equivalent benefits, compensation, and conditions of employment.
2. The worker has a responsibility to provide the employer with reasonable notice of the leave (at least 30 days when foreseeable).
3. The employer has the right to require medical certification to support the worker's claim for leave related to health conditions of self or a family member; the Department of Labor has devised a "Certificate of Health Care Provider Form" to obtain medical certification (available at http://www.dol.gov/esa//whd/fmla/index.htm -form).
4. The employer has a responsibility to keep and maintain records regarding compliance with the act; they must also conspicuously post a notice containing information about the FMLA.

F Several states have their own legislation governing family and medical leave.

G The USDL's Employment Standards Administration, Wage and Hour Division administers and enforces FMLA.

Definition: Serious health condition

A "Serious Health Condition" means an illness, injury impairment, or physical or mental condition that involves one of the following:

1. *Hospital Care*

   Inpatient care (i.e., an overnight stay) in a hospital, hospice, or residential medical care facility, including any period of incapacity[1] or subsequent treatment in connection with or consequent to such inpatient care.

2. *Absence Plus Treatment*

   A period of incapacity[1] of more than three consecutive calendar days (including any subsequent treatment or period of incapacity relating to the same condition), that also involves:

   (1) Treatment[2] two or more times by a health care provider, by a nurse or physician assistant under direct supervision of a health care provider, or by a provider of health care services (e.g., physical therapist) under orders of, or on referral by, a health care provider; or

   (2) Treatment by a health care provider on at least one occasion that results in a regimen of continuing treatment[3] under the supervision of the health care provider.

3. *Pregnancy*

   Any period of incapacity due to pregnancy, or for prenatal care.

4. *Chronic Conditions Requiring Treatments*

   A chronic condition that:

   (1) Requires periodic visits for treatment by a health care provider, or by a nurse or physician assistant under direct supervision of a health care provider.

   (2) Continues over an extended period (including recurring episodes of a single underlying condition).

   (3) May cause episodic rather than a continuing period of incapacity (e.g., asthma, diabetes, epilepsy).

5. *Permanent/Long-term Conditions Requiring Supervision*

   A period of incapacity[1] that is permanent or long-term due to a condition for which treatment may not be effective. The employee or family member must be under the continuing supervision of, but need not be receiving active treatment by, a health care provider. Examples include Alzheimer's, a severe stroke, or the terminal stages of a disease.

6. *Multiple Treatments (Non-Chronic Conditions)*

   Any period of absence to receive multiple treatments (including any period of recovery therefrom) by a health care provider or by a provider of health care services under orders of, or on referral by, a health care provider, either for restorative surgery after an accident or other injury, or for a condition that would likely result in a period of Incapacity[1] of more than 3 consecutive calendar days in the absence of medical intervention or treatment, such as cancer (e.g., chemotherapy, radiation), severe arthritis (physical therapy),

[1] "Incapacity" for purposes of FMLA is defined to mean inability to work, attend school, or perform other regular daily activities due to the serious health condition, treatment therefor, or recovery therefrom.

[2] Treatment includes examinations to determine if a serious health condition exists and evaluations of the condition. Treatment does not include routine physical examinations, eye examinations, or dental examinations.

[3] A regimen of continuing treatment includes, for example, a course of prescription medication (e.g., an antibiotic) or therapy requiring special equipment to resolve or alleviate the health condition. A regimen of treatment does not include the taking of over-the-counter medications such as aspirin, antihistamines, or salves; or bed-rest, drinking fluids, exercise, and other similar activities that can be initiated without a visit to a health care provider.

VII The Department of Transportation

A **The U.S. Department of Transportation (DOT), established by Congress in 1966, is charged with ensuring a fast, safe, efficient, accessible and convenient transportation system to meet the needs of the American people.**

1. The DOT has thirteen individual operating administrations, including the Federal Motor Carrier Safety Administration (FMCSA), established January 1, 2000 (Public Law No. 106-159, 113 Stat.1748). The FMCSA was formerly part of the Federal Highway Administration.
2. The FMCSA's primary mission is to reduce crashes, injuries, and fatalities involving large trucks and buses.
3. Provisions from Section 391.41 of the FMCSA may affect occupational and environmental health nursing practice. Physical examinations are required for persons who drive commercial motor vehicles (i.e., hold a commercial driver's license [CDL]).
   a. In general, the following guidelines establish what constitutes a commercial vehicle:
      1) Weight over 26,000 pounds;
      2) Used to transport more than 16 persons; or
      3) Used to transport hazardous materials.
   b. Guidelines developed by the FMCSA for medical examinations for drivers of commercial motor vehicles are available at http://www.fmsa.dot.gov.rulesregs/fmcsr/medical.htm.
   c. Advanced-practice nurses, in accordance with applicable state laws, may perform physical examinations for drivers of commercial motor vehicles. (Chapter 11 provides a definition of advanced practice.)

B **The DOT administers the Omnibus Transportation Employee Testing Act of 1991 (CFR 49 Part 382.101), which requires alcohol and drug testing of safety-sensitive employees in the aviation, motor carrier, railroad, and mass-transit industries (Table 3-1).**

1. Testing is performed under the following circumstances:
   a. Preemployment (for drugs only)
   b. Postaccident
   c. Reasonable suspicion
   d. Return to duty and follow-up testing
2. In 1994, the DOT published rules (49 CFR Part 40) mandating prevention programs for drug and alcohol misuse; they were revised in 1999.
3. The DOT's rules establish procedures for drug testing and breath alcohol testing.
4. All drug and alcohol testing results and records are maintained under strict confidentiality by the employer, the drug-testing laboratory, and the medical review officer.
5. See Chapter 16 for a detailed description of drug and alcohol programs and services.

C **The FMCSA, through the Office of Hazardous Materials Safety, develops and recommends regulatory changes governing the transportation of hazardous materials, including hazardous waste.**

TABLE 3-1

Safety-sensitive employees covered by the Department of Transportation (DOT) Omnibus Transportation Employee Testing Act of 1991

DOT/industry	Covered safety-sensitive employees
Federal Highway Administration (FHWA)/Commercial	Holders of commercial driver's licenses; commercial vehicle drivers
Federal Aviation Administration/ Aviation	Flight crews, attendants, instructors, air traffic controllers, aircraft dispatchers, maintenance personnel, screening personnel, ground security
Federal Railroad Administration/ Railroads	Hours of Service Act employees, engine, train, and signal services, dispatchers, operators
Federal Transit Administration/ Mass Transit workers	Vehicle operators, controllers, maintenance workers
Research and Special Programs Administration/Pipelines	Operations, maintenance, emergency response personnel
United States Coast Guard*/ Maritime	Crew members operating commercial vessels

Source: US DOT, 1994.

*Limited rules that require drug testing and post-accident testing.

VIII Clinical Laboratory Improvement Amendments (CLIA)

A **CLIA sets forth the quality standards for laboratory testing.**

1. A laboratory is defined as any facility that performs laboratory testing on human specimens and provides information used for the diagnosis, prevention, and treatment of disease or assessment of health.
2. The purpose of the CLIA is to ensure the accuracy, reliability, and timeliness of patient test results, regardless of where the test is performed.
3. CLIA regulations establish the testing requirements for laboratory testing with more stringent requirements for more complex tests.

B **CLIA requirements apply if occupational and environmental health nurses perform laboratory testing, other than drug testing, in their facility.**

1. Urine testing (e.g., sugar, pH, protein) is considered "testing for medical diagnosis or treatment."
2. There are three testing categories: waived complexity testing, moderate complexity testing, and high complexity testing.
   a. *Waived testing* includes only tests that the Food and Drug Administration (FDA) or Centers for Disease Control and Prevention (CDC) have determined as simple to use with little risk of error (e.g., blood sugar testing using a glucometer approved for home use).
   b. *Moderate complexity testing* includes the subcategory of provider-performed microscopy (PPM); waived and PPM laboratories may apply directly for their certificates, as they are not subject to routine inspections.
   c. *High complexity testing* includes laboratories that perform comprehensive testing services, for example, hospital laboratories or reference laboratories.
3. Enrollment applications for the CLIA program can be obtained on line at http://www.cms.hhs.gov/clia.

C **The Centers for Medicare and Medicaid Services (CMS) oversee the CLIA program, including laboratory registration, enforcement, and approval of providers. However, other agencies have CLIA responsibilities, for example:**
1. The FDA is responsible for test categorization (e.g., approving home testing devices).
2. The CDC is responsible for providing scientific and technical support/consultation to CMS.

IX Documentation

Documentation is the written communication of information that is the basis of the legal occupational and environmental health record.

A **The purposes of documentation are as follows:**
1. Provide information to improve the quality of care and to assist in planning care; for example, the measures that have been implemented and the results of those measures
2. Serve as a means of communication among health professionals
3. Provide a means to audit the quality of care and adherence to established policies and procedures
4. Establish a baseline by which to gauge improvement or worsening of the client's condition and can be used for comparison should a subsequent injury occur
5. May be used as the basis for retrospective, current, or prospective research
6. Provide information that can be used for worker education and counseling

B **Documentation has several characteristics that must be considered.**
1. Documentation must be complete: if it wasn't written, it wasn't done. Effective documentation includes the following basics:
   a. Each page of the worker health record must be identified with the worker's name and another unique identifier if one is used. Special care must be taken when different clients have the same name.
   b. The date (including year) and time must be noted.
   c. The signature of the person who wrote the note must be clearly identified.
   d. Original signatures must be maintained on computer-generated notes or password signatures instituted.
   e. Entries made via an automated information system must have safeguards so documentation cannot be changed.
   f. Documentation must be legible.
   g. Entries must be permanent; black ink should be used for all handwritten entries in the health records, because other colors may not produce legible photocopies.
   h. Entries should include normal and abnormal findings.
   i. Worker questions or comments about instructions given or in response to care must be included.
2. Health documentation should be presented in a concise, descriptive manner, using accepted health abbreviations and terminology.
   a. The SOAP (Subjective, Objective, Assessment, Plan) format is one recommendation (AAOHN, 2004b) (Table 3-2).
   b. An expanded version of SOAP is SOAPIE (I=implementation; E=evaluation).

3. Errors or changes to manual documentation (hard-copy) should be corrected using the SLIDE rule (Baker, 2000).
   a. Draw a Single Line through the error, leaving the original entry legible.
   b. Initial the strike through and write "error" above the notation. White-out and other correction techniques should never be used.
   c. Date when the correction was made, including the year.
   d. Explain why the correction was made (if correction is other than a spelling or word correction).
4. Corrections should be made as soon as possible after the error is noticed. No corrections should be made after there is notice of possible litigation.
5. Stereotypes, generalizations, and judgmental statements should be avoided.
   a. Example 1: Rather than "seems uncomfortable" ask the client to identify how much pain he or she is experiencing, using a pain scale from 1 to 10.
   b. Example 2: If a client is angry, describe the behavior, such as the words spoken (including obscenities or threats) and whether the client used a loud voice.
6. Health documentation should be contemporaneous with the assessment or done as soon afterwards as possible.
   a. Information that was inadvertently omitted should be documented as soon as possible.
   b. Late entries should be preceded by the notation "late entry."
   c. Late entries should identify the date of each entry and the date of the data being documented.

X Recordkeeping

A **OSHA recordkeeping requirements are governed by 29 CFR 1904: Recording and Reporting Occupational Injuries and Illnesses.**
1. The OSH Act requires most private sector employers with 11 or more workers at any time in a calendar year to prepare and maintain records of work-related injuries and illnesses.

TABLE 3-2

Example using the SOAP formula for occupational and environmental health documentation

Criteria	Description
Subjective assessment	Reason for visit, why the client is seeing you; location, quality, quantity, timing, setting, aggravating and alleviating factors, associated manifestations
Objective assessment	Physical examination, including inspection, percussion, palpation, auscultation; include any laboratory results; objective description of job demands or monitoring results that may affect the subjective complaint
Assessment or diagnosis	Medical versus nursing
Plan/Treatment	Diagnostic studies to be performed, medications prescribed, oral and written instructions, teaching, counseling, referral, follow-up

Source: Bickley, 2003.

2. Employers and individuals not required to maintain OSHA injury and illness records include the following:
   a. Private employers, such as self-employed individuals, partners with no employees, and employers of domestics in the employers' private residences.
   b. State and local government agencies are usually exempt; however, in certain states, agencies of the state and local governments are required to keep injury and illness records in accordance with state regulations.
   c. Low-risk industries such as financial institutions. The entire list of exempt industries can be found in the standard.
3. Covered employers must record (on the OSHA 300 Log) each work-related fatality, injury, or illness that is a new case, and meets one of the following general criteria:
   a. Results in death
   b. Results in days away from work
   c. Results in restricted work activity
   d. Involves medical treatment beyond first-aid (See Box 3-4 for a list of First Aid Treatments)
   e. Results in loss of consciousness
   f. Results in a significant injury or illness diagnosed by a physician or other licensed health care professional (e.g., punctured eardrum, fractured rib)
4. In addition to the general recording criteria, the following must be recorded on the 300 Log:
   a. All work-related needlestick injuries and cuts from sharp objects that are contaminated with another person's blood or other potentially infectious material (as defined by 29 CFR 1910.1030)
   b. Other bloodborne pathogen exposure (e.g. splash) if it results in the diagnosis of a bloodborne illness, such as HIV, hepatitis B, or hepatitis C, or meets one or more of the general recording criteria
   c. If a worker is medically removed under the medical surveillance requirements of an OSHA standard
   d. If a worker's hearing test (audiogram) reveals that the worker has experienced a work-related Standard Threshold Shift (STS) in hearing in one or both ears, and the worker's total hearing level is 25 decibels (dB) or more above audiometric zero (averaged at 2000, 3000, and 4000 Hz) in the same ear(s) as the STS
   e. If a worker has been occupationally exposed to anyone with a known case of active tuberculosis (TB), and that worker subsequently develops a tuberculosis infection, as evidenced by a positive skin test or diagnosis by a physician or other licensed health care professional
5. There are several injuries/illnesses that must be recorded as "Privacy Cases" on the 300 Log:
   a. An injury or illness to an intimate body part or the reproductive system
   b. An injury or illness resulting from a sexual assault
   c. Mental illnesses
   d. HIV infection, hepatitis, or tuberculosis
   e. Needlestick injuries and cuts from sharp objects that are contaminated with another person's blood or other potentially infectious material
   f. Other illnesses, if the worker voluntarily requests that his or her name not be entered on the log

6. Each year, covered employers must post a summary of the prior year 300 Log injuries and illnesses in a conspicuous place in the work environment. The summary (Form 300-A) must remain in place between February 1 and April 30.

7. Occupational and environmental health nurses are often responsible for ensuring that proper records are kept, and thus they must have current knowledge of recordkeeping rules and regulations of OSHA (federal and state) and other regulatory agencies.

B **OSHA has specific regulations related to the preservation of Employee Health and Exposure Records**

1. OSHA requires that certain health records must be retained for at least 30 years plus the worker's term of employment; these records include:
   a. Records of injuries that involve health treatment, loss of consciousness, restriction of work or motion, or transfer to another job.
      1) OSHA does not require first aid records (not including medical histories) of one-time treatment and subsequent observation of minor scratches, cuts, burns, splinters, and the like which do not involve medical treatment, loss of consciousness, restriction of work or motion, or transfer to another job, if made on-site by a non-physician and if maintained separately from the employer's medical program and its records (see Box 3-4 for OSHA definitions of First Aid).
      2) Retention of medical documentation demonstrating nursing care is strongly recommended.
   b. Worker medical records are defined as a record concerning the health status of a worker, which have been established or maintained by a physician, nurse, or other health care personnel. The health records of a worker who has worked for less than one year need not be retained beyond the term of employment if they are provided to the worker upon termination of employment.

2. A worker's exposure records and analyses using the health and exposure records are to be kept for at least 30 years beyond the worker's term of employment. Exposure records include the following:
   a. All records of environmental (workplace) monitoring or measurement, including toxic agents, air quality, and physical agents (e.g., noise).
   b. Records reporting the results of any biologic monitoring.
   c. Material Safety Data Sheets related to the exposure.
   d. Chemical inventory or any other record that reveals the identity (e.g., chemical, common, or trade name) of a toxic substance or harmful physical agent and where and when the substance is (or was) used.

3. Biologic-monitoring records must be kept as specified by OSHA standards.

4. Records may be preserved in any manner (including microfilm) as long as the information contained in the record is preserved and retrievable. NOTE: Chest x-ray films shall be preserved in their original state.

C **The application of some 'best practices' can assist the occupational and environmental health nurse to achieve effective record keeping.**

1. The worker health record may consist of both occupational and nonoccupational health data; the philosophy of the health service determines whether nonoccupational care is provided.

2. It is desirable to separate nonoccupational data from occupational data.

> ### BOX 3-4
> *OSHA definition of first aid*
>
> Using a nonprescription medication at nonprescription strength (for medications available in both prescription and nonprescription form, a recommendation by a physician or other licensed health care professional to use a nonprescription medication at prescription strength is considered medical treatment for recordkeeping purposes)
>
> Administering tetanus immunizations. (All other immunizations, such as hepatitis B vaccine or rabies vaccine are considered medical treatment.)
>
> Cleaning, flushing or soaking wounds on the surface of the skin
>
> Using wound coverings such as bandages, Band-Aids™, gauze pads, etc.; or using butterfly bandages or Steri-Strips™ (other wound closing devices such as sutures, staples, etc., are considered medical treatment)
>
> Using hot or cold therapy
>
> Using any nonrigid means of support, such as elastic bandages, wraps, nonrigid back belts, etc.
>
> (devices with rigid stays or other systems designed to immobilize parts of the body are considered medical treatment for recordkeeping purposes)
>
> Using temporary immobilization devices while transporting an accident victim (e.g., splints, slings, neck collars, back boards, etc.)
>
> Drilling of a fingernail or toenail to relieve pressure, or draining fluid from a blister
>
> Using eye patches
>
> Removing foreign bodies from the eye using only irrigation or a cotton swab
>
> Removing splinters or foreign material from areas other than the eye by irrigation, tweezers, cotton swabs or other simple means
>
> Using finger guards
>
> Using massages (physical therapy or chiropractic treatment are considered medical treatment for recordkeeping purposes)
>
> Drinking fluids for relief of heat stress

3. The record may include the following information:
    a. Pre-placement or post-offer examinations
    b. Surveillance evaluations (e.g., annual audiometric examinations and fitness for duty examinations)
    c. A job hazard analysis
    d. Job physical and occupational requirements
    e. Work injury/illness and follow-up care
    f. Diagnostic procedures
    g. Functional capacity evaluations
    h. Medications administered
    i. Consent forms, progress notes, and recommendations
    j. Treatment of injuries and illnesses (occupational and nonoccupational, if indicated)
    k. Other nonoccupational information such as the following:
        1) Health promotion and disease prevention activities, such as cholesterol or blood pressure screening

2) Primary health care services

3) Follow-up drug testing related to substance abuse treatment

4) Chronic health care monitoring (e.g., blood pressure, glucose monitoring)

4. A written policy for the management, access, and retention of individual health records should be in place; the policy should address the following issues:

   a. Where and how records are stored and secured

   b. Managing records when a worker resigns, transfers, or is terminated

   c. Mechanism for worker access and consent for disclosure

   d. Mechanism for release of information on a need-to-know basis; for example, information on work restrictions

5. Workers' health records should be maintained in a secure place (i.e., locked files) in the exclusive custody and control of company occupational health professionals.

6. Administrative records may be retained or discarded.

   a. Examples of administrative records that should be retained indefinitely include:

      1) All versions of policy and procedure manuals

      2) All versions of approved treatment protocols

      3) Equipment calibration records

   b. Examples of administrative records that may be discarded consistent with company policy include:

      1) Daily logs

      2) Monthly reports

      3) Financial records

XI Access to Employee Medical and Exposure Records

A **OSHA Access to Employee Exposure and Medical Records Standard (29CFR1910.20) requires that the worker or the worker's representative have access to records according the following guidelines:**

1. Access will be provided in a reasonable manner and place.

2. Records will be provided free of charge, and within 15 working days of the initial request.

3. The employer must make provisions for copying of records.

(NOTE: Although this standard uses the term *medical records*, these records may also contain health information that is non-medical in nature; thus in this publication, these records are called health records except when reference is made to published documents that use the term *medical record*.)

B **The worker should sign a written consent before health information is released (Fig. 3-1 presents a sample authorization letter); the authorization must include the following information:**

1. What records are to be released, including dates of services

2. The purpose of release

3. To whom the records are to be released

4. Period of time for which authorization is valid

5. Date of authorization

6. Authority by which a person is requesting records

7. Identifying data of worker, including date of birth and social security number

---

AUTHORIZATION FOR RELEASE OF MEDICAL INFORMATION

I, _____ (full name of employee) _____ hereby authorize

_____ (full name of company/employer) _____ to furnish to:

[name]

[address]

[telephone number]

☐   All information regarding my health conditions, including communicable illnesses, drug use
or abuse, drug/alcohol treatment and psychiatric treatment.
[Strike through the information that you do not want released]

☐   All information regarding any work-related and nonwork-related injuries or disease for which
I have consulted you or received your services.

☐   The following information:

_____

_____

You are instructed to release all records from __(date)__ through __(date)__ . I hereby release you from
any and all restrictions imposed by law in disclosing or revealing any professional record, or
communication in accordance with this release.
    A copy of this signed authorization for release of medical records shall be considered
effective and valid as the original. This authorization shall be valid and in force for _(amount of time)_
from the authorization date.

_____   _____
Authorization Date   Signature

_____   _____
Date of BIrth   Address

_____   _____
Social Security Number   City, State, Zip Code

FIGURE 3-1 *Sample authorization letter*

Courtesy Lori Coyle and Ted Kurt

8. Signature of the person requesting records

C **In all cases, the occupational and environmental health nurse should make
every attempt to obtain an authorization for release of health records, even
when a request for health records is made via subpoena.**

1. The authorization for release of medical records must specify whether information obtained from other sources may be released.
2. If there are concerns with such a request, the nurse should consult with
legal counsel regarding applicable state law governing access to health
records.

D **Under no circumstances should the original health record, reports, or x-rays
be released to the worker or representative before consulting with corporate
legal counsel.**

E If it is believed that access to information contained in the records regarding a special diagnosis of a terminal illness or a psychiatric condition could be detrimental to the worker's health, the employer may choose one of the following courses of action:

1. Inform the worker that access will be provided only to a designated representative of the worker having special written consent
2. Deny the worker's request for direct access to this information only

F The occupational and environmental health nurse should notify the designated employer representative whenever there is a nonroutine request for records; for example, when the request references a legal matter or an attorney requests them.

G An employer may withhold trade secret information but must provide information needed to protect worker health; when it is necessary to release a trade secret, the employer may require a written agreement as a condition of release.

H Each worker must be notified of the following information when beginning employment and at least annually thereafter:

1. The existence, location, and availability of any records covered by the OSHA Access to Employee Exposure and Medical Records Standard (29 CFR 1910.20)
2. The person responsible for maintaining and providing access to records
3. Right of access of the worker or a designated representative to these individual health and exposure records

I All health and exposure records subject to 29 CFR 1910.20 must be transferred to the successor employer, to preserve and maintain these same records.

XII HIPAA (Health Insurance Portability and Accountability Act, 1996)

A The Health Insurance Portability and Accountability Act of 1996 was designed to address industry inefficiencies related to health insurance plans and to protect health care coverage for millions of workers and their families.

1. HIPAA law is organized into the following five titles.
    a. *Title I:* Health care access, portability, and renewability, which focuses on allowing persons to qualify immediately for comparable health insurance when they change employment
    b. *Title II:* Preventing health care fraud and abuse and providing for administrative simplification that reduces the costs and administrative burden of health care by providing electronic standards to be used throughout the health care industry
    c. *Title III:* Tax-related health provisions, which address various issues, including medical savings and long term services and contracts
    d. *Title IV:* Application and enforcement of group health plan requirements and clarification of continuation of coverage requirements
    e. *Title V:* Revenue offsets, which address company owned life insurance and treatment of individuals who lose citizenship
2. HIPAA includes important new protections for workers through several provisions.
    a. It limits exclusions for preexisting conditions.

   b. It prohibits discrimination against workers and dependents based on their health status.
   c. It guarantees renewability and availability of health coverage to certain employers and individuals.
   d. It protects many workers who lose health coverage by providing better access to individual health insurance coverage.

B **HIPAA's Privacy Rule became effective in April, 2003; the Privacy Rule provides new rights for healthcare consumers to protect their health information, access to that information, and the use and disclosure of health information.**

   1. The privacy rule provides that "covered entities" may not use or disclose protected health information (PHI), except as allowed by the HIPAA Privacy Rule for treatment, payment, or health care operations, or under a specific authorization from the individual who is the subject of the PHI, or for "Public Policy Exceptions."
      a. Protected Health Information (PHI) is health plan information that:
         1) Identifies an individual
         2) Relates to the individual's health, health care treatment, or health care payment
         3) Is maintained or disclosed electronically, by paper, or orally.
      b. Occupational and environmental health nurses need to determine whether they are considered "Covered Entities" (Short, 2003). The three categories of covered entities are:
         1) Healthcare providers (providers of health care services who conduct certain financial and administrative transactions electronically (e.g. filing claims, coordinating benefits, checking claim status, eligibility inquiries, etc.)
         2) Healthcare clearinghouses (billing services, contractors, others who process data or transactions from other covered entities)
         3) Health plans (individual and/or other group plans that pay the cost of medical care; Insured and Self-Insured).
   2. Plans covered by the Privacy Rule include:
      a. Medical insurance plans (including prescription drug benefits)
      b. Dental insurance plans
      c. Vision insurance plans
      d. Health care flexible spending accounts
      e. Employee assistance programs (EAP) to the extent that they offer medical care
   3. Plans not covered by the Privacy Rule include:
      a. Disability benefit plans
         1) Short-term disability
         2) Long-term disability
         3) Accidental death and dismemberment (AD&D) a type of supplementary insurance
      b. Workers' compensation
      c. Dependent care spending accounts
      d. Life insurance
      e. Other work-life benefits (adoption assistance, tuition reimbursement, etc.)

C **Occupational and environmental health nurses must also determine what role, if any, they have regarding health insurance/health benefit plans,**

whether insured or self-insured; situations where an occupational and environmental health nurse is a "covered entity" are as follows (Short, 2003):

1. Involved in "prior authorization" for care
2. Performs "disease management" for the plan
3. Performs health risk assessments (HRAs) for the plan
4. The computer system contains information that comes from the plan (e.g. medical information, demographics)
5. Provides services *and* submit bills to the plan
6. Provides case management for persons covered by the health plans

D Occupational and environmental health nurses (and others) who work with health plan operation and PHI must be "fire-walled" from the rest of the Company.
1. Workers outside of the unit cannot access PHI from the fire-walled unit.
2. The unit must comply with the privacy rule.

E If an occupational and environmental health nurse is subject to HIPAA as a covered entity, he or she must (Short, 2002):
1. Notify workers of their privacy rights and how their information can be used
2. Obtain specific client authorization to use or disclose PHI for all purposes other than treatment, payment, or healthcare operations, and "Public Policy Exceptions"
3. Protect PHI from inadvertent misuse and disclosure
4. Train staff in appropriate administrative, physical and technical safeguards to protect PHI; beginning in April 2005 covered entities must also comply with a detailed HIPAA security rule that regulates the retention and transmission of PHI in electronic form
5. Limit PHI disclosure to the "minimum necessary" to achieve the purpose, except in limited circumstances
6. Permit individuals to review and amend health information
7. Maintain an accounting of persons to whom PHI has been disclosed
8. Appoint a "privacy officer"
9. Establish Business Associate contracts (See XII.F.)
10. Comply with more stringent state laws

F Occupational and environmental health nurses may be considered a "Business Associate" of a Covered Entity. For example, an independent nurse case manager working for a covered entity (e.g., health insurer) would be considered a business associate and would need to sign an agreement to protect PHI in accordance with the Privacy Rule.

G Even if they are not covered entities, occupational and environmental health nurses are affected by HIPAA regulations when they obtain PHI from other health care providers who are covered entities (Short, 2003).
1. Covered health care providers will require worker authorization for release of:
   a. Short-term disability and long-term disability information
   b. Pre-placement medical information
   c. Information on workers covered by the Family and Medical Leave Act and the Americans with Disabilities Act
   d. Fitness for duty medical information
2. Employers can mandate "blanket" authorizations as a condition of employment.

3. If exams are performed in-house, authorizations are not needed.

4. Covered health care providers should require HIPAA authorization forms.

5. Covered health care providers should not require worker authorization for release of workers' compensation information as permitted by state law.

6. Covered health care providers should limit workers' compensation information to the minimum necessary if the state law requires.

7. Authorization is not required for:
   a. Medical surveillance to comply with OSHA
   b. Workplace injury/illness information needed for OSHA requirements (e.g., recordkeeping)

8. Covered health care providers must provide written notice to the worker that medical surveillance data will be disclosed to the employer. (Notice may be posted at worksite, if service is provided there.)

9. Employers are not "Covered Entities" (although their "Health Plans" are)

10. Worker records (including worker health records held in the occupational health department) are excluded from the definition of PHI.

11. Once an employer receives worker-related PHI, it is no longer protected by the Privacy Rule.

12. HIPAA does not regulate health information in the possession of non-covered entities. See http://www.cms.hhs.gov/hipaa for additional information.

XIII Overview of Workers' Compensation

A **The workers' compensation system was designed to compensate workers for work-related injuries and illnesses.**

1. Workers' compensation benefits generally include the following:
   a. Income replacement (i.e., indemnity benefits) for workers who are unable to work because of injury or illness
   b. Support for dependents in the event of occupation-related death
   c. Hospital, medical, and funeral expenses
   d. Incidental expenses such as travel and parking, which may be covered in some jurisdictions

2. In general, workers' compensation laws hold that employers must assume costs of work-related injuries and illnesses without regard to fault (e.g., worker or employer negligence).

3. In exchange for providing workers' compensation benefits, the employer is usually immune from further legal action.

4. All states and the District of Columbia have workers' compensation laws that apply to workers within their respective jurisdictions.

5. Federal civilian workers are covered by federal laws.

6. Courts in each jurisdiction interpret the language of their workers' compensation statute.

7. Workers' compensation laws are generally administered by commissions or boards.

B **Compensable injuries and illnesses are defined by statute in each jurisdiction. In most statutes, workers' compensation benefits are limited to accidents and illnesses "arising out of and in the course of employment" (U.S. Chamber of Commerce, 2003).**

1. Although workers' compensation laws initially had no provision for work-related illnesses, all states recognize responsibility for them.

2. Most statutes do not provide compensation for illnesses that are "ordinary diseases of life," or one that is "not peculiar to or characteristic of the employee's occupation" (U.S. Chamber of Commerce, 2003).
3. Identifying work-related illnesses can be complex and very difficult because of the following factors:
   a. Time elapsed between exposure and onset of illness
   b. Insidious onset of the illness
   c. Multifactorial nature of the illness
   d. Obscurity of exposure because of the inability to detect low levels of toxic substances

XIII Overview of Workers' Compensation Benefits

A **In most jurisdictions, unlimited medical benefits (e.g., hospital care, medications, physician visits, rehabilitative therapy, etc.) are provided by statute.**
1. Many states use managed care concepts to affect workers' compensation benefits and control workers' compensation medical costs.
2. There are jurisdictional differences regarding who can choose the health care provider for the injured or ill worker.
   a. In many states, workers are allowed free choice of treating health care professionals.
   b. In other states, the employer chooses the provider, or workers are limited to choosing from a panel of providers.
3. The employer usually has the right to have the worker examined by a physician of the employer's choice.
4. The employer can generally use an independent medical evaluation, whereby a physician who is not the treating physician evaluates the worker and provides an opinion regarding the following issues:
   a. The worker's health condition in general
   b. Whether the worker can return to work
   c. Recommendation regarding physical limitations
   d. The length of time the worker will be off work
   e. Recommendation of current and future treatment
   f. The etiology (causation) of the health condition
   g. A determination as to whether the worker has reached maximum medical improvement

B **Income benefits (i.e., *indemnity benefits*) may not be payable until a waiting period has been met.**
1. If the worker remains off work for days or weeks, most statutes provide payment of income benefits retroactive to the date of injury.
2. Income benefits are generally based on a percentage of the injured worker's average weekly wage.
3. Many statutes provide income benefits based on a schedule for specific losses (e.g., loss of a limb).
4. Many statutes pay income benefits based on the worker's percent of impairment that results from the injury or illness.
5. Income benefits are generally based on whether the disability is temporary or permanent (i.e., payment for a number of weeks or for life).
6. Definitions of disability are determined by jurisdictional statute. The most common workers' compensation disability classifications[*] are the following:

a. *Temporary total disability*—a condition in which a worker, because of an occupational injury or illness, is unable to return to any type of continuous gainful employment

b. *Temporary partial disability*—a subcomponent of total temporary disability, wherein the worker is not medically fixed and stable but can return to "light" work at a lower wage than before he or she was injured

c. *Permanent total disability*—a condition that permanently and completely incapacitates a worker, preventing the worker from ever performing gainful employment

d. *Permanent partial disability*—a condition that results in the permanent loss of a body part or a lasting impairment that has been deemed unlikely to improve

C **Many statutes include specific provisions for rehabilitation of ill or injured workers (including vocational rehabilitation).**

D **Most jurisdictions require employers to obtain workers' compensation insurance and prove financial ability to assume the risk of worker injury.**

1. States that require workers' compensation insurance through a monopolistic state fund include North Dakota, Ohio, Washington, and West Virginia.

2. Many large corporations prefer to "self-insure" (i.e., assume their own financial liability for workers' compensation).

   a. Most states in the United States allow self-insurance in some form (e.g., individual company/group).

   b. Companies that self-insure usually use the services of a third party administration (TPA) to manage their workers' compensation benefits.

XIV Professional Position on Ethics

A **AAOHN Standards of Occupational and Environmental Health Nursing, Standard XI, Ethics: The occupational and environmental health nurse uses an ethical framework for decision making in practice (AAOHN, 2004c).**

1. Occupational and environmental health nurses are confronted with complex ethical dilemmas that require careful communication with company management and the recipients of care.

2. An ethical framework provides the guidelines within which the nurse makes ethical judgments.

3. The occupational and environmental health nurse is an advocate for clients to receive accessible, equitable, and quality health services, including a safe and healthful work environment.

B **The AAOHN Code of Ethics (AAOHN, 2003) provides the ethical framework to guide the conduct of the occupational and environmental health nurse (Appendix VII).**

XVI Ethics: Definitions and Principles

A **Definitions assure a common understanding of ethical terms.**

1. *Ethics* is the philosophic study of conduct and moral judgment.

2. *Morals* are principles of right and wrong.

3. *Morality* is society's expectation as to what people should or should not do.

---

* These definitions are from Washington State Department of Labor and Industries, 1994. Readers are advised to check the terms and definitions in their respective jurisdictions.

    4. *Value* is an expression of worth or goodness.

    5. *Moral justification* is the reason for conduct.

B **Ethical principles underpin ethical practices.**

    1. *Autonomy* means self-governance—the ability to make individual decisions and choices, to act, and to think; self-determination.

    2. *Nonmaleficence* is the principle of doing no harm to others.

    3. *Beneficence* is the principle of doing good for others.

    4. *Distributive justice* means that benefits should be equally distributed and equally shared in pursuit of the following three types of equality:

       a. Equality of moral worth

       b. Equality of opportunity

       c. Equality of outcome

C **Other principles important to occupational and environmental health nursing practice include the following:**

    1. *Confidentiality* is the implicit promise that information divulged to another will be respected and not released or repeated (see Case Study 1).

    2. *Veracity* is truthfulness.

    3. *Honesty* means freedom from deceit.

    4. *Promise-keeping* is the act of following through on a pledge.

    5. *Integrity* refers to unimpaired moral principles.

XVII Ethical Conflicts

A **Assuring workers' and others' confidentiality is an important ethical responsibility.**

    1. Employers are charged with the responsibility for maintaining the occupational health and safety records of their workers.

    2. The occupational and environmental health nurse, who is an agent of the employer, is charged with providing occupational health services to workers and maintaining health records; the occupational and environmental health nurse has a duty to accomplish the following:

       a. Document care or services provided to a client

       b. Maintain the confidentiality of the client's health records

    3. If asked to divulge information contained in a worker's health record or to provide health records, the occupational and environmental health nurse should consider the following issues:

       a. For what purpose is the information being sought?

       b. Is the requested information work-related?

       c. Who is requesting the information?

       d. Is the requested information aggregate data or individual data?

       e. Why was the information gathered?

       f. Is the information being sought pursuant to an authorization for release of health records signed by the worker?

    4. Unauthorized release of health records could result in personal liability, suspension of license to practice nursing by the state agency responsible for regulating the practice of nursing, or termination of employment by the employer.

B **Conflicts of interest and other ethical dilemmas may arise in workplaces.**

    1. The occupational and environmental health nurse has multiple roles in the workplace, including worker, health care provider, client advocate, and

Case Study 1: Confidentiality

N.O. Moore, an occupational and environmental health nurse at E.Z. Con, Ltd., performed spirometry testing and respirator fit testing for Joe Cool. This was Mr. Cool's pre-placement evaluation at E.Z. Con. During the initial evaluation, Ms. Moore noted that Mr. Cool had smoked two packs of cigarettes daily for the past 25 years, and that he was an HVAC (heating, ventilation, and air conditioning) specialist. Mr. Cool admitted that he used to smoke 2-6 joints of marijuana per day, but stopped 10 years earlier. Ms. Moore talked with Mr. Cool about his smoking, risk factors for disease, and environmental hazards at E.Z. Con.

- Two years later, Ms. Moore received several letters in the mail and several phone calls about Mr. Cool. The first letter, from an attorney who said that he represented Mr. Cool, requested Mr. Cool's medical records from E.Z. Con. An authorization signed by the attorney was enclosed.
- The second letter, from Mr. Risk at ABC Company, requested a copy of Mr. Cool's medical records at E.Z. Con. An authorization signed by Joe and dated 2 days before Ms. Moore received the letter was enclosed.
- The third letter, from Mrs. Cool, stated that Mr. Cool had died of a mesothelioma 3 months earlier and requested his medical records from E.Z. Con. An authorization signed by Mrs. Cool was enclosed.
- Ms. Snoopy from personnel called Ms. Moore and instructed Ms. Moore to make a copy of Mr. Cool's medical records for the vice president. Snoopy said that she would be down to get the records in 15 minutes.
- An attorney from H.E.L.P, E.Z. Con's corporate counsel, called and demanded a copy of Mr. Cool's medical records.

What does N.O. Moore do?
Answer: No one gets these records.

1. The authorization to release medical records must be signed by the person or a legal representative. In this case, because a person who is now deceased signed the form, the signature is not valid. Note: Mrs. Cool stated that Joe died 3 months ago.
2. Mrs. Cool, as Joe's widow, is not his "legal" representative. If the authorization had been signed Charity Cool, Administrator of the Estate of Joe Cool, then Mrs. Cool would legally be able to act in Joe's place.
3. Ms. Snoopy has no right to these medical records; neither does the vice president.
4. H.E.L.P. knows better than to request these medical records without a signed authorization

Ms. Moore has no knowledge about why everyone wants these records. If the inquiry from E.Z. Con's attorney was the result of a Mr. Cool's workers' compensation claim filed against E.Z. Con, then E.Z. Con would have a right to these medical records. However, if E.Z. Con is not a named party in the lawsuit or administrative claim, then the medical records must remain confidential.*

*NOTE: While it does not apply in this case, an authorization for release of psychiatric, substance abuse or communicable illness documentation must specifically authorize the release of the specific records and is separate from a general release of medical records. Although N.O. Moore did not provide substance abuse treatment, some legal counsel might require this special disclosure despite the fact that this incidental disclosure does not require a special release and does not rise to the same level of scrutiny as would a substance abuse program or a psychiatric counseling program.

NOTE: Remember to consult your jurisdictional statues and case law to determine how you should handle these situations because every jurisdiction may be different.

coworker; these multiple roles can result in ethical dilemmas that require choosing between two or more compelling ethical or moral values.

2. The occupational and environmental health nurse may be asked to provide the employer with information about the health needs of workers for use in

Case Study 2: Ethics

Nancy Cohn is an occupational and environmental health nurse for a large manufacturing company. The company is self-insured for worker short-term disability (STD) benefits. It is Ms. Cohn's responsibility to obtain medical information and approve/deny STD. The medical information is provided by the worker's attending physicians. The form used to obtain the medical information is signed by the worker and includes a specific consent to release pertinent information to his employer. On a regular basis, Ms. Cohn provides company management with a list of workers who are off work on STD and estimated return to work dates.

Ms. Cohn's recently hired environmental health and safety (EHS) manager, Steve Manager, requests that Ms. Cohn forward all completed STD medical information forms with him so that he can verify how Ms. Cohn is managing the program. Ms. Cohn refuses the request, citing legal and ethical issues. The company attorney is consulted who opines that there is nothing legally preventing release of the information since the worker has signed a consent for release of the information to the company.

Is there a legal issue?

Answer: There is no federal issue here. HIPAA is not a factor. However, depending on the specific jurisdictional requirements set forth in the nurse practice act, there may be language governing the nurses' release of this documentation.

What if any, is the ethical issue?

Answer: Responsibility to maintain confidentiality of personal health information as outlined in the AAOHN/CMSA's Joint Position Statement on confidentiality of health information (2003).

What are some suggestions for dealing with the issue?

Answer: Offer to have a nurse from another company location review the records. Have the workers sign a consent to release the forms to the Manager. Have the forms returned to the EHS Manager.

What could have been done to prevent the situation?

Answer: Adoption of a Company policy regarding the confidentiality of the STD information and parameters under which information is released is strongly recommended. In addition, the worker release form should be modified to include a statement that limits release of the medical information to the Company occupational and environmental health nurse.

Source: Strasser, 2004

developing health benefit plans, planning health education programs and services, and identifying work site health issues.

    a. The occupational and environmental health nurse may be involved in prioritizing program needs.

    b. The occupational and environmental health nurse may participate in the decision-making process regarding allocation of scarce economic and personnel resources among work site health programs and services.

3. The occupational and environmental health nurse may provide non–work-related health care, such as periodic health assessments and screening programs and services.

    a. The nurse must document the results of these evaluations and retain such documentation as health records.

    b. The nurse has an ethical and legal duty to maintain the confidentiality of the worker's non–work-related health information.

c. Release of non-work-related health records requires an authorization for release of health records signed by the client whose records are being released.

REFERENCES

American Association of Occupational Health Nurses (AAOHN). (1994). *The Americans with Disabilities Act* [AAOHN Advisory]. Atlanta, GA: AAOHN Publications.

American Association of Occupational Health Nurses (AAOHN) (2003). *Code of ethics and interpretive statements*. Atlanta, GA: AAOHN Publications.

American Association of Occupational Health Nurses (AAOHN)/Case Management Society of America (CMSA). (2003). Role of occupational and environmental health nurses and nurse case managers in protecting confidentiality of health information [Position Statement] Atlanta, GA: AAOHN Publications.

American Association of Occupational Health Nurses (AAOHN). (2004a). Advisory: *Best practices in an occupational health and safety program: Voluntary protection program (VPP) model*. Atlanta, GA: AAOHN Publications.

American Association of Occupational Health Nurses (AAOHN). (2004b). *AAOHN occupational health and safety service recordkeeping and record retention.* [Foundation Blocks] Atlanta, GA: AAOHN Publications.

American Association of Occupational Health Nurses (AAOHN). (2004c). *AAOHN standards of occupational and environmental health nursing*. Atlanta, GA: AAOHN Publications.

Americans with Disabilities Act. (1990). P.L. 101-356, 42 U.S.C. §12101 et seq.

Baker, S. K. (2000). Minimizing litigation risk: Documentation strategies in the occupational health setting. *AAOHN Journal, 48*(2), 100-105.

Bates, B. (1995). *A guide to physical examination and history taking*. Philadelphia: Lippincott.

Bickley, L.S. (2003). *Bates' guide to physical examination and history taking.* Philadelphia: Lippincott, Williams, and Wilkins.

Equal Employment Opportunity Commission. (1992). *A technical assistance manual on the employment provisions (Title I) of the Americans with Disabilities Act*. EEOC-M-1A. Washington, DC: 1192: U.S. Government Printing Office.

Short, L. A. (2002) HIPAA: Do you know where you fit?. *AAOHN News 22* (8).

Short, L. A. (2003) HIPAA in a nutshell. *AAOHN News* Vol.22 (9). September 2002.

Strasser, P.B. (2004). Ensuring confidentiality of employee health information—developing policies and procedures, *AAOHN Journal 52*(4), 149-153.

Strasser, P. B. (2004). Management File: Ensuring confidentiality of employee health information: Developing policies and procedures. *AAOHN Journal 52*(4), 149-153.

U.S. Chamber of Commerce. (2003). *The 2003 analysis of workers' compensation laws*. Washington DC: U.S. Chamber of Commerce.

U.S. Department of Transportation (DOT). (1994, February 3). *FHWA transportation facts*, Washington, DC: Office of Public Affairs.

Washington State Department of Labor and Industries. (1994). *Industrial insurance: glossary*. Olympia, WA: State of Washington Department of Labor and Industries.

OTHER RESOURCES

Commission on Accreditation of Rehabilitation Facilities (CARF). (1992). *Standards manual for organizations serving people with disabilities*. Tucson, AZ: CARF.

DiBenedetto, D. V. (1995). *OEM occupational health & safety manual* (2nd ed.). Boston: OEM Press.

Knoblauch, D. J. & Strasser, P. B. (2002). Managing employee health problems:

Optimal use independent medical evaluations. *AAOHN Journal, 50*(12), 549-552.

Levy, B. S., & Wegman, D. H. (2000). *Occupational health: recognizing and preventing work-related disease and injuries* (4th ed.). Boston: Little, Brown and Company.

Mappes, T. A., & DeGrazia, D. (1996). *Biomedical ethics* (4th ed.). New York: McGraw-Hill.

Papp, E. M., & Miller, A. S. (2000). *Screening and surveillance: OSHA's medical surveillance provisions. AAOHN Journal, 48*(2), 59-72.

Pryor, E. S. (1990). Flawed promises: A critical evaluation of the American Medical Association's guides to the evaluation of permanent impairment. *Harvard Law Review, 103,* 964.

Rogers, B. (2003). *Occupational and environmental health nursing concepts and practice.* (2nd ed.). Philadelphia: Saunders.

Shrey, D. E., & Lacerte, M. (1995). *Principles and practices of disability management in industry.* Winter Park, FL: CR Press.

Tate, D. (1992, June). Workers' disability and return to work.. *American Journal of Physical Med. & Rehabilitation, 71,* 92-96.

CHAPTER

4

Economic, Political, and Business Forces

DEBORAH V. DIBENEDETTO

Economic, political, and business forces (including that of managed care) shape the way business is conducted in the national and global marketplaces. It is essential that occupational and environmental health nurses understand the basics of the economic, political, and business forces and trends that affect the business environment in which they practice. This chapter presents an overview of these trends and discusses how they can affect occupational and environmental health nursing practice.

I Introduction to Economics

A *Economics* **is concerned with the way in which limited resources are allocated; specifically, it involves the following:**
  1. Allocation and management of the income and expenditures of a household, business, community, or government
     a. Production, distribution, and consumption of wealth
     b. Satisfaction of the material needs of people
  2. The study of the world economy (essentially a macroeconomic survey)
  3. Societal establishment of economic systems that serve as a means of achieving the society's economic goals

B **Knowledge of key economic terms provides a foundation for understanding economic conditions.**
  1. *Consumer Price Index (CPI)*—Measures price changes of goods consumed by an urban family of four on a moderate income
  2. *Disposable income (DI)*—The gross national product (GNP) minus depreciation, business and personal taxes, and transfer payments (such as social security or welfare payments); "the money in people's pockets" to spend as they want
  3. *Federal Reserve Discount Rate*—The rate at which the Federal Reserve Bank lends funds to its member banks
  4. *Gross domestic product*—Measures value of all goods and services produced within a nation's borders regardless of the nationality of the producer
  5. *Gross national product (GNP):* Monetary value of the total annual flow of goods and services in a nation's economy
     a. GNP is the primary indicator of the national economy.
     b. GNP measures production in the economy by aggregating all goods and services produced by their current prices; for example, bushels of fruits or numbers of automobiles sold.

c. GNP measures only goods and services that have a market.

d. International comparisons of GNP are difficult.

e. GNP does not measure quality of life.

6. *Microeconomics*—Deals with the economic behavior of individual units such as consumers, firms, and resource owners

7. *Macroeconomics*—Concerned with the behaviors of economic aggregates, such as the gross national (domestic) product (national income), consumption, the level of employment, investment, money supply, innovation, and international trade and production relationships

8. *Net national product*—The GNP less capital consumption allowance (allocated costs for depreciation of capital equipment)

9. *Political economy*—A term used to describe the influence of political and social institutions on the aggregate economy

10. *Prime rate*—The interest rate that banks charge to their commercial customers (those with good credit ratings and lowest risk) for short-term loans

11. *Producer Price Index (PPI)*—Measures the wholesale price of goods

C *Major economic systems* **include capitalism, socialism, and communism.**

1. *Capitalism*—Allows private ownership of property; income from property or capital accrues to the individual or firms that accumulate it and own it; firms are relatively free to compete with others for their own economic gain; the profit motive is basic to economic life

2. *Communism*—Production systems are government or state owned, and production decisions are made by official policy and not directed by market action

3. *Socialism*—An economic system in which government owns or controls many major industries, but may allow markets to set prices in many areas

D *Economic indicators* **measure the relative standing of one economic system (country) versus that of another.**

1. Economic indicators include the gross national product (GNP), net national product, and disposable income (DI).

2. Price indicators that reflect a nation's economic standing include the consumer price index (CPI) and the producer price index (PPI).

E *Labor-force statistics* **measure how many noninstitutionalized people are currently working at paid jobs or are willing to work; the** *labor force* **is the employable population of the economy.**

1. Persons in the military, jails, hospitals/sanitariums (patients), and full-time students are excluded in calculations of the labor force.

2. Labor-force statistics that include military personnel are also published.

3. Unemployment statistics indicate the number of people looking for paid work and point to changes in the labor market.

F *Interest rates* **are a percentage of a sum of money charged for its use; two important interest rates are the prime rate and the Federal Reserve discount rate.**

G *Balance of trade* **refers to the net value of a country's imports and exports of merchandise.**

1. The balance of trade consists of transactions in merchandise (automobiles, computers, etc.).

2. When a country exports more than it imports, it has a surplus, or *favorable,* balance of trade.

3. When a country's imports predominate, the balance of trade is in deficit and is called *unfavorable.*

II Economic State of the Nation

A During the 1980s, America's economy grew or "expanded" because of the following:

1. Decreased taxation (tax cuts) on business and citizens
2. Deregulation of businesses such as telecommunications, air travel, banking, and many others
3. Increased consumer spending, investment, and construction
4. The beginning trend of privatizing government services toward the end of the 1980s

B The government release of money to the private sector, along with deregulation of business, made the 1980s the longest period of peacetime growth (Bagby, 1995).

C Government cuts in spending did not keep pace with the growth of the national economy.

1. Tax cuts had a negative impact on government revenue.
2. Planned spending and reform of national entitlement programs, such as Medicare/Medicaid and Social Security, were not politically supported.
3. Entitlement program cuts were not large enough to cover the reduction in tax revenue.
4. American government continued to spend more than it took in; this increased deficit spending by the government, resulting in high deficits.

D The United States went from the largest creditor nation to the largest debtor nation in the global economy.

E Negative effects on Americans living with high national budget deficits include the following (Bagby, 1995):

1. Higher interest rates
2. Less money for investment
3. Lower economic growth rate
4. Less revenue to pay interest on debt
5. Debtor status to foreign countries
6. Lower sales of exports
7. Long-term decrease in the standard of living

F By the end of the 1980s, the American economy was in a recession.

G In the 1990s, the inflation rate fell and the U.S. became more competitive in the worldwide marketplace; this resulted in a period of expansion and economic growth.

H In the 2000s, it is projected that the amount and intensity of competition worldwide will increase, augmented by the use of the Internet (Dent, 2000).

I In the coming decades, there will be an increase of multinational companies and an expansion of career and investment opportunities around the world.

III The Impact of Economics on the Individual

A **Unstable, poorly functioning economies produce the following results:**
1. People have greater difficulty finding jobs that match their abilities and education.
2. Continually rising prices reduce the value of savings, thus affecting the ability of people, especially retirees, to survive.
3. Company managers may have difficulty obtaining a sufficient quantity or quality of materials at a reasonable price.
4. Companies may have difficulty distributing their products and finding buyers able to purchase them.
5. Investment opportunities may be hard to find.
6. Expending accumulated personal assets may be very difficult, because available goods and services may be limited or of poor quality.

B **In a thriving economy, individuals and society as a whole benefit from the efficient production of goods and services.**
1. People are working (society may be at the level of full employment, and unemployment levels are low).
2. Families are receiving income and consuming goods and services that they need or want.
3. Economic progress gives people access to technologically advanced products.
4. A strong market for technologically advanced products stimulates research and investment for further technologic progress.
5. A well-functioning economy is attractive to foreigners for investment of capital or purchasing goods.
6. A stable, advancing economy aids social progress in the following ways:
   a. More students pursue higher levels of education.
   b. Although students are absent from the work force while in school, they enter the work force with a higher level of skill and knowledge.
   c. Well-educated workers function at a higher productivity level and thus benefit the economy.

C **A thriving economy allows managers to accomplish the following:**
1. Plan production and personnel programs and services with reasonable confidence that they will reap the benefits of the economy and projections for sales, productivity costs, and profits
2. Evaluate company and individual performance factors that have an impact on their "bottom line" without being hindered by an unstable economy
3. Expand businesses or add personnel to payroll
4. Provide benefits and services to employees while meeting shareholders' expectations for profit or return on investment (ROI)

D **A well-run economy facilitates the production and exchange of goods and services.**

E **The low unemployment that results from a thriving economy can result in the following:**
1. A change in the way companies staff their workplaces (U.S. Department of Labor, Bureau of Labor Stastistics [USDL BLS], 2001)
   a. The number of outsourced temporary workers increased 580% between 1982 and 1998.
   b. In 2001, 8.6 million workers considered themselves independent contractors; about 13 million people work under alternative employment

arrangements as independent contractors, temporary help workers, contract workers, or on-call workers (USDL BLS, 2001).
   2. Increasing options available to workers
      a. Businesses may have difficulty hiring and retaining skilled workers.
      b. The hiring of less-skilled workers may diminish the quality of services and products.

IV Changes in the National Economy

The transition in the national economy is from protected markets to international competition.

A Economic competitiveness depends on a nation's financial, industrial, and demographic characteristics, such as its unemployment rate, GNP, per capita income, average hours and conditions of work, and distribution of wealth.

B The economic competitiveness of a nation also depends on the ability of its individual businesses to sell their goods and services at a profit in domestic (national) and foreign markets.

C America's ability to prosper depends on the ability of U.S. companies to produce and market goods and services that can compete successfully in terms of price, quality, innovation, customization, and serviceability with those of other nations.

V Factors Affecting National and Global Competitiveness

(Potter & Youngman, 1995)

A After World War II, America became the leading economic power, partly because of the destructive impact of the war on the economies of Japan and Europe.
   1. Postwar benefits, such as the GI Bill, provided housing and educational opportunities to returning veterans, thus creating a competitive labor force, boosting the construction industry, and encouraging local community development.
   2. National and global economies and industrialization surged from 1953 to 1975, increasing world industrial output an average of 6% a year.
   3. The postwar economic boom in the United States was facilitated by the deregulation of industry and by industrial developments and manpower planning that occurred during the war.
   4. Business, no longer hampered by wartime government constraints, returned to free markets and focused on meeting consumers' (rather than the government's) needs.

B During the immediate postwar decades, the world was divided into domestic and international marketplaces.
   1. U.S. companies produced primarily for domestic or regional markets with minimal competition from imports and few multinational companies.
   2. American companies led the industrialized markets with increasing technologic advances, mass production, and higher workers' wages through the 1970s.
   3. Government regulation and collective bargaining added to costs of American businesses.

4. Europe, Japan, and the Pacific Rim countries, fully rebuilt after World War II, became increasingly competitive with the United States in the world market.

C **Customers at home and abroad have become "global shoppers," seeking the best product at the most affordable price without regard to the country in which it was produced.**

D **Imports to the United States grew 260% between 1975 and 1993, the increase fueled by increased American purchasing power.**

E **U.S. exports account for the following economic benefits:**
   1. One out of every six American jobs in manufacturing
   2. $115 billion annually in services
   3. One-sixth of all U.S. agricultural production
   4. Almost 25% of America's gross domestic product (GDP)–over $1 trillion per year

F **The nation's economic status is affected by a multitude of conditions and circumstances.**
   1. Declining economic competitiveness means potentially fewer jobs, increased unemployment, lower per capita income, and larger budget deficits.
   2. The economy entered a recession and business retrenched during the 1970s, affecting manufacturing by decreasing mass production, job creation, wages, and employment levels.
   3. The national economy expanded during the 1980s, but American manufacturing lost its competitive edge to foreign competitors who could produce goods at a lower cost than American companies.
   4. The United States is no longer primarily an industrialized nation, a producer of manufactured goods; its economy depends more and more on the production of services and technology.
   5. Industries are looking to place manufacturing, high tech, and some customer service jobs "offshore" in countries where wages and operating costs are less to decrease expense and increase shareholder value (DiBenedetto 2004).

G **Since the 1990s, the United States has been the leading provider of services and technology (Dent, 2000).**
   1. The recent explosion of Internet use has revolutionized communications and has fundamentally altered the way people live, work, and conduct business in the national and global economies.
   2. The economic competitiveness of the United States has increased through the use of Internet technology, which has resulted in a huge array of customized goods and services at increasingly affordable prices.
   3. The vast increase in the use of technology to conduct business and communicate with others in "real time" increases competition and the ability to generate income and wealth.

H **The "information revolution," which began in the 1990s, will continue in the 2000s, with vast changes as business-to-business transactions become electronic and based on Internet technologies.**

VI International Trade Status of the Nation

A **Presently, the United States has a trade deficit.**
   1. The United States imports more than it exports.
   2. U.S. consumers buy more foreign products than foreigners buy U.S. goods.

B Reasons for this trade imbalance include the following:

1. Some foreign countries have high trade barriers, making it difficult for the United States to sell products there.

2. The U.S. dollar has been high compared to other currencies, making it expensive for foreigners to buy American and inexpensive for Americans to buy foreign.

3. U.S. products are less competitive than foreign products in terms of price and availability.

4. U.S. services (such as architecture, engineering, and consulting) account for billions of dollars in trade, but are not accounted for in calculating the U.S. trade deficit.

C The United States continues to produce one fourth of the world's gross national product.

VII The Global Marketplace

A The global economy is becoming an integrated marketplace and is influenced by a variety of economic and political forces, such as the following:

1. General Agreement for Trade and Tariffs (GATT)

   a. GATT, which was created after World War II, works to reduce trade barriers and promote free trade among its member nations in the Free World.

   b. In 1994, the member nations of GATT agreed to create the World Trade Organization, a more comprehensive and powerful organization to govern global trade in goods and services.

2. Unification of Europe to form the European Economic Community

3. End of the Cold War and subsequent decline of communism

4. North American Free Trade Act (NAFTA)

   a. Established in 1994, NAFTA lowered trade barriers and opened the borders of Canada, the United States, and Mexico to almost limitless trade.

   b. NAFTA's long-term goal is to remove barriers to trade extending all the way from Alaska to Argentina.

5. Increased economic growth of the Pacific Rim countries

B Since the terrorist attacks that occurred in September 2001, there has been an increased shift towards national and global security and national defense efforts.

1. The United States and other countries have banded together to wage the war in terrorism.

2. The Homeland Security Act of 2002 established the Department of Homeland Security.

3. Issues related to terrorism and national defense will continue through the 21st century.

C The world is moving toward "free trade," that is, trade without taxes or tariffs.

D Fewer products are being produced entirely within any single nation; the world is moving toward a single economy—a unified marketplace (Naisbitt & Aburdene, 1990; Dent, 2000).

E Economic and political forces are shaping a new world.

VIII Implications for the Occupational and Environmental Health Nurse

A The occupational and environmental health nurse is a company's primary resource regarding health care issues and the delivery of both occupational and non-occupational health services.

1. Occupational and environmental health nurses ensure that the work force is fit, healthy, and medically capable of performing work assignments, thus adding to the company's and the nation's productivity and ultimately to the GNP.

2. With an increasing percentage of temporary, contingent, and mobile workers, occupational and environmental health nurses will be required to be more creative and innovative in their efforts to ensure that all workers receive appropriate occupational health and safety services.

3. The role of the occupational and environmental health nurse will expand or contract throughout the business cycle and during periods of economic uncertainty (i.e., business contraction or expansion).

B Occupational health practice is shifting from the manufacturing sector to the service and technology sectors, and is expanding to include international issues of health and safety.

C As the work force expands past national borders (i.e., workers transfer to work sites in foreign countries), the occupational and environmental health nurse will be responsible for:

1. Ensuring the health of expatriates and their dependents; occupational and environmental health nursing duties include the following:
   a. Immunizations for international travel
   b. Access to quality health care abroad
   c. Health education
   d. Psychologic support systems (for example, access to employee assistance programs)

2. Helping identify international health and safety needs of the global work force

3. Identifying national and international regulatory compliance issues that will affect the work force, such as family leave and occupational health laws, homeland security, and issues related to the nation's health in times of turbulence and warfare.

(Chapter 16 presents a sample international travel program.)

IX Business Trends

A Megatrends (large social, economic, and technologic trends) that shaped the 1980s in business include the following (Naisbitt and Aburdene, 1990):

1. Shift from an industrial society to an information society
2. Forced technology to high tech/high touch; for example, interactive technology
3. National economy to a world economy
4. Short-term to long-term planning
5. Centralization to decentralization of company/business lines/units
6. Institutional help to self-help
7. Representative democracy to participatory democracy
8. Hierarchies to networking teams

9. Movement of business from northern states to southern states to save on labor and operating costs

10. Movement from "either/or" to multiple options

B **During the economic expansion in the 1980s, businesses invested, acquired additional product lines, and increased their work forces.**

1. Many businesses established operations in southern states, where operating costs were lower.

2. Companies established decentralized business operations wherein operating divisions became dedicated "strategic business units," accountable for their own profits and losses.

3. Businesses merged "horizontally," acquiring companies that enhanced existing product lines.

4. During the latter part of the 1980s, the economy contracted, and business responded by:

    a. Divesting noncore or nonessential business units and product lines

    b. Downsizing work forces through layoffs or reorganizations

    c. Initiating vertical mergers (businesses acquiring similar businesses)

C **The technology explosion of the 1990s created eight critical technology trends that will change the way employers and consumers work and live in the 2000s (Dent 2000):**

1. Vastly expanded computer power

2. Mass adoption of portable and home personal computers

3. Increased computer literacy among all age groups

4. Evolution of computers so they become simple and affordable appliances and everyday work tools

5. Linkage of microprocessor-embedded home and business products through the Internet

6. Rapid movement of consumers "on line"

7. Expansion of the communication bandwidth

8. Object-oriented programming for customized software

D **Business issues into the twenty-first century include (DiBenedetto (2004):**

1. Financial pressures: doing more with less to increase shareholder value and return on investment

2. Myriad data systems that require centralization to provide appropriate business information to management

3. The exporting of service jobs and manufacturing to third world and developing countries

4. An aging workforce

5. Explosion of health care, pharmacy, and workers' compensation costs

6. Mergers and acquisitions

7. Outsourcing of staff functions such as human resources, safety, and health

8. Increased concern for personal and business safety in light of terrorist attacks on September 11, 2001

9. Work-life balance for workers

X Major Business Issues

A **Increased federalism or regulatory constraints on business include mandatory compliance with regulations set forth by the following:**

1. Occupational Safety and Health Act of 1970

2. Department of Transportation regulations

3. Environmental Protection Agency (EPA) regulations
4. Employee Retirement Income Security Act of 1974
5. Consolidated Omnibus Budget Reconciliation Act of 1986
6. Family Medical Leave Act of 1993
7. Americans with Disabilities Act of 1990
8. State workers' compensation statutes
9. Homeland Security Act of 2002
10. Health Insurance Portability & Accountability Act (HIPAA) of 1996

B Costs of social insurance programs (Social Security, Medicare, Medicaid) have shifted from government to privately funded sources.

C Worker health and welfare benefits, such as workers' compensation and non-occupational health and disability have increased.

D Employers' trends affecting business include the following:
1. Shift toward managed care and consumer-driven health care for health benefit plans
2. Increased cost sharing of health care expenses and benefits with workers through higher deductibles and coinsurance rates, increasing workers' out-of-pocket expenditures
3. Increased involvement of workers in health care decisions
4. Aggressive negotiation with health providers and packaging of provider services
5. Aggressive management of health care costs through utilization review, second opinions, preadmission certification, concurrent review, case management, disease management, and retrospective reviews
6. Increased communication with workers, their dependents, and retirees regarding health care costs and their role as informed consumers
7. Encouragement of managed care enrollments
8. Establishment of wellness programs and services
9. Emphasis on balancing worker and family work/lifestyle issues such as elder care, childcare, work-life balance
10. Movement toward a "24-hour" system of health care (i.e., the integration of occupational and non-occupational medical care), with a focus on "total health management"
11. Shift toward integrated disability (both workers' compensation and non-occupational disability) and related health management programs and services
12. Combating *presenteeism,* a term used by human resources professionals and many consultants to describe circumstances in which workers come to work even though they are ill, posing potential problems of contagion and lower productivity (DiBenedetto 2004)
13. Addressing absenteeism
    a. On any given day as much as 35% of an employer's workforce may be absent due to scheduled or unscheduled reasons
    b. The major reasons cited for unscheduled absences include: personal illness (36%), family reasons (22%), personal needs (18%), entitlement mentality (13%), and stress (11%)
14. The use of onsite health clinics has been found beneficial as a cost saving and work-life balance measures both short-term and long-term investment in managing worker health and productivity (DiBenedetto, 2004).

E **Several issues affect workers' compensation benefits (DiBenedetto, 1999, 2004).**
1. Workers' compensation constitutes about 3% of total national medical expenditures; however, 11 million workers suffer work-related injuries resulting in $111 billion in payments for medical care, wage replacement, and disability payments.
2. More than 50% of payments ($111 billion) is associated with the payment of lost wages, and the remainder represents the cost of workers' compensation medical care (1997).
3. *Direct* costs of workers' compensation include medical care and indemnity (wage replacement) payments.
4. *Indirect* costs include lost productivity, required replacements, worker overtime, training, accident investigation, and broken equipment.
5. Identification and correction of the root causes of workers' compensation claims will facilitate a safer workplace and decrease both workers' compensation claims (medical and indemnity costs), thus increasing work-force productivity.

F **Methods being used by businesses to control the cost of workers' compensation include the following (DiBenedetto, et al., 1996, DiBenedetto, 2004):**
1. Pre-claim strategies, such as:
   a. Assignment of responsibilities
   b. Communications
   c. Occupational health and safety programs and services
   d. Injury prevention programs and services
   e. Development of job responsibilities (essential functions and physical requirements)
   f. Return-to-work programs and services
   g. Identification of modified or transitional work assignments
   h. Third party administrator (TPA) performance standards
   i. Medical and case management requirements
   j. Negotiated discounts of fee schedules and managed medical care arrangements
2. At-claim strategies, such as:
   a. Immediate reporting of accidents to management and the carrier or TPA
   b. Timely accident investigation
   c. Claim setup and initiation of medical and case management
   d. Use of evidence-based disability duration guidelines
   e. Use of evidence-based treatment guidelines or protocols
   f. Use of independent medical examinations
   g. Use of functional ability testing or functional capacity examinations
   h. Fraud investigation
   i. Establishment of appropriate claim reserves
3. Postclaim strategies, such as:
   a. TPA audits
   b. Utilization review
   c. Quality assurance reviews
4. Additional trends include the integration of workers' compensation, non-occupational disability and health care management to promote total health management, or an integrated approach to health and productivity management to conserve costs and facilitate the injured worker's return to work.

XI Implications for Occupational and Environmental Health Nursing

(DiBenedetto, 2004)

A The occupational and environmental health nurse plays a primary role in helping the work force attain its maximum level of health and thus adds to work-force productivity.

1. Occupational and environmental health nurses perform health care and management functions that vary according to the work setting, the employer's needs and expectations, the company philosophy, the regulatory requirements that govern occupational health care, safety, and workers' compensation in that particular industry.

2. Occupational and environmental health nurses are increasingly involved in worker benefits; they evaluate sponsors and benefit components, arrange for second opinions, educate workers regarding lifestyles and life skills, and integrate health promotion activities to include the needs of families.

3. Occupational and environmental health nurses are assuming a greater role in establishing and directing integrated disability management and return-to-work programs and services to increase the health, safety, and productivity of the work force.

B The occupational and environmental health nurse may have the following specific responsibilities:

1. Establish and implement health- and productivity-related policies and procedures

2. Develop and maintain the company's regulatory compliance programs and services related to OSHA, EPA, DOT, ADA, FMLA, HIPAA and workers' compensation requirements

3. Prevent both occupational and non-occupational injury and illness through health promotion and health education activities

4. Provide workers' compensation and non-occupational case management (also referred to as integrated disability management, health and productivity management); coordinate independent health examinations; arrange for second-opinion examinations and functional ability examinations; and perform case management functions to facilitate early return to work of ill and injured workers

5. Identify trends and issues that will impact worker health and productivity

6. Identify real and potential hazards in the workplace by conducting facility assessments and report those conditions to appropriate members of management for correction

C The role of the occupational and environmental health nurse and funding for occupational health and safety programs and services will expand or contract throughout the business cycle.

1. Many companies continue to outsource occupational health and safety-services; many occupational health providers are now contract providers or vendors.

2. As the work force contracts through downsizing and layoffs, workers are more likely to file for workers' compensation or disability; some claims for on-the-job injuries may be fraudulent.

XII Health Care Reform and Managed Health Care

A The major arguments for health care reform are the following:
1. The delivery of care is bogged down in administration and insurance underwriting.
2. Health care costs are escalating.
3. At least 44 million Americans lack health insurance or are underinsured.

B Health reform components that have broad support include the following:
1. A standard minimum benefit package
2. Insurance market reform
3. Health plan "report cards"
4. Consumer choice of plans
5. Voluntary purchasing pools

C Major components of health care reform proposals have included insurance market reforms, cost-containment mechanisms, managed care, and subsidies for low-income persons.

D Past proposals recommended financing health care reform through employer or individual premium mandates or from voluntary plans based on the then-current health care system.

E Federal efforts to mandate health care reform failed to pass Congress in 1994.

F Currently, market-driven reforms have moved the delivery of health care from "free choice" to managed care.

XIII Overview of Managed Care

A *Managed care* is a broad concept generally applied to "prepayment arrangement, negotiated discounts, and agreements for prior authorization and audits of performance" (Madison & Konrad, 1988, in Wassel, 1995).

B Managed care plans generally provide some restrictions on the traditional unlimited access to providers and payment of reasonable and customary charges for their health care services (Wassel, 1995).

C Managed care plans place responsibilities on consumers and providers in the form of a binding contract (Wassel, 1995).

D A managed care plan is any form of health plan that initiates selective contracting between providers, employers, or insurers to channel workers/clients to a specified set of cost-effective providers (a provider network). These providers have procedures in place to ensure that only medically necessary and appropriate use of health care services occurs.

E Three basic types of health care delivery systems under managed care arrangements are the health maintenance organization, preferred provider organization, and point-of-service plan (Wassel, 1995).
1. A *health maintenance organization (HMO)* provides a specified scope of services or benefits to members for a fixed fee.
   a. There are four types of HMOs: staff, group, network, and independent-practice associations.
   b. HMOs provide 10% to 40% savings over traditional health plans.

2. A *preferred provider organization (PPO)* provides greater consumer choice through use of a limited provider panel, and uses negotiated fee schedules, utilization review, and the physician-as-gatekeeper to hold down costs.
   a. In exchange for reduced rates, providers often receive expedited claim payments or a reasonable market share.
   b. Workers have financial incentives to use PPO providers.
3. A *point-of-service plan (POS)* is a health benefit plan through which several different types of insurance coverage are available. The worker chooses the insurance plan and provider at the time health care services are sought.
   a. POS plans provide incentives for workers to choose cost-effective providers.
   b. If the worker does not use managed care providers, he or she bears the extra cost of service.

F The *24-hour* model of health care incorporates occupational (workers' compensation) and non-occupational (disability) health care into one health care delivery system to improve continuity of care, manage and reduce claim costs, minimize redundancies in coverage, simplify adjudication, and reduce administrative efforts and costs; approaches to 24-hour care include the following (Abbott, 1994):
1. 24-hour medical coverage, in which health benefits for all accidents or injuries fall under an integrated health plan. Disability or lost-time benefits would be paid by workers' compensation.
2. 24-hour disability coverage, in which disability benefits for both occupational and non-occupational concerns would be paid from an integrated plan, but health payments would still be divided.
3. Integrated 24-hour medical and disability coverage, in which medical and indemnity payments would be integrated under one plan.
4. *Accident only* and *sickness only* medical programs and services may also exist as a subset to these three major categories.

G Managed workers' compensation is characterized by negotiated fee schedules, capitated rates, and the use of PPOs and other provider arrangements.
1. *Integrated disability management (IDM)* is a comprehensive approach to integrating all disability benefits, programs, and services to help control the employer's disability costs while returning the worker to work as soon as possible and maximizing the worker's functional capacity (Mercer, 1995).
2. *Total Health Management or Health and Productivity Management* is the next phase of employers managing the health, safety and productivity of their workforce. Its is the logical extension of IDM efforts, which also focus on early identification of the potential for disease (through the use of health risk appraisals), health counseling, early medical intervention and rehabilitation for occupational and non-occupational conditions which impact worker health, presenteeism, well-being, and the "bottom-line" (DiBenedetto, 2004)

XIV Quality Controls in Managed Care
(Employee Benefit Research Institute, 1995)

A Maintaining the quality of health care is Americans' primary concern in the changing health care system.

B Concern over rising health care costs has led private employers and public programs and services to adopt various strategies to manage health care costs.

C The aim of all these strategies is to purchase the highest quality health care at the lowest cost.

D Defining and measuring health care quality are controversial and costly endeavors.

E *Health care quality* can be viewed narrowly as *clinical effectiveness.*

F Health care quality can be viewed in a broader sense as all the attributes of medical care that clients value.

XV Judging Standards of Care

The following private organizations independently review quality standards in hospitals and other institutions and provide accreditation of those organizations.

A Joint Commission for Accreditation of Healthcare Organizations

B Health Care Financing Administration

C National Committee for Quality Assurance

D Accreditation Association for Ambulatory Health Care

E Utilization Review Accreditation Commission

XVI Defining and Evaluating Quality Outcomes

A Managed care relies on monitoring physicians' treatment patterns (through utilization review, physician profiling, and case management) and changing providers' financial incentives.

B Health Plan Employer Data and Information Set (HEDIS) was established by the private sector (several employers and managed care organizations in 1989) to help large purchasers of health care judge the comparative value of competing health care plans. HEDIS has the following characteristics:
 1. Provides a core set of performance measures that can be adapted to serve the needs of other purchasers
 2. Provides benchmarks for performance in specific areas such as health plan quality, access and client satisfaction, membership and utilization, finance and management, and activities
 3. Relies primarily on structural and process measures of quality; major outcome measures are client satisfaction and readmission rates for major disorders

C Many analysts believe that the future evolution of the health care delivery system will be driven by the development of measures of the quality of care.

D Donabedien (1988) classified attempts to measure quality of care as studies of structure, process, and outcome.
 1. *Structure* refers to attributes of care, such as caregiver's qualifications and resources available at the site of care.
 2. *Process* examines the caregiver's activities, decisions made at various points in an episode of illness, and appropriateness of care.
 3. *Outcome* measures the effects of care on health status and client satisfaction.

XVII Implications for Occupational and Environmental Health Nursing

(DiBenedetto et al., 1996, 2004)

A **Occupational and environmental health nurses are providing case management services, return-to-work planning, and management of integrated disability and workers' compensation services.**

1. As market-driven health care reform continues, the role and scope of occupational and environmental health nursing will expand into the managed care arena as an integrated model that combines both workers' compensation and disability management.
2. Occupational and environmental health nurses may be involved in the assessment, evaluation, and implementation of managed health care arrangements, programs, and services.
3. Occupational and environmental health nurses will provide value-added knowledge and services as managed care vendors expand services into the occupational health and managed workers' compensation markets.

B **Occupational and environmental health nurses will increasingly become involved in managed health care benefits for the following:**

1. Employers
2. Workers *and their dependents*
3. Retiree populations whose benefits are paid by employers
4. Managed health care vendors/organizations

C **Occupational and environmental health nurses may become the liaison between employer benefit plans and managed care organizations, thus facilitating lines of communication, professional cooperation, benefit services, and health care delivery.**

REFERENCES

Abbott, R. K. (1994, Sept/Oct). 24 hour medical care: A primer. *Innovations in human resources,* 12-14.

Bagby, M. E. (1995). *The first annual report of the United States of America: An account to American citizens of where we stand economically, socially, and internationally.* New York: Harper Business.

Dent, H. S., Jr. (2000). *The roaring 2000s.* New York: Simon and Schuster.

DiBenedetto, D. V. (1999, June) Workers' compensation managed care. *OEM report 13*(6), 41-48.

DiBenedetto, D. V. (2004, January) Absenteeism in the Workplace: Contributing Factors and Management of Lost Work Time. *OEM Report 18*(1), 1-3.

DiBenedetto, D. V., Harris, J.S, & McCunney, R.J. (1996). *Occupational health & safety manual,* (2nd ed.). Beverly Farms, MA: OEM Press.

Employee Benefit Research Institute (EBRI). (1995, March). *Measuring the quality of health care* [*EBRI Brief No. 159*]. Washington, DC: EBRI.

Madison, D.L., & Konrad, T.R. (1988). Large medical group-practice organizations and employee physicians: A relationship in transition. *Milbank Memorial Quarterly, 66*(2), 240-282.

Mercer, W. (1995). *The language of managed disability.* New York: Mercer/Met Disability.

Naisbitt, J., & Aburdene, P. (1990). *Megatrends 2000: Ten new directions for the 1990s.* New York: William Morrow & Company.

Potter, E.E., & Youngman, J.A. (1995). *Keeping America competitive: Employment policy for the twenty-first century.* Lakewood, CO: Glenbridge Publishing Ltd.

U.S. Department of Labor Bureau of Labor Statistics (**2001**). Report on the American Workforce. Washington, D.C.: U.S. Department of Labor.

Wassel, M.L. (1995). Occupational health nursing and the advent of managed care: Meeting the challenges of the current health care environment. *AAOHN Journal, 43*(1), 23–28.

OTHER RESOURCES

DiBenedetto, D.V. Principles of Workers' Compensation and Disability Case Management (1997-2004), Battle Creek, MI: DVD Associates LLC.

Donabedien, A. (1988, Spring). Quality assessment and assurance: Unity of purpose, diversity of means. *Inquiry, 25,* 173–192.

Epping, R.C. (1995). *A beginner's guide to world economy.* New York: Vintage Books.

Heilbroner, R., & Thurow, L. (1994). *Economics explained: Everything you need to know about how the economy works and where it's going.* New York: Touchstone.

Katzenbach, J.R, & Smith, D.K. (1994). *The wisdom of teams: Creating the high performance organization.* New York: Harper Business.

McRae, H. (1994). *The world in 2020: Power, culture and prosperity.* Boston: Harvard Business School Press.

Peters, T. (1992). *Liberation management: Necessary disorganization for the nanosecond nineties.* New York: Fawcett Columbine.

Traska, M.R. (1995). *Managed care strategies 1996.* New York: Faulkner and Gray.

5

Scientific Foundations of Occupational and Environmental Health Nursing Practice

JACQUELINE AGNEW

The science and practice of occupational and environmental health nursing are based on a synthesis of knowledge gained from multiple disciplines. It is essential that occupational and environmental health nurses understand the principles of the sciences that provide the theoretic, conceptual, and factual framework of the profession. In addition to the nursing and occupational and environmental health sciences (e.g., toxicology, industrial hygiene, and ergonomics), effective practice in this field requires knowledge and understanding of the public health (e.g., environmental health and epidemiology) and social/behavioral sciences. This chapter provides an introduction and overview of these foundation disciplines.

Nursing science

I Nursing Science in the Context of Public Health

A In the mid-1800s, Florence Nightingale (1820-1910) established public health as an important focus for nursing.

1. She emphasized the need for nurses to improve environmental conditions to protect the health of clients, thus laying the foundation for occupational and environmental health nursing.
   a. The major focus of her work was preventive rather than curative health service.
   b. She used statistical techniques to demonstrate the relationship between unsanitary conditions and preventable deaths.
   c. She developed a recordkeeping system that enabled her to improve the conditions in hospitals.
2. According to Nightingale, the five elements necessary for good health are: pure air, pure water, efficient drainage, cleanliness, and light.
3. She encouraged the development of nursing theory and research; her major influence was on nursing education.

B Current approaches to occupational and environmental health nursing can be viewed according to a model of public health developed by the Section of Public Health Nursing of the Minnesota Department of Health (Keller et al., 2004).

1. The Intervention Wheel, a revision of the Public Health Intervention Model, describes the application of nursing practice to populations, including workers, their families, and communities (Figure 5-1).
2. The Intervention Wheel is based on the actual work performed by public health nurses, including nurses in worksite practice settings.
3. According to this model, population-based practice focuses on populations, relies on community assessments, considers all determinants of health, emphasizes prevention, and intervenes at multiple levels.

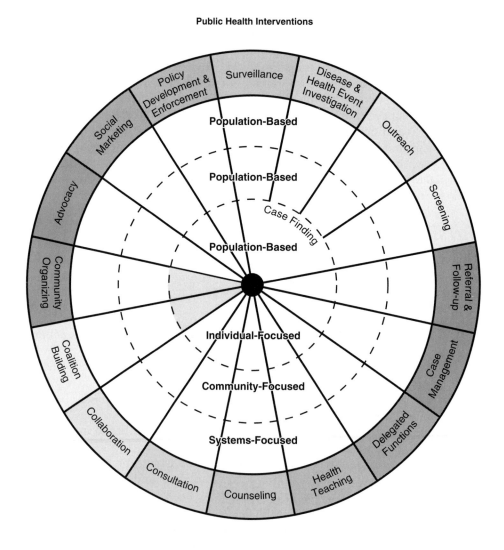

Public Health Interventions

March 2001

FIGURE 5-1 *Public health intervention wheel (Minnesota Department of Health, Division of Community Health Services Public Health Nursing Section) 2001*

4. Three levels of practice are identified: community, systems, and individuals/family.
5. Public health practice is described by 17 types of interventions, grouped into five general areas, termed "wedges":
   a. Surveillance, disease and other health event investigation, outreach, screening, and case finding
   b. Referral and follow-up, case management, and delegated functions
   c. Health teaching, counseling, and consultation
   d. Collaboration, coalition building, and community organizing
   e. Advocacy, social marketing, and policy development and enforcement

II Evolution of Occupational and Environmental Health Nursing Practice

A *Nursing, Health and the Environment* **(Institute of Medicine [IOM], 1995) is a landmark publication that defines and describes the role of nurses in environmental health. According to this publication:**
1. Environmental health is the "freedom from illness or injury related to exposure to toxic agents and other environmental conditions that are potentially detrimental to health."
2. Three themes are related to nursing and the environment:
   a. The environment is a primary determinant of health, and environmental health hazards affect all aspects of life and all areas of nursing practice.
   b. Nurses are well positioned to address environmental health concerns of individuals and communities.
   c. There is a need to enhance the awareness of and emphasis on environmental threats to the health of populations served by all nurses, regardless of their practice arena.

B **The expertise and competencies of occupational and environmental health nurses are relevant to the protection of health and safety in community settings and work settings (American Association of Occupational Health Nurses, 2003).**

C **Some of the most significant environmental conditions that are capable of harming the health of humans are experienced at work, where exposures are often higher than in other settings; the working population (population at risk) is characterized by the following:**
1. Generally healthy enough to hold a job
2. Of working age
3. Often of childbearing age

D **Occupational and environmental health nursing interventions should be population-based, supported by evidence, and reflect best practices.**

E **Occupational and environmental health nurses perform interventions depicted by the Intervention Wheel model; as examples:**
1. Nurses who establish, publicize, and monitor heavy metal screening programs and registries, followed by case finding, are performing surveillance, investigation, outreach, and screening functions at system, community, and individual levels.
2. Referral, case management, and delegated functions are accomplished at all three levels when occupational and environmental health nurses work with

health departments, worker populations, and high risk individuals to identify cases of tuberculosis, prevent further spread of the disease, and ensure treatment for those who are infected.

3. Teaching, counseling, and consultation take place through nursing activities aimed at informing health care providers and members of rural communities about risks of agricultural hazards and health effect prevention.

4. Partnerships with local health departments, community organizations, neighborhood residents, and parents to create safe play areas for urban children address the intervention areas of collaboration, coalition building, and community organizing

5. The areas of advocacy, social marketing, and policy development are exemplified by nursing practices that promote and enforce employer policies to prevent the transmission of workplace hazards into the home environment. Requirements might include provision of clothing changes, shower facilities, and worker training.

F **Several factors determine the health of individuals and populations (US Department of Health and Human Services, 2000).**
1. *Biological* factors include genetic background as well as physical and mental health status.
2. *Behaviors* occur in response to an individual's experiences and may either cause biological changes or be influenced by biology. For example, smoking (behavior) may cause lung disease (biology); fair complexion (biology) may lead to avoidance of sun exposure (behavior).
3. The *social environment* includes interaction with others, housing and community services, and institutions such as school and places of worship. The social environment profoundly influences health and can affect behavior and the biological status of populations.
4. The *physical environment* can be the source of exposure to harmful agents: chemicals, pathogens, or physical hazards. Alternatively, the physical environment can be protective or encourage positive behaviors such as exercise.
5. Additional determinants of health are: (1) policies and interventions that relate to health behaviors and health outcomes; and (2) *access to quality care*, which is essential for optimizing the health of all.

G **Workers and communities face multiple workplace hazards that place them at risk.**
1. A *hazard* is defined as a substance capable of causing harm (Chapter 1 describes categories of hazards).
2. *Risk* is the probability that harm will occur.

H **A systematic understanding of the relationships among health determinants and the principles that govern the association between hazards and health effects provides a basis for preventing morbidity and mortality and promoting health in a broad range of settings.**
1. Workers, work-related exposures, and work environments illustrate one domain in which these principles apply.
2. The influence of industrial conditions on family and community members is another example of health and environment interactions.
   a. Families can be exposed to toxins transported home on workers' bodies or belongings.
   b. Industrial waste or effluent can reach the community.

3. Approaches to risk assessment and principles of health protection similar to those used in the workplace can be used to protect the health of communities faced with natural or manmade hazards in media such as food, air, soil, and water.

I The chief disciplines that assist the occupational and environmental health nurse to understand the agent-host-environment relationship are epidemiology, toxicology, and industrial hygiene; these are described in the following sections.

Epidemiology

III Overview of Epidemiologic Terms and Principles

Epidemiology is the public health science that is fundamental to describing and understanding relationships among agents, hosts, and their environments.

A Definitions related to epidemiology are as follows:
1. *Epidemiology* is the study of the distribution and determinants of health-related states or events in specified populations, and the application of this study to the control of health problems.
2. *Incidence rate* is an epidemiologic term that describes the occurrence of new disease or injury per unit of time among persons at risk (Rothman & Greenland, 1998a).
   a. The numerator includes only new cases of disease during a given time period; the denominator includes everyone at risk of developing the disease during that period.
   b. Incidence, therefore, measures the probability (or risk) of developing disease.
   c. Incidence rates are useful for tracking trends in the development or resolution of disease.
3. *Prevalence* is an epidemiologic term that describes the proportion of the population with the condition at a given point in time or during a given time period.
   a. The numerator includes new and existing cases; the denominator includes all who are at risk of developing the disease, including those who have it.
   b. Prevalence measures the current burden of disease and is useful for measuring and projecting health care and health resource needs.

B Examples of applications of epidemiologic research include:
1. Controlling infectious diseases, such as tuberculosis among migrant farm workers
2. Controlling the effects of chemical hazards, such as asbestosis, mesothelioma, and lung cancers related to exposure to asbestos
3. Understanding genetic susceptibility to disease, such as coronary heart disease or cancer, which often result from a combination of hereditary and environmental factors
4. Understanding the effects of nutritional status, such as the link between a calcium intake and osteoporosis
5. Linking pathogens to specific disease processes, such as West Nile virus and its pattern of occurrence among humans
6. Identifying risk factors for illness or injury, such as work factors that lead to back injuries in health care workers

C **Epidemiology has great relevance to occupational and environmental health nursing.**
1. It serves as a tool for recognizing, identifying and preventing hazardous exposures.
2. Findings from epidemiologic studies of worker and community populations are often reported in the occupational and environmental health literature.
3. Epidemiologic studies help occupational and environmental health nurses provide high-quality health services.

IV Measures of Association

Evaluation of associations among exposures and health outcomes is central to epidemiology; criteria to evaluate causality based on an observed association include the following (Rothman & Greenland, 1998b):

A The strength of the association
1. The strength of the association refers to the degree of correlation between the exposure and disease.
2. It is important to remember that weak associations do not necessarily rule out a causal relationship between the exposure and disease.

B Consistency of the association
1. Similar findings result across several studies of the same association.
2. Conclusions are similar despite the use of different study designs, under different conditions, and in different populations.

C Temporality of the association
1. Studies demonstrate that the cause (exposure or independent variable) precedes the effects (disease or dependent variable) chronologically.
2. Temporality cannot be evaluated with a cross-sectional study.

D Dose-response relationship
1. As the degree of exposure increases, the risk for developing the outcome increases.
2. Lack of a dose-response relationship does not rule out a causal relationship.

E Plausibility of the association
1. The association is consistent with a plausible biologic explanation.
2. Knowledge of the natural history of the disease and results of animal and other laboratory experiments need to be considered.
3. Sometimes there is not enough scientific evidence to draw conclusions about biological plausibility.

V Sources of Epidemiologic Data

A **Population-based health outcome data are available through a variety of public and private agencies; data include:**
1. Census data (U.S. Census Bureau)
2. Vital statistics (U.S. Census Bureau)
3. National health surveys (National Center for Health Statistics)
   a. Population-based studies such as the National Health and Nutrition Examination Surveys and the National Health Interview Survey are conducted regularly.

b. Mandatory reporting systems capture data such as OSHA-recordable illnesses and injuries (Bureau of Labor Statistics).
4. Disease and death registries (e.g., from state and federal agencies or medical centers)

B **Exposure data are often more difficult to obtain, especially in environmental and occupational settings.**
1. Examples of exposure data are air monitoring data and biomarkers of exposure.
2. Data can be obtained from exposure registries such as those maintained for heavy metal exposure, certain pharmaceutics, and needlestick injuries.
3. Exposure status is sometimes estimated indirectly from information such as occupational history, dietary history, or location of residence.

VI Comparisons of Rates

A *Relative risk* (also known as *rate ratio*) is a measure of the relationship between two incidence rates, that of the exposed and that of the unexposed population.

B An *odds ratio* is a good estimate of relative risk, but is derived from case control or cross-sectional studies.

C *Attributable risk* is a measure of the difference between two rates, one for the exposed and one for the unexposed populations. It describes the increased amount of risk attributed to the exposure.

VII Types of Rates

Box 5-1 presents examples of the following rates.

A *Crude rates* are based on the actual number of events for a given time period but do not reflect true differences in risk among subgroups in the population.

B *Characteristic-specific rates* allow one to compare rates for similar subgroups of two or more populations (e.g., age-specific or gender-specific rates).

BOX 5-1

Using crude, specific, and adjusted rates to describe a health problem—an example

- *Crude Rates:* The crude rates of lung cancer in a population will not reflect the fact that older individuals are at higher risk for lung cancer. To look at the association between smoking and lung cancer, it would not be appropriate to compare crude rates of lung cancer in groups of smokers and non-smokers who differ in age distribution.

- *Specific Rates:* Rates of lung cancer could be computed for age-specific groups, perhaps by decade of age, to examine differences in lung cancer rates by age.
- *Adjusted Rates:* The age-adjusted rates of lung cancer in the smoking and nonsmoking groups could be compared to examine the question of an association between smoking and cancer.

C *Adjusted* (or *standardized*) *rates* reflect population differences by taking into consideration the distribution of important characteristics that may affect risk (e.g., age-adjusted rates).

VIII Inferential Statistics

Inferential statistics, which are taken from a sample of a population, are used to make inferences about the entire target population (Eisen & Wegman, 2000)

A A *hypothesis* is a supposition, resulting from observation or reflection.
1. A hypothesis leads to predictions that can be tested.
2. Hypothesis testing involves conducting a test of statistical significance and quantifying the degree to which sampling variability may account for the observed results.

B Some well-known tests of statistical significance include the t-test and chi-square test.

C A *p-value* is a quantitative statement of the probability that the observed difference (or association) in a particular study could have happened by chance alone.
1. $p < 0.05$ means that the probability that the observed difference occurred by chance is less than 5%.
2. $p < 0.05$ is a frequently used level for referring to an association as statistically significant.

D A *confidence interval* describes the magnitude of the effect and the inherent variability in an estimated statistic.
1. A confidence interval indicates the stability of the true rate or other statistic that describes a population.
2. A 95% confidence level means that there is a 95% probability that the true rate of an observation lies within the calculated interval.

E The *power* of a study is its likelihood of detecting a real association if one exists; power is affected by the following four variables:
1. The magnitude of the effect (or association) or difference
2. The variability of the measures of interest
3. The level of statistic significance selected (alpha)
4. The size of the sample studied
   a. Larger sample sizes increase the stability of measurements made in an epidemiologic study.
   b. Power calculations based on the above variables suggest the appropriate sample size needed for an epidemiologic study.

IX Overview of Study Designs

Chapter 17, Section V.G, presents additional information.

A *Experimental designs* are preferred for determining causality about study designs.
1. In an experimental study, the investigator assigns the exposure (or putative cause) to the study subjects.
2. *Randomized clinical trials* and *intervention studies* are examples of experimental designs.
3. Experiments are limited by ethical constraints; that is, purposeful exposures of study subjects are not always appropriate

B *Nonexperimental designs* that attempt to simulate the results of an experiment (had one been possible) are primarily *descriptive studies* or *analytic* (ex post facto) *studies.*

1. *Descriptive studies* generate hypotheses and therefore are not intended to determine causality.

   a. A *cross-sectional study* examines the relationship between diseases (or other health-related characteristics) and other variables of interest as they exist in a defined population at one point in time.

   b. An *ecologic study* looks at the group rather than the individual as the unit of analysis, usually because information is not available at the individual level.

2. *Analytic studies:* the investigator systematically determines whether risk of or a health-related condition is different for exposed and nonexposed individuals.

   a. A *cohort study* (also called a *prospective study* or *longitudinal study*) is an analytic study in which persons who are initially free of the disease (or outcome) but vary in one or more factors (such as exposure or potentially protective factors) are followed over a period of time for the occurrence of the disease (or outcome).

   b. In a *case-control study,* a group of persons with a disease (cases) are compared with a group without the disease (controls) to study the characteristics (such as exposure) that might predict, cause, or protect against the disease.

3. Table 5-1 lists advantages and disadvantages of cohort, case-control, and cross-sectional study designs.

X Bias and Confounding in Epidemiologic Studies

Identification of associations that are not real is usually the result of biased study methods or the presence of confounding variables (Greenland & Rothman, 1998).

TABLE 5-1

Advantages and disadvantages of various designs of nonexperimental epidemiologic studies

Study design	Advantages	Disadvantages
Cohort or prospective	Good for study of rare exposures Allows classification of exposure before disease develops Can determine incidence of disease Can determine true relative risk Can follow multiple outcomes	Lengthy Large sample size required Generally expensive Potential for subject loss to follow-up
Case-control	Good for study of rare outcomes Can estimate relative risk by odds ratio Takes less time Less expensive Requires smaller sample size Can look at multiple risk factors	Exposure histories may be difficult to construct Recall bias can be a problem Must select appropriate control group
Cross-sectional	Generates hypotheses Useful in study of exposures that do not change (e.g., blood type)	Cannot determine causality Current exposure does not represent relevant past exposure

Source: Rothman & Greenland, 1998b.

A *Bias* refers to systematic error in an epidemiologic study that results in an incorrect estimate of the association between exposure and risk of disease.

1. Selection bias
   a. This type of bias occurs when the identification of subjects for inclusion in the study, on the basis of either exposure (cohort study) or disease (case control study) status, depends in some way on the other axis of interest.
   b. Selection bias can result from differential surveillance, diagnosis, referral, or rates of participation of individuals in the study.
2. Information (or observation) bias
   a. This type of bias results from systematic differences in the way data on exposure or outcomes are obtained from various study groups.
   b. Examples of information bias are recall bias, interviewer bias, loss of subjects to follow-up over time, and misclassification (Table 5-2).
3. Study results may be biased either toward or away from the null hypothesis—or in both directions.

B *Confounding* results when the estimate of the effect of the exposure of interest is distorted because it is mixed with the effect of an extraneous factor; in occupational epidemiology studies, age, gender, and smoking status are often important confounding variables.

C Methods to avoid and manage study biases and confounding include the following:

1. A strict study protocol with attention to how subjects are selected for study is a means of avoiding study bias in the design phase of the study.
2. Systematic, standardized data collection techniques that are consistent for all study participants will help avoid bias in the data collection phase.
3. Confounding can be avoided by making comparisons only among individuals with the same level of the confounding variable; this is also known as *controlling for the effect of the confounding variable.*

TABLE 5-2

Types of bias in epidemiologic studies

Type of bias	Description
Information	Exposure and outcome data are ascertained differently from study groups.
Recall	Individuals with negative outcomes are more likely to remember and report exposure.
Interviewer	Interviewers' prior knowledge of outcome status affects ascertainment of exposure information in interview.
Lost to follow-up	Prospectively, those with negative outcomes may be lost to follow-up at greater rate than controls.
Misclassification	Ascertainment of either exposure or outcome status is incorrect for some subjects.
Selection	Entry into study or control group is affected by factors related to exposure (case-control) or outcome (cohort).
Self-selection	Individuals' participation is affected by their knowledge of disease or exposure status.

  a. In the design phase, matching subjects is a way to control for confounding.
  b. In an experimental study, confounding is avoided by randomization of treatment between cases and controls.
  c. In the analysis phase, confounding can sometimes be handled by stratifying or adjusting.
  d. Subjects who are lost to follow-up should be evaluated to assess whether they differ in important characteristics from those who have remained in the study.

XI Screening

Screening is the practice of testing people who are as yet asymptomatic; its purpose is to classify them with respect to their likelihood of having a disease.

A **An implicit assumption of screening is that early detection will help prevent death or disability. Criteria for screening include the following:**
  1. A recognizable presymptomatic stage of disease must exist.
  2. An effective treatment must be available.
  3. The screening test should have sufficient validity.

B **A sufficiently valid screening test is one that is highly sensitive and specific.**
  1. *Sensitivity* is the ability of a test to identify correctly those who have the disease; a sensitive test yields few false negatives. Sensitivity is an especially important trait for initial screening tests, so that most of the population who truly have the disease or condition will be included in follow-up measures.
  2. *Specificity* is the ability of a test to identify correctly those who do not have the disease; a specific test yields few false positives.
  3. Sensitivity and specificity do not change when the prevalence of the disease in the population changes.

C **The *predictive value* of screening tests is the ability to predict disease status from test results.**
  1. *Positive predictive value* is the likelihood that an individual with a positive test truly has the disease.
  2. *Negative predictive value* is the likelihood that an individual with a negative test does not have the disease.
  3. Levels of predictive value change when the prevalence of a disease in a population changes.
    a. As the prevalence of a disease in a population increases, the positive predictive value of the test will increase.
    b. However, as the prevalence increases, the negative predictive value will decrease.

D **Screening can be done for disorders related to work-site exposures or to nonoccupational causes.**
  1. OSHA standards require periodic screening of some workers (Papp and Miller, 2000).
    a. Examples are workers exposed to asbestos, cadmium, or cotton dust.
    b. This type of screening is generally called *medical surveillance* in OSHA standards.
  2. Screening for early detection is done for diseases such as breast cancer, prostate cancer, and colon cancer.

Toxicology

XII Overview of Toxicologic Terms and Principles

Toxicology is the study of the adverse effects of chemicals on biologic systems (Frumkin & Melius, 2000).

A A *target organ* is the organ that is selectively affected by a harmful agent.

B A chemical is toxic—that is, it can cause harm—if all of the following five conditions are met:
1. Its properties make it capable of producing harm
2. It is present in sufficient amount
3. It is present for sufficient time
4. It is delivered by an exposure route that allows it to be absorbed
5. It reaches the target body organ(s)

C *Toxic agents* can be classified by their form of action on biologic systems.
1. *Asphyxiants* deprive the body tissue of oxygen.
   a. Simple asphyxiants displace oxygen and cause suffocation; examples are carbon dioxide, nitrogen, and argon.
   b. Chemical asphyxiants prevent oxygen use by the cell, even when enough oxygen may be present; examples are carbon monoxide and cyanide.
2. *Corrosives* cause irreversible tissue death; ozone and acids are examples of corrosives.
3. *Irritants* cause temporary, but sometimes severe, inflammation of the eyes, skin, or respiratory tract; an example is ammonia.
4. *Sensitizers* cause allergic reactions after repeated exposure; examples are nickel and toluene diisocyanate (TDI).
5. *Carcinogens* are capable of causing cancer; examples are asbestos, coal tar, and vinyl chloride monomer.
6. *Mutagens* are toxins that cause changes to the genetic material of cells that can be passed on to future generations; known human mutagens include ethylene oxide and ionizing radiation.
7. *Teratogens* cause malformations in an unborn child; some teratogenic agents are organic mercury compounds, ionizing radiation, and some pharmaceutics.
8. Toxins may have more than one form of action and may act at more than one site. For example, formaldehyde is irritating to the eyes and respiratory tract, can irritate and sensitize the skin, and is suspected of being a carcinogen.

D Assessing the characteristics of exposure considers the following:
1. The *dose* of an agent is the amount that reaches the target organ.
   a. The dose is usually impossible to determine accurately.
   b. The dose is usually estimated by measuring the amount administered (as with drugs) or the amount in the environment to which a person has been exposed (as with work-related exposures or levels in media such as air, water, or food).
   c. Another means of estimating dose is by measuring biomarkers in body tissues as indicators of levels of the agent within the body or early physiologic changes due to exposure.
   d. Vapors or gases in the environment are usually expressed as parts per million (ppm).
   e. Solids (dusts or fumes) are expressed according to their weight per volume of air, usually as milligrams per cubic meter (mg/m^3).

f. Higher concentrations of substances are generally absorbed in greater amounts.

g. Longer or more-frequent periods of exposure also lead to greater absorbed doses.

2. Acute and chronic exposures

a. *Acute exposure* occurs when exposure is short-term and absorption is fairly rapid.

b. *Chronic exposure* refers to longer duration or repeated periods of contact.

c. In general, acute toxic exposures tend to be at higher levels, and chronic exposures occur at lower concentrations.

3. *Guidelines and standards* that serve to evaluate the seriousness of an exposure.

a. Examples of workplace guidelines are *threshold limit values;* examples of workplace standards are *permissible exposure limits* (described in detail in Section XXII).

b. Guidelines and standards indicate upper limits of exposure concentrations that are not felt to pose a danger to workers who are exposed over normal work hours.

c. Published limits cannot be viewed as definitely "safe" levels.

d. Guidelines and standards may be controversial because of a lack of scientific data, lack of agreement over the levels associated with health effects, and the reality that levels that protect most individuals may yet affect susceptible subgroups.

XIII Major Exposure Routes

There are three major routes of exposure (Lippmann, 2000).

A *Inhalation:* **This is the most important route of exposure in the occupational environment, because it is the most common route by which occupational exposures are absorbed.**

1. Most absorption takes place in the alveoli, where blood flow is high and close to the inhaled air; to reach the alveoli, the substance is generally a gas or a particulate ranging in size from approximately 1 to 10 microns in diameter.

2. Absorption by inhalation is influenced by the rate and depth of respirations; thus individuals performing heavy physical labor may absorb substances at a higher rate.

3. Although the lung may serve as the target organ of some inhaled toxins, other substances gain entry through the lungs but exert their effect elsewhere in the body; examples are solvents and carbon monoxide, which have systemic effects.

B *Cutaneous:* **The skin does provide a barrier to most substances, but its effectiveness as a barrier varies according to its condition, site, and the properties of the chemical agent.**

1. Some substances cross the epidermal layer or enter through hair follicles.

2. Some substances may enter by the trauma of injection or impalement; this mode of entry is less common.

3. In general, gases penetrate most freely, liquids less freely, and solids that are insoluble in water or fats do not penetrate the skin.

4. Longer contact promotes higher levels of absorption.

5. Damage to the epidermal cells by chemicals or trauma, such as abrasions, can promote its further absorption.

6. Clothing or gloves can trap substances and lead to longer exposure periods.

C *Ingestion:* **In the occupational setting, ingestion is the least common route of entry. However, ingestion increases in importance in the case of other types of environmental exposures, such as food, water, and substances encountered through hand-mouth activity.**

1. Caustic or irritant chemicals, if ingested, can have a direct adverse effect on the gastrointestinal tract.

2. Some toxins act systemically following their absorption.

3. Smoking or eating at work sites can lead to consumption of toxins by way of contaminated hands, food, or smoking materials.

XIV The Dose-Response Relationship

This describes the relationship between the level of exposure (dose) and the resulting toxic effects (response) in a susceptible population of humans or experimental animals (Lippmann, 2000).

A **Higher doses are generally associated with responses in a greater proportion of individuals.**

B **Identification of a dose-response relationship lends support to a theory that a substance causes a given effect.**

C **Dose-response curves provide a basis for evaluating a chemical's relative toxicity.**

1. Terms that describe toxicity of a substance are *lethal dose, 50%* (LD_{50}) and *lethal concentration, 50%* (LC_{50}).

2. These terms refer to the dose (LD_{50}) or concentration (LC_{50}) that produces death in 50% of a group of experimental animals.

3. These indices are smaller for more-toxic agents. For example, the LD_{50} of acetone is 5,340 mg/kg, whereas hydrogen cyanide, a much more toxic compound, has an LD_{50} of 0.5 mg/kg

4. Animal studies are useful because they provide information about potential toxic effects or target organs in humans; however, they must be interpreted cautiously because of the many differences in response that exist among species.

XV Nature of Effects

A **The effects of toxins with long latency periods may not be apparent until years after the exposure period.**

B **Work-related exposures commonly consist of chemical mixtures (McCauley, 1998); this is a concern because interactive effects may occur with two or more concurrent exposures.**

1. *Synergistic effects* are effects caused by exposure to more than one toxin that surpass the sum of the separate effects of those toxins.

2. *Antagonism* between toxins results in an overall effect that is less than the sum of their separate effects.

3. *Potentiation* means that a chemical has no adverse effect on its own, but its presence increases the effect of another substance or makes that substance capable of exerting an effect. Potentiation is often seen with carcinogens.

XVI The Fate of Toxins in the Body

Once toxins are absorbed, their fate in the body varies (Frumkin & Melius, 2000):

A **Excretion involves the elimination of the material from the body (Arble, 2004).**

1. Some chemicals are excreted unchanged into expired air, urine, feces, bile, or perspiration.
2. Other avenues of excretion include milk, spinal fluid, saliva, and hair.
3. Most chemicals and their metabolic products are excreted through the kidney/urine pathway.

B **Transformation is a process that results in a substance being changed in some way.**

1. Chemicals may be transformed into substances that can be excreted by a process called *biotransformation*.
2. Products of biotransformation may be either less toxic or more toxic than their parent chemical.
3. This is an important concept when individuals differ in the rate at which they metabolize substances, because this rate can affect individual susceptibility to a toxin.

C **Several factors affect the excretion of substances.**

1. Many agents are not metabolized or excreted immediately, but instead are deposited in body tissue and slowly released and excreted over time.
2. *Half-life* is the term that describes the time it takes for one half of the total absorbed amount to be eliminated from the body.
3. The length of the half-life depends on the agent and the tissue in which it is stored; for example, the half-life of lead is more than 20 years in bone, compared with about 25 to 30 days in blood.

XVII Endogenous and Exogenous Host Factors

These factors can influence susceptibility and the magnitude of the toxic response.

A *Endogenous* **factors are inherent to the individual and are beyond the control of that individual.**

1. *Gender* may influence susceptibility to some toxins, although the cause of this difference is not well understood in all cases.
   a. Some cancers and other diseases are associated with gender.
   b. Women have a greater proportion of body fat and therefore may accumulate more lipid-soluble toxins than men.
   c. Other differences in metabolism, anthropometry, and genetic types may account for varying susceptibility to toxins.
2. *Genetic differences* may cause variation in metabolism, detoxification, excretion, and cellular response to toxins.
3. *Aging* is related to rate and efficiency of metabolism, levels of organ function, and patterns of excretion.
   a. Age-related factors may increase toxic responses among older adults.
   b. Similarly, children may experience increased susceptibility because of their higher respiratory and metabolic rates, less mature nervous systems, and immature livers, which lack the detoxification mechanisms of adults.
   c. Children are also more susceptible than adults to some cancers because they are growing and their cells are dividing more rapidly.

d. Pregnant mothers may be exposed to work-site agents that have the potential to cause perinatal malignancies or developmental disorders.

4. *Health conditions* can increase individual susceptibility to toxins; for example, heart disease can influence effects of exposure to asphyxiants that affect oxygen availability or utilization.

B **Individuals may be able to exert some control over *exogenous* factors, because those factors are related to behavior or environmental conditions.**

1. *Nutrition* factors, such as deficiencies, can enhance or inhibit absorption or toxic responses.

2. *Obesity* may promote more storage of lipid-soluble substances.

3. *Lifestyle* factors such as smoking or alcohol consumption increase overall chemical exposures that must be handled by the body and may increase susceptibility due to debilitation.

4. *Stress* can have an effect on the function of some organs, such as those of the cardiovascular, immune, and gastrointestinal systems.

5. Some adverse health conditions are temporary and manageable but may affect an individual's vulnerability to toxins.

NOTE: Table 5-3 presents some major effects seen in various body systems and gives examples of work-site exposures that cause them.

XVIII Examples of Exposures and Their Effects

Exposures may be classified in many ways, such as by their chemical properties (e.g., metals) or by their action (e.g., asphyxiants). This section presents some of the major groups of work-site toxins with information about selected examples (Sullivan and Kreiger, 2001).

A **Metals are elementary substances that have specific properties, including opacity, conductivity, and ductility.**

1. Arsenic, in the inorganic form, is found in operations such as mining, smelting, and electronics manufacturing and in products such as pesticides, paints, and wood preservatives.

a. It is important to distinguish inorganic arsenic, which is toxic, from organic arsenic, which is not toxic but is found in foods such as seafood; dietary seafood can lead to high total arsenic levels in urine without any threat to health.

b. Acute arsenic exposure leads to gastrointestinal symptoms, abdominal pain, and sometimes a garlic odor on the breath. This may progress to renal failure, shock, encephalopathy, and death.

c. Chronic arsenic toxicity can lead to hyperpigmentation of the skin, hyperkeratosis, dermatitis, and skin cancer. A sign of arsenic exposure is the presence of Mee's lines, which are transverse white lines on the fingernails.

d. Multiple systems can be affected by arsenic.

1) Arsenic can cause a sensorimotor polyneuropathy, often noted in the hands and feet.

2) Vascular effects can simulate Raynaud's syndrome or lead to gangrene of the extremities.

3) Liver effects include cirrhosis and angiosarcoma.

4) Respiratory effects include lung cancer.

5) Anemia or leukopenia may result from bone marrow suppression.

e. The treatment for arsenic toxicity is chelation.

TABLE 5-3

Potential toxic effects by system, with examples of toxins

System	Effects	Sources of exposure
Respiratory	Irritation	Hydrogen chloride, ammonia
	Sensitization	Isocyanates
	Fibrosis	Silica, asbestos, beryllium
	Carcinogens	Asbestos, arsenic, chromium VI
Dermatologic	Irritation	Acetone, carbon disulfide
	Corrosive burns	Alkali, hydrogen fluoride
	Sensitization	Chromate, nickel
	Carcinogenesis	Ultraviolet light, arsenic
Nervous system	Depression/altered consciousness	Carbon monoxide, solvents Lead, mercury, manganese
	Behavior and mood disturbance	Lead, solvents Toluene, mercury
	Cognitive disturbance	Carbon monoxide, manganese, pesticides
	Cerebellar impairment	
	Parkinson-like effects	
	Peripheral neuropathy	Acrylamide, *n*-hexane, methyl *n*-butyl ketone
Hearing and vision	Acid burns of eyes	Hydrochloric and tannic acid
	Alkali burns of eyes	Sodium hydroxide, calcium oxide
	Blindness	Methanol
	Deafness	Noise
Hematopoietic	Bone marrow suppression	Ionizing radiation, benzene
	Red cell lysis	Arsine, trinitrotoluene (TNT), naphthalene
Hepatic	Necrosis	Carbon tetrachloride, chloroform, tetrachloroethane
	Cirrhosis	Carbon tetrachloride
	Malignancy	Vinyl chloride monomer
Renal and Bladder	Nephrotoxicity	Heavy metals, carbon tetrachloride, chloroform
	Renal cancer	Coke oven emissions
	Bladder cancer	Benzidine, B-naphthylamine
Reproductive	Decreased sperm production	Ionizing radiation, heat
	Decreased female fertility	Ionizing radiation, carbon disulfide
	Spontaneous abortions	Ethylene oxide
	Congenital defects	Rubella, varicella

    f. The OSHA standard for inorganic arsenic requires medical surveillance for exposed workers.

2. Beryllium is currently found in metal alloys, tools, and instruments, particularly in the aerospace industry, but was once used in manufacturing fluorescent lights and nuclear weapons.

    a. Acute toxicity to beryllium is a result of hypersensitivity of the lungs or mucous membranes.

    b. Allergic and irritant contact dermatitis with skin ulceration may also occur.

    c. Chronic beryllium disease, berylliosis, is marked by granulomas of the skin, lungs, and other organs. Other signs are dyspnea, cough, anorexia, fatigue, weight loss, and arthralgias.

    d. For more information about beryllium exposure, see AAOHN's Foundation Blocks (http://www.aaohn.org/).

3. Cadmium is found in battery manufacturing, electroplating, welding, and zinc and lead smelting. Cadmium is also present in cigarettes.
    a. The primary route of cadmium exposure is inhalation.
    b. Acute cadmium exposure can lead to metal fume fever or pulmonary edema.
    c. Cadmium causes renal failure, resulting from proximal renal tubular damage.
    d. Cadmium also causes osteomalacia, emphysema, and possibly lung and prostate cancer.
    e. The OSHA standard for cadmium-exposed workers requires, among other tests, medical surveillance for blood and urinary cadmium levels and urinary $Beta_2$-microglobulin.

4. Chromium is found in metal alloys, tanning and dye operations, and chromium plating; welding can also be a source of exposure.
    a. The principal forms that cause toxicity are trivalent and hexavalent chromium.
    b. Chromium exposure occurs through inhalation and absorption through cracks in the skin.
    c. Skin and mucous membrane exposure can lead to deep, painful ulcers and perforation of the nasal septum.
    d. Chronic exposure can lead to asthma or allergic contact dermatitis.
    e. The hexavalent form of chromium can cause lung cancer.

5. Lead exposure can arise from a number of sources. Examples include the manufacture or use of lead solder, paint, alloys, and ceramics, smelting, demolition, and radiator repair operations. The more common form of lead encountered today is inorganic lead; the organoleads were formerly used as gasoline additives.
    a. Lead is a significant environmental toxicant found in residential paint and soil, and is used in hobbies such as stained glass work and soldering.
    b. Routes of exposure to lead are inhalation and ingestion.
    c. Most lead is stored in the bone, but the toxicity of lead is related to the amount that reaches target organs.
    d. Gastrointestinal effects of lead such as constipation and abdominal colic are sometimes mistaken for other problems like appendicitis.
    e. Lead causes central nervous system effects, such as memory deficits, and mood disturbances, such as irritability and depression.
    f. Lead toxicity results in peripheral neuropathy that primarily affects motor nerves.
    g. Lead exposure can result in renal failure, gout, and possibly hypertension.
    h. Reproductive effects of lead include sperm abnormalities and effects on the fetus that can lead to spontaneous abortion or developmental delays in childhood.
    i. The OSHA standard for lead-exposed workers specifies medical surveillance requirements and medical removal criteria.
    j. The treatment for lead toxicity, in addition to removal from exposure, consists of chelation.
    k. AAOHN has developed a Lead Surveillance Screening Program (2003) available at http://www.aaohn.org./

6. Mercury is found in many products and processes, including the manufacture and repair of medical instruments, pesticides, and the preparation of dental amalgams. Organic mercury accumulates in fish.
    a. The three forms of mercury differ by mode of exposure and effect. Exposure to elemental mercury, the form used in thermometers, occurs through inhalation; inorganic mercury compounds are absorbed through the gastrointestinal tract and lungs; organic mercury is ingested.
    b. The classic triad seen with elemental and inorganic mercury toxicity are tremor, gingivitis, and personality changes that include shyness, paranoia, and labile mood.
    c. Stomatitis and dermatitis may also be present.
    d. Mercury exposure can cause renal dysfunction.
    e. A distal peripheral neuropathy can also result from mercury exposure.
    f. Organic mercury toxicity has been associated with ingestion of fish contaminated with methyl mercury.
    g. Organic mercury toxicity in adults has been associated with neurobehavioral changes, ataxia, tremor, and constriction of the visual field and has caused severe central nervous system defects in unborn children.
    h. Chelation is sometimes used to treat elemental and inorganic mercury toxicity.
7. Manganese exposure occurs during work activities such as mining, production of alloys, and use of agrochemicals. In several countries, it is contained in the gasoline additive commonly known as MMT (methylcyclopentadienyl manganese tricarbonyl) and can be present in car emissions.
    a. Although manganese is an essential dietary element, it causes health effects with high levels of exposure.
    b. The primary route of exposure to manganese is inhalation, but contamination of soil, dust, and food leads to risk of ingestion.
    c. Manganese is a known neurotoxin, causing psychologic and neurobehavioral disturbances, as well as Parkinson-like signs and other movement disorders (Levy & Nassetta, 2003).
    d. Exposure *in utero* has recently been implicated in impaired psychomotor development during early childhood (Takser, et al., 2003).

B **Respirable dusts are solid particles that are capable of being suspended in the air and ultimately inhaled into the body.**
1. Asbestos has been used for pipe and furnace insulation, tiles, automobile and train brakes, and other heat-resistant products; health risks occur when asbestos fibers become airborne.
    a. Different types of asbestos are associated with differently shaped fibers; the most common type in the United States is chrysotile.
    b. Pleural effusions and pleural plaques are seen with chronic asbestos exposure.
    c. Asbestosis is characterized by interstitial fibrosis.
    d. Mesothelioma occurs only with asbestos exposure and can affect the pleura or peritoneum; the latency period is 30 to 40 years.
    e. Bronchogenic carcinoma also can be caused by asbestos; the risk is much greater if a person exposed to asbestos also smokes.
    f. Asbestosis is possibly associated with cancers of the gastrointestinal tract.
    g. There is an OSHA standard that requires medical surveillance for asbestos-exposed workers.

2. Coal-dust exposure occurs primarily in coal mining.
   a. Coal-dust exposure causes coal workers' pneumoconiosis, also known as *black lung*.
   b. Changes are first noted on chest radiographs, starting in the upper lobes and resulting in progressive massive fibrosis.
   c. Coal-dust exposure is also associated with bronchitis and emphysema (chronic obstructive pulmonary disease).
   d. Coal dust may be associated with gastric cancers.
   e. Medical surveillance for underground coal miners consists of chest radiography and spirometry evaluations, administered as part of the Coal Worker's X-Ray Surveillance Program.
3. Silica exposure occurs in sandblasting, manufacturing of glass and pottery, mining of stone, and foundries.
   a. Acute, high-level exposure to silica leads to a severe alveolar consolidation process known as *acute silicoproteinosis or acute silicosis*.
   b. Silicosis is characterized by nodules in the upper lung lobes.
   c. Silicosis can be slowly progressive or can lead to progressive massive fibrosis.
   d. Silicosis puts an individual at increased risk for tuberculosis.
   e. Those with silicosis should be screened annually for tuberculosis.

C **Solvents are capable of dissolving other substances.**
1. Solvents are a diverse category of chemicals, defined by their ability to dissolve other substances; some are chemical reactants.
2. Many solvents are lipid soluble and can cross cell membranes easily.
3. Solvents generally have short half-lives in the body; they are metabolized in the liver and excreted through exhalation or in the urine.
4. Acute health effects of solvent exposure include central nervous system effects such as dizziness, confusion, convulsions, coma, and death.
5. Aspiration of solvents can sometimes lead to chemical pneumonitis, which can be fatal; this is the main risk when petroleum distillates are ingested.
6. Chronic health effects associated with solvents can include neurobehavioral dysfunction, peripheral neuropathy, liver disease, renal disease, dermatitis, and reproductive disorders.
7. Benzene is an aromatic hydrocarbon found in the petrochemical industry and as a component of gasoline.
   a. Chronic exposure to benzene can cause acute myeloblastic leukemia, aplastic anemia, and cytopenia.
   b. The OSHA standard for benzene-exposed workers includes requirements for periodic complete blood counts with criteria for follow-up and referral.
8. Carbon disulfide is sometimes used as a grain fumigant; exposure also occurs in the manufacture of rayon and rubber.
   a. Skin or eye contact with carbon disulfide can cause severe chemical burns.
   b. Chronic exposure to carbon disulfide can lead to nervous system effects of peripheral neuropathy, Parkinson-like effects, cranial neuropathies, and optic neuritis.
   c. Vascular effects of carbon disulfide include accelerated atherosclerosis with hypertension, elevated cholesterol, and changes in retinal blood vessels.
   d. Carbon disulfide is a reproductive toxin that causes decreased and abnormal sperm and increased risk of spontaneous abortions.

9. Ethylene oxide is used as a sterilant in hospitals; other exposures occur in industry.
   a. Acute toxic effects of ethylene oxide exposure include irritation of the eyes and respiratory tract and burns.
   b. Chronic exposure leads to neurotoxic and reproductive effects and possibly to chromosomal changes and leukemia.
   c. The OSHA standard for ethylene oxide includes medical surveillance requirements.
   d. Exposure-prevention efforts have included improvements in sterilization equipment and ventilation.

10. Formaldehyde exposure occurs in laboratories, during use of formaldehyde resins in particle board and other building materials, and in paper, rubber, and dye manufacturing.
    a. Acute exposure to formaldehyde leads to irritation of the upper and lower respiratory tract.
    b. Chronic formaldehyde exposure is linked to asthma and allergic dermatitis.
    c. Formaldehyde causes nasal cancer in animal models and is a possible human carcinogen.
    d. The OSHA standard for formaldehyde has medical evaluation requirements that include periodic administration of a questionnaire.

11. n-Hexane is used in thinners, glues, and the manufacture of rubber.
    a. n-Hexane causes a sensorimotor polyneuropathy.
    b. The toxic metabolite of n-hexane is 2,5-hexanedione.
    c. The distal portions of long nerves, such as those of the extremities, are most susceptible.
    d. The pattern of sensory loss is that of stocking-glove (feet/ankles and hands/wrists), and motor function is also impaired.
    e. After exposure ceases, the neuropathy often continues to worsen before improving; residual signs and symptoms may persist.

12. Methylene chloride is used as a degreaser and is the active agent in furniture strippers.
    a. Acute exposure to methylene chloride leads to central nervous system depression.
    b. Methylene chloride is metabolized to carbon monoxide; toxic effects are associated with this asphyxiant.
    c. The OSHA standard for methylene chloride requires medical surveillance.

13. Toluene has been used as a substitute for benzene and is used in many household products, including inks, aerosol paints, and dyes.
    a. Toluene is an irritant of the respiratory tract, causes central nervous system depression, and is toxic to the fetus.
    b. Toluene products, such as spray paint, are favored by solvent abusers. Long-term, high doses of toluene, such as those experienced by chronic abusers, are associated with severe neurobehavioral dysfunction, and cerebellar signs such as ataxia and poor coordination; abusers also commonly die from cardiac arrythmias.
    c. A major metabolite of toluene is hippuric acid; medical surveillance is based on urinary hippuric acid levels.

14. Trichloroethylene is commonly used in degreasing operations.
    a. High exposure levels cause liver and kidney toxicity.

   b. The metabolite dichloracetylene causes trigeminal neuropathy with facial numbness and masseter muscle weakness.

   c. Trichloroethylene may also cause optic neuropathy and may be linked to ventricular arrhythmias.

   d. Symptoms are worse in the presence of ethanol; the combination of ethanol and trichloroethylene may cause what is known as the *degreaser's flush*.

D **Pesticides are designed to destroy pests such as insects, nematodes, and rodents and have the potential to cause harmful effects in humans.**

   1. Pesticides are a potential toxin for agricultural workers, home pesticide users, and workers who manufacture these agents.

   2. Organophosphates are one class of pesticide; it includes parathion and malathion.

      a. These pesticides inhibit acetylcholinesterase, allowing the accumulation of acetylcholine at synapses.

      b. Parasympathetic responses include <u>d</u>iarrhea, <u>u</u>rination, <u>m</u>iosis, <u>b</u>ronchospasm, <u>e</u>mesis, <u>l</u>acrimation, and <u>s</u>alivation ("DUMBELS") and bradycardia.

      c. Nicotinic responses include weakness, paralysis, muscle twitching, and tachycardia; central nervous system effects range from excitation to depression to seizures.

      d. Death is caused by respiratory failure.

      e. Treatment for organophosphate toxicity is atropine and 2-PAM (pralidoxime).

      f. Medical surveillance includes plasma and red blood cell cholinesterase levels.

   3. Carbamates are a class of pesticide that includes aldicarb and carbaryl.

      a. Their action is similar to that of organophosphates, but symptoms are less severe and of shorter duration.

      b. The treatment is atropine, but not 2-PAM.

   4. Organochlorines include the well-known examples of chlordane and DDT (dichlorodiphenyl-trichloroethane).

      a. Organochlorines are very persistent in the environment.

      b. In humans, these pesticide are stored in fat; consequently, they have a long half-life in the body.

      c. Because of their toxicity and persistence, carbamates are not commonly used at this time.

      d. Acute toxic effects are related to the nervous system and include weakness, paresthesias, mental status changes, and seizures.

      e. Chronic toxic effects include liver, kidney, and possibly carcinogenic outcomes.

E **Asphyxiants are substances that deprive the tissues of oxygen.**

   1. Asphyxiants are inhaled and result in hypoxia or anoxia; angina and adverse effects to a fetus are other potential consequences.

   2. Simple asphyxiants displace oxygen in the atmosphere; oxygen is then unavailable to the body.

      a. Examples are carbon dioxide, argon, methane, and nitrogen.

      b. Treatment for exposure to simple asphyxiants is oxygen.

   3. Chemical asphyxiants interfere with the body's ability to transport or use oxygen.

4. Carbon monoxide (CO) is an example of a chemical asphyxiant; sources are incomplete combustion and methylene chloride metabolism.
   a. CO binds to hemoglobin; the affinity of hemoglobin for CO is much greater than it is for oxygen.
   b. The transport of oxygen is therefore inhibited.
   c. Long-term central and peripheral nervous system effects can result from acute exposure to CO.
   d. The treatment is oxygen, sometimes under hyperbaric conditions.
5. Hydrogen cyanide is another example of a chemical asphyxiant.
   a. Sources of hydrogen cyanide exposure are pesticides, gold and silver purification, combustion of some synthetic materials, and chemical processes.
   b. Hydrogen cyanide is characterized by an odor of almonds that many people cannot detect.
   c. Hydrogen cyanide inhibits cellular enzymes, preventing the use of oxygen for energy production.
   d. Treatment includes the administration of oxygen and the use of cyanide kits that include nitrites and thiosulfate; these help to bind and detoxify cyanide.

Industrial hygiene

XIX Overview of Industrial Hygiene

Industrial hygiene refers to the anticipation, recognition, evaluation, and control of environmental factors or stresses arising in or from the workplace, which can cause injury, sickness, impaired health and well-being, or significant discomfort among workers or among citizens (Smith & Schneider, 2000).

A The field of industrial hygiene draws on knowledge from many scientific disciplines, including engineering, physics, chemistry, and biology.

B Professional organizations for industrial hygienists include the American Industrial Hygiene Association and the American Conference of Governmental Industrial Hygienists (Appendix I).

XX Sources of Information to Facilitate Hazard Recognition

A *Qualitative assessment* of the work site requires the following:
   1. Communication with key personnel, such as plant management representatives and supervisors, to learn about materials and processes
   2. Communication with other occupational and environmental health professionals to learn about health problems that may be related to exposure
   3. Communication with workers and their representatives to learn about their perceptions of exposure

B *Observational assessments,* are achieved through strategies such as walk-through surveys, focused inspections, and job-hazard analyses. (Chapter 10 describes these and other strategies in detail.)

C Material safety data sheets (MSDSs) provide the following information (US Department of Labor [USDL], OSHA, 1998):
   1. Identification of the material
   2. Hazardous chemicals and their common names

3. Physical and chemical properties
4. Routes of exposure
5. Acute and chronic health effects
6. First aid information
7. Exposure limits
8. Precautions for safe handling and use
9. Control measures
10. Organization responsible for preparing MSDSs and contact information

D **Some caveats are in order when using information provided in MSDSs (Beach, 2002).**

1. The quality of MSDSs is variable; the information is sometimes outdated and unclear, and may be inconsistent with the same materials from different manufacturers.
2. Recommended protective measures need to be considered in the context of the specific material's actual use and the control measures in effect.
3. An MSDS for a mixture may not include all chemical components, particularly if their concentration is low or if they are not recognized as hazardous.

XXI Sampling Methods

Approaches for estimating the dose of an exposure received by workers include personal and environmental *sampling* and biologic and medical *monitoring* (Lippmann, 2000). Chapter 10 provides additional details regarding sampling and monitoring methods.

A **Some sampling techniques measure exposure before absorption has occurred.**

1. Approaches to workplace sampling depend on the type of agent and the route by which it is absorbed by workers (Smith & Schneider, 2000).
   a. *Skin wipes* and *cloth patches* measure amounts of materials that have come in contact with the skin.
   b. *Noise dosimeters,* worn near the worker's ear, record work-site noise levels.
   c. *Airborne contaminants* can be assessed by means of personal monitoring at the worker's breathing zone or environmental monitoring in the work area.
2. Several important factors govern whether the sampling results truly represent worker exposure (Gross and Morse, 1996).
   a. The location of the sampling device with regard to the worker and source of contaminant should be based on worker location and movements.
   b. The workers to be sampled usually are those who are most highly exposed.
   c. Timing of sampling should take into account seasonal changes, shifts, unintentional releases, and other sources of variation.
   d. Length of sampling time generally represents a full shift.
   e. The number of samples depends on the type of instrumentation, concentration of the contaminant, and purpose of sampling.

B **Biologic and medical monitoring identify the presence of a chemical in the body following exposure.**

C **Exposure records are extremely important and must be maintained for at least 30 years.**

XXII Airborne Contaminants

Levels of airborne contaminants can be compared with the following guidelines and standards.

A **Permissible exposure limits (PELs) are developed by OSHA.**
1. PELs are promulgated by OSHA and are legally enforceable.
2. PELs are 8-hour, time-weighted averages of airborne exposure.

B **Threshold limit value (TLV) guidelines are developed by the American Conference of Governmental Industrial Hygienists (ACGIH).**
1. TLVs are published annually by that organization (Appendix I).
2. TLVs are 8-hour, time-weighted averages, with the following exceptions:
   a. *Ceiling levels,* or uppermost TLV levels, cannot be exceeded.
   b. *Short-term exposure levels* are the maximum, 15-minute, time-weighted averages permitted over a workday, with at least 60 minutes between successive exposures.

C **Recommended exposure levels (REL) are developed by the National Institute for Occupational Safety and Health (NIOSH); these levels are the exposures that, in the judgment of NIOSH, will not cause adverse health effects in most workers.**

XXIII Control Strategies for Occupational Exposures

Approaches to eliminating or reducing exposure to hazardous substances at the work site are ordered into a *hierarchy* based, in general, on their degree of overall effectiveness.

A *Engineering controls* **are the preferred way to reduce or eliminate exposures and include measures designed to enclose or isolate operations, improve ventilation, or removal or substitution of toxic materials.**

B *Administrative controls* **also minimize exposure and include monitoring or surveillance programs, worker rotation, and training to address work practices.**

C *Personal protective equipment* **such as ear plugs and muffs, safety goggles, gloves, coveralls, and respirators, are considered the least-preferred control strategy.**

Ergonomics

This section provides a general overview of ergonomics. A sample ergonomics program and more details about ergonomics and work-related musculoskeletal disorders are presented in Chapter 16.

XXIV Overview of Ergonomic Terms and Principles

The term *ergonomics* (sometimes known as *human factors*) refers to the study of the interaction between humans and their work (Konz & Johnson, 2000).

A **The term literally means the *laws* (from the Greek word *nomos*) *of work* (*ergos*).**

B **The field of ergonomics is multidisciplinary, involving health professionals, engineers, behavioral scientists, physiologists, and others.**

C Its purpose is to prevent acute and chronic injuries, make work sites comfortable, enhance productivity, reduce fatigue and errors, and promote job satisfaction.

D Proper job design can make jobs appropriate for workers of both sexes and all ages; considerations are given to size, strength, visual capacity, hearing, capabilities, and limitations.

E Ergonomics seeks to fit the job to the person rather than the person to the job.

XXV Work-Related Musculoskeletal Disorders

A Several *musculoskeletal disorders* can be caused or aggravated by work-site factors (NRC, 2001).

1. Affected tissue structures include muscles, tendons, ligaments, peripheral nerves, blood vessels, joints, cartilage, and bones.
2. Problems occur in the upper and sometimes lower extremities, cervical spine, and lower back; symptoms of musculoskeletal disorders include pain, swelling, erythema, numbness, and paresthesia.

B The major work-site risk factors for work-related musculoskeletal disorders of the upper extremities are repetition, force, mechanic stresses, awkward postures, low temperatures, and vibration (NIOSH, 1997). The goal in task and tool design is to avoid or minimize these risk factors.

1. *Repetition* refers to the performance of the same or similar tasks again and again; for example, if one work cycle (a series of motions that is then repeated) lasts less than 30 seconds, or if, in the case of cycles lasting several minutes, there are subcycles that constitute more than 50% of the overall cycle, the job is generally considered repetitive
2. *Force* is exerted in tasks that require lifting weights, handling heavy tools, pinching with the fingers, or applying other grips while working.
3. The combination of repetition and force is particularly associated with carpal tunnel syndrome (NIOSH, 1997).
4. *Mechanical stress* refers to the forces that result from a worker's direct contact with work surfaces or tools.
5. The *compressive forces* that result from striking objects with hand-held tools or from leaning against hard surfaces or corners on work tables can lead to nerve compression disorders.

C Work frequently requires workers to assume awkward positions for prolonged periods or repetitive shorter periods; deviation from neutral posture has been identified as a risk factor for injury, as illustrated by the following (NIOSH, 1997):

1. Cervical spine injury—caused by extreme neck flexion and twisting
2. Back injury—caused by twisting at the waist; lifting with legs straight; bending and reaching repetitively; maintaining awkward postures for long periods; carrying, pulling, pushing, or lifting heavy objects from below the knees or above the shoulders; or lifting weight beyond one's capabilities
3. Shoulder injury—caused by raising the arm or elbow above midtorso without support, reaching behind one's body
4. Forearm/elbow injury—caused by repeated rotation (i.e., supination and pronation)

5. Wrist/hand injury—caused by repeated wrist flexion and extension, holding the hand in ulnar deviation

D *Vibration* **caused by power tools or other work equipment can adversely affect the upper extremities.**

E **Whole-body vibration, such as that experienced by drivers of trucks and heavy equipment, can affect the back, lower extremities, and possibly shoulder and neck.**

F *Cold environmental conditions* **have an effect on manual dexterity and muscle strength and may directly or indirectly cause hand disorders.**

XXVI High-Risk Jobs

Several types of jobs are considered particularly high risk in terms of ergonomic exposures:

A **Office work presents ergonomic hazards that are associated with equipment as well as with characteristics of the overall working environment.**
   1. Work with technology such as computers may require individuals to assume static or awkward positions for typing if workstations are not properly adjusted.
   2. Other conditions in the office environment that can introduce hazards include poor lighting, obstructions in walkways, slippery floors, and heavy objects.

B **Manual materials handling is a part of many jobs, from loading trucks and moving heavy goods to working in grocery stores.**
   1. In addition to repeated bending, lifting, and twisting, this work sometimes involves exposure to vibration.
   2. The risks of back injury are high for these types of jobs.

C **Assembly work is often machine-paced, giving the worker little control over the speed at which he or she works.**
   1. Repetitive motions tend to be characteristic of assembly work.
   2. Sometimes work is performed in static or awkward postures or with poorly designed tools.

XXVII Evaluating Risk Factors

Various methods can be used to evaluate work sites for ergonomic risk factors; each approach has its advantages and disadvantages.

A *Interviews or questionnaires* **ask workers directly about their work.**
   1. Advantages: Workers have the most complete view of their tasks throughout all work periods. This method may reveal factors that might not otherwise be noted.
   2. Disadvantages: There may be high variability in the way workers report their perception of work performance; reports may be incomplete or biased.

B *Observation and use of checklist* **involves observing workers while they work and noting any risk factors.**
   1. Advantages: Observers using the same methods will look at all workers in the same way and thus introduce less variability; this method is fairly efficient—that is, one observer evaluates many workers in their work setting.

2. Disadvantages: People may change the way they behave when they are under observation; the limited time period for observation may cause some risk factors to be missed; and observers must be trained to be accurate and consistent.

C *Videotaping and analysis* **is done by taping the worker on the job and later conducting a detailed analysis of motions and other risk factors.**
1. Advantages: Analysis is recorded and does not rely on one person's assessment; tape can be repeated, slowed, or frozen to evaluate details of work tasks; measurement of time and motion can be highly accurate.
2. Disadvantages: Videotaping requires expensive equipment and experienced personnel; behavior may change during taping; only a small window of worker's time is recorded, and therefore it is not useful for evaluating highly variable tasks.

XXVIII Ergonomic Improvements

Some considerations and guidelines for analyzing or designing jobs are as follows (National Research Council, 2001).

A General environment: Provide adequate illumination, comfortable levels of temperature and humidity; good visibility of labels and signs; and clear, audible auditory signals.

B Workstations and chairs: These should be adjustable to accommodate workers of different sizes.

C Layout: Place tools, controls, and materials in front of the worker to prevent twisting, reaching, and bending; keep work space free of obstacles.

D Postures: Avoid static postures; locate and orient work to promote neutral positions.

E Repetition: Engineer the product or process to reduce repetition; vary tasks; rotate workers to different jobs; allow rest time.

F Forces: Reduce the size and weight of objects held; use power grips rather than pinch grips; balance tools; provide correctly fitting gloves (not tight or bulky); sharpen tools often.

G Mechanical stresses: Ensure that handles on equipment fit the worker's hands; pad or eliminate sharp edges.

H Vibration: Eliminate vibrating tools if possible; isolate sources of vibration; keep tools and equipment properly maintained; maintain even floor surfaces to reduce vibration from driving; reduce driving speeds of vehicles such as forklifts.

I Lifting: Reduce size and weight of tools and objects that are lifted often; use mechanic lifting devices; use gravity to move work; raise the work (or lower the operator); provide grips and handles; reduce friction where objects are slid from one point to another; increase friction when objects are held; evaluate lifting tasks according to NIOSH lifting guidelines (NIOSH, 1994, http://www.cdc.gov/niosh/94-110.html)).

J Work organization: Staff adequately, alternate physically demanding and mentally demanding tasks vary the rate and nature of tasks as much as possible; provide breaks (more-frequent short breaks are generally better than less frequent long breaks).

Injury epidemiology

XXIX Occupational Injury Epidemiology

The study of the natural history of injuries helps to define the host, agent, vector, and environmental (psychosocial and physical) factors that contribute to injury.

A Characteristics of occupational injury are as follows:

1. Occupational injuries are not random events.
2. Injuries are predictable and preventable.
3. Injuries result when energy is exchanged in a manner and dose sufficient to overcome the host's threshold of resistance in the presence or absence of certain environmental conditions (Table 5-4).

B The following are examples of sources of injuries:

1. *Mechanic or kinetic energy*—Impact of an object, dashboard, floor, knife, noise, extreme air pressure (explosion)
2. *Thermal energy*—Steam, flame, hot substances, and lasers
3. *Electric energy*—Man-made sources, such as high-tension wires, and natural sources, such as lightning
4. *Radiation*—Both ionizing and nonionizing, including sunlight, radioactive minerals, and radiotherapeutic devices, implants, and pharmaceutics
5. *Chemical energy*—Effects of acids, bases, poisons/toxins, and irritants
6. *Absence* of energy-producing mechanisms necessary to sustain life, such as absence of respiration secondary to drowning

C The energy-exchanging event causing an injury can be studied as a sequence of interactions viewed in pre-event, event, and post-event phases.

XXX Countermeasures

Strategies that are effective in preventing or reducing the extent of injuries were identified and categorized by William Haddon (1963; 1979) as control *countermeasures* (Table 5-5).

TABLE 5-4

Example of risk factor analysis for injury occurrence: a fracture

Host	Injury	Agent	Vector	Exposure event	Physical environment	Sociocultural environment
Individual • Age • Sex • Health status • Physical condition	Fracture	Kinetic energy	Cement floor	Slip and fall	Oil, grease, dirt, and water on floor; painted cement floor; equipment and supplies on floor; lighting; integrity of floor	Attitude toward housekeeping; costs associated with injuries and lost time not accounted for under department budget

TABLE 5-5

Haddon matrix: case example of control countermeasures—slips and falls on the same level in a maintenance area

Phase	Human factors	Environmental and engineering factors	Social, legal, and political factors
Pre-event	• Shoes—nonskid soles • Safety training—increase awareness • Establish work practices, including housekeeping	• Nonskid floor (paint, strips) • Oil/grease absorbing material for spills • Good lighting • Proper storage and use of equipment and supplies	• OSHA inspections and regulation compliance • Safety audit • Risk management—insurance losses and litigation
Event	• Padded clothing • Optimal physical condition of workers	• Energy absorbing floors (with nonskid surface) • Emergency notification system	• Injury investigation, reporting, and tracking • Coordination of medical care
Post-event	• Effective first-aid response • Interaction with ambulance and hospital emergency services	• Prompt access to work location • Access to first-aid equipment and supplies	• Emergency response system—triage, first aid, evacuation, and definitive medical care

Source: Haddon, 1963 and 1979. In Hayes, 1990.

A Pre-event countermeasures include:
1. Preventing the creation of the workplace or community hazard
2. Reducing the severity of the hazard
3. Preventing the release of the hazard
4. Modifying the rate of release of the hazard
5. Separating the hazard from the individual

B Event countermeasures include:
1. Placing a physical barrier between the hazard and the person
2. Modifying the basic qualities of the hazard
3. Increasing the individual's resistance to injury

C Post-event countermeasures include:
1. Rapidly evaluating the injury that has occurred or is occurring, preventing continuation of the injury, and mitigating or halting the extension of its effects.
2. After stabilizing the injured party, providing definitive medical and surgical treatment and rehabilitative and reconstructive care, with a goal of restoring the worker to an optimal level of functioning.

XXXI Implications for Occupational and Environmental Health Nurses

A An understanding of occupational injury epidemiology will enable occupational and environmental health nurses to analyze, characterize, and minimize the potential for injury in their work setting.

B The occupational and environmental health nurse can use injury prevention and control principles to study, prevent, and control the occurrence of injury-producing events and the extent of injury.

Social and behavioral sciences

XXXII Effects of Social Conditions and Behavior on Health

Social and behavioral sciences examine the influences of social milieus and lifestyles on their health.

A Modern approaches to health services have been influenced by a variety of factors.
1. Life expectancy has substantially increased.
2. Patterns of disease have changed; the leading causes of death have shifted from infectious diseases to chronic diseases, often related to behaviors and environmental factors.
3. Traditional approaches such as the medical paradigm are not responsive to many modern-day health problems.

B Research in the behavioral sciences has examined the relationship between human behavior and the occurrence of illness and injury.
1. The behavior of individuals and groups is complex, and understanding behavior is a complicated process.
   a. People often make choices that they know are not good for their health (e.g., not wearing hearing protection).
   b. The key to effecting behavioral change is understanding the human thought processes that affect behavior (e.g., ear plugs are not comfortable).
   c. Focusing on behavioral strategies may result in healthier behavioral choices (e.g., allowing worker participation in selection of hearing protection devices).
   d. Behavioral approaches to research may also facilitate a better understanding of the neurologic and behavioral effects of certain exposures (to lead, for example).
2. Many theories and models have been developed to help us understand behavior. Chapter 14 presents examples of behavioral theories and models.
   a. These theories and models explain why people behave as they do.
   b. They provide a rich source of ideas that can be used to further our understanding of behavior.
   c. They enable health care providers to develop more effective interventions.

C Research in the social sciences has examined the contribution of social environments to the occurrence of illness and injury.
1. There is increased recognition of the relationship of social phenomena to health and illness outcomes.
2. Examples of social indices that may affect occupational health include rates of violence, divorce, and unemployment and the degree to which individuals have care-giving responsibilities or hold multiple jobs.
3. The provision of appropriate health services depends on complete understanding and appreciation of the nature of work and the social context of the workplace.

D Unique attributes of social and behavioral sciences include the following:
1. Qualitative techniques, which are more likely to be used for collecting data
2. Quality of life, which is an important outcome for the social and behavioral sciences; quality of life considers emotional, social, intellectual, physical, and spiritual health

XXXIII Health Promotion and Risk Reduction

Health promotion and risk reduction require an understanding of the psychosocial determinants of health (Glasgow, Lichtenstein, & Marcus, 2003).

A There is a need to develop organizational "healthy policy" as a strategy to improve workers' health.
1. Healthy policy facilitates and supports healthy behaviors.
2. Health-promoting and health-damaging policies of organizations are likely to receive increased scrutiny in the coming years (Oldenburg, Sallis, Harris & Owen, 2002).
3. Organizational change is a critical factor in achieving a healthy occupational environment.

B An important area that would benefit from the attention of the social and behavioral sciences is health promotion that reduces the effects of occupational and environmental exposures. The true benefit of this approach may only be apparent after several years.

C Social and behavioral sciences can identify and examine factors that threaten the health of workers.
1. The psychosocial environment of the workplace plays a critical role in the occurrence of occupational injury and illness. (See Chapter 15: Managing psychosocial factors in the occupational setting.)
2. The organization of work is influenced by the ideologies, values, and beliefs of people within the organization (managers and workers) and outside of it (scientists and government); these ideologies affect the social dimensions of the workplace.
3. The organization of work has been identified as a research priority by NIOSH (NIOSH, 1996).
4. Implementing strategies based on findings from social and behavioral investigations is likely to result in cost savings to employers and a better quality of life for workers.

REFERENCES

American Association of Occupational Health Nurses. (2003). Competencies in occupational and environmental health nursing. *AAOHN Journal, 51*(3), 290-302.

Arble, J. (2004). Toxicology Primer: Understanding workplace hazards and protecting worker health. *AAOHN Journal, 52*(6), 254-261.

Beach, J. (2002). The problem with material safety data sheets. *Occupational Medicine, 52*(2), 67-68.

Eisen, E. A, & Wegman, D. H. (2000). Epidemiology. In B. S. Levy and D. H. Wegman (Eds.), *Occupational health: rec-ognizing and preventing work-related disease and injury* (4th ed., pp. 143-160). Philadelphia: Lippincott, Williams & Wilkins.

Frumkin, H., & Melius, J. (2000). Toxins. In B. S. Levy and D. H. Wegman (Eds.), *Occupational health: recognizing and preventing work-related disease and injury* (4th ed., pp. 309-333). Philadelphia: Lippincott, Williams & Wilkins.

Glasgow, R. E., Lichtenstein, E., & Marcus, A. C. (2003). Why don't we see more translation of health promotion research to practice: Rethinking the efficacy-to-effectiveness transition. *American Journal of Public Health, 93*(8), 1261-1267.

Greenland, S., & Rothman, K. J. (1998). Measures of effect and measures of association. In K. J. Rothman and S. Greenland, (Eds.), *Modern Epidemiology* (2nd ed., pp. 47-64). Philadelphia, PA: Lippincott-Raven.

Gross, E. R., & Morse, E. P. (1996). Overview of industrial hygiene. In B.A. Plog, J. Niland, & P.J. Quinlan (Eds.), *Fundamentals of industrial hygiene* (4th ed., pp. 453–483). Itasca, IL: National Safety Council.

Hayes, W. (1990). Nursing advances in occupational injury prevention and control. In J.M. Radford (Ed.), *Recent advances in nursing (26). Occupational health nursing*, Edinburgh, Scotland: Churchill, Livingstone.

Institute of Medicine. (1995). *Nursing, health, and the environment* (A.M. Pope, M.A. Snyder, & L.H. Mood, Eds.). Washington, DC: National Academy Press.

Keller, L. O., Strohschein, S., Lia-Hoagberg, B., & Schaffer, M. A. (2004). Population-Based Public Health Interventions: Practice-Based and Evidence-Supported. Part I. *Public Health Nursing, 21*(5), 453-468.

Konz, S., & Johnson, S. (2000). *Work design: Industrial ergonomics* (5th ed.). Scottsdale, Arizona: Holcomb Hathaway Publishers.

Levy, B. S., & Nessetta, W. J. (2003). Neurologic effects of manganese in humans: A review. *Int J Occup Environ Health, 9*(2), 153-161.

Lippmann, M. (2000). Characterization of chemical contaminants. In M. Lippmann (Ed.). *Environmental toxicants: Human exposures and their health effects* (2nd ed., pp. 1-29). New York: John Wiley & Sons.

McCauley, L. A. (1998). Chemical mixtures in the workplace: Research and practice. *AAOHN Journal, 46*(1), 29-40.

National Research Council (NRC), National Academy of Sciences (NAS) (2001). Interventions in the workplace. In Panel on Musculoskeletal Disorders and the Workplace, *Musculoskeletal disorders and the workplace: Low back and upper extremities*. (pp. 310-329). Washington, D.C., National Academy Press.

National Institute for Occupational Safety and Health (NIOSH). (1994). *Applications manual for the revised NIOSH lifting equation..* (DHHS (NIOSH) publication 94-110): U.S. Department of Health and Human Services. Available at http://www.cdc.gov/niosh/94-110.html.

National Institute for Occupational Safety and Health (NIOSH). (1996). *National occupational research agenda*. (DHHS [NIOSH] Publication No. 96-115). Atlanta: U.S. Department of Health and Human Services.

National Institute for Occupational Safety and Health (NIOSH). (1997). *Musculoskeletal disorders and workplace factors. A critical review of epidemiologic evidence for work-related musculoskeletal disorders of the neck, upper extremity, and low back.* (DHHS [NIOSH] Publication No. 97-41). Cincinnati: U.S. Department of Health and Human Services.

Oldenburg, B., Sallis, J. F., Harris, D., & Owen N. (2002). Checklist of health promotion environments at worksites (CHEW): development and measurement characteristics. *Am J Health Promot, 16*(5), 288-99.

Papp, E. M., & Miller, A. S. (2000). Screening and surveillance: OSHA's medical surveillance provisions. *AAOHN Journal, 48*(2), 59-72.

Rothman, K.J., & Greenland, S. (1998a). Measures of disease frequency. In K.J. Rothman and S. Greenland, (Eds.), *Modern epidemiology* (2nd ed., pp. 29-46). Philadelphia, PA: Lippincott-Raven.

Rothman, K. J., & Greenland, S. (1998b). Causation and causal inference. In K. J. Rothman and S. Greenland. (Eds.), *Modern epidemiology* (2nd ed., pp. 24-26). Philadelphia, PA: Lippincott-Raven.

Smith, T. J. & Schneider, T. (2000). Occupational hygiene. In B. S. Levy and D. H. Wegman (Eds.), *Occupational health: recognizing and preventing work-related disease* and injury (4th ed., pp. 161-180). Philadelphia: Lippincott, Williams & Wilkins.

Sullivan, J. B., & Krieger, G. R. (2001). *Clinical environmental health and toxic exposures*. (2nd ed.) Baltimore: Lippincott Williams & Wilkins.

Takser, L., Mergler, D., Hellier, G., Sahuquillo, J., & Huel, G. (2003). Manganese, monoamine metabolite levels at birth, childhood psychomotor development. *Neurotoxicology, 24*, 667-674.

U.S. Department of Health and Human Services. (2000). *Healthy people 2010: understanding and improving health*, Washington D.C. Available at http://www.osha.gov/Publications/osha3084.pdf.

U.S. Department of Labor, Occupational Health and Safety Administration (1998). (p. 7) Chemical Hazard Communication, OSHA 3084 (revised 1998).

CHAPTER

6

Environmental Health

Barbara Sattler and Jane Lipscomb

The environment is one of the primary determinants of individual and community health. Nurses must understand the mechanisms and pathways of exposure to environmental health hazards, basic prevention and control strategies, the interdisciplinary nature of effective interventions, and the role of research and advocacy. Diagnosis, treatment, and prevention of environmentally related diseases are critical, as are history taking, exposure assessment, risk communication, required reporting, and advocacy.

Environmental health comprises those aspects of human health, including quality of life, that are determined by physical, chemical, biological, and social and psychologic problems in the environment. It also refers to the theory and practice of assessing, correcting, controlling, and preventing those factors in the environment that can potentially adversely affect the health of present and future generations (World Health Organization, http://www.who.int/phe/en/).

I Introduction

A The environment is a major concern in the 21st century.
1. Tens of thousands of synthetic chemicals that did not exist before the 1940s have been introduced into the environment.
2. Synthetic chemicals can be found in food, air, soil, and water—in workplaces, schools, homes, and communities.
3. Synthetic chemicals can be found within human bodies (including breast milk) in measurable amounts.
4. To date, there is limited information regarding the human health effects associated with many of the synthetic chemicals in our environments (EPA, 1998).
5. Publicly accessible toxicity data are *not* available for 71% of the 3,000 high-production industrial chemicals (EPA, 1998).

B The magnitude of environmental health issues is of increasing concern.
1. Chemical exposures have become an increasingly serious problem in the United States.
   a. Of the top 20 environmental pollutants that were reported to the Environmental Protection Agency (EPA) in 1997, nearly 75% were known or suspected neurotoxins; this accounted for more than a billion pounds of neurotoxins being released into the air, water, and land.
   b. 1.2 billion pounds of pesticide products are intentionally and legally released each year in the United States.

    c. More than 50% of Americans live in an area that exceeds current national ambient air quality standards for ozone, nitrous oxide, sulfuric oxide, and particulates.

    d. Forty states have issued one or more health advisories for mercury in their waterways; ten states have issued advisories for *every* lake and river within their borders.

    e. Mobile sources (motor vehicles) are the number one cause of air pollution in the United States.

    f. Antibiotics, 17b-estradiol (estrogen-like chemical), caffeine, and acetaminophen have been found in measurable quantities in the nation's streams.

    g. *Consumer Reports* (1998) tested leading-brand beef baby food and measured dioxin levels that exceeded the EPA allowable quantities by 100 times.

    h. Thirty million Americans drink water that contains contaminants which exceed one or more of the EPA safe drinking-water standards. Contaminants include lead, other heavy metals, nitrites, dioxin, hydrocarbons, pesticides, radon, and cyanide. (Some of the contaminants are naturally occurring, but are nonetheless toxic.)

2. There are multiple human health concerns associated with environmental exposures.

    a. Combinations of commonly used agricultural chemicals, in levels typically found in groundwater, can significantly influence the immune and endocrine systems and neurologic function in laboratory animals.

    b. Thirty-seven pesticides registered for use on food are neurotoxic organophosphates.

    c. It has been estimated that radon may be responsible for about 20% of lung cancers among nonsmokers (Zenz, 1994).

    d. Several pesticides and herbicides have been linked to leukemia.

    e. Endocrine disrupters are a diverse group of compounds that include plasticizers, polychlorinated biphenyls, many pesticides, and dioxins.

       1) These compounds are so pervasive that studies have shown them to appear in 95% of the population.

       2) When exposure to these chemicals occurs very early in life, these compounds have the potential to disrupt critical endocrine pathways with the possibility of causing adverse effects to the reproductive, neurologic, and immunologic systems.

       3) Dioxins (a group of chemicals) mimic estrogen.

    f. Poor indoor and outdoor air quality increases asthma's severity.

    g. The environment has a principal role in causing cancer.

C Chemical, biological, and radiologic risks exist in environments in which people live, work, play, and learn.

1. The relationship between environment and health is determined by host factors such as age, gender, genetic makeup, underlying diseases, dose-response factors, and the length of time exposed. Chapter 5 provides additional information about toxicology.

2. Chemical and radiologic exposures can be cumulative. Occupational and environmental health nurses must assess a person's total exposure to environmental risks in order to understand and address potential health threats.

3. Very specific gestational ages can be associated with exquisite vulnerability to the effects of certain toxic chemicals.
4. As in occupational health, environmental health is based on a public health model with an emphasis on prevention.
   a. Preventive interventions in environmental health include pollution prevention, product design, engineering controls, purchasing choice, and education.
   b. Additionally, access to information via labeling and other forms of "right to know" create opportunities for informed decisions.
5. Although U.S. environmental standards (e.g., EPA, OSHA) are "health-based," they often are not sufficiently protective of our most vulnerable populations.
   a. Standards are often based on the health risks to an otherwise healthy, 70 kilogram (154 pound), white male.
   b. The standards may not provide sufficient protection to pregnant women and fetuses, young children, the frail and the elderly, or the immuno-compromised.

II Environmental Health Assessment

A Potential environmental exposures and environmentally related diseases can be assessed individually or on a community-wide basis.
1. Individual environmental health assessments should take into account all of the potential exposures that a person may have in the home, workplace, school, and community.
   a. The National Library of Medicine's *ToxTown* provides easily accessible, peer-reviewed information about the potential health hazards in our environments (available in Spanish).
      1) *ToxTown* covers a broad range of information about health risks associated with: factories, farms, homes, offices, schools, drinking water, recreational water, pests, vehicles, hazardous waste sites, airplanes, construction, and EMFs (electric and magnetic fields).
      2) Within *ToxTown*, there is a database of likely chemical exposures associated with an extensive list of specific job categories.
      3) Household product information, including auto products, landscape/yard, home maintenance, pet care, arts and crafts, personal care, and cleaning products can be found on: http://www.household.nlm.nih.gov/.
   b. The Children's Health and Environment Coalition provides high quality information regarding children's exposures; their *e-house* website specifically provides information about home-related environmental health risks.
   c. The EPA website provides a range of environmental exposure information.
      1) *EnvironFacts* (www.epa.gov/enviro.em/) provides geographically-related information.
      2) *EnviroMapper* (www.epa.gov/enviro/html.em/) provides air, water, and hazardous waste site information by location/region.
   d. The Children's Environmental Health Network has developed a health assessment tool for children (http://www.cehn.org).

e. The University of Maryland's website, *EnviRN*, has a home assessment survey that includes information about the health implications of environmental exposures. (http://www.envirn.umaryland.edu/)

f. The Agency of Toxic Substances and Disease Registry, an agency within the Centers for Disease Control and Prevention (CDC), has created ToxFacts, which provide excellent toxicologic information on chemicals that are commonly associated with environmental health risks. (http://www.atsdr.cdc.gov/toxfaq.htm.)

2. Community environmental health assessments identify potential exposures in water (including drinking water), air (including indoor air), dust (including lead-based paint particles), soil (including exposures from current and previous land use), and radiation (ionizing and nonionizing).

a. There is no single source for environmental assessment information, and often there is no community-specific information.

b. Assessments may depend on extrapolating from aggregate national, statewide, county, or metropolitan exposure data.

3. A geographic information system (GIS) is a method for assessing community risks to environmental exposures and potential health problems.

a. GIS consists of computerized mapping of graphically related data. Environmental exposure and health status data can be entered and thus evaluated for geographic relationships. These data can also be presented in map form.

b. More information on GIS may be obtained from http://www.gisportal.com/, the Agency for Toxic Substances and Disease Registry, or geography departments in universities.

4. An essential competency for environmental health assessments is knowledge of the federal, state, and local health and environmental statutes, regulations, and practices regarding what data are collected and how they are accessed.

B **Epidemiology and toxicology are the principal sciences used to determine the relationship between environmental exposures and health outcomes. Chapter 5 provides an overview of these sciences.**

1. Environmental epidemiology uses epidemiologic techniques to examine environmental exposures.

a. Analytical studies (cohort and case control) are often the design of choice in environmental health; experimental studies are rarely done, because it is unethical to intentionally expose individuals or communities to environmental hazards.

b. Cluster investigations are often used to respond to community concerns about an excess of cancer or birth defects.

1) These investigations usually render negative or equivocal results.

2) Cluster investigations are most convincing when the disease in question is rare and very specific for the putative etiologic exposure, as is the case in asbestos causing mesothelioma.

c. Limitations are inherent in environmental epidemiology.

1) Exposures are often poorly defined and measured.

2) A very limited understanding of the health effects of mixed exposures makes studying the most common type of environmental exposure situations particularly challenging.

3) Often a relatively small number of individuals (e.g., a community) constitute the study populations, yielding limited statistical power to detect an association between exposures of concern and health effects.

4) A lack of understanding about variability in the susceptibility of segments of the populations (e.g., the poor, children, elderly) limits the ability to compare findings across studies.

5) The long latency between many environmental exposures and the evidence of chronic disease, in particular cancer, creates additional challenges to exposure assessment.

2. Environmental toxicology is the science that examines the toxic effects of agents on the environment.

a. Toxicology, which is the science that investigates the adverse affects of chemicals on health, is similar to pharmacology (Table 6-1).

b. The effects of hazardous chemicals can be either immediate (acute) or long-term, or can present after a latency period often associated with cancer outcomes.

c. Host factors must be considered when looking at hazardous chemicals. Such factors as age, sex, genetics, weight, drugs that the person may be taking, and pregnancy status may affect the therapeutic or toxic effect of a drug or a chemical.

d. Hazardous chemical exposures are often *involuntary*.

TABLE 6-1

Comparison of pharmacology and toxicology

Pharmacology	Toxicology
Pharmacology is the scientific study of the origin, nature, chemistry, effects, and use of drugs.	*Toxicology* is the science that investigates the adverse effects of chemicals on health.
Dose refers to the amount of a drug absorbed from an administration.	*Dose* refers to the amount of a chemical absorbed into the body from a chemical exposure.
A drug can be administered one time, short-term, or long-term.	*Exposure* is the actual contact that a person has with a chemical. Exposure can be one-time, short-term, or long-term.
A *dose-response curve* graphically represents the relationship between the dose of a drug and the response elicited.	A *dose-response curve* describes the relationship of the body's response to different amounts of an agent such as a drug or toxin.
Routes of administration are oral, intramuscular, intravenous, subcutaneous, dermal, topical.	*Routes of entry* are ingestion, inhalation, dermal absorption.
With drugs there are therapeutic responses (desirable) and side effects (undesirable).	In toxicology, only the toxic effects are of concern. *Toxicity* is the ability of a chemical to damage an organ system, disrupt a biochemical process, or disturb an enzyme system.
Beyond the therapeutic dose, a drug may become toxic.	
Potency refers to the relative amount of drug required to produce the desired response.	The *potency* of a toxic chemical refers to the relative amount it takes to elicit a toxic effect compared with other chemicals.
Biologic monitoring is done for some drugs: clotting time is monitored in clients on anticoagulants like warfarin. Actual drug levels are measured for some drugs, such as digoxin.	*Biologic monitoring* is done for some toxic exposures, such as blood lead levels or metabolites of chemicals such as cotinines for environmental tobacco smoke.

Sattler, 1998.

e. The regulatory process by which a drug comes to the market includes several stages of animal and human testing. The U.S. regulatory process for hazardous chemicals that are not foods or drugs requires virtually no original testing.

f. Few of the chemicals in widespread use today—even those regularly found in human tissue, including umbilical cord blood and amniotic fluid—have been submitted to any testing to determine their possible neurologic, reproductive or developmental impacts.

g. The European Union has adopted a more comprehensive chemicals policy, known as REACH—which stands for Registration, Evaluation and Authorization of Chemicals—that is requiring more pre-market testing and disclosure than currently exist in the United States (See Box 6-3 and Section VIII A 8).

III Children and Environmental Health

A **Children have unique risks related to environmental exposures.**

1. The metabolic and physiologic processes of children differ dramatically from those of adults. Their skin, respiratory, and gastrointestinal absorption of toxic materials is greater than that of adults.

2. Children's normal exploratory behavior (e.g., hand-to-mouth activity and crawling) increases opportunities to ingest toxicants such as lead-based paint.

3. Children in developed countries spend 90% of their time in homes, day-care centers, schools, motor vehicles, and other indoor environments.

   a. These environments often have a large number of chemicals and pollutants from tobacco smoke, building materials, consumer products, pets, insects and other pests, mold, inadequately ventilated cooling and heating devices, and the influx of outdoor air pollutants.

   b. The concentration of indoor pollutants can be 4 to 10 times more than outdoor pollutants.

4. Children born today will cumulatively have more exposures to toxic chemicals throughout their lifetime than children born in earlier times.

5. Exposure to environmental toxins can disrupt and cause permanent damage to the developing nervous, immune, and respiratory systems of the unborn and young children.

6. Young children's exposure to toxic chemicals in their diet is substantial—from pesticide residues on apples and other fruits/vegetables, lead in drinking water, and polychlorinated biphenyl(s) and dioxins in breastmilk.

B **Children have not routinely been included in risk assessment, and most environmental health regulations are based on studies of adult males. Humans' developmental stages can create varying degrees of vulnerability to toxic chemicals, even in healthy humans.**

C **There is increasing evidence that a wide range of reproductive disorders, including male and female infertility, menstrual irregularities, spontaneous abortion or fetal loss, major and minor birth defects, and developmental abnormalities, may result from human exposure to any of a number of toxic substances.**

D **Many environmental hazards affect children.**

1. Ten million U.S. children live within four miles of a toxic waste dump, thus creating increased potential for hazardous chemical exposures via air, drinking water, or direct contact with the contamination.

2. One million children in the United States exceed currently acceptable levels of lead in their blood (10 μdl); this exposure may be associated with a range of health effects, including behavioral (e.g., violent behavior) and cognitive effects.

3. Environmental tobacco smoke is responsible for 7 million lost school days by children.

4. Epidemiologic studies suggest a relationship between nitrates in drinking water and juvenile diabetes.

5. Many children are exposed to toxins from manufacturing plants in their neighborhoods; for example, 20% of the children in Arkansas who live near an herbicide manufacturing plant had herbicide residues in their urine.

6. Asthma is the number one reason that children miss school and are hospitalized in the United States.
   a. The Centers for Disease Control has calculated that over 5 million children under the age of 18 are affected by asthma in the United States.
   b. Indoor triggers for asthma include second-hand smoke, dust mites, cockroach feces and exoskeleton dust, mold, and pets.
   c. Outdoor triggers include ozone, nitrogen oxides, diesel exhaust and pollen.

7. Children can be exposed directly by contact to arsenic-treated (chromated copper arsenate) wood (often referred to as "treated wood" or "pressure treated wood") in play structures, decks, and other items; the arsenic can leach into the groundwater which, in turn, may be a source of drinking water.

8. Developing lungs are more sensitive to the effects of ozone (See Section XI, A2f).

9. Pollutants (especially mercury) in some fish can cause developmental problems.

10. There is increasing evidence that toxic chemicals affect the brain and can play a role in brain disorders:
    a. **Lead** exposures during infancy and childhood can cause attention problems, hyperactivity, impulsive behavior, reduced intelligence quotient (IQ), poor school performance, aggression, and delinquent behavior.
    b. **Mercury** easily crosses the placenta and disrupts many steps in brain development. Even exposures at relatively low levels to a pregnant woman can impair the IQ, language development, visual-spatial skills, memory, and attention of her child. As with lead, the "safe" level of mercury keeps dropping the more mercury is studied.
    c. **Manganese** is essential to health at low levels in the diet, but elevated levels of manganese are associated with various disorders.
       1) High levels of manganese in hair are associated with attention deficit hyperactivity disorder (ADHD).
       2) Laboratory experiments in animals link manganese with hyperactivity; it is also associated with Parkinson's disease.
    d. **PCBs** (polychlorinated biphenyls), industrial chemicals that are now banned but persist in the environment, especially in fatty tissue, can impair reflexes and IQ, delay mental development and the development of motor skills, and are associated with hyperactivity.
    e. **Tobacco smoke and nicotine** are among the best-studied agents for their effects on the developing brain. Children born to women who smoke during pregnancy are at risk for IQ deficits, learning disorders, and attention deficits.

f. **Bisphenol A** alters the expression of genes that are important for long-term memory formation and for early brain development.

g. **Perchlorate**, a rocket fuel that now contaminates drinking water in many communities in the western United States, interferes with thyroid hormone control of brain development in mice.

h. **Solvents** such as toluene cause learning, speech, and motor skill problems in children.

IV Environmental Justice and Advocacy

A *Environmental justice* refers to the "fair treatment for people of all races, cultures, and incomes, regarding the development of environmental laws, regulations, and policies" (http://www.epa.gov/swerosps/ej/index.html).

1. The environmental health status that poor communities experience is subject to the compounding effects of poor housing, poor nutrition, poor access to health care, unemployment, underemployment, and employment in the most hazardous jobs.

2. The environmental risk burden is generally greater for minorities and those who are economically disadvantaged, because they are exposed to a greater number and intensity of environmental pollutants in food, air, water, homes, and workplaces.

3. The National Health and Nutrition Exam Study results indicate that minority women have higher levels of toxic chemicals in their bodies than do white women.

4. Information sharing may be inadequate or less effective in economically disadvantaged communities as a function of language and literacy issues, including the challenge of understanding technical language in warning signs and other right-to-know materials.

5. Indicators of increased risk include:
   a. Proximity to hazardous waste sites, polluting industries, and incinerators.
   b. Substandard housing that may have friable asbestos, deteriorating lead paint, yards with contaminated soil, pests, pesticides, and mold.

6. Federal mandates to address environmental justice include:
   a. Environmental Justice Act (1993)
   b. Executive Order 12898 (1994): Federal Actions to Address Environmental Justice in Minority Populations

7. The passage of federal legislation resulted in the development of policies to more comprehensively reduce the incidence of environmental inequity by mandating that every federal agency act in a manner to address and prevent environmental illnesses and injuries.

8. In 1994, the National Environmental Justice Advisory Council was created as a federal advisory committee to the EPA to convene community, governmental, and business constituents to assess environmental justice issues and make recommendations to the Administrator of the EPA.

B *Advocacy* and *environmental justice* are interrelated concepts of critical importance to the field of environmental health and to occupational and environmental health nurses.

1. *Case advocacy* refers to the process of advocating for individual clients and families to solve problems and secure needed services.

2. *Class advocacy* is aimed at changing policy, institutional systems, and norms, laws, or patterns of resource allocation to improve the health of the group or community.

a. *Collaborative approaches* (e.g., membership on planning and advisory committees) are characterized as citizens and authorities working collaboratively to reach an agreed-upon goal.

b. *Campaigning approaches* (e.g., lobbying) require that citizens or professionals work singly or collectively to persuade authorities (lawmakers and regulators) that new problem definitions and solutions are needed.

c. *Contest strategies* (e.g., protest marches) involve citizens organizing to force attention to community problems that they feel are being ignored or mishandled by authorities.

d. *Legal remedies* include activities such as class action suits.

3. Nurses are often the primary health care providers in poor and disenfranchised communities; advocacy on behalf of such communities is critical to improving the health of these communities.

V Risk Assessment, Risk Management, and Risk Communication

Risk is the probability of undesirable effects (or unhealthy outcomes) arising from exposure to a hazard. Risk assessment, risk management, and risk communication are critical strategies for dealing with environmental risks.

A *Risk assessment* **refers to the use of available information to evaluate and estimate exposure to a substance and the resulting adverse health effects.**

1. Formal risk assessment is used by almost all federal regulatory agencies.

   a. This should be distinguished from nursing assessments used to identify health risks.

   b. Risk assessment is formulaic and virtually always depends on estimates for each of the following four steps:

      1) *Hazard identification* relies on toxicologic and epidemiologic studies of the potential of a substance to cause harm.

      2) *Dose-response evaluation* measures whether the harm increases with increasing doses of the substances.

      3) *Exposure assessment* involves measuring the amount of the chemical or other harmful substances to which a population is exposed with a goal of estimating the dose.

      4) *Risk characterization* involves estimating the public or environmental impact or problem.

   c. Estimations of risk can be widely diverse, depending on who is doing the risk assessment.

2. The context in which risk assessment is typically used is in policy and regulatory development, during which time political and economic interests are likely to be equally important variables influencing the final policy or standard.

B *Risk management* **is the process of evaluating alternative strategies for reducing risk and prioritizing or selecting among them.**

1. Risk management strategies often involve policy development; this may include regulatory, legislative, and voluntary options and may be targeted at the company-institution level; at the local, state, national governmental level; or at international level, such as with the Kyoto Agreement (Box 6-1).

2. Environmental engineering can be a critical tool in risk management.

3. Engineering strategies to control exposure to environmental hazards are similar to the industrial hygiene "hierarchy of controls;" they include

elimination of the exposure through substitution of products or processes, as well as the following:

   a. Reduction of pollution at its source (source reduction)
   b. Waste minimization
   c. Reuse, recycling
   d. Emissions control
   e. Waste cleanup

4. Risk-management strategies should always include involvement of all stakeholders regarding the nature of risk and the costs and benefits of proposed risk-management options.
5. Coalition building and community action are vehicles to successful risk management.
6. Legal remedies may be used to manage risk in combination with the above strategies.
7. Community members should always be "at the table" regarding decisions that are being made about their risks.
8. The *Precautionary Principle* assumes that where there are possible threats of serious or irreversible damage, lack of scientific certainty shall not be used as a reason for postponing measures to prevent risks. (In 2003, the American Nurses' Association adopted the *Precautionary Approach*, based on the Precautionary Principle, as the primary tenet on which they will base their environmental health policy/advocacy work) (Box 6-2).

BOX 6-1

KYOTO agreement

The United Nations Convention on Climate Change

The Kyoto Agreement (also referred to as *Kyoto Protocols*) is a framework laid down by 38 developed countries to prevent global warming. At a summit held in 1997, the nations joining the treaty agreed to reduce their emission of greenhouse gases by the year 2012. Greenhouse gases trap heat within our planet's atmosphere and cause an increase in global temperatures. While different countries have committed to varying levels of reduction, average emission cuts by the Kyoto Agreement are calculated to be about 5.2%.

Under the Convention, governments:

- Gather and share information on greenhouse gas emissions, national policies and best practices

- Launch national strategies for addressing greenhouse emissions and adapting to expected impacts, including the provision of financial and technologic support to developing countries
- Cooperate in preparing for adaptation to the impacts of climate change

The reduction of emissions is grouped into two classes of greenhouse gases. The first class relates to carbon dioxide, nitrous oxide, and methane. Reductions made to these gases are compared to 1990 emission levels. In the latter class are hydrofluorocarbon gases, perfluorocarbons, and sulphur hexafluoride. Under the terms of the agreement, cuts made to these gases are based on 1995 emission levels. **The United States is not among the signatories of the Kyoto Agreement.**

BOX 6-2

Precautionary principle

In 1998, a consensus-building conference was convened at the Wingspread Conference Center that resulted in the adoption of a "Precautionary Principle," which is based on the following statement:

"When an activity raises threats of harm to the environment or human health, precautionary measures should be taken even if some cause and effect relationships are not fully established scientifically."

All statements of the Precautionary Principle contain a version of this formula: *When the health of humans and the environment is at stake, it may not be necessary to wait for scientific certainty to take protective action.* The Precautionary Principle is based on the common sense idea behind many adages: "Be careful." "Better safe than sorry." "Look before you leap." "First do no harm."

"Precautionary principle" is a translation of the German *Vorsorgeprinzip. Vorsorge* means, literally, "forecaring." It carries the sense of foresight and preparation—not merely "caution." The principle applies to human health and the environment. The ethical assumption behind the Precautionary Principle is that humans are responsible to protect, preserve, and restore the global ecosystems on which all life, including our own, depends. When evidence gives us good reason to believe that an activity, technology, or substance may be harmful, we should act to prevent harm. If we always wait for scientific certainty, people may suffer and die and the natural world

may suffer irreversible damage.

The Precautionary Principle is most powerful when it serves as a guide to making wiser decisions in the face of uncertainty. *Any action that contributes to preventing harm to humans and the environment, learning more about the consequences of actions, and acting appropriately is precautionary.*

Precaution does not work if it is only a last resort and results only in bans or moratoriums. It is best linked to these implementation methods:

- Exploring *alternatives* to possibly harmful actions, especially "clean" technologies that eliminate waste and toxic substances
- Placing the *burden of proof* on proponents of an activity rather than on victims or potential victims of the activity
- Setting and working toward *goals* that protect health and the environment
- Bringing *democracy and transparency* to decisions affecting health and the environment

(The previous statements were abstracted from the Science and Environmental Health Network's website: http://www.sehn.org regarding the Precautionary Principle, 2005.)

In 2003, the American Nurses Association adopted the "Precautionary Approach" as a guiding tenet for their environmental health policy and advocacy work. This Precautionary Approach is based on the Wingspread definition of the Precautionary Principle described above.

C *Risk communication*, in the context of environmental health, is the art of communicating about the potential health risks associated with environmental exposures.

1. There are four elements to consider in risk communication: the message, the messenger, the audience, and the context.

   a. Considerations related to the *message* include:

      1) Environmental health risks are often difficult to define.
      2) Exposures may be difficult to characterize.
      3) The exposed population can be very diverse in age and many other important variables.
      4) Exposures will always include multiple chemicals, whereas most scientific investigation is primarily about individual chemicals and rarely chemical mixtures.
      5) Sometimes scientific evidence is inconclusive or nonexistent.

   b. Characteristics of the successful *messenger* include:

      1) The messenger must be perceived as trusted and credible. Nurses are considered highly credible and trustworthy sources of information within the community.
      2) The messenger must be prepared to communicate with empathy and care when the message evokes hostile emotions.

   c. Characteristics of the *audience* include:

      1) Audiences bring individual biases to any forum in which environmental health risks might be discussed.
      2) Audience's distrust of the messenger may be based on their feelings about whom the messenger represents (e.g., government, industry, or an environmental organization).
      3) An audience may trust or distrust a messenger based on his or her age, race, sex, etc.

   d. Considerations related to *context* are as follows:

      1) Risk communication does not occur in a vacuum; it often occurs when there has been a perceived environmental health threat such as a

TABLE 6-2

Factors that affect perceptions of risk

Risks may be *perceived* as less or more risky based on the following attributes:

Less risky	More risky
Voluntary	Involuntary
Familiar	Unfamiliar
Controllable	Uncontrollable
Controlled by self	Controlled by others
Not memorable	Memorable
Not dread	Dread
Chronic	Acute
Diffuse in time and space	Focused in time and space
Not fatal	Fatal
Immediate	Delayed
Natural	Artificial
Individual mitigation possible	Individual mitigation impossible
Detectable	Undetectable

Source: Sandman, 1993.

potentially contaminated water supply, an accidental release of a hazardous chemical, or a newly identified hazardous waste site adjacent to a daycare center.

2) The conditions and context will influence the audiences' ability to listen and trust.

3) The media can play an important part in a community's understandings and biases regarding environmental risk.

2. Risk communication is affected by risk perception. Table 6-2 lists factors that affect the perceptions of risk.

3. The Environmental Protection Agency has created a list of 7 Cardinal Rules for Risk Communication.

   a. Accept and involve the public as a legitimate partner.
   b. Plan carefully and evaluate your efforts.
   c. Listen to your audience.
   d. Be honest, frank, and open.
   e. Coordinate and collaborate with other credible sources.
   f. Meet the needs of the press.
   g. Speak clearly and with compassion.

VI Federal Agencies

A **The Environmental Protection Agency (EPA) and its counterparts at the state level are the primary regulatory agencies responsible for environmental protection and the protection of health from environmental risks.**

1. The EPA was established by Congress through the 1970 *National Environmental Policy Act* to permit coordinated and effective governmental action on behalf of the environment. Major environmental statutes include:

   a. *Clean Air Act*—Regulates air emissions from area, stationary, and mobile sources. The 1990 reauthorization requires Risk Management Plans whereby industry must identify the "worst case" scenario for hazardous chemicals that they transport, use, or dispose.

   b. *Clean Water Act*—Sets basic structure for regulating pollutants in U.S. waters

   c. *Federal Insecticide, Fungicide, and Rodenticide Act* —provides control of pesticide distribution, sale, and use. Requires registration of all pesticides; requires farmers and utility companies to register their pesticide use; requires applicators to take registration exams; and requires labeling.

   d. *Safe Drinking Water Act*—Establishes safe drinking water standards for owners and operators of public drinking water. The 1996 reauthorization requires that owners/operators annually provide their customers with a Consumer Confidence Report that summarizes exceedences in drinking water standards and the associated health risks.

   e. *Resource Conservation and Recovery Act*—Regulates the generation, transportation, treatment, and storage of hazardous waste. The 1986 reauthorization allowed the EPA to address underground storage tanks, as well.

   f. *Toxic Substances Control Act*—Gives the EPA the ability to track the 80,000+ industrial chemicals produced by or imported into the United States.

   g. *Comprehensive Environmental Response, Compensation, and Liability Act*— Established a tax on the chemical and petroleum industry to be used on hazardous waste sites. This was commonly known as "Superfund." The reauthorizations of Superfund created more emphasis on human health threats, provided community "right to know," and established state and local emergency planning committees.

h. *National Environmental Education Act*—Created a structure for more coordinated environmental education efforts. The Act established the National Environmental Education and Training Foundation, which has addressed environmental health learning needs of health professionals.

i. *Pollution Prevention Act*—Focuses industry, government, and public attention on reduction of pollution: production, operation, and raw materials use. It also includes energy efficiency, recycling, source reduction, and sustainable agriculture.

j. *Food Quality Protection Act* (amended the Food, Drug, and Cosmetic Act)—Requires new safety approaches to pesticides used on foods that result in "reasonable certainty of no harm." It called for explicit consideration of pesticide effects on children.

2. The EPA endeavors to abate and control pollution systematically by properly integrating a variety of research, monitoring, standard setting, and enforcement activities.

3. The EPA coordinates and supports research and antipollution activities by state and local governments, private and public groups, individuals, and educational institutions.

4. The EPA also reinforces efforts among other federal agencies to monitor and control the impact of their operations on the environment.

5. Each state has a designated agency that is responsible for regulatory oversight of all environmental regulations and standards that are set by the EPA. States can promulgate regulations and standards as long as they are at least as effective as the federal standards.

6. Environmental statutes and regulations may be promulgated and implemented on a federal, state, or even local level. For instance, zoning, which is a local decision-making activity, can have profound influence over land use and associated human health and well being.

7. Most environmental statutes are media-specific, such as air, water, soil, or food.

8. The EPA, like all major federal agencies, has 10 regional offices around the country.

9. Most environmental protection laws are reauthorized by Congress every 5 years.

B **Numerous other federal agencies address issues related to the environment, including air, water, soil, and food, as well as safety and health in the workplace. Appendix I provides addresses of agencies.**

1. Other major federal agencies have become increasingly involved in the impact of the environment on the health of the public. Examples of this environmental health involvement include the following:

a. The *Department of Transportation* (DOT) regulates hazardous materials transportation.

b. The *Department of Agriculture* (USDA) is responsible for food and agricultural health and safety.
   1) Its Food Safety Administration regulates pesticides, hormones, and antibiotics used in the food supply.
   2) Its Food, Nutrition and Consumer Services is responsible for ensuring access to nutritious, healthful diets for all Americans, through food assistance and nutrition education for consumers.

c. The *Food and Drug Administration* (FDA) inspects food and drug manufacturing plants and warehouses; collects and analyzes samples of foods, drugs, cosmetics, and therapeutic devices for adulteration and mis-branding; and enforces the Radiation Control Act as related to consumer products. With the USDA, the FDA collects information about food required by a number of regulations.

d. The *Department of Energy* (DOE) regulates industry involved in energy research and production, and manages many national energy research facilities and the nuclear weapons production sites. It is responsible for providing a framework for a balanced, comprehensive national energy plan.

  1) The Office of Environment, Safety and Health of the DOE provides independent oversight of departmental execution of environmental and occupational safety and health, nuclear and non-nuclear safety, and environmental restoration.

  2) The Office of Environmental Management provides program policy development and guidance for the assessment and cleanup of inactive waste sites and facilities and for waste management operations.

e. The *Department of Defense* (DOD) addresses environmental health concerns associated with defense-related activities. Some of the most contaminated landsites in the United States are owned and operated by the DOD and the DOE.

f. The *Nuclear Regulatory Commission* (NRC) licenses, inspects, and regulates civilian use of nuclear energy to protect health and safety and the environment. This is achieved by licensing persons and companies to build and operate nuclear reactors and other facilities and to own and use nuclear materials.

g. The *Occupational Safety and Health Administration* (OSHA) was created within the Department of Labor under the Occupation Safety and Health Act (OSH Act) of 1970 to promulgate and enforce national occupational health and safety standards (Chapter 3).

h. Many smaller federal agencies have activities directly related to health and the environment, such as the *National Oceanographic and Atmospheric Agency, National Weather Service,* the *United States Geographic Services,* and the *National Chemical Safety Board.*

C **The U.S. Department of Health and Human Services (DHHS) is the department of the federal executive branch most concerned with the nation's human health concerns. The public health infrastructure is vital to environmental health. Within DHHS, the following sub-agencies focus on environmental health:**

1. The *Centers for Disease Control* (CDC) composes the prime public health agency concerned about human health. Within the CDC structure are:

a. *National Center for Environmental Health*—Promotes health and quality of life by preventing or controlling disease, injury, and disability related to the interactions between people and their environment outside the work place.

b. *Agency for Toxic Substances and Disease Registry* (ATSDR), now part of the CDC—Responsible for environmental health-related issues associated with actual or potential exposure to hazardous substances from waste sites, unplanned releases, and other sources of pollution in the environment.

1) ATSDR's mission is to prevent or mitigate adverse human health effects and diminished quality of life resulting from exposure to hazardous substances in the environment.
2) ATSDR's activities include public health assessments, health investigations, exposure and disease registry, emergency response, toxicologic profiles, health education, and applied research.
3) ATSDR's Environmental Health Nursing Initiative is a collaborative effort to increase and sustain environmental health knowledge and skills in nurses and other health professionals.

c. The *National Institute for Occupational Safety and Health* (NIOSH)—Established by the OSH Act to conduct research on occupational diseases and injuries, responds to requests for assistance by investigating problems of health and safety in workplaces, and recommend standards to OSHA.

2. The *National Institute of Environmental Health Sciences* (NIEHS)—The principal federal agency for biomedical research on the effects of chemical, physical, and biologic agents on human health and well-being.

a. NIEHS supports research and training focused on harmful agents in the environment and the associated health effects. It supports basic and applied research, environmental justice projects, and community-based participatory research.

b. Research forms the basis for preventive programs and actions for regulatory agencies. (Note: within the EPA, there is an Office of Research and Development that also provides extramural research grants to universities and research institutions.)

3. The *Consumer Product Safety Commission*—Provides information on health and safety effects related to consumer products, including chemical hazards in consumer products, such as arsenic in treated wood.

4. The *Health Resources and Services Administration*—The part of DHHS responsible for insuring that the workforce includes the right number of professionals/technicians, etc., properly qualified to attend to the country's health needs. HRSA has provided universities (including schools of nursing) with grants to build capacity in environmental health.

VII Public Health Infrastructure

While the federal agencies are primarily responsible for setting exposure limits on environmental health risks, it is the public health infrastructure at the local, state, and federal levels that principally establishes the health surveillance systems, investigates population-based health problems, and creates the programmatic responses for environmentally-related health problems.

A The Centers for Disease Control and state and local health departments (and the Indian Health Services) make up the greatest part of the public health infrastructure addressing environmental health.

B There is extreme variability in the level of environmental health programming between state health departments and between local health departments from area to area. State and local budgets, state and local mandates, and leadership within the agencies, among other factors, can influence this variability.

C The National Center for Health Statistics implements the National Health and Nutrition Exam Survey.

1. The National Health and Nutrition Exam Survey (NHANES) is a population-based survey designed to collect information on the health and nutrition of the U.S. household population.

2. In 2000, in addition to the survey and medical exam, they took blood and urine samples to assay for the presence of 116 chemicals that are known to be toxic. The results show that children and women have higher levels, on average, than adult men and that minorities have higher levels than whites.

D There is a significant deficit in both public health tracking and environmental exposure tracking which, in combination, hinders us from understanding the relationship between environmental health outcomes and environmental exposures.

VIII Accessing Information and the "Right to Know"

A Access to information about environmental risks in our food, water, and soil is provided through a variety of agencies via an array of federal and state statutes.

1. A range of environmental right-to-know statutes and regulations exist; the mandatory labeling of commercial food products is an example of a consumer right-to-know requirement.
   a. Access to information about food is provided by a number of regulations, implemented by the USDA and FDA.
   b. This information includes the ingredients, nutritional content, and in some instances health-related information, such as the designation that a food is *organic*.
   c. It is equally important to note what is *not* required on the label. The following are examples:
      1) Pesticide use during the growing of produce
      2) Pesticides in animal feed for livestock
      3) Nontherapeutic antibiotics in animal feed for livestock, including poultry and aquaculture (fish farms)
      4) Genetically modified organisms (GMOs) or genetically engineered organisms in our produce or processed food

2. Access to information about water is provided under two statutes: the Clean Water Act and the Safe Drinking Water Act.
   a. The Clean Water Act was promulgated to protect the nation's waterways, whereas the Safe Drinking Water Act protects drinking water from its source to the tap.
   b. Through the Safe Drinking Water Act, residents who purchase water from a water provider have the right to know what is in their drinking water.
   c. Annually, as part of the drinking water right-to-know regulations, the water utility must provide a "consumer confidence report" (CCR) or "right-to-know" report listing the contaminants (chemical, biologic, and radiologic) that have exceeded EPA standards within the last year and their probable sources.
      1) The source of the drinking water should also be included in the CCR.
      2) The source can be groundwater or surface water. If surface water, the body or bodies of water must be named. Many of the public drinking water suppliers have submitted their CCRs to the EPA, and the information is displayed on the EPA website.

3. Industrial contaminants that are released into the air or water are reportable, based on the chemical and its quantity, under the community

right-to-know component of the Superfund Amendments and Reauthorization Act (SARA).

　　a. SARA requires polluters to report certain effluents and emissions for the Toxic Release Inventory (TRI).

　　b. TRI data are displayed on the EPA's EnviroFACTS website. An excellent source of this information has been created by Environmental Defense, which takes the TRI data, allows it to be queried by zip code, and provides the associated toxicologic and human health risk information in a readily accessible format (http://www.scorecard.org/). This is an excellent source for community environmental assessments.

4. Employees have the right to know under the Hazard Communication Standard, an occupational safety and health standard regulated by OSHA (Chapter 16 provides additional information about this standard).

5. States may establish additional rights to know, such as California's Prop 65, a statute intended to protect California citizens and the State's drinking water sources from chemicals known to cause cancer or birth defects or other reproductive harm, and to inform citizens about exposures to such chemicals via labels on consumer products, inclusion of notices in mailings to water customers, posting of notices, placing notices in public news media, and the like, provided that the warning is clear and reasonable.

6. Many states have developed some form of right-to-know notification regarding pesticide application. This can be for pesticides used in homes for termite treatment, in schools, and/or for pesticide applications on lawns.

7. The 1966 Freedom of Information Act provides that any person can make requests for government information.

　　a. Citizens are not required to identify themselves or why they want the information.

　　b. Certain restrictions exist on work in progress, enforcement confidential information, classified documents, and national security information.

8. Internationally, in 2003, the European Commission adopted the Registration, Evaluation, and Authorization of Chemicals Policy (REACH), which calls for the registration of all chemicals produced or imported at quantities above 1 ton (Box 6-3).

　　a. This policy has implications for all multinational manufacturers and will undoubtedly influence future U.S. chemicals policies.

　　b. REACH is intended to increase human and environmental protection from toxic chemicals, improve the management of the risks associated with environmental toxics, and increase the health and safety information to all levels of productions during which potential for exposure exists.

　　c. REACH policies will require:

　　　　1) Registration of all chemicals manufactured or imported greater than 1 ton to a central database.

　　　　2) Data sharing of all animal studies as a way of both enhancing the development of scientific knowledge and reducing unnecessary animal testing.

　　　　3) Increased dissemination of hazard information up and down the production line.

　　　　4) Incorporating all downstream users in the information loop.

　　　　5) Evaluating and coordinating toxicity testing.

　　　　6) Requiring the "authorization" of highly toxic chemicals to confirm adequate controls and to justify that the benefits outweigh the risks.

　　　　7) Restricting or banning the use of highly toxic chemicals.

BOX 6-3

REACH

In October 2003, the European Commission presented a proposal for a complete and radical review of the European Union's chemical substances policy. The proposal sets up a comprehensive system for the registration, evaluation, and authorization of chemicals (REACH).

Objectives of REACH Policies

- Develop a new integrated and coherent chemicals policy reflecting the precautionary principle and the principle of sustainability.
- Modernize the regulatory framework to encourage innovation, competitiveness, and the efficient working of the internal market.
- Increase the safety of humans and the environment in the handling of chemicals and at the same time improve the competitiveness of the chemicals industry in Europe.
- Create a single regulatory framework called REACH (registration, evaluation and authorization of chemicals) to replace the current dual system for assessing risks of "existing" (placed on market before 1981) and new substances. Some 30,000 substances are to be assessed through the REACH process.
- Reversal of burden of proof from authorities to industry for testing and risk assessment of chemicals.

Main Elements

Registration

- All substances produced or imported in quantities of one ton or more per year will have to be registered in a central database.

- Registration is not required for substances produced and imported in quantities less than one ton, substances for use in research activities, and polymers.
- Information required will be proportional to production volumes and risks.

Evaluation

- Two types of evaluations: dossiers and substances; European member states' competent authorities can carry out evaluations of substances when they have justified reasons that there is a risk to human health or the environment.

Authorization

- Authorization will be required for highly problematic substances: CMRs (carcinogenic, mutagenic or toxic to reproduction), PBTs (persistent, bio-accumulative and toxic), vPvBs (very persistent and very bio-accumulative) and other substances with serious and irreversible effects on humans and the environment.
- Authorization will be granted to these substances if risks can be adequately controlled or on valid socioeconomic grounds if there are no technologic alternatives.

Administrative Agency

A European Chemicals Agency will be established to manage the registration database; it will also play a role in the evaluation and authorization. The new Agency will be located in Helsinki, Finland.

8) Creating Europe-wide management of the program.
9) Creating standard classifications for toxicity: carcinogens, mutagens, reproductive toxins, and respiratory sensitizers.
10) Creating Internet access to all of the above mentioned information with provisions to protect confidentiality.

Environmental health risks across settings

Individual environmental health assessment should take into account all of the potential exposures that persons may have in their homes, workplaces, schools and community. Many risks can occur in more than one setting; for example, pesticides, lead, carbon monoxide, and tobacco smoke may occur in any of these settings.

IX Environmental Health Risks in the Home
A Home environments can be affected by the following:
   1. Building products (e.g., urea formaldehyde insulation, asbestos, lead-based paint, lead pipes, lead solder, and copper chromated arsenate [for pressure treated wood])
   2. Heating, ventilation, and air conditioning (e.g., carbon monoxide, mold)
   3. Consumer products (e.g., aerosols, nail polish remover [acetone], air fresheners, and dry-cleaned clothes)
   4. Cleaning products (e.g., ammonia, chlorine)
   5. Arts/hobby activities (e.g., glues, paints, leaded solder for stained glass)
   6. Pesticides (both indoor use and outdoor use that is tracked into the home)
   7. Furnishings, including carpets
   8. Renovation and rehabilitation activities (e.g., paint removers, adhesives, and other volatile organic compounds)
   9. Contaminants that are taken home from workplaces
   10. Inappropriately handled, stored, and disposed household hazardous materials
   11. Pests (cockroaches, fleas, ticks, rodents, and dust mites)
   12. Environmental tobacco smoke
   13. Personal care products
   14. Engaging in energy conservation

B Lead in homes poses a serious hazard to family members; most often the source is lead-based paint.
   1. Fifty-two million American homes have some lead-based paint in their homes.
   2. Dust emanating from lead-based paint poses a major threat to our nation's children.
   3. Over 1 million children have elevated blood lead levels in the United States. Lead poisoning is the most preventable of the environmentally-related, childhood diseases.
   4. There are a wide array of local, state, and federal statutes and regulations regarding lead-based paint poisoning from both the housing inspection/remediation perspective and the health screening/treatment perspective.
   5. Lead-based paint was banned from indoor use in 1978.
   6. The symptoms of lead poisoning are varied; they include neurologic deficits (affecting both the peripheral and central nervous systems), renal damage,

hypertension, and reproductive problems (in both males and females). The symptoms can be permanent.

7. There is no cure for lead poisoning, only prevention and palliative care.

C **Pesticides are associated with multiple health effects.**

1. Pesticides are formulated to either kill an organism (microorganism, fungi, insect, rodent, plant) or hinder its reproduction.

2. Most pesticides in common household and agricultural use have not been fully tested for their potential to harm humans, especially their effects during the varying stages of human development (e.g., fetal, child, etc.).

3. Regular indoor or outdoor use of pesticides increases the risk of leukemia to children who reside in the home.

4. There is an association between exposure to commercially applied agricultural pesticides during a crucial period in fetal development and the likelihood of fetal death due to congenital defects.

5. Some pesticides have estrogenic properties or are otherwise endocrine disrupting; are reproductive toxicants (for males and/or females); are known to be neurotoxic; are associated with birth defects; and/or are associated with asthma.

6. Pesticide "foggers" often have persistent active ingredients that take up residence in textiles such as stuffed animals, pillows, and other items with which children may have close contact.

7. Pesticides applied to produce may pose a threat to health.

8. The 1996 Food Quality Protection Act addresses health risks associated with pesticide residues on and in food.

D **Many indoor air contaminants (chemical and biologic) can trigger asthmatic events; biologic contaminants include bacteria, mold and mildew, mites, animal hair and dander, and pollen.**

1. The Centers for Disease Control has calculated that over 5 million people under the age of 18 are affected by asthma in the United States.

2. Although genetic factors are involved, environmental factors are almost certainly responsible for the increase in asthma over the past two decades.

3. Common indoor triggers include second-hand smoke, dust mites, cockroach feces and exoskeleton dust, mold, and pets. Outdoor triggers include ozone, nitrogen oxides, diesel exhaust, and pollen. Many studies demonstrate that different constituents of air pollution can trigger asthma attacks.

4. In addition, infections, occupational exposures, some drugs (such as aspirin), and sulfites (food additives used in dried fruit, wine, dehydrated potato products, shrimp, etc.) can trigger asthma attacks.

E **Many other precautions can be taken to decrease homeowners' risks for environmental exposures.**

1. Because of high risk associated with radon, all homes should be tested for radon and, if indicated, remediated.

2. Environmental tobacco smoke is associated with a wide array of health problems. Smokers should quit or smoke outside, especially if children reside in the home.

3. Drinking water derived from private wells should be tested annually to determine its fitness for drinking.

4. Carbon monoxide detectors should be installed.

5. Furnaces and gas combustion appliances should be regularly serviced.

BOX 6-4

Integrated pest management (IPM)

IPM is a managed pest management system that:
- Eliminates or mitigates economic and health damage caused by pests.
- Minimizes the use of pesticides and the risk to human health and the environment associated with pesticide applications.
- Uses integrated methods, site or pest inspections, pest population monitoring, an evaluation of the need for pest control, and one or more pest control methods, including sanitation, structural repairs, mechanical and living biologic controls, other nonchemical methods, and, if nontoxic options are unreasonable and have been exhausted, least toxic pesticides.

(As defined by Beyond Pesticides/NCAMP on their website: http://www.beyondpesticides/infoservices/pcos/IPM.htm The EPA calls for the use of IPM in schools. Different approaches to IPM can be used in different settings, such as homes, agricultural practices, and schools.

---

6. Wood that has not been treated with copper chromated arsenate should be used for construction and household projects.
7. An integrated pest management (IPM) approach should be used when controlling pests. (IPM is an approach that considers the food, water, and breeding needs of a pest(s); it also employs the least toxic interventions (see Box 6-4).

X Environmental Risks in Schools

A On any given school day, one sixth of the U.S. population can be found in a school building.

B School environments provide many of the same risks as home environments from indoor air contaminants.
1. Schools are more likely to use industrial-strength cleaners and pest control measures that can create health risks for children.
2. Some schools have moved to the IPM approach to pest control (Box 6-4).
3. Safe and adequate drinking water and sanitary facilities are an issue in some schools.
4. The location of schools is an issue as less land becomes available for necessary school expansions in urban and even suburban areas. Expanding school property onto land with previous usage can create risks if the soil is contaminated.
5. Attention to indoor air quality in schools (particularly mold issues) is heightened by the increasing rates of children with asthma.

C Many schools, including those that are expressly vocational training schools, mimic workplaces; automotive programs, arts and science rooms, cosmetology programs, construction shops, and photography darkrooms present risks similar to their industrial counterparts.
1. As such, OSHA standards should be met and the industrial hygiene hierarchy of controls should be applied to protect students, teachers, and school staff members from unhealthy exposures.

2. It should be recognized that children can be even more vulnerable to exposures.

D Carpeting can be the source of chemical and biologic contaminants. It is advisable to either have easily cleaned surfaces, such as tile flooring, or to have a rigorous cleaning program for carpeting to minimize unhealthy exposures.

XI Environmental Risks in the Community

A Environmental health risks in the community may derive from unhealthy air, water, or soil.

1. The Clean Air Act regulates air pollution from fixed sites and non-point (mobile) sources
2. The EPA has established six Criteria Pollutants that are used to define air quality under the National Ambient Air Quality Standards:
   a. Sulfur dioxide is produced during combustion and industrial processes.
      1) Sulfur dioxide is a major contributor to acid rain.
      2) It is associated with respiratory illness, alterations in pulmonary function, aggravation of existing cardiovascular disease, and asthma.
   b. Nitrous dioxide is produced during combustion; it affects the lungs, immune function, and asthma.
   c. Carbon monoxide is produced during the burning of fossil fuel.
      1) Carbon monoxide is substantially produced by motor vehicles.
      2) Carbon monoxide binds very effectively with hemoglobin, precluding the binding of oxygen, which results in anoxia; the most sensitive population are those with cardiovascular diseases.
   d. Particulate matter consists of liquid and solid aerosols from fuel combustion, motor vehicle exhaust, high temperature industrial processes, and incineration.
      1) Particulate matter includes dust, dirt, soot, smoke, and liquid droplets.
      2) The lungs are a prime site for damage and exacerbation of underlying disease; the size of the particle determines the deposition in the lungs.
   e. Lead in the aerosolized particulate matter is from industrial processes and incineration; lead is toxic to the nervous, immune, cardiovascular, and reproductive systems, as well as damaging to heme synthesis and to the kidneys.
   f. Ozone is an odorless, colorless gas composed of three atoms of oxygen. Ozone occurs both in the Earth's upper atmosphere and at ground level. Ozone can be good or bad, depending on where it is found. Ozone is categorized as "good" ozone or "bad" ozone.
      1) The "good" ozone occurs at a layer in the stratosphere about 10-25 miles above the earth, and it serves to protect us from the most damaging UV rays. It has been damaged significantly by chlorofluorocarbons (CFCs).
      2) The "bad" ozone is ground level ozone that is created by reaction of hydrocarbons, which include volatile organic compounds (VOCs) and nitrogen oxides in the presence of sunlight.
         • The VOCs are emitted from a wide range of sources: dry cleaners, cars, chemical manufacturers, paint shops, and many others.
         • The prime target organ for ozone is the lung, where it causes damage, diminishes lung function, and sensitizes the lung to other irritants.

- The burning of fossil fuel (e.g., in diesel engines, industrial boilers, and power plants) and waste incineration are two other major contributors.
    3) Bad, ground-level (manmade) ozone can irritate the respiratory system, aggravate asthma, reduce lung function, and inflame and damage the lung epithelium.
3. Health effects associated with air pollution include asthma and other respiratory diseases, cardiovascular diseases (including hypertension), cancer, immunologic effects, reproductive health problems (including birth defects), and neurologic problems.
4. Adverse health effects have been found at levels below the EPA air quality standards. The elderly and those with chronic pulmonary and/or vascular diseases appear to be at increased risk for mortality from short-term increases in both indoor and outdoor air pollution.
5. There are a range of persistent bioaccumulative toxics (PBTs) that are airborne during some part of their "fate and transport" from agricultural use or industrial processes, or as unintentional by-products of industrial and other processes.
    a. The U.N. has identified 12 particularly toxic chemicals in its Stockholm Treaty, calling for their ban for ways in which to diminish their occurrence. The Stockholm Treaty is sometimes referred to as the POPs –(persistent organic pollutants) Treaty. The new term, *persistent bioaccumulative toxins* (PBTs), is also associated with this treaty.
    b. Eight of the 12 toxic chemicals are pesticides: aldrin, chlordane, DDT, dieldrin, endrin, heptachlor, hexachlorobenzene, and mirex. The other four include two industrial and two industrial by-products resulting from industrial processes and waste incineration (including medical waste incineration).
        1) Incinerated hospital waste is a major source of dioxin in the United States because of the heavy reliance on polyvinyl chlorides in the health care industry.
        2) These carcinogens are also endocrine disrupters, and are considered by the EPA to be reproductive toxicants.
    c. Coal-fired power plants are the greatest source of mercury pollution.

B **Industrial sites (old and current) are sources of air, water, and soil contamination.**
1. Such sites may be designated Brownfields or Superfund sites.
    a. *Brownfields* are abandoned, idled, or underused industrial and commercial facilities where expansion or redevelopment is complicated by real or perceived environmental contamination (EPA definition).
    b. *Superfund* hazardous waste sites are sites that have been identified by the EPA as the most seriously contaminated in the nation. The National Priorities List (NPL) is a compilation of the most serious sites that are targeted for cleanup under Superfund.
2. The Superfund and Brownfield designations are derived from federal and state environmental statutes and are applied when a site is environmentally compromised and creating a health risk.
3. Under both Superfund and Brownfields laws, community members have the right to know and the right to involvement in the assessment phase, selection of remediation, and involvement in reuse decision, as well as any long-term monitoring for the site.

C Safe and reliable drinking water is a basic requirement.

1. Approximately half of the country derives its drinking water from groundwater (via wells), and the other half from surface water (reservoirs, lakes, and rivers).

2. Public water suppliers must test their final water product for approximately 80 EPA-designated contaminants as per the Safe Drinking Water Act.
   a. The results of testing must be reported to consumers annually.
   b. There is no federal regulation requiring individual residents to test their personal wells from which they derive their drinking water (though it is recommended to do so).

3. Our drinking water sources (both ground and surface) may be contaminated by industrial waste streams, waste injection, pesticides, or fertilizer run-off. Superfund sites often cause groundwater contamination. The most common groundwater contaminant from Superfund sites is trichloroethylene, a carcinogen.

4. Each state must have a plan for protecting its sources of drinking water.

5. The U.S. Geologic Service has measured acetaminophen, caffeine, codeine, and 17-b estradiol in our nation's streams.
   a. These are derived primarily from human waste.
   b. In addition, antibiotics have been measured in aquifers near hog "factories" and concentrated animal feed organizations (factory farms or intensive livestock production operations that are owned by large corporations).

6. Some drinking water contaminants can be naturally occurring, such as radon and arsenic.

7. Some drinking water contaminants occur cyclically with the use of agricultural chemicals, such as atrazine-contaminated groundwater during the growing season. Atrazine is an herbicide used to kill weeds, primarily on farms, but has also been used on highway and railroad rights-of-way. It has been observed in animals to cause liver, kidney, and heart damage. The EPA now restricts how atrazine can be used and applied; only trained people are allowed to spray it.

8. Leaking chemical storage tanks (both above ground and underground) pose hazards to the soil and groundwater, almost always associated with the potential for human health risks.

9. When selecting a water treatment option, such as a filtration system for home use, it is essential to first determine the contaminants that are present in the water (i.e., pathogenic microbes, heavy metals, VOCs) and *then* choose a treatment system that will remedy your specific problem.

D Global warming is an international concern.

1. The earth's temperature is rising as a function of accumulated, manmade "greenhouse" gases, including carbon monoxide, methane, and nitrous oxide.

2. The earth's temperature has risen .6 degrees Celsius since 1800 and is projected to rise between 1.4 and 5.8 degrees C. in the next 100 years. This projection includes climatic changes and the associated rising of sea level.

3. The United Nations–sponsored Kyoto Agreement calls for international cooperation in cutting greenhouse emissions by employing cleaner technologies. Russia has recently signed on to the agreement, as have most industrialized countries; however, the United States has not.

E **Agricultural and food production practices can result in health threats.**

   1. The use of pesticides in plant production can leave potentially hazardous residues on fruits and vegetables.
   2. Much of the meat and poultry in the United States is treated with antibiotics.
       a. More than 50% of the antibiotics sold in the United States are used in animal feed to improve animal growth, not for disease prophylaxis.
       b. Many of the antibiotics are similar to or the same as the ones used for the treatment of human infections.
       c. Antibiotics are being detected in soil and water.
       d. This use of antibiotics in animal feed for the purpose of growth promotion may lead to the development of antibiotic-resistant strains of bacteria that could threaten human and animal health; well over half the beef and pork in the United States is raised by using subclinical doses of antibiotics.
       e. No labeling is required to let consumers know whether antibiotics have been used in their meats or poultry.
   3. In 1990, the Organic Foods Production Act was passed to establish national standards governing the marketing of certain agricultural products to assure consumers that products labeled as "organic" meet a consistent standard and to facilitate commerce in organically produced fresh and processed food.
   4. Supersized farms, such as the concentrated animal feed organizations (CAFOs)—particularly for raising hogs—create a range of environmental challenges, such as huge animal waste ponds that are sufficiently hazardous to be regulated by the EPA.
       a. Farming operations of this scale threaten the local ecology and are not sustainable.
       b. In recent decades an alarming number of smaller, sustainable farms (mostly family farms) have been lost and replaced by these very large farming operations.
   5. Herbicides, pesticides, and fertilizers that are used in home gardens and in agricultural settings can leach into the groundwater and/or run off onto surface water. This can result in contamination of drinking water sources, compromise recreational waters, and contaminate and injure the flora and fauna that reside in the water.
   6. The use of fertilizers near waterways can cause runoff that results in eutrification—the result of an imbalance of nutrients in the water. Such eutrification is thought to contribute to algae blooms, such as the *Pfiesteria* that threatens human and ecologic health.
   7. Use of genetically modified organisms in agriculture is a controversial subject. The unfolding of this issue merits vigilance for environmental health nurses.
   8. Many of the persistent organic compounds, such as dioxins and several pesticides that contaminate the air and water, are found at detectable levels in the fatty tissues of beef, pork, and poultry and in dairy products.
   9. Advocating for organic foods that have been grown in a sustainable manner is a sound public health approach.

F **Fish also contain many of the pollutants that wind up in the water.**

   1. Mercury is of particular concern, especially in large fish that are high on the food chain, such as tuna and swordfish.

2. The EPA and the FDA both have fish alerts for women of child-bearing ages, counseling them to limit their fish consumption of certain fish to one portion a week.

XII Industrial Pollutants

A Industrial exposures of concern to surrounding communities include potentially hazardous chemicals that are emitted into the air and water and may be a source of environmental degradation and/or health threat within a community.

B Occupational and environmental health nurses can serve a vital role in protecting communities that have industrial sites.
1. Sharing the company's planning efforts for anticipated and accidental chemical releases will create better communications and trust with the community.
2. Occupational and environmental health nurses should establish relationships with public health, school nurses, and other nurses in the community to promote communication regarding industrial activities that may pose a health risk to the surrounding community.
3. Occupational and environmental health nurses should serve on state and local emergency planning committees (which are required in every jurisdiction in the United States by federal statute), state source-water protection planning boards (for drinking water protection), state environmental justice commissions (at least 20 states have one), and other public forums regarding environmental health protection.

C Information regarding chemical releases from industrial sites is available via the Environmental Defense web site: http://www.scorecard.org./.

D The EPA provides information collected by its Toxic Release Inventory database via the EPA web site: http://www.epa.gov./

Nurses' roles in environmental health

The following section describes findings and recommendations from the Institute of Medicine report, *Nursing, Health and the Environment* (IOM, 1995). These recommendations are directed to all nurses and should be considered essential minimal competencies for all nurses practicing in the field of occupational and environmental health.

XIII General Environmental Health Competency for Nurses

All nurses should have the following competencies (IOM, 1995):

A Understand the scientific principles and underpinnings of the relationship between individuals or populations and the environment, including the following:
1. The basic mechanisms and pathways of exposure to environmental health hazards
2. Basic prevention and control strategies
3. The interdisciplinary nature of effective interventions
4. The role of research

B Assess and refer, using the following strategies:

1. Successfully completing an environmental health history
2. Recognizing potential environmental hazards and sentinel illnesses
3. Making appropriate referrals for conditions with probable environmental etiologies
4. Accessing and providing information to clients and communities, and locating referral sources

C Demonstrate knowledge of the role of advocacy (case and class), ethics, and risk communication in client care and community intervention with respect to the potential adverse effects of the environment on health.

D Understand the policy framework and major pieces of legislation and regulations related to environmental health.

XIV The Institute of Medicine's Recommendations on Nursing Practice, Education, Research, and Advocacy

A Environmental health should be reemphasized in the scope of responsibilities for nursing practice.

1. Resources to support environmental health content in nursing practice should be identified and made available.
2. Nurses should participate as members and leaders in interdisciplinary teams that address environmental health problems.
3. Communication should extend beyond counseling individual clients and families to facilitating the exchange of information on environmental hazards and community responses.
4. The concept of advocacy in nursing should be expanded to include advocacy on behalf of groups and communities, in addition to advocacy on behalf of individual clients and their families.
5. Research regarding the ethical implications of occupational and environmental health hazards should be conducted and findings incorporated into curricula and practice.

B Environmental health concepts should be incorporated into all levels of nursing education.

1. Environmental health content should be included in nursing licensure and certification examinations.
2. Expertise in various environmental health disciplines should be included in the education of nurses.
3. Environmental health content should be an integral part of lifelong learning and continuing education for nurses.
4. Professional associations, public agencies, and private organizations should provide more resources and educational opportunities to enhance environmental health awareness in nursing practice.

C Multidisciplinary and interdisciplinary research endeavors should be developed and implemented to build the knowledge base for nursing practice in environmental health.

1. The number of nurse researchers should be increased to build the knowledge base in environmental health as it relates to the practice of nursing.
2. Research priorities for environmental health nursing should be established and used by funding agencies for resource allocation decisions and to give direction to nurse researchers.

3. Current efforts to disseminate research findings to nurses, other health care providers, and the public should be strengthened and expanded.

D **Nurses should have the skills to work with the community, environmental groups, and local government, including the following activities:**
   1. Legislative lobbying
   2. Reporting community hazards
   3. Advocating for safer environments
   4. Policy implementation

E **Nurses can be involved with environmental health in other ways, such as the following:**
   1. Generating data systems for environmental assessment and outcomes, including supporting the National Children's Longitudinal Study and the efforts to create better health tracking
   2. Designing "critical paths" that include environmental assessment through incorporation of environmental health into history taking and "new client" information forms
   3. Conducting impact studies (e.g., consumer goods, land use) and intervention studies to develop an evidence base for environmental health nursing interventions
   4. Increasing the visibility of nurses in environmental health policy development and implementation by participating on governmental and nongovernmental advisory bodies, commissions, and boards; working with nursing lobbyists to affect legislative changes; working with nongovernmental organizations to develop and implement strategies for positive change; and working within our own institutions or companies to advocate for the best possible policies and practices
   5. Educating, of course, but also petitioning the political system for change. Laws can sometimes change behavior more effectively than public education (e.g., bike helmet and seat belt laws).
   6. Revolutionizing nursing education to focus more on environmental health, social justice, and critical thinking
   7. Serving as role models, and developing role expectations such that attention to environmental health is routine

REFERENCES

Agency for Toxic Substances and Disease Registry. (1992). *Taking an exposure history, Case studies in environmental health,* No. 26. Atlanta, GA: U.S. Department of Health and Human Services.

Consumer Reports. (1998). Hormone mimics hit home: Tests of plastic wraps, baby foods. *Consumer Report Online.* Available at http://www.consumerreports.org/special/consumerinterest/reports.

Environmental Protection Agency. (January, 1998). *Parent's guide to school indoor air quality.* Washington, DC: EPA.

Environmental Protection Agency. (1998). *Chemical hazard data availability study: What do we really know about the safety of high production volume chemicals?* Washington, DC: Office of Prevention, Pesticides and Toxic Substances. Available at http://www.epa.gov/opptintr/chemtest/hazchem.htm.

Institute of Medicine. (1995). *Nursing, health and the environment: Strengthening the relationship to improve the public's health.* Washington, DC: National Academy Press.

World Health Organization (WHO, 2005). Protection of human environment. Retrieved August 2005 from http://www.who.int/phe/en

Zenz, C. (1994). *Occupational medicine* (3rd ed.). St. Louis, MO: Mosby.

OTHER RESOURCES

Etzel, R. E., Balk, S. J., & the Committee on Environmental Health of the American Academy of Pediatricians. (1999). *Handbook of pediatric environmental health*. Elk Grove Village, IL: American Academy of Pediatrics.

Greater Boston Physicians for Social Responsibility and the Massachusetts Public Interest Research Group Education Fund (Greater Boston PSR and MASSPIRG). (1996). *Generations at risk: How environmental toxics may affect reproductive health in Massachusetts*. Cambridge, MA: PSR.

Lichtenstein, P., Holm, N. V., Kerkasalo, P. K., Iliadou, A., Kaprio, J., Koskenvuo, M., Pukkala, E., Skytthe, A., & Hemminki, K. (2000). Environmental and heritable factors in the causation of cancer, *New England Journal of Medicine. 343*, 78-84.

Sandman, P. (1993). *Responding to community outrage: Strategies for effective risk communication*. Fairfax, VA: AIHA Publications.

Schettler, T., Solomon, G., Valenti, M., & Huddle, A. (1999). *Generations at risk: Reproductive health and the environment*. Boston, MA: Massachusetts Institute of Technology.

Schettler, T., Stein, J., Reich, F., & Valenti, M. (2000). *In harm's way: Toxic threats to development*, a Report by Greater Boston Physicians for Social Responsibility (PSR), prepared for a joint project with Clean Water. Cambridge, MA: PSR.

Steingraber, S. (1997). *Living downstream: A scientist's personal investigation of cancer and the environment*. NY: Random House.

U.S. Department of Agriculture. (1998). *Agriculture fact book*. Washington DC: Office of Communications.

CHAPTER 7

Principles of Leadership and Management

Joy E. Wachs and Frances Childre

Occupational and environmental health nurses must have leadership and management skills to give the direction, provide the services, manage the resources, and document the outcomes related to worker health. As business and industry in America seek new solutions to the high cost of health care, these abilities enable occupational and environmental health nurse managers to promote, maintain, and restore the health of workers and positively affect corporate profits.

I Leadership

Leadership is the "desire and ability to influence others to set and achieve goals that represent the values and the motivations of both leader and followers" (Perra, 1999).

A Various leadership approaches are used in American business and industry.
1. *Tactical leadership* is demonstrated when a leader "clarifies the goal, convinces us that it is absolutely essential to achieve that goal, explains the plan and strategies, organizes and coordinates our activities, and deals aggressively with individual performance issues" (Crislip & Larson, 1994).
2. *Transactional leadership* occurs "when one person takes the initiative in making contact with others for the purpose of an exchange of valued things" (Burns, 1978).
3. *Collaborative leadership* involves a leader who can mobilize a diverse group to work with ambiguous issues and make sure the process is constructive and outcome driven (Crislip & Larson, 1994).
4. *Transformational leadership* is exemplified when "one or more persons engage with others in such a way that leaders and followers raise one another to higher levels of motivation and morality . . . ." (Burns, 1978).
5. *Servant leadership* occurs when the leader is servant first, "to make sure others' highest priority needs are being served" (Greenleaf, 1970).

B Leaders and followers have distinct but related responsibilities.
1. Leaders are responsible for the following (Depree, 1989):
   a. Defining what is (reality) and what could be (vision)
   b. Serving by enabling others to reach their potential
   c. Saying thank you for the opportunity to lead
2. Leaders need followers who demonstrate the following behaviors (Chaleff, 1998):

a. Assume responsibility through personal growth, passion, and risk-taking
b. Serve both the leader and the cause
c. Challenge themselves, the leader, and the group
d. Participate in transformation by being a catalyst, resource, and role model
e. If necessary, leave the organization to allow the organization and the follower to grow

C **Collins (2001) proposes five levels of organizational leadership.**
1. Level 1 *Highly Capable Individual*—Star employee who makes substantial contributions based on personal talents, effort, knowledge and skills.
2. Level 2 *Contributing Team Member*—Person who meets team goals by contributing individually and working well within the team.
3. Level 3 *Competent Manager*—Person who meets organizational goals by effectively organizing personnel and resources.
4. Level 4 *Executive Leader*—Person who motivates personnel to pursue a vision of what could be by performing at extraordinary levels.
5. Level 5 The *Executive*—Person who has the following qualities:
   a. Sets inspired performance standards
   b. Has ambition for his or her company(ies)
   c. Selects superb successors
   d. Wants the company to be more successful after his or her departure
   e. Takes responsibility for failure but give credit to others for success.

D **Leadership tasks include the following (Kouzes & Posner, 2003)**
1. Challenging the process to support innovation and change
2. Inspiring others to share a vision and see its exciting possibilities
3. Enabling others to act by building teams based on trust and respect
4. Modeling the way for others through personal example and dedicated execution
5. Encouraging the heart by recognizing individual and team achievements

E **Leadership requires vision and relationship (S. Chater, personal communication, 2005)**

II Vision

A **To develop a compelling vision requires creativity.**
1. Begin this process with idea immersion.
2. Allow the ideas to incubate.
3. Often this process comes to fruition when least expected.
4. The most important step in the creative process is implementing the innovation.

B **A vision is the result of a core ideology and an envisioned future (Collins & Porras, 2000).**
1. Core ideology defines what the organization represents and why the organization exists.
   a. Core values are "a system of guiding principles and tenets with intrinsic value and importance" (p. 66)
   b. Core purpose is "the organization's most fundamental reason for existence, which reflects people's idealistic motivations for doing the company's work" (p. 68)

2. Envisioned future defines what the company aspires to become, to achieve, to create—something that will require significant change and progress to attain.

   a. Big Hairy Audacious Goals (BHAG) are compelling, unifying, and engaging and require 10 to 30 years to accomplish.

   b. The vivid description paints a picture of what the company, community or world will be like when the BHAG is reached.

III Relationship

A *Organizational culture* **is "a long-term, complex phenomenon" arising from "a combination of the founders, past leadership, current leadership, crises, events, history and size," resulting in "routines, rituals and the 'way we do things'" (Clark, 2000, pp. 6-7).**

1. "Collective vision and common folklore" are a reflection of culture (Clark, 2000, p. 7).

2. Culture influences climate by impacting leaders' ideas and actions.

3. Paradigms explaining the origin of organizational culture include the following (Zamanou & Glaser, 1994):

   a. Fundamentalist: "Organizations *produce* culture."

   b. Interpretive: "Organizations *are* culture" because they are the product of interaction among people.

B *Organizational climate* **is "a short-term phenomenon created by the current leadership" and represents workers' "shared perceptions, beliefs and attitudes" (Clark, 2000, pp. 6-7).**

1. Individual and team motivation and satisfaction are influenced by what workers believe about the organization and its leadership.

2. Organizational culture and organizational climate are distinct concepts.

   a. *Organizational culture* is an anthropologic concept, is highly enduring, emerges from a historical context, is often held in workers' unconscious, and influences the organization's climate (Moran & Volkwein, 1992).

   b. *Organizational climate* is a concept of social psychology, is relatively enduring, is mediated by the organization's internal and external environments, is held in the awareness of workers, and is a manifestation of the organization's culture (Moran & Volkwein, 1992).

C **Emotional intelligence is demonstrated by how leaders handle themselves and their relationships (Goleman, 1995; Goleman, 1998; Goleman, Boyatzis & McKee, 2002).**

1. Emotional intelligence is at least as important to quality leadership as is cognitive intelligence, perhaps more so.

2. Leaders with emotional intelligence have:

   a. The drive to achieve results

   b. The ability to take initiative

   c. The skills to collaborate and lead teams

3. There are two components to emotional intelligence: personal competence and social competence.

   a. Leaders who are *personally competent* are self-aware, meaning they can read their own emotions and know their strengths and limitations as well as their self-worth and capabilities; additionally, leaders with personal competence have self-management skills, including emotional self control; clear, honest and trustworthy actions; adaptability; achievement; initiative; and optimism.

b. Leaders with *social competence* have empathy, organizational awareness, and a commitment to service; socially competent leaders also possess the ability to inspire and influence others, work collaboratively, offer others development opportunities, have a network of relationships, are a catalyst for change and elegantly resolve conflicts.

4. Many of these competencies are needed in the strategic planning and change processes.

IV Strategic Planning

Strategic (long-range) planning sets the course for the organization.

A **A clearly articulated vision results in the development of purpose, mission, and goals.**

1. The vision, philosophy, mission statement, goals, and objectives of occupational health services should reflect those of the greater organization (Yoder-Wise, 1999).

2. Vision statements describe the future of the organization and provide a context for the philosophy and mission statements (Yoder-Wise, 1999).

3. The philosophy in an occupational health unit should articulate the following:
   a. The inherent worth of individual workers to the company
   b. A commitment to quality care based on standards of nursing practice
   c. An expectation that nursing practice be research-based
   d. An emphasis on health-promotion and risk-reduction services
   e. An emphasis on continuing education and appropriate certifications

4. The mission aims to promote, protect, and restore the health of workers.

5. Goals and objectives clarify the essential actions necessary to achieving the philosophy and mission (Yoder-Wise, 1999), such as programs and services provided and resources used.

6. The philosophy, mission, goals, and objectives need to be developed by management and staff of the health unit, approved by upper management, and revised periodically to fit the ever-changing business environment.

B **The strategic planning process must accomplish the following (Yoder-Wise, 1999):**

1. Assess the internal and external environments
2. Identify strengths and weaknesses as well as threats and opportunities
3. Identify strategies
4. Implement prioritized strategies
5. Evaluate activities and outcomes

C **The goals of strategic planning include the following (Yoder-Wise, 1999):**

1. Improved likelihood of success in achieving goals and outcomes
2. Effective and efficient use of resources
3. Creative vision for the future direction of the occupational health unit

D **Planned change can be approached from a linear or nonlinear frame of reference (Yoder-Wise, 1999).**

1. *Linear change* is a systematic process used in organizations to facilitate needed, semi-permanent change through mutual goal setting between worker and the change agent (Lewin, 1951).

a. The role of the occupational and environmental health nurse as an agent for change includes the following:
   1) Identifying problems
   2) Assessing the forces that will drive or restrain the change
   3) Determining costs and benefits of the change
   4) Establishing a helping relationship with management and workers
   5) Ensuring that the change will last until it is time to change again
   b. Planned change may relate to programs, services, staffing, facilities, cost containment, or health outcomes of workers.

2. Chaos theory and learning organization theory are examples of nonlinear change models (Wheatley, 1992; Senge, 2000).
   a. Organizations are analogous to living organisms, not to machines that can be controlled linearly (Senge, 2000).
   b. People in organizations "seek to create a world in which (they) can thrive" by working from the inside, identifying needs, applying experience and perceptions, enlisting support, and creating their own solutions (Wheatley, 1999, p. 153).

V Management Theories: Historical Perspective

A **Management theories are statements predicting which actions will lead to what results—and why (Christensen & Raynor, 2003).**
1. Research and theory can provide guidance and direction to managers.
2. In management research, breakthroughs in predictability occur when researchers identify the causal mechanism that ties actions to results, and describe the circumstances in which that mechanism does and does not result in success (Christensen & Raynor, 2003).
3. A theory that helps one manager succeed can be fatal for another operating under different conditions. Good theories are contingent on circumstances (Christensen & Raynor, 2003).

B **Management theories were first articulated in the early 1900s.**
1. Key theorists were Frederick W. Taylor, Frank and Lillian Gilbreth, and Henry Gantt (Sullivan & Decker, 1997; Allen, 1998).
   a. Taylor's definitive studies examined the time and motion details of a job to increase worker productivity.
   b. The Gilbreths focused on dividing work into its fundamental elements in order to streamline the process as a whole.
   c. Gantt focused on motivational schemes, emphasizing the greater effectiveness of incentives for good work. He also developed the Gantt chart, which is used to schedule overlapping tasks over a specified time period.
2. The 1900s were a period of scientific management.

C **Management theories in the 1920s were characterized by bureaucracy and universalism.**
1. *Bureaucracy* was promoted as the most rational structure for large organizations (Allen, 1998).
2. *Universalism* was a process approach to management, encompassing: planning, organizing, commanding, coordinating and controlling (University of Glamorgan, 1999; 2001).
3. Key theorists during this period were Max Weber and Henri Fayol.
   a. Max Weber, known as the father of modern sociology, analyzed social stratification and how it applied to power and bureaucracy (Allen, 1998).

    b. Henri Fayol promoted principles of management that were primarily task oriented, the most important being specialization of labor, unity of command and line of authority (Analytictech.com, 2005).

4. During this period, hierarchies of supervisors and managers provided direction to workers (chain of command) and workers were expected to obey supervisors, be loyal to the organization, and be rewarded for production (Sullivan & Decker, 1997).

D **The 1930s was a period that focused on human relations.**

1. A key management theorist was George Elton Mayo, known as the father of the Hawthorne studies; these experiments identified the bias that occurs when people know that they are being studied (Allen, 1998).

2. Work was considered a group activity and social interaction was viewed as important; it was believed that people worked well if they felt valued (University of Glamorgan, 1999; 2001; Accel-Team, 2004).

E **Management theories in the 1950s focused on motivation.**

1. Abraham Maslow, a key theorist of this period, researched human behavior and developed the hierarchy of needs (Accel-Team, 2004).

    a. Maslow ranked these needs in order of importance: physiological, safety, love, esteem, and self-actualization.

    b. Management reward systems were developed to satisfy these needs.

2. Frederick Herzberg, another key theorist, developed the hygiene theory (Accel-Team, 2004).

    a. This theory stated that the worker's environment, such as physical surroundings, can cause a worker to feel dissatisfied with his job; for a worker to be happy, the physical surroundings cannot cause discomfort.

    b. Satisfaction with the job environment leads to the higher motivators: achievement, recognition, growth/advancement, and interest in the job.

F **During the 1960s, several behaviorist theories were introduced.**

1. Douglas McGregor introduced Theory X and Theory Y (Grohar-Murray & DiCroce, 1992).

    a. In Theory **X,** people intensely dislike working and must be "coerced, controlled, and directed" by management in doing the work required.

    b. In Theory **Y,** people enjoy work and are "self-directed, responsible, and capable of solving their own problems."

2. Chris Argyris (1960) focused on organizational and individual goals and values and posited that if humanistic values are adhered to, trusting, authentic relationships will develop, increasing interpersonal competence, inter-group cooperation, and flexibility, resulting in increased organizational effectiveness (Accel-Team, 2004).

3. Rensis Likert (1967) conducted much research on human behavior and posed that the organization making the greatest use of human capacity is one that has "highly effective work groups linked together in an overlapping pattern by other similarly effective groups" (Accel-Team, 2004).

    a. He identified a continuum of management systems that included exploitive-authoritative, benevolent-authoritative, consultative, and participative-group.

    b. The Likert scale is a rating method that uses a continuum from "strongly agree" to "strongly disagree," or "always" to "never" that is frequently used in studies and in evaluation surveys.

4. Edgar Schein (1961) is one of the pioneers of the concept of corporate culture; he is particularly well known for his work on motivation and the "psychological contract"; i.e., the understandings that exist between employer and employee and vice versa (Emerald, 2000).

5. Victor Vroom (1964) developed expectancy theory, which is a mathematical model that focuses workers' motivation: workers believe there is a positive correlation between efforts and performance, favorable performance results in a desirable reward, the reward satisfies an important need, and the need is strong enough to make the effort worthwhile (Green, 2000).

G **During the 1970s, there was a focus on the concepts of strategic management (University of Glamorgan, 1999).**

1. Strategic management included setting measurable objectives for staff and assessing achievement, decentralization, managing in turbulent times and competitive advantage.

2. The term *management by objectives* became popular during this time.

H **During the 1980s, empirical approaches emerged.**

1. William Ouchi (1981) developed Theory Z, a method that combined American and Japanese managing practices.

2. The centerpiece of Theory Z are the concepts of "collective decision making, long-term employment, slower promotions, indirect supervision, and holistic concern for employees" (Tappen, 1989).

I **Contemporary theories of management attempt to explain and interpret the rapidly changing nature of the current business environment.**

1. Contingency Theory "asserts that when managers make a decision, they must take into account all aspects of the current situation and act on those aspects that are key to the situation at hand" (McNamara, 1999).

2. Systems Theory suggests that a system has inputs, processes, outputs and outcomes. Systems share feedback among each of these four aspects and recognize the interrelations of the parts, for example, coordination of engineering with manufacturing, supervisors with workers (McNamara, 1999).

3. Chaos Theory suggests that systems naturally go toward more complexity, and as they do, they become more susceptible to cataclysmic events, and must expend more energy and build structure to maintain the complexity, thus making them susceptible to a system split, combining with another system or disintegration (McNamara, 1999).

4. Business Process Reengineering (BPR) focuses on redesigning work processes in an effort to reduce specific resource needs and the work force with an ultimate reduction in overhead costs (DeCock & Hipkin, 1997).

5. Total Quality Management is a model of customer-supplier relationship that helps establish requirements and increase customer satisfaction. There are five pillars of quality: customer focus, total involvement, measurement, systematic support, and continuous improvement (Organizational Dynamics, 1991).

6. Empowerment proposes that workers are authorized to do their work without the need to seek approval from their supervisor.

VI The Management Process

A The *management process* is a sequence of steps or a course of action that operationalizes how leaders exert influence (Wenek, 2003).

B The Task Cycle® is a useful framework for the management process, because it relates competencies to operational performance and interpersonal relations.

C The Task Cycle® is "a logical sequence of steps essential to directing the performance of tasks" consisting of six phases (Wilson, 1990):
1. Making goals clear and important
2. Planning and problem solving
3. Facilitating the work of others
4. Obtaining and providing feedback
5. Monitoring and adjusting the process
6. Reinforcing performance

The following sections describe these six phases of the Task Cycle® in detail.

VII Phase 1 of Task Cycle®: *Making Goals Clear and Important*

A Managers operationalize the leader's mission and vision into measurable goals.
1. Goal-setting must be realistic, yet challenging; enthusiastic, yet disciplined.
2. Qualities of a good goal are: S.M.A.R.T., P.U.R.E AND C.L.E.A.R (Box 7-1).

B *End goals* serve as the final objective to be achieved.
1. These goals are in alignment with the organizational mission, vision, and purpose. They provide the inspiration.
2. End goals are collective goals and do not lend themselves to individual control (Whitmore, 2002).

C *Performance goals* also need to be established.
1. The performance goal defines the specifications for achieving the end goal.
2. Identifying the performance level that gives a high probability of reaching the end goal is largely within the manager's control and provides a means of measuring progress (Whitmore, 2002).

D End goals and performance goals should be communicated as part of the leadership vision, using all means available (Kotter, 1995).
1. In routine communication about a business problem, discuss how proposed solutions do or do not support the goals.
2. Use department meetings to relate progress on goals as part of an exciting overall vision.

BOX 7-1
Qualities of an effective goal

Specific	Positive	Challenging
Measurable	Understood	Legal
Attainable	Relevant	Environmentally Sound
Realistic	Ethical	Agreed
Time-Phased		Recorded

Source: Whitmore, 2002

3. In regular coaching sessions, discuss how an employee's behavior helps or hinders goals
4. Use newsletters, meetings, and internal management courses as mechanisms to communicate goals.
5. "Walk the talk." Consciously attempt to model behavior that supports the goals.

E The goals need to be translated into results by the following (Forsberg, 1996):
1. Meeting the established timelines
2. Implementing action steps needed to achieve the goals
3. Eliminating barriers to achievement
4. Optimizing the mix of personnel who contribute to the achieving results

VIII Phase 2 of Task Cycle®: *Planning and Problem-Solving*

A The generic task for the planning and problem-solving phase is to determine "How do I do it?"
1. Planning is developing a strategy and schedule (action steps) for meeting goals.
2. Problem solving involves analyzing circumstances or factors, and the issues they create, which affect whether goals are successfully met.
3. The skill set for this phase includes project management, budgeting, critical thinking, and decision-making.

B *Project Management* is the process of planning and managing project tasks and resources, and communicating the progress and the results (Perce, 1998).
1. A project is a set of activities that has a starting point, an end point, and performance criteria expectations for a specific outcome; it often has time and budget constraints (Eichenberger, 1997; Perce, 1998).
2. Project management is "getting the job done on time, within budget, and according to specifications" (Eichenberger, 1997). Tools to enhance efficiency of projects include:
   a. Work breakdown structure—a visual representation of each task
   b. Gantt chart—a list of tasks on the y axis plotted against time on the x axis
   c. Critical Path Method Program Evaluation and Review Technique (CPM/PERT chart)—identifies the sequence of activities that require the greatest expected amount of time (Perce, 1998)
3. Problem analysis methods include (Perce, 1998):
   a. Gap analysis to analyze and identify the gap between project plans and results
   b. Fishbone diagram, which is a display of all the causes of the problem (the ribs of the fish) and the effect of the problem (the fish's head)
   c. Pareto chart, which is a series of bars whose heights reflect the frequency or impact of causes of problems
   d. Pie chart, which displays the causes of a problem once it has been identified
4. Problem solving is focused on trying to solve the immediate problem identified: "the gap between "what is" and "what should be"" (Yoder-Wise, 1999); the problem-solving process includes the following steps:
   a. Defining the problem with adequate, creative, new or alternative definitions and representations

    b. Gathering and analyzing data

    c. Developing multiple possible solutions

    d. Selecting a solution

    e. Implementing the solution

    f. Evaluating the outcome

    g. Possibly further trials of other potential solutions

    h. Adopting the answer to the problem

C *Budgeting* **is part of a management control process for allocating financial resources for a given time period. The occupational health unit manager has the primary responsibility for controlling the occupational health unit budget.**

1. Budgets usually fall within one of three categories: operating, capital expenditure, and financial budgets.

    a. *Operating budgets* consist of a forecast of expected revenues and expenses, presumably under efficient operations (Kaplan & Norton,, 2000).

    b. *Capital expenditure budgets* portray the organization's planned and approved capital expenditures for a period from one to ten years; e.g., equipment or facility renovation.

    c. *Financial budgets* project cash flow statements, balance sheets and statements of sources and uses of funds (Barrett & Fraser, 1977).

2. Several methods can be used for budgeting.

    a. The *incremental or historical budget method* begins with the previous year's budget and adjusts each line item to fund existing programs and services; it is often tied to the inflation rate or another global financial measure.

        1) *Advantages:* the historical foundation requires little need to justify continuing services and programs; it works well in a stable environment.

        2) *Disadvantages:* resources may be lost if not used in a given year; thus there may be an incentive to overspend the budget to justify the need for increases the next year; it encourages lack of accountability and efficiency and it does not allow for budgeting of strategic initiatives.

    b. The *zero-based budget method* forecasts revenues and expenses solely on future events and expectations (Byrne, 2003); it requires annual justification for each program and service in terms of outcome and cost.

        1) *Advantages*: it requires annual analyses of all occupational health programs and services to evaluate their productivity and cost; it works well during times of rapid change or volatility (Byrne, 2003).

        2) *Disadvantage*s: extra time is required to produce the analyses and provide prioritized alternatives for each program and service.

D **The budgeting process includes the following steps:**

1. Analysis of historical data

    a. Was the previous fiscal plan adequate?

    b. Can any trends be identified?

    c. In what areas were there significant variances?

    d. Should previous budget allocations be redistributed?

2. Identification of needs or emerging trends that can positively or negatively affect the planned budget

    a. Are general market factors affecting the base cost of needed resources?

b. Is a change occurring (e.g., new technologies, expansion of worker base, new compliance regulations) that may require the allocation of additional resources or possibly reduce the cost of operations?

3. Developing operating assumptions, that is, defining expectations for the coming year and providing a framework for designing and selling the budget; assumptions should define either continuation of existing services or anticipated new services

4. Designing the budget according to the common language or format used in the company; operating budgets are typically organized into categories, such as:
   a. Materials and supplies
   b. Personnel/ staffing
   c. Benefits
   d. Contracted services; e.g., waste management, maintenance, Employees Assistance Programs, Third Party Administrator
   e. Programs, e.g., medical surveillance, health promotion

5. Selling the budget: The budget's fundamental rationale of needs and assumptions forms the basis for selling the plan to management; value can be demonstrated by using the following:
   a. Comparison of the costs of providing services in-house with the price of outsourcing to community providers
   b. Utilization statistics
   c. Return on investment in the form of calculating productivity saved by having health services on site (e.g., average salary of labor category times number of hours workers on average would use to seek health care off site)
   d. Case management productivity savings in early return to work

6. Monitoring and controlling the actual budget via variance analysis and critical performance reports. Pitfalls to controlling a planned budget include:
   a. Turnover of staff
   b. Unanticipated training needs
   c. Litigation
   d. Changes in regulatory requirements
   e. Unexpected budget cuts

E Other planning and problem-solving skills needed to lay a foundation for the management process include critical thinking, effective decision-making and ethical considerations.

1. *Critical thinking* is the "intellectually disciplined process of actively and skillfully conceptualizing, applying, analyzing, synthesizing, or evaluating information gathered from, or generated by, observation, experience, reflection, reasoning, or communication, as a guide to belief and action" (Paul, 1995).

2. Critical thinking links creativity to decision making and problem solving.

3. *Decision making* is "a purposeful and goal directed effort using a systematic process to choose among options" (Yoder-Wise, 1999); there are two broad approaches to decision making: inquiry and advocacy (Garvin & Roberto, 2001).
   a. "*Inquiry* is an open process designed to generate multiple alternatives, foster the exchange of ideas, and produce a well-tested solution."
   b. *Advocacy* is a process in which participants approach decision making as a contest. They are passionate about their preferred solutions and the goal is to present a compelling case.

4. The continuum of decision making may decision range from an independent decision to a group decision.
5. Whether an independent or group decision, it should be matched to the problem, time frame, and the level of group commitment.
6. Cognitive conflict can deliver high quality decisions (Garvin & Roberto, 2001).
7. Increasing cognitive conflict requires:
   a. Vigorous debate
   b. Prohibiting language that increases defensiveness
   c. Assigning people to tasks without consideration of traditional loyalties
   d. Shifting individuals out of well-worn grooves
   e. Challenging stalemated participants to revisit key information
8. The hallmark of decision making is "the identification and selection of options" (Yoder-Wise, 1999).
9. The incorporation of ethics into decision making can improve the functioning of an organization and ultimately can maximize corporate profits (Key & Popkin, 1998).
   a. The organization may wish to serve the following interests:
      1) Private interests (e.g., providing a healthy and safe work environment for all workers)
      2) Public interests (e.g., proper disposal of hazardous waste for the entire community)
   b. These identified interests should be analyzed in terms of moral, social, and legal responsibilities.
   c. Processes whereby an understanding of various interests and responsibilities become part of any decision making within the organization should be created (Key & Popkin, 1998).
10. The occupational and environmental health nurse manager has daily opportunities to incorporate ethics into decisions made regarding the health and safety of workers; examples include:
    a. Confidentiality of health-related documents and interactions
    b. Recommendations regarding random or for cause drug testing
    c. Return to work policies
    d. Employee assistance program evaluation

IX Phase 3 of Task Cycle®: *Facilitating the Work of Others*

A The generic task in Phase 3 is: "How do I carry out the plan?"
1. Managers facilitate the work of others by mentoring, modeling and challenging.
2. The skill set for Phase 3 includes hiring the right people (recruitment and retention), mastering management styles, staff development, and networking.

B Hiring the right people is fundamental to accomplishing the task; however, *recruitment and retention* is a major challenge for modern day employers; factors that contribute to recruitment challenges include:
1. Baby boomers are turning 50 at the rate of 11,000 per day; yet the age cohort right behind them is one of the smallest ever.
2. The absolute number of workers age 25 to 34 has declined about 12% since 1990 and will continue to fall for several more years (Harvard Management Update, 1999a, 1999b).

C Managers need to be strategic in their efforts to recruit and retain applicants, especially in a limited labor market (Harvard Management Update, 1999a, 1999b). Box 7-2 provides a list of possible strategies.

D On-line recruiting has become more common and is often the preferred approach, as it potentially reaches a large quantity of people around the world in a timely manner. Methods may include the following (Harvard Management Update, 2000):
1. Determine demographics of types of people that the company wants to hire, then go to web sites frequented by those groups.
2. Post job openings (with specific job descriptions) and job application process on the company's own website.
3. Link company website to other useful sites that give applicants information on the region, cost of living, average salaries, average home price, etc.
4. Provide a fill-in-the-blank application on the company website to encourage more immediate response from those interested.

E Despite the popularity of on-line recruiting, it has limitations (Thaler-Carter, 1998).
1. It may be overwhelming to both applicants and recruiters as the number of Internet sites expands.

BOX 7-2

Recruitment strategies

1. Comb online employment sites
2. Step up on-campus efforts
3. Pay referral bonuses to workers who recommend new hires (Make sure workers are kept up-to-date on hiring needs.)
4. Consider customers as a recruiting source
5. Consider weekend hires, simulations, and temp-to-perm strategies for the selection process
6. Institute "staying bonuses" and incentive plans with multi-year vesting schedules
7. Map out short-term career paths that provide variety and challenge to young workers
8. Flexible benefit plans (some offer home and auto insurance)
9. Providing family-centered benefits that allow workers to balance home and work obligations
10. Part-time work, job sharing
11. Telecommuting
12. Released time for community projects
13. Phased retirement
14. Institute variable pay incentives
15. Develop accommodating retirement policies that encourage older workers to remain in or rejoin the work force (Powell, 1998; Steinhauser, 1998)
16. Provide family-centered benefits that allow workers to balance home and work obligations
17. Enlarge the entry-level pool by considering demographic groups traditionally avoided: high school drop-outs, welfare recipients, and people with or without disabilities who have never had a job. *Caveat*—develop training for those new to the workforce

Source: Harvard Management Update, 1999a, 1999b.

2. There is the potential for breach of confidentiality when resumes are shared among recruiters via the Internet.

3. Only those with Internet access join the applicant pool.

4. There is likely to be a large number of applicants, many of whom are unqualified or uninterested.

F **Extensive research has been conducted on the efficacy of various methods used to evaluate applicants, including different forms of interviews, reference checks, psychologic or personality tests, physical ability, and graphology; evaluation methods must have the following characteristics (Fernandez-Araoz, 1999):**

1. They must be linked to actual job requirements.

2. They must be reliable and valid.

3. They must be predictive of worker success in a particular job.

G **Résumés provide a summary of the applicant qualifications.**

1. The résumé may be organized chronologically or functionally (Amann, 1997).

2. A general résumé needs customizing for any specific job position (Yate, 2001).

3. A cover letter should tie the accomplishments documented in the résumé to the opportunities detailed in the position announcement.

4. The standard length of a résumé is two pages, unless the potential employer requests specific data to be presented for the particular opportunity (Yate, 2001).

5. Résumés should avoid listing irrelevant responsibilities or extraneous data that do not relate to the job objective.

H **Research has demonstrated that structured interviews are the most reliable of all popular techniques for predicting performance (Fernandez-Araoz, 1999).**

1. Structured interviews consist of a list of well-prepared questions that are designed to reveal the candidate's competencies as they relate to the requirements of the job.

2. Structured interviews should be conducted by more than one person in the organization. *Caveat*: Each interview must be truly independent.

3. The best predictor of future performance is past behavior.
   a. Sample questions use phrases like: *Describe a time, Tell me about a situation when, Give me an example, How have you been involved?*
   b. Ask questions to get at HEAR: **h**istory, **e**xamples, **a**ctions taken, **r**esults of action

4. To avoid embellishment of the truth, drill down for details about how a candidate handled a particular situation. Ask definitional questions that test the candidate's knowledge of a specific topic (Harvard Management Update, 2001).

5. Absolute questions, such as "What are your strengths and weaknesses?" generate opinions and should be understood as such (Fernandez-Araoz, 1999).

6. Avoid the "halo effect"—letting one positive characteristic outshine them all.

I *Reference checks* **mean little if only general opinions are solicited. The following steps should be followed to obtain a meaningful reference (Fernandez-Araoz, 1999).**

1. Describe the open job and its challenges.

2. Ask for details about how the candidate faced similar challenges in his or her current or last position

3. Always ask, "Would you hire this person again?" It is difficult to answer this question in an untruthful way (Howe, 2003).

4. Verify the facts on a candidate's resume.

5. Try to speak with someone you know and trust who actually knows the candidate.

J **Management or leadership styles enable the process by influencing the thoughts and actions of other people. Using a combination of management styles achieves the best results (Goleman, 2000).**

1. The authoritative or "Come with me" style is future-focused, as opposed to looking backward.
   a. It works best when a business or department is adrift; changes require a new vision, or a new direction is needed.
   b. It is used to motivate people by helping them understand how their work fits into the larger vision; it positively affects every aspect of climate.
   c. A drawback is that it does not work well with a highly experienced team of experts.

2. The democratic/participatory style asks the question, "What do you think?"
   a. It works well to generate new and fresh ideas. For it to be successful, followers must be competent and informed enough to offer sound advice.
   b. It forges consensus through getting people's ideas and commitment about how decisions affect their goals and how they do their work.
   c. A drawback is that it can be used to put off a crucial decision, or can create dependence on meetings; people can end up feeling leaderless.

3. The affiliative style focuses on "People coming first."
   a. It works best when one is motivating people during stressful circumstances or when there is a need for increasing morale.
   b. It creates harmony, emotional bonding, trust and loyalty. This style encourages habitual risk taking and innovation.
   c. A drawback is that it can allow poor performance to go uncorrected; mediocrity may be tolerated.

4. The pace-setting style makes the statement: "Do as I [the expert] do."
   a. It works well with very skilled, highly motivated workers who need little direction and allows full utilization of talents.
   b. It requires an awareness of the level of competence and personal integrity of workers.
   c. There are several potential drawbacks:
      1) It may can because of lack of direction.
      2) Workers can become overwhelmed with the constant demand for excellence.
      3) Flexibility can evaporate.

5. Coaching is a "Try this" style.
   a. It works best to improve performance and develop long-term strengths.
   b. It focuses on personal development of the worker; the receiving employee must be open to it and desire to improve his or her own performance or develop new abilities.
   c. It is not effective with those who are resistant to change; it is time-consuming; managers must have the expertise to help the worker.

6. The coercive style is also authoritarian: "Do what I tell you."
   a. It works best with problem workers, in a crisis or emergency, when a leader is trying to jump-start a turn-around, or to make a dramatic culture change.
   b. This style decreases flexibility, discourages generation of new ideas, and diminishes feelings of ownership.

K **Staff development activities include mentoring, training, coaching, and team building.**

1. Mentoring is a process whereby a seasoned, skilled, and influential worker (mentor) commits to a long-term relationship with a novice worker (mentee) for the purpose of enhancing the career of the mentee (Carey & Campbell, 1994; Hensler, 1994; Ondeck & Gingerich, 1994).
   a. The word *mentor* derives from the Greek roots meaning "counsel," "remember," and "endure."
   b. "Mentors don't solve problems; they step forward, when asked, and provide resources and help" (Cooper & Sawaf, 1997).
   c. The mentoring process can be either formal (managed by the organization) or informal (spontaneous relationship) and is marked by four stages: initiation, cultivation, separation, and redefinition (Shaffer, Tallarica, & Walsh, 2000; Bartlett, 1995; Burgess, 1995; Hernandez-Piloto Brito, 1992).
   d. Mentoring is directed at ensuring professional competency.
   e. Mentoring is used to prepare occupational and environmental health nurses to effectively apply nursing and occupational health and safety principles in an occupational setting.
   f. Mentoring relationships are crucial to the development of leadership personalities and should be directed to both those on an established career track and to those with the least power in order to encourage the creative process (Zaleznik, 2001).

2. Training is a more structured process of preparing staff to meet the needs of the organization.
   a. A goal of training is to develop multi-skilled, multi-disciplined workforces.
   b. Training begins with orientation to the department and the position.
   c. Training activities can include on-site, in-house presentations; on-site, vendor-generated seminars; off-site offerings; or independent study.
   d. Training activities are initiated on the basis of the individual needs of staff members, annual performance appraisals, changes in job requirements, identified service or product innovations, and organizational needs.
   e. Training may be directed to the occupational and environmental nurse; or training may be that which the occupational and environmental nurse provides to others.
   f. Training priorities may result from legislative mandates, such as the ADA, Drug Free Workplace Act, or OSHA rule making.
   g. Training should be linked to the organization's strategic goals, in order to foster a sustainable and productive workforce.

3. Coaching is "a system that *grows* people by enabling them to learn through guided discovery and hands-on experience" (Renke, 1999).
   a. "A coach is not a problem-solver, a teacher, an advisor or even an expert; he or she is a sounding board, a facilitator, a counselor, an awareness raiser." (Whitmore, 2002).

b. Coaching is the means of generating responsibility, self-motivation, and awareness to enhance performance.

c. The ideal coach is: patient, detached, supportive, interested, a good listener, perceptive, aware, self-aware, attentive, retentive (Whitmore, 2002).

d. Coaches facilitate self-discovery via the following methods:
   1) Listening for meaning rather than words
   2) Engaging in expert question-asking
   3) Encouraging critical thinking
   4) Sharing relevant experiences

4. Team building is important when tasks are complex and work requires a collaborative effort.

   a. The more the workers in a group need the input of other members, the greater the need for team building.

   b. A question is: Do workers individually or collectively provide the final value to the client or customer? If collectively, team building is crucial.

   c. Characteristics of a team include:
      1) Shared agreement on a common vision or goal
      2) Recognizing interdependence and the contribution of each individual or discipline
      3) Engaging in a common code of conduct
      4) Sharing rewards

   d. Tools to enhance teamwork include, but are not limited to:
      1) Behavior-style inventories, for example:
         • Meyers-Briggs, which is used to identify workers' personality preference from 16 different possibilities (http://www.myersbriggs.org/)
         • Hemann Brain Dominance Survey, which is used to determine workers' preferred thinking approach: emotional, analytical, structural, or strategic (http://www.hbdi.com/)
      2) Regular staff meetings with time allotted to acknowledge team-member strengths
      3) Bi-annual strategic meetings
      4) Physical activity (e.g., ropes course, interdepartmental sports)
      5) Celebrations for not only work well done, but also personal events and holidays

   e. Team building results in mutual respect and appreciation of each member's contribution.

   f. One goal of team building is the creation of empowered teams whose members demonstrate the following qualities (Renke, 1999):
      1) They focus on results.
      2) They are risk-takers who make mistakes and learn from them.
      3) They communicate effectively to build coalitions and networks.
      4) They lead.
      5) They are creative and visionary.

   g. Because teams take a long time to develop into efficiently functioning entities, the stability of team membership and frequent opportunities for team members to collaborate are important.

   h. Interdependent interactions require trust, an affinity for working with other people, a balance of inner strength and other-directedness, and a tolerance for conflict (Drexler & Forrester, 1998).

   i. Interdisciplinary occupational health and safety teams may include an occupational and environmental health nurse, occupational physician, industrial hygienist, safety manager, ergonomist, human resources representative, toxicologist, and others.

   j. The coordination of the interdisciplinary team is often the responsibility of the occupational and environmental health nurse manager.

5. The key to mentoring, training, and coaching is motivation.

   a. *Motivation* is an "intrinsic drive" or "fuel for performance" resulting from an individual's instincts, needs, and actual or expected rewards; it determines an individual's behavior (Tappen, 1989; Sullivan & Decker, 1997).

   b. Worker motivation is driven by three beliefs (Green, 2000):

     1) "I can do it."—Confidence

     2) Trust that the organization or manager will give the employee what his or her performance merits

     3) The outcomes tied to performance will be satisfying

   c. Motivation is stimulated by others, including managers, mentors, or a work team.

6. Workers and managers must evaluate staff development in terms of the following:

   a. The identified skills or abilities gap

   b. The desired behavior change as a result of the training

   c. The desired improvement in knowledge, skills, or attitudes

   d. The usefulness to the organization of the knowledge, skills, or attitudes to be taught

L **Networking is a process of developing and using personal contacts to mutually exchange information, advice, or moral support on an informal or voluntary basis.**

1. In a business environment, effective networking reflects reciprocal trust, a functional feedback system, common goals or purposes, and positive interdependence of members among each other (The Center for Healthcare Leadership, 2000).

2. Methods of networking include the following:

   a. Identify essential contacts in the organization and in the community

   b. Make a list of needs that others in the organization could fill

   c. Volunteer to serve on committees/projects in the organization

   d. Become involved in community activities, such as serving on health-related advisory boards, attending community events, or joining professional organizations

   e. Seek a mentor within the organization

   f. Serve as a mentor

3. Networking is beneficial not only for the occupational and environmental health nurse manager, but also for the organization.

   a. It helps to recruit and retain workers

   b. It increases visibility within the community and is excellent publicity for the organization

X Phase 4 of Task Cycle®: *Obtaining and Providing Feedback*

A **The generic tasks for Phase 4 are to determine "How am I performing?" and to track and share information.**

B **The skill set includes: communication (listening, negotiation and conflict resolution, effective writing), and the performance management process.**

C Listening is a valued communication skill for managers and leaders; if a manager is a good listener, he or she can accept ideas, criticism, and other feedback that can improve the organization and create an atmosphere of excellence and caring (Smith, 1998).

1. Obstacles to effective listening include the following:
   a. Multiple demands on occupational and environmental health nurses
   b. Biases and beliefs, especially among diverse groups (Tannen, 1994)
   c. Misunderstanding the meaning or tenor of words
   d. Differences in the rates of speech and listening
   e. The need to solve the problem rather than listen to the person
2. Effective listening requires the following:
   a. Encouraging the speaker to continue the interaction through the use of nonverbal communication, and asking occasional questions to keep track of what is being said
   b. Listening for others' observations, feelings, needs, and requests (Rosenberg, 1999)
3. The listening role is a powerful one, often making the difference in whether or not agreements can be reached and work can be accomplished.

D Negotiation and conflict resolution are communication skills that are most effective when both parties have moderate to high levels of emotional intelligence:

1. Emotional intelligence consists of self-awareness, self-regulation, motivation, empathy, and social skills.
2. The most common sources of conflict are personal differences, religious differences, political differences, cultural differences, and external environmental stressors.
3. There are many ways to resolve conflicts: surrendering, running away, overpowering your opponent with violence, filing a lawsuit, etc.
4. Approaches to conflict resolution include the following (Orchard, 1998):
   a. *Competition:* The manager "overpowers the opposition" to meet his or her needs or goals.
   b. *Accommodation:* The manager is more concerned with working relationships than with outcomes and thus will allow others to achieve their goals.
   c. *Avoidance:* The manager refuses to address the issue.
   d. *Compromise:* The manager attempts to find a "middle ground"—a mutually acceptable solution that partially satisfies both parties.
   e. *Collaboration:* All parties work together to find the most satisfying solution for everyone involved.
5. Negotiation is "the art of letting them have your way". "Understanding your counterpart's interest and shaping the decision so the other side agrees for its own reasons is the key to jointly creating and claiming sustainable negotiation" (Sebenius, 2001).
6. Principled negotiation is a method designed to decide issues on their merits rather than on a process of haggling (Fisher & Ury, 1991).
7. Successful negotiation requires the following (Fisher & Ury, 1991; Fisher & Ertel, 1995, Kirby, 1997):
   a. Clarify each party's interests and desires rather than stated positions; search for underlying interests
   b. Brainstorm as many possible solutions and alternative results as possible to meet the needs

    c. Develop a best alternative or action to take if negotiations fail (BATNA—best alternative to a negotiated agreement)

    d. Use effective communication and build relationships; get to know the other parties in other frameworks outside of the negotiating arena

    e. Identify issues to be included in an agreement and define steps to reach that agreement

E **Day-to-day communication is handled with meetings, e-mails, and in writing.**

1. Meetings are a means of disseminating information, brainstorming, planning, problem solving, making decisions or motivating (Wachs, 1992).

2. Keys to an effective meeting include the following (Wachs, 1992; Amann, 2000):

    a. Establish the need for and purpose of the meeting. Ask: Is the meeting really necessary?

    b. Determine who needs to attend the meeting. Ask: Who has the information to make informed decisions? Who has the ability to allocate resources and initiate action? Who has the responsibility for the meeting outcome?

    c. Draw up an agenda that describes the who, what, when, where, and why of the meeting and circulate it before the meeting, if possible.

    d. Do not run the meeting, facilitate it: Solicit a note taker and a timekeeper; establish a "parking lot" for items to be discussed later; summarize often.

    e. Use technology needed to help convey information: videoconferencing, web conferencing in real time, internet for audiovisuals, digital whiteboards.

    f. Close the meeting: Summarize issues, action items to be completed, and next steps.

    g. Distribute the minutes or a written summary of the meeting to all participants and other interested parties.

3. E-mail is used as a primary vehicle for business. In addition to knowing the policies of the organization, appropriate use of e-mail includes the following (Strasser, 2003):

    a. Decide whether e-mail is the correct method for the communication; uncertainty leads toward person-to-person communication.

    b. Be discreet, professional, aware of the tenor of the message, and careful what you say and how you say it—it cannot be taken back.

    c. Consider who will receive the message or response based on "need to know" and action expected.

    d. Construct messages in the same manner as a properly composed business letter.

    e. Do not send urgent messages via e-mail.

4. Business writing conveys information, presents facts and conclusions, and motivates or persuades.

    a. The primary audience of the written document makes decisions and acts on the information; the secondary audience needs to know the data.

    b. An effective document is clear, concise, grammatically correct, and visually appealing, and requests action within a time frame (Crowe, 1999); use the style common to the organization.

5. Quarterly and annual reports can be used to document productivity, quality of services, and progress toward goal attainment.

   a. Quarterly or monthly reports should include the following:
1) Utilization statistics and identified trends
2) Status of progress on agreed upon goals and objectives
3) Performance metrics
4) Activity update to include programs, services and initiatives, along with outcome data
5) Safety and Medical Surveillance activities, as applicable
6) Report of financial measures: workers' compensation data, short-term disability data, budget projections versus actual expenditures, return on investment data
7) Human resource summary (e.g., hires, vacancies)
8) Staff-development activities
9) Staff participation in interdepartmental and interdisciplinary activities
10) Trends related to injuries and illnesses

   b. Annual reports provide an overview of accomplishments during the past year and include the following (Amann, 2000b):
1) Goals and vision established for the current year and the outcome
2) Summary of financial status and measures
3) Demonstration of changes in levels and impact of services as compared to previous years
4) Identified trends
5) Summary statistics; may include injury and illness rates, disability data, utilization data
6) Summary of major milestones or accomplishments

F The *performance management process* at the macro level is an opportunity to evaluate conformance of the occupational health unit's services to pre-established requirements; at the individual level, it is an opportunity for the worker and manager to discuss development goals and jointly create a plan for achieving them within the context of organizational goals.

1. Performance appraisals are based on position descriptions, particularly job responsibilities, and standards of performance.
   a. Position or job descriptions are a statement of what the worker agrees to accomplish in exchange for being paid, and serve the following purposes (Harvard Management Communication Letter, 2001):
1) As the basis for developing staff by providing the milestones to be reached as the term of employment plays out
2) As the foundation for performance appraisals (i.e., the measurement of workers' job performance quality and productivity)
3) To describe the company culture and help everyone involved understand the mission, culture, needs and goals of the company
4) As an opportunity to re-evaluate what the job role should really be
5) To form the basis of a legal termination of employment

   b. Position descriptions should describe the results that are desired and the key competencies of the position in behavioral terms. Example: The term "team player" translates to: "The ability to:
1) Build group identity and commitment; or
2) Share credit for work well done; or
3) Draw all members of the team into active and enthusiastic participation" (Fernandez-Arraoz, 1999).

   c. Position descriptions should have the following characteristics:

1) Include the emotional intelligence competencies critical to getting the work done (Fernandez-Arraoz, 1999)
2) Distinguish among credentials, skills and traits that are the *minimum* level required to do the job, to the degree that if the job requirements changed overnight, a new hire would be able to manage in the short-term (Harvard Management Communication Letter, 2001)
3) Comply with current practice standards and with all legal restrictions and apply to the requirements of getting the job done, to include both physical and mental demands
4) Be results-oriented, describing what the worker is to accomplish, rather than listing a percentage of time a worker should be spending performing a certain function

2. Performance appraisal methods include verbal feedback, corrective demonstration, conferences, memos, and other forms of communication.
3. Standards of performance "specify for the employee the conditions that will exist when the job is done to the manager's satisfaction" (Webb & Cantone, 1993).
4. Each job responsibility should have a companion performance standard; examples of performance standards are as follows:
   a. Provides professional nursing care appropriate to worker needs
   b. Identifies worker health needs accurately, using health history and physical assessment skills for 95% of the workers who present in the occupational health unit
   c. Following signed protocols, prescribes appropriate treatment to meet identified health needs for 100% of workers who present in the occupational health unit
5. Documenting progress toward standards of performance is important; it serves to justify salary increases and promotions.
   a. Begin with annual self-appraisal of accomplishments and contributions.
   b. Determine the single most important message to send to the worker about performance over the past year and deliver it.
   c. Write an objective assessment, using concrete terms ("Does not meet expectations" vs. "Needs improvement"), of worker performance based on data collected throughout the year.
   d. Provide time for discussion with a core message of strengths, needs for immediate improvement, and opportunities for development.
   e. Tell the truth (Falcone, 1999; Grote, 1998; Amann, 1996).
   f. Act and make a change, when the performance management process is unsuccessful with an individual.
   g. Evaluate the efficacy of computer-assisted performance appraisal systems in providing objective, timely assessments and stimulating worker behavioral change (Flowers, Tudor, & Trumble, 1997).
6. Continuous quality improvement (CQI), as a performance management tool, focuses on work processes and outcomes.
   a. The quality improvement process is a disciplined, ongoing process for producing outputs and preventing errors in products and services.
   b. W. Edwards Deming's quality program, called the *Deming Cycle*, includes the following steps (Deming, 1986):
      1) Plan a work process.
      2) Do or implement a work process.
      3) Check or measure a work process.

4) Act on results to continuously improve the process.

   c. Philip B. Crosby's program is based on organizational development, with the following absolutes for quality management (Crosby, 1979):

     1) Conformance to organizational requirements

     2) Prevention of potential problems

     3) Zero defects in products or services

     4) Determination of the cost of quality

7. Other sources of information that can be used to evaluate the performance of occupational health services include customer satisfaction surveys of workers who use health services, conformance to organizational goals and standards, community resources, vendors, professional colleagues, and occupational health unit staff (Wells, 1999; Eckes, 1994; Weber, 1995).

XI Phase 5 of Task Cycle®: *Monitoring and Adjusting the Process*

A The generic tasks of Phase 5 are: "How do I fix my mistakes? How do I exercise positive control to serve the commitments made?"

B The elements of Phase 5 are: policies and procedures, outcomes management, and benchmarking.

C Policies and procedures lay the foundation for quality programs and services and provide uniform ways of responding to situations and meeting organizational challenges (Ebaugh, 1998).

1. Policies and procedures, which are often developed as a result of problems in the workplace or regulatory mandates, should be handled as follows:

   a. They must be developed through collaborative efforts, requiring the participation of all affected parties and the approval and support of management.

   b. They must be reviewed and revised regularly.

   c. They should be deleted once they have outlived their usefulness (after careful consideration).

2. A policy is a statement that establishes an organization's position on a particular issue, serving as a guideline for decision-making and action (Amann, 2001; Ebaugh, 1998); it should accomplish the following:

   a. Provide direction for goal attainment

   b. Define the scope of the occupational health unit's activities and to whom they apply

   c. Be clear, flexible, and consistent

3. Procedures are the specific chronologic steps necessary to operationalize policy.

   a. Procedures include a purpose, responsibilities, specific steps, expected results, documentation, and other considerations (Ebaugh, 1998).

   b. Not all tasks performed in the occupational health unit require a procedure; if the task is a common one that staff members are all familiar with, writing a procedure is not necessary.

4. Once the policies and procedures are developed and approved, they should be:

   a. Disseminated to affected workers through an employee handbook, newsletters, payroll stuffers, closed-circuit television, or by in-house computer networks when available

    b. Stored in a manual in an easily accessible location, or on a local area network
    c. Reviewed and revised on a regular schedule
    d. Used to monitor on-going operations

D *Outcomes management* **is "the systematic approach to evaluate, through process, all steps leading to a result (outcome) and proactively use the information at the front end to design and implement best practices" (Kosinski, 1998).**

1. Outcomes management is used to measure the following:
   a. The cost versus benefit of programs and services
   b. The effect of programs and services on organizational profit margin
2. To design an effective outcomes management programs and services, execute the following steps:
   a. Determine the issues of concern and what outcomes should be measured or evaluated.
   b. Compare the identified outcomes to be measured with the operational needs of the organization.
   c. Assess current resources and additional needs to determine which outcome measures are within the feasible scope of the programs and services.
   d. Form an outcomes management team that is multi-functional.
   e. Describe expected results based on appropriate benchmarks (past performance or goals for future performance) (Kosinski, 1998).
3. Collect data from more than one source and by more than one method if possible.
4. Keep the project design focused on high-priority issues with a clear understanding about what is being evaluated and why (Kosinski, 1998).
5. Use results to modify and develop best practices, and to establish occupational and environmental health benchmarks.

E *Benchmarking* **is an explicit, evidence-based method for evaluating and improving processes and systems (AAOHN, 1999). It is the "continuous process of measuring a company's products, services, and practices against industry leading competitors" (Collins, 1995) and "against industry's best practice" (Landwehr, 1995).**

1. The purposes of benchmarking include the following (Beasley & Cook, 1995):
   a. Modifying organizational culture or climate
   b. Fostering competition
   c. Creating an awareness of the quality standard within the industry
   d. Measuring productivity and performance quality
   e. Setting performance standards
   f. Managing the organization to achieve the best results
2. The benchmarking process includes the following steps (Iacobucci & Nordhielm, 2000; Brown, 1995; Collins, 1995; Murray & Murray, 1992; Landwehr, 1995; Bergman, 1994):
   a. Planning: deciding which processes will be benchmarked and what the assessment activities will be
      1) A method for doing this would be to list each step of the client's or customer's experience from the initial recognition of need to the final follow-up after the service is delivered.
      2) Determine which factors most influence the client's perception of value at each step of the experience.

   b. Developing assessment tools and assessing internal functioning
   c. Identifying organizations that are models of excellence for each factor, no matter what industry they are in, and sharing information and data
   d. Analyzing data: identifying performance gaps between the study company and the benchmark companies
   e. Changing: using the data to unfreeze workers to accept the need for modification in the work process under review and then implement the change based on the benchmark criteria
   f. Monitoring: overseeing the change process, of course, but also recalibrating benchmarks at regular intervals
3. Benchmarking has some potential problems, such as the following (McWilliams, 1995):
   a. Failure to appreciate that organizations are unique in ways that may affect the legitimacy of the comparison
   b. The need for common definitions of processes and criteria
   c. The need to be the best, no matter what the cost
   d. Reluctance to use quality interventions other than benchmarking
4. Benchmarks common to occupational and environmental health practice are:
   a. Frequency and severity of claims
   b. Lost-time cases and days
   c. Lag time between incident and report
   d. Medical to indemnity ratio
   e. Individual costs to total claim costs
   f. Cost of claims per worker
   g. Cost of claims per $1,000 revenue
   h. Cost of claims as a percent of payroll

XII Phase 6 of Task Cycle®: *Reinforcing Performance*

A The generic task for Phase 6 of the process is to share rewards for achievement of results.

B It is important to visibly recognize worker contributions to a common vision (Kouzes & Posner, 1987).
1. Effective recognition comes from someone held in high esteem, such as one's manager.
2. Timing is important. The sooner workers' performance is recognized, the clearer the message is received and the more likely the desired performance will be repeated (Nelson, 2003).
3. Recognition is most powerful when contingent upon desired behavior and performance.
4. Match the reward to the person.
5. Match the reward to the achievement.
6. Be creative. Reward staff for unique approaches to occupational health unit problems.
7. Institute recognition rituals.
8. Celebrate when people are promoted (Herman & Gioia, 2000).

C Several types of rewards and recognitions are effective (Nelson, 2003). They include:
1. Basic praise: personal praise, written praise, public praise, and electronic praise

2. Management support and involvement: asking workers for their opinion, involving workers in decision-making, giving workers authority to do their job, supporting workers when they make a mistake
3. Flexible working hours
4. Learning and development opportunities
5. Manager availability and time

XIII Power: Concern for Influencing People

A Managers must possess a high need for power—that is, a concern for influencing people.

B The need must be disciplined and controlled so that it is directed toward the benefit of the institution as a whole and not toward the manager's personal aggrandizement or need to achieve (McClelland & Burnham, 2002).

C The most important determining factor of high morale is that a manager's need for power be higher than his or her need to be liked.

D Managers with high power motivation balanced by high controlled action care about the institution and use power to stimulate their workers to be more productive.

E An effective manager recognizes that things get done in an organization only if they influence the people around them.

F Occupational and environmental nurse managers must assess their own need for power and achievement and become aware of power bases in order to implement decisions regarding the health and safety of workers (Box 7-3).

BOX 7-3

Sources of power

- **Legitimate power** or authority arises from one's position within the organization.
- **Referent power** or charisma comes from one's personality and other personal characteristics; confidence, controlling emotions, and dress may all contribute to referent power.
- **Reward power** is based on one's ability to reward others, for example, with merit pay increases and worker recognition.
- **Expert power** allows the occupational and environmental health nurse manager to make health care decisions because

others recognize a nurse's special knowledge, skills, and abilities.
- **Connection power** is created when individuals work together, as when health and safety professionals collaborate with human resources staff (Ellis & Hartley, 1991).
- **Information power** is held by those who control and possess information; they are often more powerful than those who need the information but are barred from access to it (Ellis & Hartley, 1991).
- **Coercive power** is often used by authoritarian managers to control the behavior of others through fear, threats, and punishment.

XIV The Image of the Occupational and Environmental Health Nurse

The occupational and environmental health nurse should be seen as a competent businessperson who has particular expertise in health and safety.

A *Image* **is created through the display of personal characteristics and interpersonal skills.**
   1. Personal appearance plays a major role in the occupational and environmental health nurse's image.
   2. Professionalism displayed through interactions with workers, managers, and community members attests to the positive image of nurses.
      a. A nurse's caring and competence are often evaluated by workers and managers.
      b. Dealings with community providers, vendors, and other business people will color the community's perception of not only an individual occupational and environmental health nurse but of nurses in general.
   3. The occupational and environmental health nurse can also positively affect the image of nurses by engaging in the following activities:
      a. Publishing articles in the organization's newsletter and the community newspaper
      b. Belonging to professional organizations such as AAOHN
      c. Recognizing and publicizing excellence among staff members (Brown, 1995)

B **The image of the occupational and environmental health nurse relates directly to the nurse's influence and ability to promote health and safety in the organization.**

XV Customer Service

Successful occupational health organizations are likely to have a culture that supports customer service.

A **Managers anticipate and respond to internal and external customer needs, recognizing the importance of positive customer relationships with business goals.**

B **Keys to positive customer interaction include the following (Stauffer, 2001; Stauffer, 1999):**
   1. Address all customer service issues fully, resolving them completely.
   2. Respond to a complaint with follow-up questions to get at underlying needs.
   3. Ensure that front-line workers have the information, authority, tools, and know-how to solve customer's problems.
   4. Determine what customers want from health services, not what health services would like them to want.
   5. Identify what customers *will* want and strategize ways to give it to them.
   6. Do not assign blame. Take responsibility for solving a problem.
   7. Respond with positive, truthful alternatives to a complaint.
   8. Value the customer who complains, so that problems can be solved.
   9. Conduct customer service surveys both informally and formally.

REFERENCES

Accel-Team. (2004). Employee motivation, the organizational environment and productivity. Retrieved on November 15, 2004, from http://www.accelteam.com/humanrelations/hrels_05_herzberg.html.

Allen, G. (1998). Management History. Retrieved on November 15, 2004, from http://ollie.dcccd. edu/mgmt1374/book_content s/1overview/management_history/mgmt_history.htm.

Amann, M. (1996). Performance management. Part 2: Performance review and appraisal. *AAOHN Journal, 44,* 421-422.

Amann, M. (1997). Business skills for occupational health nurses: Preparing the perfect resume. *AAOHN Journal, 45,* 107-108.

Amann, M. (2000). Combining technology and skill to ensure effective meetings. *AAOHN Journal, 47*(8), 367-369.

Amann, M. (2000b). The annual report: Documenting organizational results. *AAOHN Journal, 47*(11), 509-511.

Amann, M. (2001). The policy and procedure manual—keeping it current. *AAOHN Journal 48*(2), 69-71.

American Association of Occupational Health Nurses (AAOHN). (1999). *Success tools: Developing business expertise—strategies for thriving & surviving in business.* Atlanta, GA: AAOHN Publications.

Analytictech.com (2005). Henri Fayol. Retrieved February 20, 2005, from http://www.analytictech.com/mb021/fayol.htm.

Barrett, M. E., Fraser, L. B. (1977, July-August). Conflicting roles in budgeting for operations. *Harvard Business Review, 55*(4), 137-144.

Bartlett, R. C. (1995). The mentoring message. *Chief Executive, 101,* 48-49.

Beasley, G., & Cook, J. (1995). The "what," "why," and "how" of benchmarking. *Agency Sales, 25*(6), 52-56.

Bergman, R. (1994). Hitting the mark. *Hospitals and Health Networks, 68*(8), 48-51.

Brown, S. (1995). Measures of perfection. *Sales & Marketing Management, 147*(5), 104-105.

Burgess, L. (1995). Mentoring with the blindfold. *Employment Relations Today, 21*(4), 439-444.

Burns, J. M. (1978). *Leadership.* New York: Harper & Row.

Byrne, A. (2003). Realistic Budgeting. Retrieved September 26, 2004, from http://www.charityvillage.com/cv/research/rim11.html.

Carey, S. J., & Campbell, S. T. (1994). Preceptor, mentor and sponsor roles: Creative strategies for nurse retention. *Journal of Nursing Administration, 24*(12), 39-48.

Chaleff, I. (1998). *The courageous follower.* San Francisco: Berrett-Koehler Publishers.

Christensen, C. M., & Raynor, M. E. (2003). Why hard-nosed executives should care about management theory. *Harvard Business Review OnPoint, 81*(9), 66.

Clark, D. (2000). Concept of leadership. Retrieved October 9, 2004, from http://www.nwlink.com/donclark/leader/leadcon.html.

Collins, J. (2001). *Good to great.* New York: HarperBusiness.

Collins, J. C., & Porras, J. L. (1996). Building your company's vision. *Harvard Business Review, 74*(5), 65-77.

Collins, M. J. (1995). Benchmarking with simulation: How it can help your production operations. *Production, 107*(7), 51-52.

Cooper, R. K., & Sawaf, A. (1997). *Executive EQ. Emotional intelligence in leadership organizations.* New York: The Berkley Publishing Group.

Crislip, D. D., & Larson, C. E. (1994). *Collaborative leadership.* San Francisco: Jossey-Bass Publishers.

Crosby, P. B. (1979). *Quality is free.* New York: New American Library.

Crowe, R. (1999). Business writing: A necessary skill for occupational and environmental health nurses. *AAOHN Journal, 47,* 383-385.

DeCock, C., & Hipkin, I. (1997). TQM and BPR: Beyond the beyond myth. *Journal of Management Studies, 34,* 661-675.

Deming, W. E. (1986). *Out of the crisis.* Cambridge, MA: MIT-CAES.

Depree, M. (1989). *Leadership is an art.* New York: Dell Publishing.

Drexler, A. B., & Forrester, R. (1998). Interdependence: The crux of teamwork. *HRMagazine, 43,* 52-62.

Ebaugh, H. (1998). Defining the scope of occupational health services: Effective policy and procedure development. *AAOHN Journal, 46,* 547-553.

Eckes, G. (1994). Practical alternatives to performance appraisals. *Quality Progress, 27(11),* 57-60.

Eichenberger, J. (1997). Project management for occupational health nurses. *AAOHN Journal 45(12),* 607-608.

Emerald Now. (2000). Spotlight on Edgar Schein. Retrieved February 20, 2005, from http://juno.emeraldinsight.com/vl=12843246/c l=36/nw=1/rpsv/now/archive/mar2000/spotlight.

Falcone, P. (1999). Rejuvenate your performance evaluation writing skills. *HRMagazine, 44,* 126-136.

Fernandez-Arraoz, C. (1999, July-August). Hiring without firing. *Harvard Business Review, 77(4),* 109-120.

Fisher, R., & Ertel, D. (1995). *Getting ready to negotiate.* New York: Penguin Books.

Fisher, R., & Ury, W. (1991). *Getting to yes.* New York: Penguin Books.

Flowers, L. A., Tudor, T. R., & Trumble, R. R. (1997). Computer assisted performance appraisal systems. *Journal of Compensation and Benefits, 12,* 34-35.

Forsberg, K., Mooz, H., Cotterman, H. (1996). *Visualizing Project Management.* New York: John Wiley & Sons, Inc.

Garvin, D. A., & Roberto, M. A. (2001, November 1). What you don't know about making decisions. *Harvard Business Review, 79(8),* 108.

Goleman, D. (1995). *Emotional intelligence.* New York: Bantam Books.

Goleman, D. (1998). *Working with emotional intelligence.* New York: Bantam Books.

Goleman, D. (2000, March-April). Leadership that gets results. *Harvard Business Review, 78(2)* 78-90.

Goleman, D., Boyatzis, R., & McKee, A. (2002). *Primal leadership. Realizing the power of emotional intelligence.* Boston, MA: Harvard Business School Press.

Green, T. (2000). *Motivation management.* Palo Alto, CA: Davies-Black Publishing.

Greenleaf, R. K. (1970). *The servant as leader.* Indianapolis, IN: Robert K. Greenleaf Center for Servant Leadership.

Grohar-Murray, M. E., & DiCroce, H. R. (1992). *Leadership and management in nursing.* Norwalk, CT: Appleton & Lange.

Grote, D. (1998). Painless performance appraisals focus on results, behaviors. *HRMagazine, 43,* 52-58.

Harvard Management Communication Letter. (2001). *21st century job descriptions.* Boston, MA: Harvard Business School Publishing.

Harvard Management Update. (1999a). *Managing the labor shortage: Part 1. How to keep your 50-somethings.* Boston, MA: Harvard Business School Publishing.

Harvard Management Update. (1999b). *Managing the labor shortage: Part 2. Finding—and keeping—good young employees.* Boston, MA: Harvard Business School Publishing.

Harvard Management Update. (2000). *Online hiring? Do it right.* Boston, MA: Harvard Business School Publishing.

Harvard Management Update. (2001). *Interview questions that hit the mark.* Boston, MA: Harvard Business School Publishing.

Hensler, D. J. (1994). Mentoring at the management level. *Industrial Management, 36(6),* 20-21.

Herman, R. E., Gioia, J. L. (2000). *Employer of choice.* Winchester, VA: Oakhill Press.

Hernandez-Piloto Brito, H. (1992). Nurses in action: An innovative approach to mentoring. *Journal of Nursing Administration, 22(5),* 23-28.

Howe, T. (2003). Ten steps to successful interviewing. Retrieved September 26, 2004, from http://www.charityvillage.com/cv/research/rhr7.html.

Iacobucci, D, Nordhielm, C. (2000, November-December). Creative benchmarking. *Harvard Business Review, 78(3),* 24-25.

Kaplan, R. S., Norton, D. P. (2000). Linking strategy to planning and budgeting. *Balanced Scorecard Report, May 15,* Boston, MA: Harvard Business School Publishing.

Key, S., & Popkin, S. J. (1998). Integrating ethics into the strategic management process: doing well by doing good. *Management Decision, 36,* 331-338.

Kirby, W. H. (1997). Negotiation. Retrieved on October 7, 2004, from http://www.uwsp.edu/education/Wkirby/ntrprsnl/negot.htm.

Kotter, J. P. (1995, March-April). Leading change: Why transformation efforts fail. *Harvard Business Review, 73(2),* 59-66.

Kouzes, J. M., & Posner, B. Z. (1987). *Leadership challenge*. Palo Alto, CA: TPG/Learning Systems.

Kosinski, M. (1998). Effective outcomes management in occupational and environmental health. *AAOHN Journal, 46*, 500-510.

Landwehr, W. R. (1995). Focus on benchmarking: Achieving world-class maintenance and superior competitive performance. *Plant Engineering, 49*(7), 120-121.

Lewin, K. (1951). *Field theory in social sciences*. New York: Harper & Row.

McClelland, D. C., Burnham, D. H. (2002). Power is the great motivator. *Harvard Business Review Best of HBR, January, 2003*. Boston, MA: Harvard Business School Publishing.

McNamara, C. (1999). Brief overview of contemporary theories in management. Retrieved September 27, 2004, from http://www.managementhelp.org/mgmnt/cntmpory.htm.

McWilliams, B. (1995). What's wrong with benchmarking? *CFO, 11*(5), 105-106.

Moran, E. T., & Volkwein, J. F. (1992). The cultural approach to the formation of organizational climate. *Human Relations, 45*(1), 19-47.

Murray, J. A., & Murray, M. H. (1992). Benchmarking: A tool for excellence in palliative care. *Journal of Palliative Care, 8*(4), 41-45.

Nelson, B. (2003). Five questions about employee recognition and reward. *Harvard Management Update, September 1*. Boston, MA: Harvard Business School Publishing.

Ondeck, D. A., & Gingerich, B. S. (1994). The mentoring relationship. *Journal of Home Health Care Practice, 6*(4), 1-7.

Orchard, B. (1998). Creating constructive outcomes in conflict. *AAOHN Journal, 46*, 302-313.

Organizational Dynamics, Inc. (1991). *The Quality Advantage*. Burlington, MA: Organizational Dynamics, Inc.

Paul, R. W. (1995). *Critical thinking: How to prepare students for a rapidly changing world*. Santa Rose, CA: Foundations for Critical Thinking.

Perce, K. H. (1998). Project management skills. *AAOHN Journal, 46*(8), 391-403.

Perra, B. M. (1999). The leader in you. *Nursing Management, 30*, 35-38.

Renke, W. J. (1999). Manage like a coach not a cop. *Balance, 3*, 24-26.

Rosenberg, M. B. (1999). *Nonviolent communication*. Del Mar, CA: PuddleDancer Press.

Sebenius, J. K. (2001). Six habits of merely effective negotiators. *Harvard Business Review OnPoint, March 1, 2002*.

Senge, P.M. (2000). Leadership in living organizations. In F. Hesselbein, M. Goldsmith, & I. Somerville (Eds.), *Leading beyond the walls* (pp. 73-90). San Francisco: Jossey-Bass Publishers.

Shaffer, B., Tallarica, B., & Walsh, J. (2000). Win-win mentoring. *Nursing Management, 31*, 32-34.

Smith, P.M. (1998). *Rules & tools for leaders: A down-to earth guide to effective managing*. Garden City Park, NY: Avery Publishing Group.

Stauffer, D. (1999). The art of delivering great customer service. *Harvard Management Update, September 1*. Boston, MA: Harvard Business School Publishing.

Stauffer, D. (2001). What customer-centric really means: Seven key insights. *Harvard Management Update, August 1*. Boston, MA: Harvard Business School Publishing.

Strasser, P. (2003). Electronic Mail Communication. *AAOHN Journal, 51*(12), 504-506.

Sullivan, E.J., & Decker, P. J. (1997). *Effective leadership and management in nursing*. Menlo Park, CA: Addison-Wesley.

Tannen, D. (1994). *Talking from 9 to 5*. New York: Avon Books.

Tappen, R. M. (1989). *Nursing leadership and management: Concepts and practice*. Philadelphia: F.A. Davis

Thaler-Carter, R.E. (1998). Recruiting through the web: Better or just bigger? *HRMagazine, 43*, 61-68.

The Center for Healthcare Leadership. (2000). *LEAD: Guide to Development*. Atlanta, GA: Emory Healthcare.

University of Glamorgan. (1999, 2001). Management styles. Retrieved November 15, 2004, from http://www.comp.glam.ac.uk/teaching/ismanagement/manstyles-t6.htm.

Wachs, J. E. (1992). Facilitating an effective meeting. *AAOHN Journal, 40*(6), 294-296.

Webb, P. R., & Cantone, J.M. (1993). Performance evaluation: Triumph or torture? *Journal of Home Health Care Practice, 5*(2), 14-19.

Weber, A. J. (1995). Making performance appraisals consistent with a quality environment. *Quality Progress, 28*(6), 65-69.

Wells, S. J. (1999). A new road: Traveling beyond 360-degree evaluation. *HRMagazine, 44,* 82-91.

Wenek, K. W. J. (2003). Defining Effective Leadership in the Canadian Forces: A Content and Process Framework. Kingston, Ontario: Canadian Forces Leadership Institute.

Wheatley, M. J. (1992). *Leadership and the new science.* San Francisco: Berrett-Koehler.

Wheatley, M. J. (1999). Good-bye, command and control. In F. Hesselbein & P.M. Cohen (Eds.), *Leader to leader* (pp. 151-162). San Francisco: Jossey-Bass Publishers.

Whitmore, J. (2002). *Coaching for Performance: Growing People, Performance and Purpose.* London: Brealey, Nicholas Publishing.

Wilson, C. L., O'Hare, D., Shipper, F. (1990). Task Cycle Theory: The Processes of Influence. In K. E. Clark, & M. B. Clark, (Eds.), *Measures of Leadership* (pp. 185-204). West Orange, NJ: Leadership Library of America, Inc.

Yate, M. (2001). *Cover letters that knock 'em dead.* Holbrook, MA: Adams Media Corporation.

Yoder-Wise, P. S. (1999). *Leading and managing in nursing.* St. Louis, MO: Mosby.

Zamanou, S., & Glaser, S. R. (1994). Moving toward participation and involvement. *Group & Organization Management, 19*(4), 475-502.

Zaleznik, A. (1992, March-April). Managers and leaders: Are they different? *Harvard Business Review,* 70(2), 126-135.

CHAPTER

8

Information Management in the Occupational Health Setting

MARY C. AMANN AND DONNI TOTH

The ability to collect, store, access, and manage information efficiently is critical to the successful delivery of health services. An increase in the volume and complexity of information that must be managed in the modern day workplace requires new organizational skills and the use of advanced technologic tools. This chapter provides an overview of some of the many systems, programs, and techniques that can help the occupational and environmental health nurse effectively manage information, and describes how these systems can be used to optimize service delivery.

I Introduction to Nursing Informatics

A *Nursing informatics* **is defined as "a combination of computer science, information science and nursing science designed to assist in the management and processing of nursing data, information and knowledge to support the practice of nursing and the delivery of nursing care" (Graves & Corcoran, 1989, p. 227).**
1. The American Nurses Association (ANA, 2001) states that:
   a. "Nursing informatics facilitates the integration of data, information and knowledge to support patients, nurses and other providers in their decision-making in all roles and settings."
   b. "This support is accomplished through the use of information structures, information processes, and information technology."
2. Nursing informatics consists of management and processing components.
   a. The *management* component of informatics is the functional ability to collect, aggregate, organize, move, and represent information in an economical, efficient way that is useful to the users of the system.
   b. The *processing* component of informatics refers to the transformation of data into information and of information into knowledge.
3. Factors that necessitate more efficient management of information include the following:
   a. An increase in health-related legislation with requirements for the protection of information and for extensive recordkeeping, tracking, reporting, and documentation
   b. The rapid emergence of new health issues requiring immediate action

215

c. The changing demographics of client populations that may include workers who are older, more mobile, working from home, caring for family members, working multiple jobs, sharing jobs, or engaging in activities that may compound the effects of work on health

d. The more global nature of businesses, resulting in widely dispersed workers and customers

e. An expectation that the occupational and environmental health nurse will work collaboratively as part of multidisciplinary teams to address complex health issues in the workplace

f. A need to justify occupational health services as a worthwhile expenditure in a competitive market

g. The need to operate occupational health programs and services as a "business"

B **The occupational and environmental health nurse applies the principles of nursing informatics in the following activities:**

1. Assessing the needs of workers for services, education, and surveillance programs

2. Developing interventions that are appropriate for the client audience

3. Evaluating services to ensure quality of care and desired outcomes

4. Disseminating information to workers, peers, managers, and others in a timely, efficient manner

5. Ensuring compliance with all regulations and legislation that affect the occupational health service and the corporation

6. Conducting research

7. Accessing and using information from expert sources to support decision making

C **Information management systems can be applied to all aspects of the occupational health service, including the following:**

1. Developing and managing budgets

2. Selecting, training, and managing the performance and professional development of staff members

3. Overseeing the physical plant from which services are delivered

4. Anticipating, acquiring, and managing the resources required to deliver effective services

5. Producing and presenting reports that help business leaders make informed decisions

6. Developing and implementing policies that protect the health of workers

7. Developing and implementing protocols and standards of practice that ensure consistent delivery of goal-oriented services

II Tools Available to the Occupational and Environmental Health Nurse

A *Occupational health information management systems* **are computerized programs that provide a mechanism to collect, access, and use large amounts of information from many different sources in a single repository. They may be designed to be client-centered or site-management systems, or a combination of both.**

1. *Client-centered systems* facilitate the development of an electronic medical record that tracks health experiences of an individual from placement through the period of employment and for the period of retention as

required by the Occupational Safety and Health Administration (OSHA) (AAOHN, 2002); information maintained in a client-centered system includes the following:
  a. Preplacement health evaluations
  b. On-the-job injury treatment documentation
  c. Clinic visit notes
  d. Work restriction management records
  e. Disability case management notes
  f. Exposure documentation
  g. Participation in workplace surveillance programs
  h. Assignment and fitting of personal protective equipment
  i. Examination and test results
2. *Site-management systems* enable the occupational health professional to document activities related to a physical work environment, a corporation, or some geographical region; examples of the type of data captured by a site-management system include the following:
  a. Industrial hygiene sampling activities and results over time
  b. Exposures and actions taken
  c. OSHA recordkeeping
  d. Equipment calibration and maintenance records
  e. Vendor, supplier, and community provider lists
  f. Motor vehicle accident records

B *Combination systems* **are usually modular in design, and thus can be tailored to the specific needs of the organization.**
  1. These systems enable occupational health professionals to select, purchase, and implement those functions that are most applicable to their specific needs.
  2. Because of the expanding role of the occupational and environmental health nurse and the need to manage many different types of data, combination systems are increasingly preferred.

III Selecting and Implementing Information Management Systems

A **The American Nurses Association Taskforce on Nursing Information Systems has described the essential characteristics of effective health information systems (Zielstorff, Hudgings & Grobe, 1993); they must have the following characteristics:**
  1. Be flexible to meet changing requirements, such as incorporating new functionality to help track workers in a new exposure group
  2. Be compatible and able to integrate with other internal and external systems, such as Personnel or Human Resources
  3. Have a simple, logical approach to language and codes, including minimal technical jargon
  4. Support the work of the nurse without increasing effort, including eliminating double entry of the same data
  5. Provide useful outputs, such as reports, letters, and notices that the nurse develops
  6. Be cost efficient and cost beneficial to the organization and the user
  7. Ensure sustained performance with minimal downtime and ensure that data are easily recovered in the event of system failure

8. Ensure system security that prevents unauthorized entry or access to health information

9. Ensure data integrity that prevents loss, changes, or corruption of information captured in the system

10. Ensure confidentiality of sensitive information recorded by a health professional regarding the health status of a client

B **Other characteristics that are important to include in systems include:**

1. A standardized vocabulary and coding system

2. Drop-down lists to force consistency among users and avoid errors in data entry

   a. A drop-down list is a field that contains a list of selectable options.

   b. A user of a drop-down list can select an entry from the list by clicking the "down arrow" to the right of the field and highlighting the selection.

C *Selection* **of an occupational health information system must be a well-organized, thoughtful process that involves the input of any individual or group who will be using, interfacing with, or supporting the system.**

1. Typical team members participating in the selection process might include the following:

   a. Occupational and environmental health nurses

   b. Other occupational health professionals who may be users, that is, occupational physicians, industrial hygienists, safety professionals, employee assistant personnel, and others

   c. A management representative

   d. A person assigned from the corporate information systems department

   e. Representatives from the human resources or personnel department

2. The following steps will provide a framework for the team:

   a. Identify and define the information needs of users, other departments, and the company.

      1) List all services and functions to be supported by the system.

      2) Develop workflow diagrams for each process (Fig. 8-1).

      3) Identify the data needs for each step in the diagram (e.g., forms, questionnaires, notices, reports) (Fig. 8-2).

      4) Specify all interfaces and information exchanges required for each work process.

      5) Specify the methods of communication required for each interface (e.g., automatic fax, e-mail, hard-copy mail).

      6) Develop a list of all requirements and assign priorities for each function (Fig. 8-3).

   b. Determine whether to develop the system internally or purchase a commercial product.

   c. If the decision is made to purchase a commercial product, initiate the following activities to research suppliers and products:

      1) Attend trade shows and vendor exhibits at conferences such as the AAOHN Symposium & Expo.

      2) Network with occupational and environmental health nurses who are users of automated systems.

      3) Review the literature on specific products in journals, newsletters, and web sites.

      4) Invite vendors to demonstrate software products, using the list of functionality and specifications generated by the selection team.

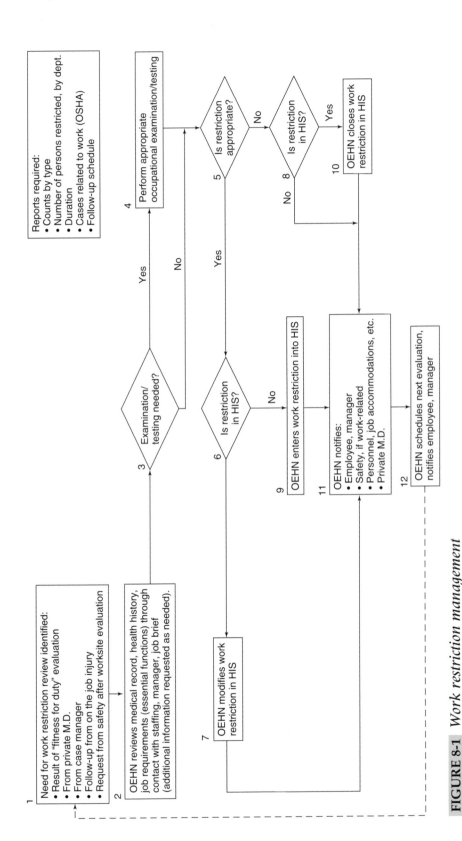

FIGURE 8-1 *Work restriction management*

OEHN, Occupational and environmental health nurse; *HIS*, health information system.

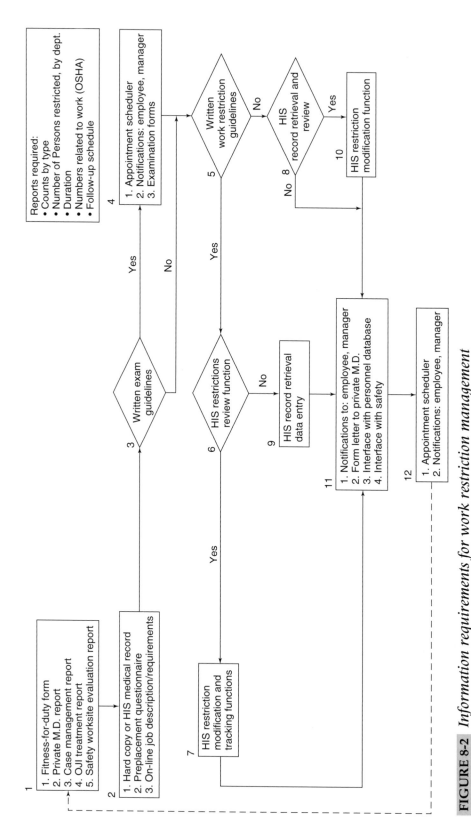

FIGURE 8-2 *Information requirements for work restriction management*

OJI, On-the-job injury; *HIS*, health information system; *OSHA*, Occupational Safety and Health Administration.

Function	Priority	System 1 Score/ weighted score		System 2 Score/ weighted score		System 3 Score/ weighted score	
Windows based							
Utilizes company network and platform							
Imports demographics from HR							
Ad hoc reporting							
User-defined standardized reports							
User-defined selection lists							
User-generated letters, notices, forms, questionnaires							
Schedules appointments							
Maintains activity log by site, staff, etc.							
Contains standards lists, ICD, MSDS							
Tracks costs/savings							
Archives records							
Provides on-line help for users							
Maintains vendor/provider lists							
Internet enabled							
E-mail connected							
Produces charts/graphics							
Interfaces with laboratory							
Instrument interfaces (audio, PFT)							
Word processing editing							
Search engine							
Preplacement Questionnaire/form							
Notices							
Establishes evaluation by job title							
Employee health record Encounters							
Clinical notes							
Procedures							
Allergies/serious health problems							
Medical Surveillance Target groups by risk							
Exam protocols/test panels							
Tracks exam/test results							
Imports environmental monitoring							
Imports job description, physical requirements							
Tracks equipment calibration records							
Hearing conservation program							
Respiratory protection program							

FIGURE 8-3 *Occupational health system review grid. Using a scale of 1 (least) to 5 (greatest), indicate the priority of each function to you. Give each system a score according to its ability to perform each function; then multiply the score by the priority to arrive at a weighted score for each function.*

HR, Human resources; ICD, international classification of diseases; MSDS, material safety data sheets; PFT, pulmonary function testing. PVT MD, private medical doctor; IME, independent medical examiner; FMLA, Family and Medical Leave Act; DOT, Department of Transportation; HR, human resources; TWA, time-weighted average.

Continued

Function	Priority	System 1 Score/ weighted score		System 2 Score/ weighted score		System 3 Score/ weighted score	
Immunization/vaccination records							
BBP required forms							
Titer results							
Prophylaxis records							
Notification of boosters/doses							
Captures serum information							
Motor vehicle accidents							
Accident details							
Claim details							
Costs to the company							
Employee training							
Documents course, attendance, hrs.							
Schedules							
Notifies							
Generates rosters							
Case management							
Case profile							
Duration guidelines							
PVT MD/IME reports							
Workers compensation history							
Rehab record							
Tracks costs							
Tracks days lost/restricted days							
Records FMLA criteria							
Drug testing							
Produces random selection							
Notifies employee/supervisor							
Records results							
Produces DOT reports							
Work restrictions							
Automatic re-evaluation notification							
Lists essential functions by job							
Transmits info to HR database							
Notifies employee/supervisor							
Calculates restricted work days							
Exports restricted day count to OSHA log							
Industrial hygiene							
Tracks sampling by area, employee							
Calculates exposure levels, TWA							
Security							
Multi-level password protected							
Audit trails for all files and records							
Encryption/coding capability							
Time lock for changes to records							
Audits							
Standard forms							
Schedule of locations/areas							
Produces randomized site selection							
Generates supervisor report							

FIGURE 8-3—*cont'd Occupational health system review grid.*

Function	Priority	System 1 Score/ weighted score		System 2 Score/ weighted score		System 3 Score/ weighted score	
System management System cost, license fee, # user fee							
Module/feature costs							
Cost of required hardware							
Cost of on-going support							
User training							
System documentation,							
User training manuals, job aids							
User groups							
Loss of customizations with upgrades							
Designated customer rep							
Response to change requests							
Health promotion Lists programs							
Captures roster/attendance							
Tracks individual attendance over time							
Distributes notices							
Captures costs							
Information technology Compatibility							
Networking capability							
Firewall issues							
Expandability							
Internet connectivity							
Ability to export to other programs							
Total of weighted scores for complete grid							

FIGURE 8-3 —*cont'd*

     5) Interview customers of specific software programs regarding functionality and support provided by the vendor.

    d. Prepare and submit a business case justifying the purchase or development of an electronic health information system.

D *Implementation* **of an occupational and environmental health information system can be facilitated by using project management techniques and tools (Chapter 7 describes the principles of project management). The following strategies will help ensure that the process of implementation is well organized and that all possible barriers have been anticipated.**

    1. Widely publicize the purchase and planned implementation.

    2. Secure the commitment of top-level management, unions, and other authority figures.

    3. Develop policies and procedures for appropriate use of the system.

    4. Appoint a lead representative to work directly with the system vendor/developer.

    5. Secure a designated representative from the company information systems department.

6. Establish evaluation criteria, including the following:
   a. Cost savings versus expenditures
   b. Time savings
   c. Improved communication between departments
   d. Improved access to critical information for professional decision making
   e. More-useful reports
   f. Increased satisfaction of users
7. Determine and institute measures to ensure security (e.g., passwords for users).
8. Provide ways to obtain and maintain appropriate hardware and software.
9. Ensure that users have basic computer skills; if not, institute tutorials or workshops.
10. Train one or more users to be "super users" who can support others during implementation and troubleshoot problems.
11. Test the system thoroughly, using scenarios developed by team members and ensuring that all functionality is utilized.
12. Establish a pilot program at a single location and document the experience thoroughly.
13. Implement the system on a limited basis (e.g., one function or one location at a time).
14. Have users keep a log of their progress, issues, and problems.
15. Have regular meetings to debrief workers and resolve issues as they occur.
16. Monitor direct and indirect costs associated with implementation.

IV The Internet

A **The *Internet* is a worldwide network of computers and users who are able to communicate using standardized protocols.**
1. Many forms of media, including voice, graphics, sound, video, and data can be transmitted among different users, user sites, machines, and networks of machines.
   a. The Internet (originally called the ARPANET or Advanced Research Project Agency Network) was created in 1969 for the purpose of communicating research data among four universities.
   b. The World Wide Web (www) is a widely used protocol, developed much later, that allows users to move freely from one site to another.
2. *Protocols* are sets of rules or common directions for accomplishing a task; the following protocols are commonly used on the Internet:
   a. TCP/IP (Transmission Control Protocol/Internet Protocol) is the suite of protocols that are required for Internet use.
   b. SMTP (Simple Mail Transfer Protocol) is the protocol used to send electronic mail via the Internet.
   c. POP has the following two meanings:
      1) *Point of presence* refers to a location where a user connects to a network, usually a city and often with dial-up phone lines. Internet customers should clarify with their Internet service provider if connecting using the assigned POP will require a long distance phone call.
      2) *Post Office Protocol* refers to the way e-mail software retrieves mail from a mail server.
   d. FTP (File Transfer Protocol) is a very common method of moving files from one site to another (e.g., accessing material from a library or catalog, or downloading software).

    e. HTTP (Hypertext Transfer Protocol) is the most important protocol used on the www, because it allows files to be moved across the Internet using hypertext, or the language that makes it possible to call up and display another site simply by selecting it.

    f. HTTPS (Hypertext Transfer Protocol—Secured) indicates that an HTTP site has had a level of security applied by software that limits access and protects information transmitted by users

3. There are other important terms that one needs to know to understand and use the Internet to its fullest potential, including the following:

    a. *HTML* (Hypertext Markup Language) is a coding language.

        1) *Hypertext* enables words, symbols, graphics, sound and video files, and other items to be linked to other sites or items within a site.

        2) Selecting hypertext items allows users to "navigate" or "surf" from site to site in a nonlinear way.

    b. *Bandwidth* is the amount of data that can be transmitted at once.

    c. *Bits* are the smallest unit of computerized data (bandwidth is measured in bits-per-second).

    d. *Bytes* are a set of bits (usually 8).

        1) A *kilobyte* is 1000 bytes, and a *megabyte* is one million bytes.

        2) This metric is most often used to describe the space available on a drive or in memory.

    e. *Baud* is the speed at which a computer can send or receive bits of data.

    f. A *bookmark* (sometimes called a *favorite)* is a direct link created by the user to a site that was once visited and is likely to be visited again.

        1) Creating bookmarks is a fast, efficient way to use the browser to navigate directly to a site without searching.

        2) Occupational and environmental health nurses can use bookmarks to create directories of sites that contain commonly used information, such as the sites maintained by the Centers for Disease Control and Prevention (CDC), Occupational Safety and Health Administration (OSHA), American Association of Occupational Health Nurses (AAOHN), American Board for Occupational Health Nurses (ABOHN), and National Institute for Occupational Safety and Health (NIOSH). (Appendix IV provides the addresses for these and other Web sites.)

    g. A *browser* is a software program that is the interface between the user and the Internet and allows users to contact other Web servers.

    h. A *Web page* is a collection of resources located at a single Internet address.

    i. *Search engines* are software programs that allow users to search for sites that contain user-specified key words or phrases.

    j. A *URL* (Uniform Resource Locator) is an Internet *address;* every item on the Internet has a distinct URL. The following list explains the elements of this sample URL: http://www.cdc.gov/travel/vaccinat/htm

        1) http: The protocol necessary to access the site

        2) www.cdc.gov: the "domain" or who and what type of organization owns the site

        3) travel/vaccinat: the "path" within the site to the desired information

        4) htm: the language or coding system used in the site

B **There are several methods of finding information on the Internet.**

1. A search engine produces a list of web sites that meet user's search criteria; examples of search engines are Yahoo, Google, AltaVista, and AskJeeves.

    a. Tips for searching the Internet include:
       1) Use combinations of "key" words
       2) Use more words for better search results
       3) Try synonyms or plural forms of words if desired results are not achieved
       4) Use quotation marks to search for phrases or names
       5) Use the word "OR" in caps to expand the search
       6) Use a minus sign (–) to exclude sites or information that is not relevant (For example, "cardiac disease – pediatric" to eliminate all references to cardiac disease in children)
       7) Use multiple search engines to produce more and different results
    b. Tips for searching within sites on the Internet include:
       1) Use key words or phrases in the search box
       2) Take advantage of options to exclude words or sites from the search
       3) Use alphabetical search options to conduct topic searches when available
       4) The use of quotation marks usually specifies an exact match
       5) Utilize links in search results to go directly to the desired information
       6) Observe the "title line" in the URL box to identify where you are in the site and what search criteria are being used
       7) Note the bottom of the search result screen to determine how many documents or sites were identified that matched the search criteria.
       8) Search results are presented in order of relevance or match
  2. Other methods that can be used to find information include:
    a. Typing the URL into an address field
    b. Linking to a site by clicking on hypertext in another site
    c. Going directly to a site by means of a bookmark
    d. Selecting a site from the "history" list of previously visited sites

C **The occupational and environmental health nurse may use the Internet for the following purposes:**
  1. To obtain current information related to a health issue
  2. To stay abreast of current legislation and regulations
  3. To share experiences with other occupational health professionals
  4. To search and "shop" for products and services to meet the needs of clients
  5. To participate in research
  6. To obtain continuing education
  7. To market services to potential customers

D **Although the Internet provides a vast source of information for consumers and practitioners, there are few standards to regulate the quality of information or the credibility of the suppliers of information.**

E **The following guidelines should be used by Internet users to assess health information available on the Internet:**
  1. Authors should be clearly identified.
  2. Authors should be qualified and their credentials listed.
  3. Professional references should be listed.
  4. The site should not focus on the sale of services or products.
  5. The site owners should indicate that the information offered is not a substitute for services provided directly by a trained professional caregiver.
  6. A mechanism to request feedback or more information should be supplied.
  7. Confidentiality must be ensured to individuals requesting information.
  8. The appearance of the site should be professional.

9. Information provided should be current and the date of last revision noted.
10. Any sources of funding must be identified.
11. If the site is not supported by a government agency, it should bear a mark of recognition by one of several organizations that evaluate health information on the Internet, such as the American Nurses Association or the Health on the Net Foundation.

V Intranets

A *Intranets* **are private networks developed by companies, universities, or other agencies to provide information and services to a prescribed audience by means of the same technology used on the Internet.**

B **Companies use intranets to accomplish the following:**
1. Centralize services, such as payroll and benefits
2. Allow workers access to company news and business information
3. Distribute information in a timely, efficient manner
4. Post and maintain business directives and policies in a central location
5. Foster the sharing of information among workers, business units, and organizations within the corporation.

C **The occupational health programs and services manager may take advantage of the technology afforded by company intranets to accomplish the following purposes:**
1. Distribute health-related information to workers via department Web sites or electronic newsletters
2. Share relevant information with departments such as benefits, safety, and personnel
3. Centralize information such as health-related policies and procedures
4. Automate, expedite, and improve the accuracy of processes such as accident reporting
5. Deliver health-related training to workers, and services such as interactive health-risk appraisals
6. Provide workers with links to important Internet sites that contain relevant health and safety information
7. Communicate and share information with external suppliers of services, such as insurance carriers, laboratories, independent medical examiners, or medical supply companies

D *Extranets* **are proprietary systems that allow limited access to an Intranet.**
1. These systems are usually networks that have identified necessary interfaces and established policies and protocols to permit communication through company security mechanisms to specific areas within the Intranet.
2. Access to these specialized networks may be granted to individuals or groups such as customers, vendors, or suppliers for a variety of purposes.

VI Security

Policies and procedures should be in place to ensure that the confidentiality, integrity, quality, and security of computerized health information are maintained. Data security exists when data are protected from accidental or intentional disclosure to unauthorized persons and from unauthorized or accidental alteration (e.g., loss by physical damage such as fire, water, or electrical failure).

A A *firewall* is a security system consisting of a combination of hardware and software that limits the exposure of a computer or computer network from unauthorized access.

1. Unauthorized access may be accomplished by "hackers" (or more correctly "crackers"), who are skilled programmers with the reputation of having a mischievous bent for breaking into secured systems, sometimes with extremely damaging consequences.

2. A company uses a firewall to ensure the security of its intranet and limit access to workers only.

3. A firewall is a critical component of the company's computing security policies and practices; the firewall protects against unauthenticated interactive logins from the "outside" world.

4. The firewall provides a single point where security and audit can be imposed; it may provide summaries about:
   a. What kinds and amount of traffic passed through it
   b. How many attempts there were to break into it

5. Firewalls must be part of a consistent overall organizational security architecture. It cannot protect information from:
   a. Malicious individuals inside the network
   b. Users who reveal sensitive information inappropriately

6. The firewall cannot be relied upon as the only protection against viruses (Robertson, Curtin & Ranum, 2004)

B Viruses or malicious software (malware) are software programs capable of reproducing themselves and usually capable of causing great harm to files or other programs on the same computer. (A worm is a particular type of virus. It is an acronym for "write once, read many.") (Enzer, 2005)

1. A firewall will protect only against viruses that come from the Internet, not from other sources such as disks, CDs, etc.

2. Every vulnerable desktop should have virus-scanning software that is run when the machine is rebooted.

C Appropriate means and mechanisms should be used to protect identifiable health information (American Society for Testing Materials, 1999).

1. Use a personal identifier that is not readily linkable to other nonhealth-related databases to protect the individual's privacy

2. Apply encryption technology when transmitting data from one location to another

3. Have confidentiality agreements in place:
   a. With vendors and other business partners
   b. With staff to reinforce commitment to maintaining confidentiality

4. The health information system should:
   a. Allow users and managers to classify data for access purposes
      1) Some may have summary information, while others may hold detailed information.
      2) Policies and procedures should identify the users/roles that are authorized to read, enter, modify, amend, or download data and which data elements or data groups that person may access.
      3) Systems should be designed to verify and authenticate the identity of the user and record each access to the record/database and action taken.

    4) Periodically review the assignment of access privileges on the basis of job duties, roles, and requirements.

    5) The system should automatically record any apparent inappropriate access or breach of level of authorized access by a user and automatically notify the system's data security officer.

  b. Protect data from loss or damage by providing:

    1) Routine data back-up

    2) Storage of data in a manner that will withstand deterioration, corruption, and unauthorized destruction

    3) Physical security for appropriate components of information systems, including computer rooms, printers, network components, data archives, health record areas, printed reports, and downloaded data

    4) Alarms and alerts for hardware failures

    5) A back-up plan for system downtime

VII Office Management Programs

Office management programs represent another category of electronic tools available to the occupational and environmental health nurse.

A **Used separately or in combination with health information systems, the Internet, or company intranets, the following office management programs are invaluable when refining information management techniques:**

1. *Word processing programs,* such as Microsoft Word and WordPerfect, allow the occupational and environmental health nurse to create text documents such as letters, reports, and notices.

2. *Spreadsheet programs,* such as Excel, create files that allow large amounts of data to be captured, manipulated, and displayed in categorical fashion, such as budgets and other resource management documents.

3. *Relational database systems,* such as Access, allow information to be stored in fields and tables that can be sorted and reported in many combinations. These programs are often used to create forms and questionnaires such as health risk appraisals, training records, exposure questionnaires, and audits.

4. *Presentation programs,* such as PowerPoint, allow the occupational and environmental health nurse to create visually effective programs or slide presentations that can contain text, graphics, charts, tables, pictures, and sound. These programs are useful in developing reports, worker training programs, and professional presentations.

B *Communication systems,* **including voice and electronic mail, enable the occupational and environmental health nurse to communicate rapidly and efficiently with peers and customers. Tools within this category include the following:**

1. *Mail lists,* which allow the user to send the same message to a group of individuals simultaneously (See Box 8-1: Rules for E-mail Users)

2. *Folders,* which are repositories for saved mail messages on the same topic or from the same sender

3. *Directories,* which are electronic *address books* that enable the user of the mail system to capture and store information about individuals who are contacted often

4. *Mail system calendars,* which allow users to reserve dates and times on their personal schedules and check the availability of others for purposes of meeting planning

---

BOX 8-1

Informal Rules for E-mail Use

1. Limit copies to the people who need the information. This keeps the number of messages manageable.
2. Choose an accurate description for the subject line. This practice helps recipients to determine which messages should be read first
3. Give e-mail messages the same consideration given to business correspondence. Parties other than intended recipients may seee-mail. In an e-mail message, nothing should be written that one would not publicly post.
4. Make messages clear, short, and to the point.
5. Avoid the use of all-capital letters. This is difficult to read, and may be perceived as yelling, according to e-mail etiquette.
6. Limit abbreviations to those that are easily understood.
7. Read mail, file messages in categories, and delete messages no longer needed on a regular basis.

Source: Hebda, Czar, Mascara (1998).

---

5. *Conferencing,* which allows individuals to participate simultaneously in a telephone session and may often be used in conjunction with a computer presentation to supplement the discussion with visual media

VIII Implications for Occupational and Environmental Health Nursing

A The ability to manage information efficiently requires occupational and environmental health nurses to integrate information from many sources, including the following:

1. The client
   a. Health status
   b. Illness/injury experience
   c. Work history
   d. Intervention participation
   e. Training and education
2. The company
   a. Benefits information
   b. Salary and hours/shifts worked
   c. Job descriptions, including essential functions
   d. Insurance utilization and experience
   e. Administrative controls
3. Other occupational health and safety departments
   a. Industrial hygiene sampling activity
   b. Safety audits
   c. Personal protective equipment status
   d. Exposure history for individuals, groups, and the organization
   e. OSHA recordable injuries and illnesses
   f. Accident investigations
   g. Remediation plans and assignment of responsibility

4. Regulatory, legislative, and guideline-setting agencies
   a. Current regulations related to specific work, tasks, technology, conditions, and environmental agents
   b. Recommendations for addressing potential health and safety issues
   c. Guidelines for establishing effective programs and interventions
   d. Specifications of materials and equipment
   e. Information about specific agents, chemicals, or compounds
5. Outside providers of products and services
   a. Reports and recommendations of providers of clinical services
   b. Support for regulated programs, such as Department of Transportation (DOT) drug testing. (Chapters 3 and 16 provide additional information about such programs.)
   c. Information from suppliers of health-related equipment and supplies
6. Academic and professional organizations
   a. Current research findings
   b. Literature related to the occupational health setting
   c. Networking with peers within the specialty of occupational health
   d. Advice and consultation about specific health issues
   e. Continuing education for occupational health professionals
   f. Participation in web conferencing on major health issues, hosted by agencies such as NIOSH, CDC, and Environmental Protection Agency (EPA)

B **Occupational and environmental health nurses are often required to use a combination of tools to help manage occupational health units; these include the following:**
1. Occupational health information systems
2. The Internet
3. Intranets
4. Office management programs

C **Occupational and environmental health nurses must be attentive to the legal, ethical, and professional implications of using automated systems to manage occupational health information.**
1. To safeguard the security and integrity of health information, the occupational and environmental health nurse must accomplish the following:
   a. Develop policies and procedures regarding the use of all electronic systems and equipment, including computers, fax systems, scanners, and mail systems
   b. Require that all workers with access to health records are trained in the management of health information
   c. Establish a policy on "electronic signatures" that is consistent with company policy and state regulations
   d. Establish and impose penalties for the misuse of the information system and its contents
   e. Establish and maintain audit trails or records to monitor who accesses a record, and when and for what purpose it was accessed
   f. Back up information frequently and store backups in a separate, secure location
   g. Impose "locks" on electronic records that prevent changes to an entry after a predetermined period of time

2. To safeguard the confidentiality of worker health information, the occupational and environmental health nurse must accomplish the following:
   a. Establish and maintain lists of approved users, signatures, titles, and clearance levels, including the following information:
      1) Who may access a record
      2) Who may make an entry to a particular record
      3) Who may read a particular record
      4) Who may retrieve or transmit a record
      5) What fields within a record individuals may view
   b. Require that all workers with access to health records sign a "statement of protection of confidentiality"
   c. Block specific information or restrict access to those with a bona fide "need to know" and those on current user approval lists
   d. Establish and use client identifiers, such as worker numbers, for use during transmission of data
   e. Encode or encrypt sensitive information during transmission
   f. Use multilevel passwords to identify authorized users
   g. Change passwords often on an unscheduled basis

D **To manage the transition from manual to automated systems, the occupational and environmental health nurse must accomplish the following:**
   1. Acknowledge the philosophical as well as the technical changes required
   2. Involve as many staff members as practical in all stages of decision making, implementation, and maintenance of information management programs
   3. Assess the initial and ongoing training needs of users
   4. Recognize that different users learn and adapt at different rates
   5. Support users and provide positive feedback for progress made
   6. Monitor the benefits and savings of moving from manual to automated methods of managing information
   7. Use the technology to highlight the advances being made by the occupational health organization

E **Effective information management will increase the ability of the occupational and environmental health nurse to accomplish the following:**
   1. Manage resources more efficiently
   2. Develop more appropriate, higher-quality interventions
   3. Communicate more effectively
   4. Make better clinical decisions
   5. Stay better informed on current and emerging health and safety issues

REFERENCES

American Association of Occupational Health Nurses. (2002). *Employee health record management. AAOHN Advisory.* Atlanta, GA: AAOHN Publications.

American Nurses Association. (2001). *Scope and standards of nursing informatics practice.* Washington, DC: American Nurses Association.

American Society for Testing and Materials. (1999). Standard guide for confidentiality, privacy, access, and data security principles for health information including computer-based patient records. In *1999 Annual book of ASTM standards Volume 14.01: Healthcare informatics; computerized systems and chemical and material information* (pp. 858-865). West Conshohocken, PA: American Society for Testing and Materials.

Enzer, M. (2005). Internet literacy consultants glossary of Internet terms. Available at http://www.matisse.net/files/glossary,html.

TABLE 9-1

Structure, process, and outcomes: evaluative elements in quality assurance

Structural elements	Process elements	Outcome elements
Physical setting	Management of the	Improved health
Philosophy of health by	operation	Compliance with treatment
management, workers,	Decision-making processes	regimens
health care professionals	Collaboration	Reduced morbidity and
Organizational mission and	Nursing interventions/	mortality
structure	monitoring	Positive changes in
Unit goals and objectives	Services provided	knowledge and attitudes
Human and financial	Development of records and	about health
resources	reports	Satisfaction with service
Operational resources		quality

Source: Adapted from Rogers, 2003.

demographics; and the mission, goals, and objectives to meet the health and safety needs of the work-site community. A knowledge of the structural elements can be achieved through the following activities:

1. Review the management reporting structure; determine who supports the occupational health program and services.
   a. Determine who the occupational and environmental health nurse reports to, administratively and professionally.
   b. Participate in the formulation and implementation of administrative procedures.
   c. Participate in the development of policies and procedures applicable to health issues (e.g., return to work, case management, fitness for duty).
   d. Develop the philosophy and written goals and objectives for occupational health programs and services.
   e. Conduct periodic reviews of occupational health programs and services to ensure that goals and objectives are being met.
   f. Participate in meetings that address health issues (e.g., safety, management staff, department, and human resource meetings).
   g. Communicate clearly and in writing with management and department heads as needed.
   h. Demonstrate the effectiveness of the health services department in terms of cost, productivity, and return on investment.
   i. Communicate workplace information, distribution lists, upcoming events, and plans to the occupational health and safety staff.
2. Evaluate the suitability of physical facilities provided for occupational health programs and services; the following features are important:
   a. Central location with easy access for workers
   b. Accessible for ambulance stretchers and other wheeled traffic
   c. Sufficiently spacious to provide examination, treatment, and consultation needs
   d. Confidentiality and privacy for clients and for the nurses to complete all aspects of work (telephone consults, examinations, etc.)
   e. Entrance clearly marked "Occupational Health Services" or "Health Unit"
   f. Sink and toilet facilities available and accessible
   g. Convenient and comfortable waiting area

    h. Adequate ventilation, heating, and air conditioning
    i. Access for separate telephone lines for fax, telephone, and computer
    j. Space to maintain supplies and medical records

3. Identify supplies and equipment needed to deliver occupational health programs and services.
   a. Supplies and medications appropriate for the practice are maintained in adequate supply, stored under proper conditions, and not kept beyond expiration dates.
   b. Appropriate medical equipment (e.g., refrigerator, oxygen, otoscope, sphygmomanometers) is available and in good working condition.
   c. Equipment used in performing examinations required by OSHA (e.g., audiometric booths, spirometer) is maintained and calibrated according to federal standards.
   d. Laboratory tests (e.g., cholesterol tests, drug specimen collection) are conducted in accordance with state and federal guidelines.

4. Identify staffing requirements, qualifications, and professional development recommendations.
   a. Copies of professional licenses and required certifications are kept for all staff.
   b. Copies of updated curriculum vitae or résumés are kept on file.
   c. Occupational health staff takes advantage of opportunities to grow professionally and to advance the specialty of occupational and environmental health nursing.
   d. Attainment of occupational health nursing certification is supported and encouraged (Certified Occupational Health Nurse [COHN] or Certified Occupational Health Nurse-Specialist [COHN-S]). (Refer to http://www.abohn.org/ for certification guidelines.)
   e. Nurses' active membership and involvement in AAOHN, including attendance at local and regional or state chapter meetings, is encouraged and supported.
   f. Nurses' participation in professional development seminars designed to advance individual practice in occupational and environmental health nursing is supported and encouraged.
   g. Occupational health staff is encouraged to continue formal and informal education.
   h. Professional journals (e.g., nursing, occupational, health, and safety) and other professional resources are available.
   i. Nursing responsibilities are clearly defined in a position description.

5. Assess work-site community and ensure that programs and services, including those required by OSHA, are available to meet the needs of the workers.
   a. Work-force analyses are used to determine the number of workers and managers, median age of population, approximate distribution of population by gender, number of accommodated workers (according to Americans with Disabilities Act) on property, and health status of worker population.
   b. Health and safety hazards, specific exposures, and OSHA-required programs and services are identified (e.g., bloodborne pathogens, hearing conservation, respirator usage).

6. Develop mission, goals, and objectives that meet the health and safety of the workers and the business needs of the company.

    a. Goals and objectives need to be regularly revised and updated.

    b. Mission, goals, and objectives should reflect current issues and practices in occupational health.

B *Process elements* **include such things as the delivery of nursing clinical practice; methods used to provide services and programs; and recordkeeping and documentation development.**

  1. Nursing clinical practice is appropriate for the occupational health setting, provided that the following requirements are met:

    a. Clinical practice is consistent with the following:

      1) State nurse practice act

      2) Pharmacy and medical practice acts

      3) AAOHN Standards of Practice

      4) Published clinical practice guidelines

      5) AAOHN competencies

    b. A policy and procedure manual is written and reflects current occupational health practice.

    c. Occupational and environmental health nursing resources are used to guide clinical practice.

  2. The scope of clinical services and programs should be designed to meet the needs of the work-site community.

    a. Injury and illness management services include the following:

      1) Care and treatment of occupational injuries and illnesses

      2) Care and treatment of nonoccupational injuries and illnesses

      3) Emergency care for workers and visitors at the facility

      4) Registered nurse supervision of nursing care provided to workers

    b. To evaluate health promotion and screening programs and services, the occupational and environmental health nurse should:

      1) Determine the efficacy of health promotion programs and services that have been delivered at the work site. Examples include: back safety, ergonomics, hearing/vision conservation, occupational dermatitis and hypertension screening.

      2) Evaluate formats used to offer health promotion and health education. Examples are formal lectures, management meetings, informational pamphlet distribution, posters, and bulletin board or table displays.

    c. Case management of occupational and nonoccupational injury and illness (including absenteeism) involves the following activities (Chapter 12 provides additional information):

      1) The nurse communicates and collaborates with managers, claims administrators, workers, and medical providers to facilitate appropriate, safe, and timely return to work.

      2) The nurse is familiar with the state's workers' compensation laws.

      3) The nurse reviews health care and response to treatment, including expected normal recovery times (*The Medical Disability Advisor*, 4th edition, is a recommended resource).

      4) The nurse recommends an independent medical evaluation when appropriate.

      5) The nurse has a working knowledge of medical and health benefit programs and services offered by the employer.

      6) The nurse, together with the manager, identifies temporary modified jobs that support treatment goals.

7) The nurse maintains contact with workers who have sustained an injury or illness.

8) The nurse evaluates workers who are absent from work for more than 5 days with non–work-related illness or injury.

d. The occupational and environmental health nurse should attend meetings of the safety committee to discuss health and safety issues and to share findings and knowledge about health and safety issues.

e. OSHA surveillance programs, other required programs and services, and training sessions should be provided and completed as appropriate. Examples include hearing loss prevention programs, respirator approval (refer to current OSHA guidelines), and Department of Transportation (DOT) drug testing programs.

f. Employee assistance program (EAP) and/or referrals should be available to workers. The occupational and environmental health nurse is responsible for:

1) Identifying how EAP services are provided at the work site

2) Assessing workers and referring them for appropriate treatment

3) In some cases, delivering some components of the EAP service such as counseling, depending on the nurse's educational preparation and experience (See Chapter 14)

g. Immunization programs are offered for prevention, post exposure, and travel (e.g., hepatitis B, influenza, and tetanus).

3. Emergency response planning is increasingly important in the modern day workplace. At a minimum, an emergency response program should include a biopreparedness/disaster plan, an automatic external defibrillator (AED) program, and a first aid/responder team.

a. An emergency response/disaster/biopreparedness plan will provide guidance and direction for the program. In order to have a successful plan, the following must occur:

1) Workers responsible for coordinating and implementing the disaster plan within the facility must be identified.

2) The plan must be periodically tested and revised as needed.

3) There must be active workers' participation in the planning, implementation, testing and evaluation of the plan.

4) The plan must be coordinated with the local community, first responders, and hospital and other health centers (e.g., public health departments).

b. Automatic external defibrillators (AEDs) are used to assess a worker's heart rhythm, determine if defibrillation is needed, and then administer a proper level of shock.

1) The AED unit must be approved by the U.S. Food and Drug Administration.

2) Procedures for using the AED that meet state and local requirements are available.

3) A registered nurse should be designated as the AED program coordinator.

c. A first aid/responder team should be developed; the team may consist of workers, managers, and/or health professionals.

1) Members of the team should include workers at strategic locations and from all shifts who are able to respond to medical emergencies.

2) The first aid team should be trained to provide cardiopulmonary resuscitation (CPR) and first aid, to comply with bloodborne pathogen requirements, and to use AED equipment.

3) The first aid logs should be reviewed in order to evaluate the effectiveness and appropriateness of care provided by the first aid/responder team members.

4) AAOHN's Foundation Block: *Establishing an Automatic External Defibrillator Program (2004)* provides a detailed description of a comprehensive AED program.

4. The documentation and recordkeeping system should be regularly evaluated.

a. The quality of documentation and recordkeeping should be evaluated to be sure records are appropriate and clear and that they meet legal reporting requirements.

b. The type of system used for documentation (manual or computer) should be identified; the system should have the following characteristics:

1) Documentation is timely and complete

2) Entries on the daily log reflect accurate documentation in the health record.

3) Daily logs are used to summarize clinical activity and trends to report to management.

4) All health records are secured in a locked cabinet/area.

5) Computerized records are secured by passwords, limiting access to occupational health staff only.

6) Health records are retained according to federal law (exposure records are to be retained for 30 years; health records are retained for the duration of employment plus 30 years).

7) Disclosure of information from a worker's health record is made only with written informed consent of the individual, adhering to confidentiality and Health Insurance Portability and Accountability Act (HIPAA) guidelines (i.e., Privacy Rule).

8) Work-related injuries and illnesses are shared with the employer only on a need-to-know basis.

c. OSHA forms, training logs, and other management reports related to the following should be reviewed:

1) Bloodborne pathogens training

2) Hearing conservation programs and services

3) Respiratory protection programs and services

4) Other relevant programs

C *Outcome elements:* **Programs and services provided to an individual worker or population of workers need to be evaluated in order to determine if expected outcomes have been achieved.**

1. Health outcomes resulting from the programs and services include the following:

a. Illness and injury has been prevented whenever possible.

b. There is evidence that compliance with treatment regimens has increased.

c. Workers have increased knowledge about self-care

d. Function following injury occurrence has been restored.

1) Physical functions include ambulation, lifting, etc.

2) Psychological functions include memory, cognition, or mood

3) Social functions include interpersonal relationships and communication

4) Role functions relate to care of family members, that is, children, parent, or others

  e. Diseases, such as an infection or hypertension, are cured or successfully managed.
  f. Workers experience relief of discomfort such as:
    1) Physical discomfort, such as pain
    2) Psychologic discomfort, such as depression
2. The outcomes related to health care programs and services are compared with the costs, so that judgments about the value of the programs and services can be made for the company. Some examples follow:
  a. Work-site influenza immunization program (immunize healthy adults against influenza to reduce absenteeism)
    1) *Outcome:* The company will have a healthier work force, resulting in less absenteeism and improved productivity.
    2) *Cost savings:* A study by Nichol (AAOHN, 1999) determined a return on investment of $47/worker for their flu immunization program.
  b. Back injury prevention program (work-related back injuries account for high-volume, high-cost worker's compensation claims)
    1) *Outcome:* Use of a lift team extends beyond effect on injury and financial outcomes—these teams can be used for recruitment and retention strategies. Ultimately, a lift team helps protect a valuable resource—the health care worker.
    2) *Cost savings:* Direct and indirect medical expenses for back injuries decreased dramatically. Average cost per recordable back injury decreased from $6,294 to $1,099 (*A Lift Team Success Story*, AAOHN, 2003)
  c. Case management (workers' compensation and disability cases)
    1) *Outcome:* The most commonly reported outcome of the case management program is the workers' timely return to work. Quality outcomes such as workers' quality of life and well being after an injury and worker's satisfaction (obtained through interviews) are also important factors to report.
    2) *Cost savings:* Decreased medical costs and lost work days are reported as positive results of case-managed cases.
3. The measurement of health outcomes begins at the individual level; many individual outcomes can be pooled to assess factors of interest or need for services across worker groups.

V Methods of Evaluation

A **Several techniques may be used for gathering information. These may include:**
1. The retrospective chart audit, which:
  a. Focuses on documented evidence of nursing care provided
  b. Assumes that what is documented is what care has been performed
2. Concurrent document review which involves:
  a. A critical examination of case management (while care is in progress) and of client outcomes
  b. A review of chart, plans for care, immediate feedback
3. Interviewing, which consists of verbal interaction with workers.
  a. In order to be meaningful, the interviewer needs to clarify questions, attitudes, opinions, client satisfaction, and management understanding of health care.

   b. It is important to word questions consistently from worker to worker to decrease bias.
   4. Questionnaires, which are the most common tool used for program evaluation; it is important to write questions clearly and to provide clear directions for completion.
   5. Observations, which are important supplements to other techniques.
      a. Occupational and environmental health nursing managers may observe the delivery of health services in order to evaluate physical assessment skills, such as occupational history taking, medication administration practices, and the development of treatment plans.
      b. Worksites may be observed to identify work hazards and working conditions.
      c. Workers may be observed to determine if they are using safe work practices.
      d. Observations provide the opportunity to provide immediate feedback, validate the procedure manual for appropriateness, and to determine the relationship of outcomes to actual nursing practices.

B **The staffing and type of work environment requires consideration when conducting a quality review. (See AAOHN's** *Staffing Ratios for Occupational Health and Safety Services***) (2004).**
   1. In corporate settings with a number of nurses, a quality-assurance program can be developed by the nurses and used at several different sites.
   2. In settings where nurses work alone, develop a quality-review team of interested peers located nearby or form a team of occupational and environmental health nurses representing local AAOHN constituencies.
   3. Develop and customize an evaluation tool to identify the specific needs of your company's occupational health program.
   4. Use an evaluation tool that reflects current practice in occupational health as a framework to develop your own evaluation tool. AAOHN's *Quality Assurance Packet* (AAOHN Foundation Blocks, 2004) includes several evaluation tools, including a Site Evaluation Tool, a chart Audit Form, and an Employee Evaluation of Health Services Form.

VI Cost-Effective and Cost-Benefit Programs and Services

A **Cost evaluations can be used to determine the effectiveness and efficiency of programs and services.**
   1. Management's goal for developing or maintaining occupational health services and programs is often to contain costs.
   2. Cost-benefit and cost-effectiveness analyses can be used to demonstrate the cost effectiveness of the overall program and the cost benefit of its specific components.
   3. Health conditions and safety problems that are having a significant impact on the company's "bottom line" should be targeted for program development, followed by cost-benefit analyses.
   4. Cost-effectiveness analysis and cost-benefit analysis are convincing tools for communicating with upper management.

B **Two methods are used to analyze the monetary value of a program or service: cost-benefit analysis and cost-effectiveness analysis.**
   1. Cost-benefit analysis compares the benefits of programs and services to the costs.
   2. A cost-benefit analysis has the following characteristics:

a. Considers both costs and benefits (or outcomes) of a program in monetary terms

b. Permits a comparison between unlike elements.

c. Yields a benefit-to-cost ratio.

3. Cost-effectiveness analysis determines how effectively resources are used; it is used to demonstrate the programs' services in relation to the costs and to compare its costs with alternative approaches and its outcomes with benchmarks (Morris, Smith, 2001, p. 547).

C **There are multiple reasons for conducting cost analyses:**

1. Cost-benefit and cost-effectiveness analyses, which help determine which programs or services can produce a benefit that is greater than the cost, are helpful because many administrators are not aware of the true potential of health services or programs for the company or their workers.

2. Demonstrate short-term and long-term costs and benefits:

   a. Find cause-and-effect relationships between programs and benefits as noted above, and project how the organization can gain from effective programming in these areas.

   b. Categorize, quantify, and compare benefits and costs.

      1) *Short-term benefits* may include increased morale, productivity, and corporate image.

      2) *Long-term benefits* may include decreased health and life insurance costs, decreased workers' compensation claims, and decreased worker turnover.

      3) *Short-term costs* involve commitment of space, resources, supplies, and equipment, and organizational time and involvement.

      4) *Long-term costs* can include time for participation of management and workers and the ongoing cost of utilities and program maintenance expenses.

   c. Determine the areas of greatest program impact, such as physical impairments, workers' compensation claims, or public relations.

   d. Compare program costs with those of other current company programs and services and determine how this program compares with their costs and benefits.

   e. Ask whether the proposed health and safety program is a good investment and worthy of everyone's time and effort.

   f. A documentation of workers' compensation costs may help to demonstrate the need for work-related programs and services in the organization.

D **Steps in conducting cost-benefit and cost-effectiveness analyses include the following:**

1. Determine the program/service for financial analysis.

2. Formulate the objectives and goals of the programs and services.

3. List alternative ways objectives and goals can be achieved.

4. Determine costs/benefits for all alternatives.

5. Determine monetary values for costs/benefits, or determine outcome measures (e.g., absenteeism rates; health services utilization; changes in risk behaviors).

6. Calculate discounting.

   a. Discounting reduces future costs to their present worth.

   b. It answers the question: "What is the cost of providing this service now compared with what it will cost in the future?"

7. See AAOHN Publication, *Success Tools: Measuring and Articulating Value* (1998) for examples of determining cost-benefit and cost-effectiveness analysis.

VII Other Health and Safety Program Considerations

Occupational and environmental health nurses who are actively involved in planning and developing health and safety programs and services will need to explore many issues to ensure program success and participation.

A **Issues that should be addressed in health and safety programs and services include confidentiality, legal issues, advisory committee involvement, and management support.**

1. The confidentiality of information collected from or about workers is a major concern, especially as it relates to personal health data; workers often fear that this information may be used to punish or dismiss them or that it otherwise endangers their employment.

2. Legal concerns include the company's liability for workers if they become injured when participating in company-sponsored health programs and services such as Fun Runs and Health Fairs.

3. It is important that a health and safety advisory committee be involved in program planning, implementation, and evaluation.
   a. Labor *and* management representation and input are necessary to ensure the success of programs and services.
   b. A committee is instrumental in suggesting topics, obtaining peer support, identifying barriers, and identifying resources.

4. Management support must be garnered early in the planning stages to approve the program's financing, workers' involvement, and the program's relevance for the workplace, and to take into account other political and philosophical considerations.

B **Occupational and environmental health nurses should consider using a business approach to health and safety program development, because the language of business is more easily understood by management; in addition, a *business plan* is helpful in setting up programs and services and monitoring their success.**

1. A business plan can serve the following functions:
   a. Provide an overview of the services included in the comprehensive occupational health and safety program.
   b. Guide the program in its implementation and evaluation.
   c. Provide guidelines for identifying resources required to implement a program.
   d. Communicate ideas and approaches to management and unions.

2. A business plan should be tailored to the individual needs of the organization and the program; the basic components of a business plan are as follows:
   a. *Executive summary*. An Executive summary outlines the goals and objectives of the program and service.
      1) This is sometimes the most important section for company executives/managers to commit resources to the program or service.
      2) This summary is also an important communication tool for employees and potential customers who need to understand and get behind the purpose and ideas of the plan.
   b. *History*. A brief account of the history highlights similar programs' success at other "benchmark" companies; the concept of the program or service should be clearly explained.
   c. *Goals*. In a few short paragraphs, explain the goals of the program or service by answering the following questions:

1) How fast will the program grow?
2) Who will be the primary customers?
3) What is the program expected to achieve?

d. *Leaders.* The people responsible to implement the programs and services should be identified.
   1) Include names and backgrounds of the lead members.
   2) Describe the scope of work and the nature of tasks related to the plan, including who is responsible for each task.

e. *Program and service.* Any aspects of the program that are unique should be identified.
   1) Provide guidelines for the plan by identifying constraints, limitations, and resources; a glossary is needed so there is a common understanding.
   2) Describe how and when the plan will be implemented.

f. *Market potential.* Specifically identify who in the business will use the program or service.

g. *Marketing strategy.* Describe the methods to communicate the program/service.
   1) Advertise in print, company intranet, or web.
   2) Identify how much is needed to spend on marketing.

h. *Financial Projection.* A one-, three-, and five-year projection of costs should be provided.
   1) Identify start up costs (supplies, staff, space).
   2) Project on-going costs to maintain the program.
   3) Identify any expected revenue that would be generated by the program.

i. *Canceling/Discontinuing.* A section that lays out benchmarks that would be used to cancel/discontinue a program should be included.
   1) Include a section to identify criteria to decide if the program or service is not working.
   2) This could be based on financial costs, attendance at program, utilization of service, or consensus among the managers of the program.

3. The plan should be regularly reviewed, re-evaluated, and updated.
   a. Be ready to "expand or contract" the plan based on actual experience.
   b. Recalculate costs and time commitments.
   c. Provide cost estimates as needed for on-going budget planning cycles.

NOTE: Other useful AAOHN resources that can assist in the development of occupational health and safety programs and services include the following: AAOHN Foundation Blocks: *Guidelines: for starting an occupational health and safety service (Series II)* and *Staffing ratios for the occupational health and safety service (Series VI).*

REFERENCES

American Association of Occupational Health Nurses. (2003). Competencies in occupational and environmental health nursing. *AAOHN Journal, 51*(7), 290-302.

American Association of Occupational Health Nurses. *Foundation blocks: A guide to occupational & environmental health nursing.* Atlanta, GA: AAOHN publications:

Series I: *Quality assurance packet.* L. Green (2003).

Series II: *Guidelines for starting an occupational health and safety service.* D. Richlin & D Meske (2003).

Series V: *Establishing an automatic external defibrillator program.* D. Richlin (2004).

Series VI: *Staffing ratios for the occupational health and safety service.* D. Richlin (2004).

Series IX: *Outsource management for the occupational health service,* AAOHN. (2004)

American Association of Occupational Health Nurses. (1998). *SuccessTools: Strategies for thriving and surviving in business (Module one: Measuring and articulating value).* Atlanta, GA: AAOHN Publications.

OTHER RESOURCES

American Association of Occupational Health Nurses. (2002). *Confidentiality— Guidelines for confidentiality of health information.* (AAOHN position statement). Atlanta, GA: AAOHN publications.

American Association of Occupational Health Nurses. (2003). *AAOHN code of ethics and interpretative statement.* Atlanta, GA: AAOHN publications.

American Association of Occupational Health Nurses. (2003). Standards of occupational and environmental health nursing. *AAOHN Journal, 52*(7), 270-274.

American Association of Occupational Health Nurses. (2004). *Standards of occupational health nursing practice.* Atlanta, GA: AAOHN Publications.

American Board for Occupational Health Nurses, Inc. (ABOHN). Certification agency for occupational health nurses. Available at http://www.abohn.org/ or 888-842-2646.

Amann, M. C. (2001). The policy and procedure manual—Keeping it current. *AAOHN Journal* 49(2), 69-71.

American College of Occupational and Environmental Medicine. (1998). *Guidelines for health services in health care facilities.* Elm Grove Village, IL, ACOEM publications.

Burton, W. N., Conti, D. J., Chen, C. Y., Schultz, A. B., & Edington, D. W. (1999). The role of health risk factors and disease on worker productivity. *Journal of Occupational and Environmental Medicine, 41*(10), 863-877.

Denton, V., & Leinhart, J. (2001). Absence monitoring: A case management perspective. *AAOHN Journal, 48* (10) 465-469.

Dyck, D. (2002). Outsourcing occupational health services: Critical elements. *AAOHN Journal, 50*(2), 83-89.

Donabedien, A. (1966). Evaluating the quality of medical care. *Milbank Fund Quarterly, 44(3),* 166-206.

American Association of Occupational Health Nurses. (1999). *SuccessTools: Strategies for thriving and surviving in business (Module two: Developing business expertise).* Atlanta, GA: AAOHN Publications.

Rogers, B (2003). *Occupational and environmental health nurse* (2nd ed.). Philadelphia: WB Saunders.

Edbaugh, H. (1998). Defining the scope of occupational health services: Effective policy and procedure development. *AAOHN Journal, 46*(11), 547-554.

Gregory, J. W., Lukes, E., & Gregory, L.G. (2002). Using financial metrics to prove and communicate value to management: Occupational health nurses as key players on the management team. *AAOHN Journal, 50*(9), 400-405.

Hefti, K. S., Farnham, R. J., Docken, L., Bentaas, R., Bossman, S. & Schaefer, J. (2003). Back injury prevention: A lift team success story. *AAOHN Journal, 51*(6), 246-251.

Heirich, M., & Dieck, C. J. (2000). Worksite cardiovascular wellness programs as a route to substance abuse prevention. *Journal of Occupational and Environmental Medicine, 42*(1), 47-56.

Lukes, E., & Schiavone, G. (2001*).* Self-assurance for quality and assurance. *AAOHN Journal, 49*(1), 44-54.

Melhorn, M. L., Wilkinson, L., Gardner, P., Horst, W. D., & Silkey, B. (1999). An outcomes study of an occupational medicine intervention program for the reduction of musculoskeletal disorders and cumulative trauma disorders in the workplace. *Journal of Occupational and Environmental Medicine, 421*(10), 833-846.

Meservy, D., Bass, J., & Weldonna, T. (1997). Health surveillance : Effective components of a successful program. *AAOHN Journal, 45*(10), 500-512.

Mignone, J. & Guidotti, T. L. (1999). Support groups for injured workers: Process & outcomes. *Journal of Occupational and Environmental Medicine, 41*(12), 1059-1064.

Morris, J. A., & Smith, P. S. (2001). Demonstrating the cost effectiveness of an expert occupational and environmental health nurse: Application of AAOHN success tools. *AAOHN Journal, 49*(12), 547-556.

Nelson, Y. (2001). Roles and value added contributions of the occupational health nurse: Corporate perceptions. *AAOHN Journal, 49*(3), 121-129.

Occupational Safety and Health Administration (2000). *Screening and Surveillance: A Guide to OSHA Standards.* (OSHA 3162). Washington DC: U.S. Government Printing Office.

Papp, E. M. & Miller, A. S. (2000). Screening and surveillance: OSHA's medical surveillance provisions. *AAOHN Journal, 48*(2), 59-72.

Ranavaya, M. S. & Talmage, J. B. (2001). AMA guides to the evaluation of permanent impairment. *Disability Medicine, 1*(1), 4-5.

Reed, P. (Ed.). (2003). *The Medical Disability Advisor* (4th ed.). Boulder, CO: Reed Group, Ltd.

Reith, L. K. (2000). The occupational health service: Staffing, facilities, and equipment. *AAOHN Journal, 48*(8), 395-403.

Rogers, B. (2004). Research utilization—Putting the research evidence into practice. *AAOHN Journal, 52*(1), 12-15.

Rogers, B., Livsey, K. (2000). Occupational health surveillance, screening, and prevention activities in occupational health nursing practice. *AAOHN Journal, 48*(2), 92-99.

Rogers, B., Randolph, S. A., & Mastroianni, K. (2003*). Occupational health nursing guidelines for primary clinical conditions* (3rd ed.). Boston: OEM Press.

Salazar, M. K. Kemerer, S., Amann, M. C., & Fabrey, L. J. (2002). Defining the roles and functions of occupational and environmental health nurses: Results of a national job analysis. *AAOHN Journal, 50*(1), 16-25.

Simonowitz, J. A., (2000). The occupational and environmental health nurse and health surveillance. (Editorial). *AAOHN Journal, 48*(2), 56-58.

Stone, D. S. (2000). Health surveillance for health care workers: A vital role for the occupational and environmental health nurse. *AAOHN Journal, 48*(2), 73-79.

Strasser, P. (2001). Management file: Demonstrating the value of occupational and environmental health programs. *AAOHN Journal, 49*(12), 545-546.

Task force on Community Preventive Services (2000). Introducing the guide to community preventive services. *American Journal of Preventive Medicine. A supplement, 18*(1S), 1-142.

Tsai, J. H., Salazar, M. K., Graham, K.Y., & Grines, J. (1999). Case management for injured workers. A descriptive study using a record review. *AAOHN Journal, 47*(9), 405-415.

U. S. Department of Health and Human Services (2000). *Healthy People 2010. With understanding and improving health and objectives for improving health.* (2nd ed.). 2 vols. Washington, DC.

U.S. Government Printing Office, *November 2000 (National Health Promotion and Disease Prevention Objectives*: Occupational Safety and Health, Chapter 10.)

U. S. Department of Health and Human Services & Agency for Health Care Policy and Research. (1995). *Using clinical practice guidelines to evaluate quality of care.* AHCPR Pub. No. 95-0046, Vols. 1 and 2. Washington, DC: DHSS.

CHAPTER

10

Prevention of Occupational Injuries and Illnesses

MARILYN L. HAU

The prevention of occupational injuries and illnesses requires an in-depth knowledge of the work environment with the appropriate skills to recognize and identify actual and potential hazards, evaluate these hazards, and institute appropriate control measures. Prevention and control are on-going processes, requiring continual assessment and evaluation, and the development and refining of programs. This chapter provides a broad overview of techniques and strategies that can be adapted for a variety of health and safety programs. It is the responsibility of occupational and environmental health nurses to determine the particular needs of their organizations and to tailor those programs to their setting.

Recognition and identification

To recognize and identify occupational health and safety hazards, occupational and environmental health nurses must know their workplaces and the nature of the work performed; they also need to appreciate the unique attributes, including the risk factors, which may characterize the worker population.

I First Steps in a Prevention Program

The first two steps in a work-site program to prevent illness or injury of the workers are: (1) the recognition or anticipation of hazards, and (2) the clear identification of hazards.

A *Recognition* **is the process of detecting workplace hazards.**

B *Anticipation* **is the foresight to recognize and eliminate hazards in equipment and processes during the planning, process review, and design stages.**

C *Identification* **is the process of defining, describing, and classifying hazards.**

D *Hazard* **is "the potential for harm or damage to people, property, or the environment" (Manuele, 2003a).**

   1. Workplace hazards may be classified as physical, chemical, biologic, environmental/mechanical, and psychosocial.
   2. Recognizing and identifying hazards requires knowledge of the workers, work site, work practices and processes, and industrial materials used.
   3. Sources of information regarding hazards include knowledgeable company representatives; health and safety professionals; professional publications

and courses; and direct observation of production processes and workers' activities.

E The overall goal of a prevention program is to recognize and identify hazards, evaluate and analyze these hazards, and select and implement preventive and control measures as a continual process (Figure 10-1).

II Methods of Identifying Hazards

A A *site survey,* or *walk-through,* is a work-site inspection not related to any particular incident, work area, or piece of equipment.

1. The purpose of the site survey is to identify unsafe conditions and practices, including items not in compliance with local, state, and federal regulations, such as Occupational Safety and Health Administration (OSHA) standards (Box 10-1).
2. Types of walk-through inspections include:
   a. *Informal inspection*—Focuses on routine work, such as inspecting and testing equipment at the beginning of each shift
   b. *Formal inspection*—Performed periodically by a team of occupational health and safety professionals; scheduled at convenient times; includes a written report of findings
   c. *General inspection*—May be conducted to ensure compliance with legal requirements or for insurance purposes, corporate or union audits, and fire code compliance
3. A *site survey* follows the flow of work from the beginning to end.
4. A checklist is used to guide the inspection; inspection checklists should be site specific rather than generic.
5. Pre-inspection activities may include the following:
   a. Determination of inspection time
   b. Meeting with managers and supervisors
   c. Review of previous inspection and accident reports, material safety data sheets, and other relevant records and reports
   d. Gathering of essential personal protective equipment needed at site
   e. Gathering of checklists, sampling devices, and other items needed for the inspection

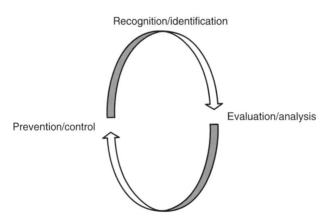

FIGURE 10-1 *Continual processes for preventing injuries and illnesses*

Source: National Safety Council, 1992.

BOX 10-1

A few examples of what to inspect during a site survey

- Atmospheric conditions: dusts, vapors, odors
- Illumination: general and work-stations
- First aid and emergency units: eye-wash stations, deluge showers
- Containers: labeling, flammable liquid, waste
- Supplies and materials: caustics, acids, poisons, compressed gases, cryogenics, oxidizers, flammable or spontaneously combustible materials
- Buildings and structures: windows, aisles, floors, stairs, exit signs
- Electrical hazards: extension cords, outlet usage, cord condition, electric gear clearance, shock hazards

- Fire fighting equipment: fire extinguishers, sprinkler systems, standpipes, accessibility, alarms, and testing procedures
- Machinery: guarding of moving parts and pinch points, barrier safety shields, proximity switches, automatic shutoffs
- Material handling: lifting devices, conveyors, lift truck operations, cranes, hoists
- Personal protective equipment: clothing, safety glasses, chemical goggles, gloves, safety shoes, hard hats
- Work practices: eating at the work-station, personal hygiene, adherence to safe operating procedures, housekeeping

Source: National Safety Council, 1992.

---

6. Inspection activities may include the following:
    a. Explanation of procedure to supervisors at inspection sites
    b. Observation of employees' work practices
    c. Recording of unsafe conditions and practices, including items out of compliance with OSHA standards
    d. Identification of problems and their causes
    e. Commendation of supervisor and workers when conditions are noted to be safe
    f. Corrective action if an immediate danger, such as a blocked exit, is noted
7. Post-inspection activities may include:
    a. Meeting with managers and supervisors
    b. Conducting a long-term analysis based on data from both current and previous inspections
    c. Preparing appropriate reports
    d. Circulating reports, which should include recommendations for possible solutions and correction priorities
8. An audit system to periodically check for corrected and unresolved problems should be established.
9. For an example of a walk-through program, see AAOHN's Foundation Block: Worksite Safety Walkthrough Program (2003a).

B *Focused inspections* **are conducted periodically for the following purposes: to inspect specific processes, equipment, or areas; to investigate an accident; to evaluate a reported health or safety hazard; or to respond to complaints of such things as a strange odor or loud noise.**

1. Individuals or multidisciplinary teams with in-depth knowledge of the process or area should conduct the inspection.
2. Critical parts or operations usually require more frequent inspections (e.g., light switches, safety valves, cables, belts, fire extinguishers, eyewash stations, or exhaust hoods).
3. Some focused inspections are legally mandated (e.g., elevators, autoclaves, and boilers).
4. A checklist can serve as a useful guide to a focused inspection (Figure 10-2).

C A *records review* or **audit may be done alone or as a supplement to other methods of hazard identification.**
1. Record audits have the following purposes:
   a. Identify work-site hazards
   b. Better acquaint the occupational and environmental health nurse with the site
   c. Provide historical data for trend analysis and epidemiologic study
   d. Ensure compliance with OSHA standards
2. Although records may indicate the absence or inadequate control of work-site hazards, the recorded information may not reflect the actual circumstance.

Electric Forklift Daily Checklist:	Truck No.:				Ser. No.:		Check before each shift.			
Date:										
Hour meter:										
Driver:										
Visual/operation checks	OK	Not OK	OK	Not OK	OK	Not OK	OK	Not OK	OK	Not OK
Obvious damage/leaks										
Tire condition										
Battery plug connect										
Warning lights										
Battery discharge meter										
Horn										
Steering										
Foot brake										
Parking brake										
Hydraulic controls										
Fork operation										
Battery water level										
Seat belts										
Fire extinguisher										
Repairs needed:										
Comments:							Add additional comments on the back			

FIGURE 10-2 *Focused checklist for electric forklift*

Source: Ohio Division of Safety and Hygiene, 1995.

3. The following records may be helpful:
   a. Records concerning production and quality-control problems
   b. Workers' compensation claims
   c. Employee assistance program utilization reports
   d. Personnel records, including absentee records and job histories
   e. Written hazard-control programs, training records, and records concerning fit-testing and distribution of personal protective equipment
   f. Safety surveys, inspection reports, and exposure monitoring reports
   g. Machine and equipment maintenance logs
   h. Emission and process records
   i. System monitoring and alarm test records
   j. Plans for disaster preparedness and emergency response
   k. Designs and reviews of new or planned facilities, processes, materials, or equipment
   l. Written complaints from workers and minutes of the safety committee meetings
   m. OSHA recordkeeping forms
   n. Other site-specific records that can be identified and examined if deemed appropriate

D *Job hazard analysis,* **also called** *job safety analysis,* **is the process of studying and recording each step of a job to identify existing and potential health and safety hazards and to determine the best way to perform the job to reduce or eliminate these hazards (Swartz, 2002). The conduct of a job hazard analysis requires the following steps:**

1. Set priorities: begin with the jobs with the highest rates of accident and disabling injuries, jobs where "close calls" have occurred, new jobs, and jobs where changes have been made in processes and procedures.
2. Assess the general conditions under which the job is performed, using a checklist if applicable. Then do the following:
   a. List each step of the job in order of occurrence as you watch the worker performing the job, recording enough information to describe each job action.
   b. Examine each step to determine the existing or potential hazards.
   c. Repeat the job observation as often as necessary until all hazards have been identified.
   d. Review each hazard or potential hazard with the worker who performs the job to determine whether the job could be performed in a safer way or whether safety equipment and precautions are needed.
   e. List exactly each new step or method, and identify exactly what the worker needs to know to perform the job safely.
3. Recommend safety procedures and corrections, including:
   a. Developing a training program
   b. Redesigning equipment, changing tools, adding guards, improving ventilation, or using personal protective equipment
   c. Reducing the necessity or frequency of performing the job
   d. Avoiding general warnings such as "be careful"
4. Repeat and revise the job hazard/job safety analysis periodically and after an accident or injury. Figure 10-3 presents an example of a job safety analysis form.
5. A job hazard/job safety analysis provides the following benefits (Swartz, 2001):
   a. Improves worker hazard awareness

Job Safety Analysis	Job:		Date:	
Title of worker who performs job:	Foreman/supervisor:		Analysis by:	
Specific work location:	Section:		Reviewed by:	
Required and/or recommended personal protective equipment:				
Sequence of basic job steps	*Potential accidents or hazards*		*Recommended safe job procedures*	

FIGURE 10-3 *Job safety analysis form*

Source: Ohio Division of Safety and Hygiene, 1995.

    b. Increases worker safety training and supervisor/worker communication

    c. Enhances identification of root causes of accidents

    d. Serves as a valuable tool for ergonomic studies

    e. Increases the thoroughness of machine inspections

    f. Helps train new supervisors in unfamiliar jobs

    g. Determines physical and mental requirements necessary for job performance, a necessity in evaluating job candidates with disabilities

E *Incident analyses* **are fact-finding procedures to identify the pertinent factors that allow accidents or near misses to occur so similar future incidents can be prevented. A** *near miss* **is an incident that could have resulted in injury or property damage under different circumstances. It should be evaluated to prevent recurrence and a more serious outcome.**

    1. The first step in an incident analysis is to identify immediate causes; this is accomplished via the following steps:

        a. Interviewing workers and collecting physical evidence, including results of any applicable drug screening or alcohol testing, as soon as possible after an accident

    b. Inspecting the scene of the accident or near miss and recording relevant details, using photographs, drawings, and measurements

    c. Interviewing witnesses in private

    d. Being alert to the possibility of attempts to hide injuries or facts because of fear of reprisal, poor evaluations, ruining safety records, discovery of substance abuse, embarrassment, or implicating others

    e. Using the company's incident investigation form to avoid omitting information

    f. Trying to quote workers' statements in their exact words

    g. Staying objective, avoiding biased statements or questions

2. Some of the "root causes" of incidents may be (AAOHN, 2001a):

    a. Lack of management support for safety

    b. Failure to positively reinforce or reward safe behaviors

    c. Lack of preventive maintenance programs

    d. Production output stressed over safety

    e. Low worker morale

    f. Unqualified trainers

    g. Lack of job safety analysis

    h. No assigned responsibility for a function

    i. Unsafe work behaviors without accident experience

    j. Peer values

    k. Poor example set by supervisors/managers

3. Workplace factors that often contribute to incidents include procedures, facilities, communication patterns, and behaviors (Box 10-2).

4. The following benefits are derived from an incident analysis:

    a. Increases health and safety awareness for workers and supervisors

    b. Establishes better rapport between the occupational and environmental health nurse, supervisor, and injured or ill worker

    c. Provides data that can be used for an overall safety program evaluation and prevention of future incidents

    d. Provides essential facts for workers' compensation, OSHA recordkeeping, and insurance claims, such as company fire insurance

F An *incident historical review* **is the compilation and analysis of incidents and near misses that have occurred over a selected period of time.**

1. Categories of incidents include the following:

    a. Incidents related to specific seasons

    b. Incidents occurring on a particular shift

    c. Incidents occurring to a specific group of workers

    d. Incidents occurring at a specific location or within a specific process

2. The review begins with an analysis of incidents and trends in incidents through review of the following relevant records:

    a. OSHA forms

    b. Safety committee minutes

    c. Accident, incident, or near-miss reports

    d. Logs of daily health service visits

    e. Other periodic reports and records of the health and safety service

    f. Comparison of incident rates with those in similar industries (Box 10-3 presents formulas for calculating incident rates.)

3. The following factors should be considered when evaluating incident trends: (Spear, 2002)

BOX 10-2

Examples of immediate causes of incidents

Procedures

Nonexistent, not followed, not trained in, not understood, not accurate, impossible to follow

Facilities/Tools/Equipment

Personal protective equipment failure, improper design, nonergonomic design, wear/deterioration, lack of proper equipment, poor housekeeping, process equipment failure, missing guards or safety devices

Hazards

Manmade, natural source, documented but not repaired, unidentified, identified but accepted, inadequately repaired, presenting a "challenge" to workers

Communication

Inadequate planning; breakdown in communication between co-workers, between workers and supervisors, or between contractor and company; confused communications; lack of warning signs; language barriers; illiteracy

Behavior

Rushed by supervision, co-worker competition, motivation to finish early, taking shortcuts, no teamwork, heavy client workload, bonus incentives, medication effects, boredom, fatalistic "it can't happen to me" attitude, unauthorized smoking/eating, inattention/distraction, fear of asking for help

Training

None, insufficient, safe work practices not addressed in training, training applied incorrectly, no hands-on training, inadequate follow-up, need for refresher training, training not site-specific

Other Factors

Fatigue, lack of sleep, illness, physical stress, repetitive motion, fright, physical incapability, disrupted circadian rhythms because of shift work

Source: AAOHN, 2001.

---

    a. Worker's attitudes and behavior: impatience, boredom, recklessness, feeling rushed (such as those paid for piecework), insufficient training, upset by shift work

    b. Management's attitudes and behavior: emphasis on production over safety, failure to identify hazards and perform corrective actions, failure to enforce safe behavior

    c. Work environment deficiencies: poor lighting, inadequate ventilation, obsolete equipment

G *Chemical inventories* **and** *material safety data sheets* **provide critical information for workers and employers.**

    1. They are required by the OSHA 29 CFR* 1910.1200 Hazard Communication Standard. (Certain laboratories are required to comply with a similar standard: 29 CFR 1910.1450, which is specific to laboratories.)

---

* NOTE: CFR refers to the Code of Federal Regulations, a compilation of final rules and regulations that are originally published in the Federal Register. The CFR is divided into 50 titles representing broad areas subject to federal regulation. Title 29 is labor; Title 40 is protection of the environment.

BOX 10-3

Incidence rate calculation

$$\text{Incidence rate} = \frac{\text{Number of new cases/year x 200,000 work hours per facility}^*}{\text{Number of hours worked at facility/year}}$$

*200,000 work hours is equivalent to 100 employees working 40 hours per week, 50 weeks per year. (Multiplying by 200,000 allows one to compare rates with those of other companies and is a more readily understood number.)

or

$$\text{Incidence rate} = \frac{\text{Number of new cases/year x 200,000 work hours}}{\text{Number of people at facility x 2000 hours}^{\dagger}}$$

---

  2. They are useful for estimating potential hazards associated with raw materials, products, and other hazardous substances present in the facility.

H *Employee perception surveys/questionnaires* **involve workers directly in hazard recognition and identification; this is important, because the worker most directly involved with the work process often provides insight not otherwise obtained.**
  1. Information obtained from surveys and questionnaires is most accurate when collected by an independent, unbiased third party.
  2. Surveys and questionnaires should consist of questions that have been researched and field-tested for reliability.
  3. Results should be shared so that all workers can benefit from their co-workers' insight; additionally, workers may wish to clarify, modify, or otherwise add to information contained in the results.

I *Process safety reviews* **consist of evaluations performed on activities involving chemicals, including using, storing, manufacturing, handling, or moving chemicals at the site.**
  1. Information is gathered on the hazards of the chemicals, technology, and equipment used in a process, allowing health and safety staff to perform the following activities:
     a. Identify the hazards of new and changed processes
     b. Evaluate processes reviewed within the past 5 years
     c. Review processes related to incidents that had a potential for catastrophic consequences
  2. Process safety reviews serve as a means of determining what could go wrong and what safeguards must be implemented to prevent hazardous chemical releases.
  3. The reviews are mandated by the EPA 40 CFR Part 68: "Worst Case Scenario" section, and the OSHA 29 CFR 1910.119: "Process Safety Management of Highly Hazardous Chemicals" for:
     a. Industries using any of more than 130 chemicals in listed quantities.
     b. Industries using flammable liquids and gases in quantities of 10,000 pounds or more.

4. Methods to determine and evaluate the consequences of the failure of engineering and administrative controls include the following (National Safety Council, 2001):
   a. *What if* is a method of thinking in which failure potentials are brainstormed and their causes and effects analyzed.
   b. *Checklists* identify the major hazards and nuisances associated with a particular material.
   c. A *hazard and operability study* (HAZOP) is a formal systematic study of a newly designed facility or operation to assess the potential of individual equipment components to fail, resulting in consequential effects on the overall facility.
   d. *Failure mode and effects analysis* (FMEA) is a "bottom-up" technique in which the failure of a particular process component is assessed for its effects on other components and on the process system as a potential source for accidents.
   e. *Fault tree analysis* is a formalized deductive technique that works backward from a defined accident to identify and graphically display the combination of equipment failures and operational errors that could have led up to the accident.
5. *Worker health and safety information,* including the health effects of chemicals and the possible need for specific exposure monitoring and first aid planning, should be evaluated.

J The *ergonomic analysis* **evaluates stresses related to the performance of work so strategies for prevention can be developed.**
1. The NIOSH Equation for Manual Lifting can be used to identify tasks having a risk of overexertion injuries and low back pain because of lifting and lowering activities.
   a. The guidelines describe an equation that is based on the following variables: horizontal distance; vertical distance; distance of lift; asymmetry of lift; coupling; frequency of lifting (refer to Garg, 1995 for lifting guidelines).
   b. The goal is to design the task so the lifting index is at or below 1.0.
2. Preventive strategies include the following:
   a. Redesigning workstations and work equipment (e.g., machine guards)
   b. Improving work environment (e.g., developing a work-rest schedule to prevent heat stress)
   c. Designing warning signs for hazardous equipment and locations
3. Effective ergonomics programs include the following (AAOHN, 2004):
   a. Surveillance strategies to assess patterns of exertion injuries
   b. Job hazard analysis/job safety analysis to identify workers at risk
   c. Job design or redesign that considers ergonomic factors
   d. Management and worker training related to the recognition and control of biochemical hazards
   e. Protocol for health management of injured workers

Hazard evaluation and analysis

The next steps for preventing injury and illness are evaluating hazards to determine to what degree a standard has been met, and analyzing identified hazards to determine how hazard controls must be prioritized in terms of human and financial resources.

III Purpose of Hazard Evaluation and Analysis

A The ultimate purpose of hazard evaluation and analysis is to control *all* hazards, existing and potential.

B Hazards that present a high probability of severe injury or illness warrant a greater priority when control measures are implemented than do potential hazards that present a remote possibility of less-severe injury or illness.

C Hazard evaluation and analysis serves as an ongoing tool to determine what is working well and what isn't, what deserves commendation, and what needs constructive correction.

D Analysis and evaluation strategies serve as guides for program implementation (Plog, 2002).

1. When exposure monitoring indicates that agent action levels have been reached, a worker health surveillance program should be implemented.
2. When worker health data suggest adverse work-site exposures, exposure monitoring may be indicated.
3. Environmental or biologic monitoring results that suggest elevated exposure may indicate the need for additional engineering and administrative control measures or for additional training in the proper use of personal protective equipment.

IV Industry Standards

Industry standards provide a guide for evaluating and analyzing hazards.

A There are two types of industry standards.

1. *Mandatory standards* that establish minimum safety program requirements and maximum levels of permitted exposures are enforced by government agencies such as the Occupational Safety and Health Administration (OSHA) and the Environmental Protection Agency (EPA).
2. *Consensus standards* are voluntary industry standards adopted by agreement among participating members.

B Standards can serve as professional yardsticks against which to measure hazard identification and prevention activities.

1. Occasionally mandatory standards quote consensus standards as their requirements.

   Example: state fire regulations that reference the National Fire Protection Association (NFPA) recommendations.

2. Standards can carry heavy weight in issues such as insurance company coverage, legal actions, grant funding, and other issues in which competency and compliance issues are involved.

   Example: the evaluation process and ratings of the Joint Committee on Accreditation of Healthcare Organizations (JCAHO) as a condition for third party cost reimbursement.

3. Trade associations, scientific and technical societies, and insurance companies may have certification or compliance requirements that industry can use as a yardstick for hazards and preventive measures.

   Example: the standard for laboratory ventilation provided by the American National Standards Institute (ANSI).

4. International associations that promulgate consensus standards, often as part of environmental treaties and quality initiatives, are the International Labour Organization and the International Organization for Standardization (ISO 9000 Series, ISO 14000).

BOX 10-4

Examples of processes affecting standards in other countries

European Directives

The Council of the European Union has issued a series of directives intended to ensure harmonization of requirements for the health and safety of individuals. The European directives set out a common framework, for member countries to implement at a national level, of laws, regulations and administrative procedures necessary to comply with their requirements. The European legal instruments can be put into five categories:

- Regulations: binding on all member states and introduced.
- Directives: establish principles that are binding on all member states and implemented in accordance with member states arrangements.
- Decisions: binding on those to whom they are addressed.
- Recommendations and Opinions: not binding, but encourage good practice.
- Action Programs: adopted by the Council; indicative of the Council's intention to take measures to achieve its objectives.

Non-European Directives

Other countries also have regulations associated with occupational health and safety issues. These regulations vary widely in nature and complexity. For example:

- China—China has a significant number of regulations associated with occupational health and safety issues. These regulations vary in different provinces and regions and can be quite complex. In addition, there are many local rules. For example, there are 807 laws, regulations, standards, and rules applicable to Shanghai City.
- Australia—In Australia, standards are determined by the individual states and territories, such as the Queensland Division of Workplace Health and Safety or the Victoria Health and Safety Organisation. A major initiative is self-regulation via a "code of practice," placing a broad duty of care on employers to provide a safe and risk-free workplace.
- Japan—Japanese regulations are determined centrally by the Labor Standards Bureau of the Ministry of Labor. An unusual feature of the Japanese system is that industrial law requires that all employed persons undergo a prescribed occupational medical examination each year (Fleming, Herzstein, & Bunn, 1997).

C **Some standards are inadequate for the following reasons:**
1. They may conflict with each other in their requirements, such as the labeling requirements of the Department of Transportation (DOT) versus those of OSHA.
2. Standards in the United States may differ from those of other countries, thus affecting international corporations (Box 10-4).
   a. The processes that are followed, the participants and their extent of involvement, and the legal structures embracing all these standards are different from those of the United States.
   b. It is essential that judgments of other countries not be based on what we have experienced in the United States.
3. Standards may not address an organization's principal risks; thus it is critical that workplaces be assessed for *all* hazards, not just those that are subject to regulation.

NOTE: AAOHN's Foundation Block (2003b) provides *A Safety Action Plan Template* that can be used for general industry and manufacturing settings.

V Risk Analysis

A **In the occupational setting, risk analysis is an interdisciplinary science that evaluates health and environmental hazards and risks that result from work-related activities.**

B **The following must be considered when evaluating the significance of hazards identified.**
1. "Low numbers of incidents and injuries do not necessarily mean a hazard-free worksite" (Manuele, 2003b).
2. A hazardous event may be rated as catastrophic, critical, marginal, or negligible in its severity; these are subjective categories based on fatalities, injury severity, and financial damage (Manuele, 2003b).
3. The likelihood of a hazardous event is estimated subjectively as frequent, probable, occasional, remote, or improbable.

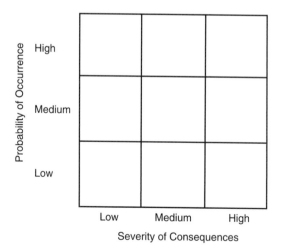

FIGURE 10-4 *Risk-analysis matrix*

> **BOX 10-5**
>
> *A formula for estimating risk score*
>
> $$R = S \times E \times P$$
>
> where R = Risk Score, S = Severity, E = Exposure, P = Probability
>
> Risk scores can be used to rank the priority of hazards. Assign a value to each variable (for example, by using a scale from 1 to 5); then multiply the potential severity of injury by the frequency of exposure by the probability of exposure to obtain a risk score estimate (Perkinson, 1995).

4. Risk analysis should consider both the probability of an incident occurring and the expected severity of adverse results, thus ranking the risks. Box 10-5 provides a formula for estimating a "risk score," and Figure 10-4 presents a risk-analysis matrix.
5. Risk analysis should define the people, property, and environment that identified hazards may affect.

C To be meaningful, the results of risk analyses must be communicated to the people they affect: the worker, health and safety professionals, and management.

VI Exposure Monitoring

Exposure monitoring is the quantitative analysis of work-site exposures to hazards that are recognized, suspected, or anticipated, based on other preliminary hazard identification methods (Weeks, Levy, & Wagner, 2004).

A Sampling is conducted for all types of exposures.
1. A sample should represent the workers' exposure or condition that is being evaluated (Plog et al., 2002).
2. When sampling, the occupational and environmental health nurse must determine:
   a. Whom to sample (those directly or indirectly exposed)
   b. Where to sample (breathing zone, hearing zone, work area, point of operation)
   c. Sampling duration or volume needed
   d. Number and types of samples needed
   e. Sampling period (e.g., day or night, summer or winter)
3. Findings should be compared to occupational health standards such as OSHA's Permissible Exposure Limits (PEL), the United Kingdom Health and Safety Executive's Occupational Exposure Limits (OEL), or the American Conference of Governmental Industrial Hygienists' (ACGIH) threshold limit values (TLVs).[*]
4. Interpretation of results must also take the following factors into account (DiNardi, 2002)):
   a. Exposure levels versus absorbed dose
   b. Sites of entry versus sites of action
   c. Combined effects of two or more substances or sources

---

[*]Many countries adopt the ACGIH TLVs as their regulatory exposure limits.

    d. Individual susceptibility

    e. Conditions of use in the work environment, including work-site controls in place

    f. Individual worker practices

5. Examples of sampling and analysis problems include the following (McDermott, 2004):

    a. Air pumps and sound-level meters that are not accurately calibrated or that spontaneously change flow rates

    b. Flow rates or exposure circumstances intentionally altered by the subject worker

    c. Color shade changes

    d. Fluctuating environmental conditions

    e. Improper timing, such as sampling when exposure levels are minimal

    f. Problems in quality control, such as failure to submit or download all recorded data or to properly store and analyze samples

B Assessment of noise exposure

1. Measurements of sound-pressure levels are expressed in terms of decibels (dB).

2. An A-weighted scale combines frequency with intensity to yield dBA measurement (Dobie, 2002).

3. Potential hearing damage can be estimated with a knowledge of the dBA sound level, the duration of exposure during a workday, and the total work-life exposure (Plog, et al, 2002).

4. Personal dosimeters integrate time and noise exposure (Plog, et al. 2002)

5. For engineering controls of noise, sound-pressure levels throughout the frequency spectrum must be measured with an octave band analyzer (Plog, et al., 2002).

6. Internationally, many noise exposure regulations are found in environmental statutes with requirements for community exposure limitations in addition to work-site restrictions.

Chapter 16 presents an example of a hearing conservation program.

C Atmospheric monitoring

1. The purpose of atmospheric monitoring is to evaluate, over a given period of time, the presence and concentration of airborne contaminants to which the worker is being exposed (McDermott, 2004).

2. Various methods used to sample gases, vapors, and particulates include the following:

    a. Dosimeter badges, which are used to evaluate a single person's exposure over time

    b. Detector or colorimetric tubes, containing a media that changes colors on exposure, using hand-operated pumps to draw air samples

    c. Electronic direct-reading instruments with sensors

    d. Filters, sorbent tubes (containing a solid that absorbs chemicals for laboratory analysis), impingers (containing a liquid media that absorbs chemicals for laboratory analysis), and other entrapment devices

3. Types of sampling procedures

    a. *Instantaneous* or "grab" sampling collects an air sample over a short period of time, ranging from a few seconds to less than two minutes.

    b. The *personal* sample consists of drawing a known volume of air through an appropriate medium located in the worker's breathing zone for a sampling period of from 15 minutes to 8 hours.

c. An *area* sample determines the source of contaminants by creating a "map" of levels present.

d. Air, chemicals, water, and soil can be monitored by *bulk* sampling.

e. *Bioaerosol* monitoring for bacteria, viruses, fungi, and other biologicals is performed by methods similar to airborne chemical contaminant monitoring (Perkins, 2003).

f. *Combustible gas indicators* are direct-reading instruments used to measure explosive levels of gases in confined spaces.

g. *Oxygen detectors* are direct-reading instruments used to evaluate the percentage of oxygen in the air, especially in confined spaces. (Safe levels established by U.S. standards are from 19.5% to 23.0% oxygen in air.) (McDermott, 2004)

4. The sense of smell or irritation of the skin, eyes, and upper respiratory system can provide valuable clues to the levels of concentration of the contaminant, but these sensory indicators are unreliable for actual concentration or presence determinations.

D **Ionizing radiation monitoring is best carried out by personal dosimetry.**

1. Thermal-luminescent dosimeters—the newest being aluminum oxide—or the older film badges are worn by workers, with collection and reading at periodic intervals based on the extent of potential exposure (Breitenstein & Spickard, 2002).

2. Swipe samples, consisting of a wet surface wipe-down and analysis, are taken for evidence of surface contamination by radionuclides (Breitenstein & Spickard, 2002).

3. Area monitoring is accomplished by measuring roentgens per day with the Geiger-Mueller instrument (Geiger counter).

4. Results of radiation measurement are compared with allowable dose standards from the Nuclear Regulatory Commission, EPA, OSHA, and other agencies that regulate radiation protection and measurement.

E **Non-ionizing radiation monitoring may also be performed (Stern & Mansdorf, 1999).**

1. Ultraviolet radiation is monitored with a radiometer to determine the effective irradiance that is either read directly or is calculated. Protection is provided by shields, sunblocks, and protective UV-absorbing eyewear.

2. Laser hazards are determined by numerical hazard evaluation techniques to determine a nominal hazard zone in which no entry or exposure should be permitted. Direct measuring is too complex and can easily result in accidental exposure to the laser beam. Protection is afforded through laser beam enclosure.

3. Radio-frequency radiation is measured with broadband receivers to determine the effectiveness of shielding.

4. Both field and personal monitors are used to measure electrical and magnetic fields found around electric welding, electric furnaces, and major utility electric utility equipment, and controlled through shielding, time, and distance.

F **Temperature monitoring identifies hazardous extremes in hot or cold environments.**

1. Potential for heat stress requires measurement of air temperature by dry-bulb measurement, humidity by natural wet-bulb measurement, and radiant heat by black-globe temperature.

2. Other considerations for measuring for heat stress include fluid and electrolyte balance, training for heat tolerance, drugs, alcohol consumption, age, obesity, and extent of clothing.

3. Proposed occupational health standards for exposure to heat consist of a sliding scale based on the wet-bulb globe temperature, differing for acclimatized and unacclimatized workers.

4. Potential for cold injury requires measurement of air temperature by dry-bulb method plus measurement of wind speed to arrive at a wind-chill factor.

5. Other considerations when measuring for cold injury include exposure to moisture, extent of clothing, and level of exhaustion.

G Surface sampling, or wipe sampling, can be performed to evaluate external surfaces and the worker's skin and clothing for chemical, radiation, and biologic contamination.

H Continuous monitors are alarm units used primarily to detect emergency conditions and trigger evacuation rather than to measure worker exposure (McDermott, 2004).

1. Monitors may detect high radiation levels, fire, smoke, flammable atmospheres, oxygen-deficient air, and toxic levels of poisonous gases such as hydrogen sulfide and carbon monoxide.

2. Stationary systems may provide real-time alarm warnings to workers in the area of a hazardous environmental condition.

3. Personal continuous monitors may be worn by workers in areas where potential releases could reach evacuation levels, such as in confined spaces.

4. Portable continuous monitors are similar to personal monitors but may have more display capability and can collect data over a period of time for a specific chemical.

VII Worker Populations Analysis

Worker populations should be viewed not just as a collection of individuals but as a single entity; worker populations include communities and subgroups of workers.

A Analyzing groups, not just individuals, can detect patterns, trends, changes, and commonalties.

1. Population data can be used to describe injury and illness trends over time, so patterns with common causes can be identified and prevented.

2. Occupational and environmental health nurses should be alert to group patterns of injury and illness, as follows:

a. If health visits reveal a cluster of illnesses or injuries, visit the work site to get an understanding of how and why these events may be happening.

b. Attempt to identify whether workers with similar complaints perform the same job, work in the same area, or have something else in common (DiNardi, 2002).

c. Monitor trends that may suggest new hazards or the breakdown of prevention and control measures.

d. Determine whether conditions are improving or worsening.

e. Identify the work-site locations involved.

f. Enlist colleagues from other disciplines (e.g., industrial hygiene, engineering), as appropriate.

B *Epidemic events* **are any marked upward fluctuation in disease and injury incidence.**
  1. Epidemics are verified when the incidence of a disease or injury exceeds what normally would be expected.
  2. An epidemic must have an agent or a cause, in addition to individuals who are susceptible to the illness or injury related to the cause.
  3. Management of an epidemic in the work setting should follow these steps:
      a. Identify the cause and/or source.
      b. Identify and arrange for treatment of clients.
      c. Institute control measures to decrease spread of contamination or risk of injury.
      d. Provide workers with appropriate health education.
      e. Establish a program of continued surveillance and monitoring for the infective agent or the source of injury.
      f. Establish a program to prevent recurrence.

C *Epidemic (mass) hysteria* **(also called *mass psychogenic illness*) is an event in which a group of workers exposed to the same stimulus exhibit common physical symptoms of psychologic origin (Blackman and Walkerdine, 2001).**
  1. Characteristics of exposure
      a. This illness occurs most often in work settings with physical and emotional stressors, such as boring, repetitive tasks, and poor rapport between the work force and company management.
      b. A noxious odor, a substance perceived as toxic, extreme heat, or loud, repetitive noises can serve as triggers.
      c. Transmission of symptoms occurs by sight, sound, or word of mouth rather than by simply being in a common exposure area.
  2. Symptom development includes the following characteristics:
      a. There is an explosive onset of symptoms whose severity is out of proportion to the apparent cause and that can disappear and return rapidly.
      b. A range of symptoms, including headache, nausea, dizziness, chills, difficulty in breathing, and other vague, subjective complaints, divert the worker's attention from hidden stress to external work-site factors.
  3. Epidemic stress may be recognized by carrying out the following activities:
      a. Carefully investigate complaints and conduct an exposure analysis of all potential toxicologic and biologic causes to rule out a physical basis
      b. Evaluate the work site for psychosocial stressors
      c. Identify workers at high risk for somatoform disorders
  4. Other considerations
      a. A careful work-site analysis should be performed; the possibility of physical symptoms must be considered even in the absence of objective findings.
      b. "Hysteria" reactions may be the result of psychosocial stressors in the workplace; this possibility should be investigated (Blackman and Walkerdine, 2001).
      c. Treatment consists of first establishing and communicating the lack of connection between the symptoms and the "trigger," then taking measures to reduce occupational stressors.

D An occupational *sentinel health event* **is a disease, disability, or untimely death that is work related.**

1. Sentinel events provide the impetus for epidemiologic or industrial hygiene studies; they serve as a warning that prevention and control strategies are needed.

2. The occurrence of sentinel health events may serve as the stimulus for hazard evaluation and reassessment of control measures.

3. The occupational and environmental health nurse may play an important role in identifying sentinel health events. It is essential that the occupational and environmental health nurse:

   a. Have a thorough knowledge of the work site and its hazards

   b. Collaborate with professional colleagues within the company when a sentinel health event is suspected

   c. Participate in continuing education efforts

   d. Maintain a high index of suspicion for the possibility of a sentinel health event ("gatekeeper" role)

   e. Refer all potentially exposed workers for further evaluation when a work-related problem is suspected

E *Multiple chemical sensitivity* **(MCS) has been described as a syndrome that may develop in one or many workers and "affect(s) multiple systems and occur(s) in multiple unrelated environments" (Levy & Wegman, 2000).**

1. Common symptoms of MCS are fatigue, headache, frequent colds, dizziness, nausea, lack of concentration, memory loss, menstrual irregularities, and visual problems.

   a. Often the MCS symptom pattern changes, with some symptoms disappearing and new ones occurring.

   b. Symptoms can produce total disability.

2. MCS is poorly understood; hence it is a highly controversial phenomenon (Heimlich, 2004).

   a. Symptoms are subjective, with no objective evidence of organ system damage or dysfunction.

   b. Health effects described as MCS are related to verifiable environmental exposure.

   c. MCS symptoms are elicited by extremely low exposures to chemicals.

   d. MCS symptoms seem to have a predictable return with environmental stimuli (Sparks, et al., 1994).

3. There is a need for epidemiologic studies and for careful environmental and occupational history taking to better understand multiple chemical sensitivity.

F **Work-site violence**

1. Because of continuing prevalence, workplace violence represents a new form of job hazard and an increased sense of worker vulnerability (Grenyer et al., 2004).

2. Workplace violence includes harassment, threats, and actual physical assaults in the work site.

3. Recognizing and understanding the potential hazard of work-site violence is a new essential assessment in industry (United States Department of Justice, 2004). Chapters 13 and 15 present additional information on workplace violence.

Prevention and control

The last steps of work-site programs are to select and implement prevention and control measures. Prevention and control of occupational hazards are central to occupational and environmental health nursing practice. The choice of a control strategy depends on the nature of the workplace, financial and technologic feasibility, work tasks, and workers. More than one approach is often required to achieve optimal health and safety.

VIII Prevention and Control Approaches That Focus on Engineering Controls

Engineering methods are the most preferred means of hazard control; engineering controls do not rely on the human behavior factor to ensure success.

A **Elimination** or **substitution** **of manual tasks and highly hazardous materials is intended to minimize the source of potential exposure by completely removing the hazardous material or replacing it with a less hazardous substitute (DiNardi, 2002).**
  1. Elimination (or substitution) is the most preferred strategy for control and the method of choice whenever possible.
  2. The benefits to health and safety of elimination and substitution often have to be weighed against the technologic and economic consequences.
  3. When using substitution, care must be taken to ensure that the replacement product does not pose other health or safety risks.
  4. Examples of elimination or substitution include the following:
     a. Removing insulation that contains asbestos fibers
     b. Using mechanical or vacuum lifting devices to replace manual lifting
     c. Using a dipping method to coat an object rather than spraying, thus reducing the danger of inhalation
     d. Substituting unbreakable acrylic or thermoplastic product for breakable glass
     e. Using a less toxic and less flammable chemical than one in current use

B **Worksite** **engineering designs** **are intended to stop hazards at their source or in the path of their transmission and are the preferred strategy when elimination or substitution is not possible.**
  1. Characteristics of workplace designs that promote occupational health and safety include the following:
     a. Appropriate lighting to enable workers to perform their tasks safely
     b. Workstations that are ergonomically designed to reduce the risk factors of repetitive motions, static or awkward postures, forceful exertions, and mechanical pressure on soft tissues
     c. Stairs or platforms with railings, guarded floor and wall openings, and proper floor finishes to reduce slips, trips, and falls
     d. Mats that are specially designed to reduce safety hazards (Box 10-6)
     e. Security designs to reduce the potential for work-site violence (e.g., bullet-proof glass, silent alarms, well-lit parking lots)
     f. Designs that consider the personal comfort of workers (Box 10-7); for example, well-designed workstations can reduce worker stress
  2. Examples of beneficial workplace designs include:
     a. *Isolation* that provides a barrier between a hazard and those who might be affected by that hazard.

BOX 10-6

Examples of mats designed to reduce safety hazards

- *Fatigue-reducing mats* lessen muscular fatigue and often reduce noise.
- *Slip-resistant mats* protect against slipping on water, oil, ice, or mud.
- *Conductive mats* dissipate static electricity in rooms with high oxygen content, sensitive electronic components, explosives, or volatile liquids.
- *Nonconductive rubber mats* are used in front of switchboards and other high-voltage locations to protect workers from electric shock.

BOX 10-7

Features of stress-reducing workplace designs

- Availability of informal and formal meeting places
- Enclosures accommodating the need for personal space
- Permission to personalize spaces
- Access to daylight/sunlight
- Incorporation of variability through artifacts and cultural symbols, colors, and textures
- Freedom from distractions; visual and auditory privacy

---

      1) Process isolation: operations handled through remote computer applications in a control room
      2) Underground tanks and isolated storage buildings for hazardous materials
      3) Noise barriers
      4) Shields that prevent exposure of nearby persons to welding arcs
   b. *Time-distance-shielding* is the most common approach to protecting workers from ionizing radiation (National Safety Council, 2001).
      1) *Time:* controlling the amount of time of exposure to the radiation source, measured in mR/hr
      2) *Distance:* remaining as far away from the radiation source as possible
      3) *Shielding:* placing a barrier impenetrable to radiation between the worker and the source

NOTE: *This includes avoiding inhalation or ingestion* of radionuclide materials found in health care and research organizations through ventilation controls or radioactive particulates through shelters in the event of radioactive fallout.

C *Automatic systems* **are systems that shut down processes or issue warnings when hazardous conditions develop. They include the following:**
   1. Fire detectors/alarms, water sprinkler systems, and gas extinguisher systems, such as halon in computer rooms

2. Safety valves, fusible plugs, and rupture discs in boilers and pressure vessels to permit excess pressure relief
3. Automatic fall-protection devices that allow normal descent by a worker in the device, but lock in the event of a rapid descent or fall
4. Circuit breakers, fuses, and other electrical current interruption devices that respond to overcurrents or overloads
5. Explosion detectors that release a suppressant to inhibit further reaction

D *Ventilation* **captures or dilutes airborne contaminants, cleaning the air before or after release (Friend & Kohn, 2003).**
1. Local exhaust systems remove contaminated air from the point of origin, away from the worker's breathing zone through a scrubber or cleaning system to the outside (Plog et al., 2002).
2. Dilution ventilation circulates fresh air into the work site to dilute the contaminant air to an acceptable exposure level (Plog et al., 2002).
3. Filtration systems clean the air before it is released back into the general ventilation or to the outside.
4. Other air cleaning methods include electrostatic precipitators, scrubbers, absorbers, and chemical reactors (Plog et al., 2002).

E *Storage* **of hazardous materials requires consideration of the properties of the material.**
1. Flammable liquids are stored using bonding and grounding to dissipate static electricity, which could ignite their vapors.
2. Special lead containers are used to store radioactive materials.
3. Explosion-proof refrigerators are used to store heat-sensitive materials or heat-reactive chemicals.
4. Air-reactive chemicals are stored under water. Water-reactive chemicals are stored dry or under oil.
5. Special storage cabinets and safety cans are used to store small amounts of flammable liquids, such as hydrocarbons, gasoline, and kerosene.
6. Puncture-proof sharps containers are used to store contaminated needles and sharps awaiting disposal as hazardous health waste.
7. Certain highly toxic specialty gases, such as silane, must be kept in special gas cabinets.
8. Only the amount of hazardous substance that will actually be used in a reasonable time should be kept.

F **Consideration must be given to the** *location* **of the equipment.**
1. Ladders are secured on wall hangers, not propped against a wall.
2. Cylinders of compressed gas, including the oxygen cylinders used by the occupational and environmental health nurse, must be kept upright and secured.
3. Fire extinguishers are mounted in specified locations with recognizable signs and color codes.
4. Products and parts are stored on racks, pallets, and other devices with specified densities, stacking limitations, and aisle-way clearances.

G *Hazardous energy control* **is used to prevent contact between the worker and hazardous energy sources.**
1. Hazardous energy sources include electricity, chemical reactivity, thermal extremes, mechanical energy, and physical energy.
2. Machine safeguarding is used to eliminate machine hazards.
   a. All moving parts on machines that create pinch points or nip points, such as pulleys, belts, chains, etc., should be guarded during operation.

Interlocks preventing machine operation during guard removal should be in place.

b. Portable power tools, lawnmowers, and grinders should also be guarded (Occupational Safety and Health Administration, 1992).

c. Methods of safeguarding machines are based on the type of operation, stock size and shape, handling method, and physical layout of the area (Occupational Safety and Health Administration, 1992).

    1) Guards are barriers that prevent access to danger areas (Figures 10-5 and 10-6).

    2) Devices such as restraints, gates, presence-sensing (optical) devices, and trip controls stop the machine if a hand or other body part is inadvertently placed in the danger area.

3. Electric shock control is accomplished through the following safeguards:

a. Proper initial installation

b. The use of grounded outlets, circuit breakers, and disconnects (devices that interrupt current flow when it exceeds the wire's capacity)

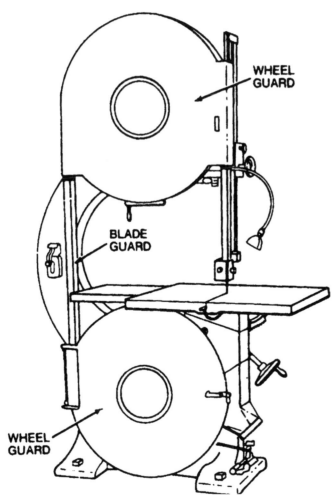

FIGURE 10-5 *Machine guard*

Source: U.S. Department of Labor, 1992.

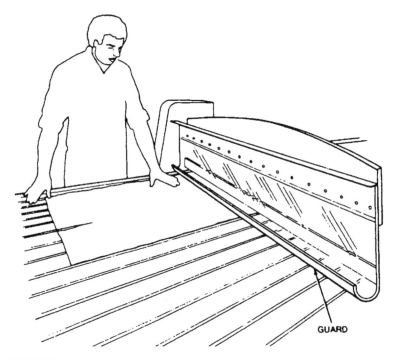

FIGURE 10-6 *Machine guard*

      c. The use of ground fault circuit interrupters
      d. Proper insulation
  4. Robots are used to perform unsafe, hazardous, highly repetitive, and unpleasant tasks.
  5. Lockout/tagout (Figure 10-7) is used to control hazardous energy sources during the service and maintenance of machinery or equipment that has exhibited unexpected startup or stored energy release (National Safety Council, 2001).
      a. OSHA 29 CFR 1910.147 Control of Hazardous Energy requires the following safety measures regarding a lockout/tagout system:
         1) Employee training
         2) Periodic inspections of the energy control program
         3) Written procedures for identifying all energy sources
         4) A tag warning system
         5) Periodic review and revision of procedures as needed
      b. All energy control devices are placed in the "off" or "safe" position, locked in that position, and tagged with a warning tag.
      c. Chemical process lines are bled out and disconnected or have a line block, called a *blank*, inserted.
      d. Upon work completion, the authorized employee will verify that the equipment has been returned to a safe state of operation before lockout/tagout devices are removed.

H *Mechanical integrity programs* **include preventive maintenance.**
  1. *Preventive maintenance* is the scheduling of planned, periodic equipment upkeep and the refurbishing, refitting, inspection, or overhaul of process

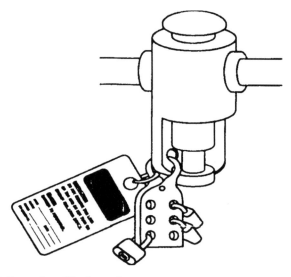

FIGURE 10-7 *Sample of lockout/tagout*

Source: U.S. Department of Labor, 1992.

units to prevent hazardous operating conditions from developing over time and after repeated use (National Safety Council, 2001).
2. Regular, periodic testing of equipment is done to compare actual to required performance measures, such as testing fire sprinkler system fire pump output monthly or measuring chemical fume hood face velocities annually.
3. Equipment deficiencies outside the acceptable limits defined by engineering standards must be corrected before further use.
4. Maintenance materials, spare parts, and equipment suitable for the process application must be maintained in inventory.

IX Prevention and Control Approaches That Focus on Administrative Controls

Administrative controls are supervisory and management practices to promote safe work behaviors that eliminate or limit hazard exposures.

A **Controlling *work practices* (the manner in which work is performed) is often an important strategy that can limit or reduce a worker's exposure to workplace hazards.**
1. Changes in work practices should be accompanied by on-site evaluations to accomplish the following:
    a. Characterize the risks inherent to the tasks
    b. Ensure that the work practice is appropriate to the task
    c. Perform a job safety analysis (JSA) on individual work tasks to identify those that may contribute to exposure (Swartz, 2002)
2. It is essential that the workers performing the job participate in the development of safe work practices to maximize the effectiveness of these strategies.
3. Barriers to the implementation of safe work practices include:
    a. Paying workers by the piece, also called piecework, which encourages workers to cut corners for the sake of production output, often sacrificing safe work practices

    b. Refusing to provide support and funding to safety programs, which undermines their effectiveness

    c. An enviroment that creates fear of harassment or violence; this can prevent the adoption of safe work practices

    d. Providing incentives that reward productivity that may lead to unsafe work practices

4. Examples of work practice modifications include:

    a. Vacuuming with equipment that has high-efficiency particulate (HEPA) filters that can keep hazardous dusts from being resuspended

    b. Wet mopping instead of sweeping, which is another way to minimize contamination from hazardous dusts and particulates

    c. Using proper body mechanics when bending or lifting, which can prevent strains and sprains

    d. The two-person concept (or "buddy system"), which is a safeguard for workers involved in hazardous operations (National Safety Council, 2001)

        1) Both persons are exposed to the same hazard simultaneously; each one monitors the other and provides assistance when needed, such as the mutual aid and surveillance employed by power company personnel on live high-voltage systems (National Safety Council, 2001)

        2) One person is exposed to the hazard, while the other acts as an attendant to observe and summon help if an emergency develops

B *Safety committees* **with well-defined missions and regular meetings promote illness and injury prevention by engaging in the following activities:**

1. Evaluating worker suggestions
2. Promoting accident prevention and safe work practices within each committee member's work area
3. Investigating reported safety deficiencies or assisting in the investigation
4. Reviewing accidents and identifying root causes and prevention methods
5. Performing walk-through surveys and safety inspections
6. Making recommendations on company safety rules
7. Assisting in safety training programs
8. Voting on safety awards recipients
9. Suggesting and promoting safety incentive programs

C *Safety training* **provides specific knowledge, instructions, and skills to enable workers to perform jobs safely while optimizing productivity and motivation (Klane, 2004).**

1. Training should be site-specific and based on needs identified during hazard identification and evaluation (Bean, 2004).
2. Training should be provided by effective trainers who are knowledgeable in the subject and available to answer questions and interpret information. Simply showing a videotape to workers is not adequate.
3. Testing and certification are methods for determining competency and ensuring safe performance of various job functions. The following are a few examples of testing and certification programs:

    a. Forklift operator training is often followed by written and performance testing to evaluate for proper, safe forklift operation.

    b. Boiler operators are licensed by the state.

    c. Drivers of certain types and sizes of vehicles must pass a commercial driver's license examination.

    d. Structural welders are usually certified in their skills by the Welder's Institute.

    e. Hazardous materials technicians are certified upon successful completion of the OSHA requirements under 29 CFR 1910.120.

  4. Training should be conducted according to adult education principles and should take into consideration language barriers and possible illiteracy.

D *Proper scheduling* **can reduce the amount of time any worker is exposed to a hazard or control the timing of the work to avoid the hazard. Examples of proper scheduling include the following:**

  1. Schedule work activities that can produce heat stress during cooler parts of the day.

  2. Schedule rotations among various job assignments, limiting exposure associated with a single job.

  3. Do not schedule workers to perform a new job assignment alone until they have demonstrated adequate job knowledge and performance.

E *Work permits* **are a system to evaluate projects for hazards, specify safe work practices, identify essential personal protective equipment and other safety measures, and provide authorization before any work is done (National Safety Council, 2001).**

  1. A Hot Work Permit is used for activities that produce sparks or flames, referred to as *hot work*.

  2. A Confined Space Entry Permit is required before working in areas defined as *permit-required confined spaces*.

    a. A *confined space* is an area that is large enough and so configured that an employee can enter and perform assigned work, but has limited or restricted means of access and is not designed for continuous worker occupancy.

    b. A *permit-required confined space* is a confined space with one or more of the following characteristics:

      1) Contains or has a potential to contain a hazardous atmosphere

      2) Contains a material that has the potential for engulfing an entrant

      3) Has an internal configuration such that an entrant could be trapped or asphyxiated by inwardly converging walls or by a floor that slopes downward and tapers to a smaller cross-section

      4) Contains any other recognized serious safety or health hazard

    c. Hazards associated with confined spaces that must be evaluated in the permitting process are hazardous atmospheres (oxygen-deficient, flammable, toxic), temperature extremes, engulfment hazards, noise, falling objects, and any other recognized serious hazard.

  3. Waste Disposal/Storage Permits may be required for environmental hazardous waste control.

  4. Excavation Permits may be necessary before digging operations are performed.

  5. Line-breaking Permits may be required before process piping is opened.

F *Housekeeping* **practices that promote safe working conditions include controlling pests; promptly disposing of waste; keeping floors clear of oil, grease, and water; preventing trip hazards; and properly storing materials, tools, and equipment. Weekly housekeeping inspections are recommended.**

G *Labeling, coding, and posting warning signs* **all help communicate safety issues throughout the work-site.**

1. Some OSHA standards require posting of warning signs in areas where hazards have been identified (e.g., noise or radiation).
2. Safety showers and eyewash stations and alarms are marked with signs and color coding to enhance visibility and rapid access.
3. Exits must be clearly identified with lighted signs; doorways that are not exits must be clearly labeled as such.
4. Color, indicators of direction of flow, and other signs mark controls, piping outlets, and pipelines.
   a. Red—fire protection equipment, danger, and "emergency stops" on equipment
   b. Yellow—trip hazards, flammable-liquid storage cabinets, and materials-handling equipment such as forklifts
   c. Green—location of first-aid and safety equipment
   d. Black on yellow—radiation hazard
   e. Bright blue—inert gases
5. Signs and maps are posted throughout the facility to mark evacuation routes and shelters. General warning signs do not substitute for safe work practices but can serve as cautions and reminders (National Safety Council, 2001).
6. Signage must be compliant with the Americans with Disabilities Act requirements, such as raised lettering or Braille, size, etc.

H *General safety promotion* **is designed to publicize, strengthen, and reinforce injury and illness prevention awareness and the attitudes that mold and strengthen it.**
1. Safety newsletters are used to relate safety information directly to each worker (Friend & Kohn, 2003).
   a. They impart information and help to boost morale.
   b. To be successful, they should put the spotlight on workers, balancing useful information with recognition of workers' accomplishments.
   c. They can promote safety contests, provide a network for news, offer a management column, and report actual incidents.
2. Bulletin boards, which should be visible to everyone, attractive, and eye-catching, can provide a variety of health and safety information.
3. Promotional posters, changed often to avoid over-familiarity, serve as visual reminders of prevention and control programs.
4. Incentive programs are used to motivate workers to work safely and prevent accidents and injuries (National Safety Council, 2001).
   a. Examples of incentive programs include the following:
      1) Contests among departments for the best safety record or best housekeeping performance
      2) Safety awards for companies and plants, offered by organizations such as local safety councils
      3) Safety patches, pins, hard-hat stickers, ball caps, and other apparel bearing positive safety messages
      4) Bonuses to workers, supervisors, and managers when targeted safety goals are reached
   b. Programs should be monitored so workers, supervisors, and managers do not attempt to hide accidents, injuries, and other events to avoid being the cause of a lost record or award.
   c. The primary focus of managers should not be numbers and statistics but rather acknowledging the excellent safety performance of workers.

5. Health-promotion programs target lifestyles to lessen workers' vulnerability to work-site exposures and to enhance their ability and capacity to perform job assignments more safely.
   a. Back strengthening through exercise programs can help reduce the incidence of back strain during materials handling.
   b. Smoking cessation programs can reduce risks of synergistic effects of cigarette smoke and asbestos exposure.
   c. Stress management programs can help workers deal with work-related stress.

I *Medical controls* **are used to prevent or reduce the effect of a hazard by reducing worker vulnerability, preventing expected illness onset, or eliminating all exposure to vulnerable workers.**
1. Removal from exposure for medical reasons may require job reassignment.
   a. Some OSHA regulations have medical removal requirements, which require removal of a worker based on biologic monitoring results before clinical health effects appear or end-organ systems are injured; these regulations include the lead and cadmium standards.
   b. Medical removal requirements may have to be employed when a worker becomes sensitized to a work-site hazardous material, such as an isocyanate or an anhydride, and cannot risk any further exposures.
2. Restricted work programs or light-duty assignments return workers gradually to the rigors of full work assignments.
3. Primary preventive measures decrease the worker's vulnerability. Examples are immunization against smallpox in biologic researchers, and administration of iodine in radiation unit workers.
4. Secondary preventive measures anticipate illness from an exposure and prevent onset, for example, using a hyperbaric chamber when deep-sea pressure with rapid ascent has occurred.

J *Emergency preparedness* **planning and response operations are control measures intended to prevent or minimize harm to persons, property, systems, and the environment in the event of a critical incident (Hau & Dierwechter, 2000).**
1. This strategy may be used for a medical emergency, fire, technologic event (such as a hazardous materials release), or civil event (such as a bomb threat).
2. Phases of an emergency preparedness operation include mitigation, planning, response, and recovery.
   a. In the mitigation phase, the attempt is made to identify and eliminate hazards that have a potential for generating an emergency.
   b. Planning is then conducted in coordination with community response agencies to prepare to bring emergency conditions under control and eventually to return to normal operations, if possible (Figure 10-8).
   c. Response is action designed to address the immediate and short-term effects of the emergency, with life safety as the priority.
   d. Recovery is action intended to address the long-term effects of the emergency, including restoration of systems, services, and functions to normal pre-emergency conditions.

K *Materials and services management* **reduces hazards by establishing effective purchasing systems and preventing substandard equipment, materials, and services from being delivered to the work site (National Safety Council, 2001).**

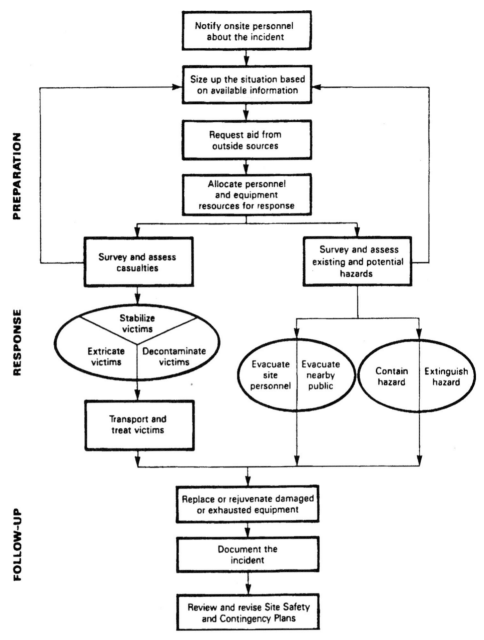

FIGURE 10-8 *Emergency response operations*

1. Training and effective systems ensure that health and safety considerations are applied to the procurement of goods and services; these systems should provide and use lists of all materials, products, machines, equipment, and chemical substances and their required specifications.
2. Goods received are inspected for package integrity and checked against approved lists to ensure proper quality and safety.
3. New equipment and materials are formally reviewed by suitably qualified personnel to identify potential loss exposure and controls to be implemented for them before purchasing.

4. Handling practices and operating and maintenance procedures are developed and communicated before new items are used.
5. Contractor safety records, health and safety programs, training records, and worker certifications are reviewed for hazard potentials and hazard prevention.

L *Environmental management systems* **are intended to reduce environmental hazards to the community and to the facility workers (Sullivan, 2003).**
   1. *Recycling programs* collect and redistribute reusable chemicals in the workplace, thereby reducing the volume of those chemicals in purchasing, shipping, handling, and waste collections.
   2. *Waste minimization programs* reduce the amount of hazardous waste being generated, resulting in less workplace hazardous materials exposures.
   3. *Collection programs* eliminate harmful workplace substances.

   Example: mercury collection programs, to eliminate breakage and consequent exposure of mercury to the air.

   4. *Emissions control engineering programs*, such as air and water toxic emissions reduction, reduce the level of exposure to these agents in both the community and the workplace.

M *Special programs* **are available to help employers meet and exceed regulatory requirements; for example:**
   1. OSHA's Voluntary Protection Program (Chapter 3)
   2. Association-sponsored programs, for example, Chemical Manufacturer's Association's "Responsible Care"
   3. Proprietary programs, for example, Dupont's "STOP" program and Det Norske Veritas' "International Safety Rating System"

X Prevention and Control Approaches That Focus on Personal Protective Equipment

Personal protective equipment (PPE) includes all clothing and accessories, worn by the worker, designed to create a barrier against work-site hazards. It is the least desirable control method because of the expense, discomfort, and enforcement problems it creates.

A **Characteristics of personal protective equipment are as follows:**
   1. Workers must be trained in the reasons for wearing PPE; what PPE to wear; how to don, use, and wear PPE; the proper care, maintenance, and useful life of PPE; and any other training requirement involving PPE.
   2. The occupational and environmental health nurse should become familiar with the details of the specific PPE used at the facility and with the requirements of the applicable OSHA standard.
      a. Typical PPE dispensed by the occupational and environmental health nurse includes eye protection, hearing protection, and skin barrier creams.
      b. The occupational and environmental health nurse must take special care to review the research and professional recommendations regarding proper PPE selections and proper fitting.

B **Regulations related to personal protective equipment provide guidance for employers.**
   1. The company is required to have a written PPE program and to provide PPE to workers. Some companies have workers contribute to the cost of prescription safety glasses and safety shoes.

2. OSHA 29 CFR 1910.132 requires a work-site hazard assessment that has the following characteristics:
   a. Includes a walk-through survey
   b. Requires written certification that the assessment has been performed
   c. Provides a mechanism for ensuring that the need for PPE has been determined and that the PPE selected is appropriate to the hazard

C **There are several types of personal protective equipment.**

1. 29 CFR 1910.133 requires protective eye and face equipment.
   a. Safety glasses with sideshields are used to protect against flying objects; they must be heat-treated and able to withstand the drop of a 5-pound lead ball without shattering.
   b. Chemical goggles, of vented and air-tight varieties, protect against chemical splashes, vapors, and gases.
   c. Ultraviolet (UV) light protection is most commonly used by welders to protect against the UV welding arc.
   d. Laser beam protection is necessary to prevent corneal and retinal injuries from exposure to laser beams.
   e. Face shields add further protection against splashes or sparks.
   f. The use of contact lenses, especially while wearing respiratory protection, is not recommended when there is concern that dirt or other debris can lodge between the lens and the pupil or that soft lenses will absorb chemical contaminants from the air.

2. Hearing protection under 29 CFR 1910.95 requires a written hearing conservation program, including hearing protection and annual audiometric testing for workers exposed to excessive noise. Chapter 16 presents an example of a hearing conservation program.
   a. Hearing protection devices include ear plugs, ear muffs, ear molds, and canal caps (Chapter 16).
   b. Hearing aids and music headphones do not protect against the effects of loud noise, even when the worker cannot hear the noise.
   c. Workers must be shown how to wear hearing protection and how to care for it, and should be observed to ensure that they are using it correctly.
   d. Changes in noise levels may require changes in hearing protection devices.

3. Hand/skin protection is required under 29 CFR 1910.138.
   a. Gloves are selected to protect against heat, cold, abrasion, and chemicals.
   b. No single glove material or fabric is effective against all chemical exposures, including latex examination gloves; selection must be made using a chemical compatibility chart from the glove manufacturer.
   c. Barrier creams are of two varieties, setting up a coating to shield the skin either against water-related exposures or against drying powder-type exposures.
   d. Tapes, similar to adhesive tape, have a gritty or rubbery external surface to protect fingers against abrasion from repeated rubbing or gripping and to aid in gripping.
   e. Sunscreen protects workers from the sun and other UV sources.
   f. Glove boxes, although not strictly PPE, are also used to protect hand exposures, particularly against biologic agents.

4. 29 CFR 1910.136 specifies safety shoes for protecting feet from being crushed and fractured.

   a. Boots are used to protect against exposure to water, chemicals, and fire.
   b. Steel-toed shoes protect the toes from hazards such as heavy rolling or falling objects.
   c. Metatarsal plates fit over the shoe and extend protection to the metatarsals from toe-injury hazards.
5. Torso protection is selected according to the specific type of hazard involved.
   a. Chemical-protective clothing may consist of aprons, coveralls, hooded suits, fully encapsulated suits with self-contained breathing apparatus, sleeves, pants, or chaps, and is selected to protect against heat, cold, abrasion, and chemicals.
   b. No single material or fabric is effective against all chemical exposures; selection is made using a chemical compatibility chart from the material manufacturer.
   c. Radiation protection is provided by lead aprons and protective suits.
   d. Thermal garments include heat-resistant firefighter gear, flash-protection garments, proximity suits for radiant heat, cooling garments and vests using ice packs or circulating cold water, and other garments to protect against extremely hot or cold conditions.
   e. Blast and fragmentation suits are used for protection against small detonations; they do not provide hearing protection.
6. 29 CFR 1910.135 specifies head protection from impact and penetration from falling and flying objects and from limited electric shock and burn hazards.
   a. Hard hats are used in areas where falling and flying objects are a hazard.
   b. Heat-resistant and chemical-resistant hoods are also used.
7. 29 CFR 1910.134 requires respiratory protection when airborne contamination exceeds the TLV or PEL and cannot be eliminated by engineering controls.
   a. Requirements include a written comprehensive respirator program with annual fit testing and worker training.
   b. Respiratory protection is of two types: *supplied air* and *air purifying*. Figure 10-9 presents examples of respiratory equipment, and Figure 10-10 provides guidelines for selecting respirators.
      1) Supplied air respirators provide clean air from either a tank (a self-contained breathing apparatus or SCBA) or an air line connected to an air supply.
      2) Air-purifying respirators use a filter or canister to remove hazards from inhaled air; they may be full-mask or half-mask.
   c. Respirator face masks must form a tight seal against the face, requiring fit testing with isoamyl nitrate or irritant smoke as a fit check, prohibiting facial hair growth over 24 hours and eyeglass sidebars underneath the mask; this includes N-95 face masks used for tuberculosis exposure protection (Figure 10-11) (Perkins, 2003).
   d. Respirators must be tested for fit by the wearer before each use.
   e. After use, respirators must be properly stored, regularly inspected, and repaired as needed; disposable respirators are not reused. (Sterns, 2004)
   f. A respirator wearer's health status must be reviewed periodically (usually annually) to assess physical and psychologic fitness for using the respiratory protection equipment.

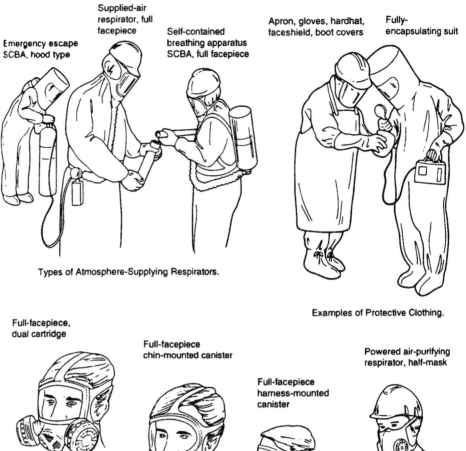

Types of Atmosphere-Supplying Respirators.

Examples of Protective Clothing.

Types of Air-Purifying Respirators.

FIGURE 10-9 *Examples of respiratory equipment*

Source: U.S. Department of Health and Human Services, 1987.

g. The type of respirator to be used depends on the type of airborne hazard. Respirator and cartridge selection is based on data from air sampling performed in an exposure monitoring program.

h. Only NIOSH-approved respirators can be worn.

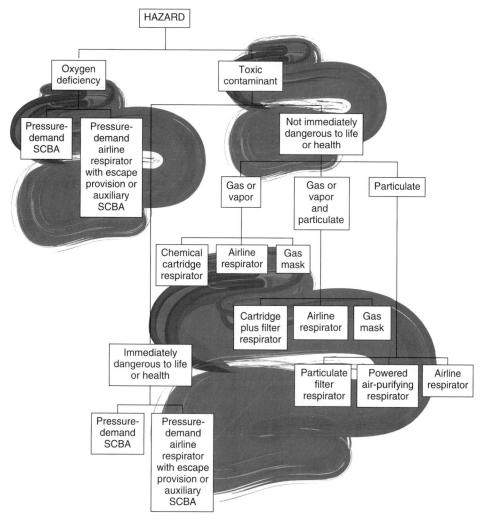

FIGURE 10-10 *Guidelines for the selection of respirators for routine use*

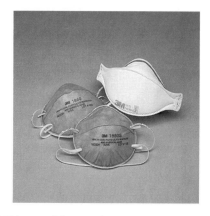

FIGURE 10-11 *N-95 Disposable respirator*

Source: NIOSH Understanding Respiratory Protection. Available at
http://www.cdc.gov/niosh/ npptl/topics/respirators/factsheets/respsars.html

     i. Escape respirator devices allow a person working in a normally safe environment sufficient time to escape from suddenly occurring respiratory hazards. They should be used for escape purposes only.

     j. Because respirators are uncomfortable or unacceptable to some workers, they may not be worn properly and thus not protect the worker from hazardous exposure.

XI Prevention and Control Programs That Focus on Comprehensive Containment Approaches

In certain work settings, risk analysis reveals new technologies and activities with hazards yet to be discovered or recognized. For example, recombinant DNA technologies and emerging infectious disease organisms are being seen in research and diagnostic laboratories (Emery & Malcolm, 1995). A thorough risk assessment must be conducted to determine a level of *containment* necessary to reduce or eliminate exposure of laboratory workers, other persons, and the outside environment to potentially hazardous agents.

A **Containment approaches include the engineering and administrative elements as well as the use of personal protective equipment.**

   1. Engineering elements include primary and secondary barriers.

     a. *Primary barriers* consist of safety equipment such as biologic safety cabinets (BSCs), enclosed containers, and other engineering controls designed to remove or minimize exposures to hazardous biologic materials.

       1) The biologic safety cabinet (BSC) is the principal device used to provide containment of infectious splashes or aerosols generated by many microbiologic procedures.

       2) Another primary barrier is the safety centrifuge cup, an enclosed container designed to prevent aerosols from being released during centrifugation.

     b. *Secondary barriers* are established through facility design and construction.

       1) Secondary barriers usually require separation of the laboratory work area from public access, availability of a decontamination facility (e.g., autoclave), and handwashing facilities.

       2) When the risk of infection by exposure to an infectious aerosol is present, multiple secondary barriers may become necessary, such as specialized ventilation systems to provide directional air flow, air treatment systems to decontaminate or remove agents from exhaust air, controlled access zones, airlocks as laboratory entrances, or separate buildings or modules to isolate the laboratory.

   2. Administrative elements include control of work practices, safety training, infectious disease committee permits, medical control, and materials and services management.

     a. "The most important element of containment is strict adherence to standard microbiological practices and techniques" (CDC & National Institutes of Health [NIH], 1999).

     b. Each laboratory must anticipate the hazards that will or may be encountered, and identify work practices and procedures designed to minimize or eliminate exposures to these hazards.

     c. Persons working with infectious agents must be trained and demonstrate proficiency in these work practices and procedures.

TABLE 10-1

Summary of recommended biosafety levels (BSL) for infectious agents

BSL	Agent	Practices	Safety Equipment (Primary Barriers)	Facilities (Secondary Barriers)
1	Not known to consistently cause disease in healthy adults	Standard microbiologic practices	None required	Open bench top sink required
2	Associated with human disease, hazard = percutaneous injury, ingestion, mucous membrane exposure	BSL-1 practice plus: • Limited access • Biohazard warning signs • "Sharps" precautions • Biosafety manual defining any needed waste decontamination or medical surveillance policies	Primary barriers = Class I or II Biologic Safety Cabinets (BSCs) or other physical containment devices used for all manipulations of agents that cause splashes or aerosols of infectious materials; PPEs: laboratory coats; gloves; face protection as needed	BSL-1 plus: Autoclave available
3	Indigenous or exotic agents with potential for aerosol transmission; disease may have serious or lethal consequences	BSL-2 practice plus: • Controlled access • Decontamination of all waste • Decontamination of lab clothing before laundering • Baseline serum	Primary barriers = Class I or II BCSs or other physical containment devices used for all open manipulations of agents; PPEs: protective lab clothing; gloves; respiratory protection as needed	BSL-2 plus: • Physical separation from access corridors • Self-closing, double-door access • Exhausted air not recirculated • Negative airflow into laboratory
4	Dangerous/exotic agents which pose high risk of life-threatening disease, aerosol-transmitted lab infections; or related agents with unknown risk of transmission	BSL-3 practices plus: • Clothing change before entering • Shower on exit • All material decontaminated on exit from facility	Primary barriers = All procedures conducted in Class III BSCs or Class I or II BSCs in combination with full-body, air-supplied, positive pressure personnel suit	BSL-3 plus: • Separate building or isolated zone • Dedicated supply and exhaust, vacuum, and decon systems • Other requirements outlined in the text

Source: Centers for Disease Control and Prevention and National Institutes of Health (1999). *Biosafety in Biomedical and Microbiological Laboratories* [BMBL] 4th ed.

    d. Baseline serums and immunizations, if available, must be offered.

    e. Strict guidelines on the shipping, packaging, and receipt of these agents must be followed, including examination of packages for leakage.

3. Personal protective equipment (PPE) is also utilized based on the hazard analysis.

    a. PPE includes gloves, coats, gowns, shoe covers, boots, respirators, face shields, safety glasses, or goggles.

    b. PPE, especially gloves, is used in combination with biologic safety cabinets.

    c. In some situations it is impractical to work in biologic safety cabinets, requiring that personal protective equipment serve as the primary barrier; examples include certain animal studies, animal necropsy, agent production activities, and activities relating to maintenance, service, or support of the laboratory facility.

B **Four different *biosafety levels (BSLs)* have been defined, which consist of combinations of administrative, engineering, and personal protective equipment approaches.**

1. "Each combination is specifically appropriate for the operations performed, the documented or suspected routes of transmission of the infectious agents, and the laboratory function or activity" (CDC & NIH, 1999).

2. The biosafety level is determined by what is known about the level of infectivity of the agent (see Table 10-1 and Figure 10-12).

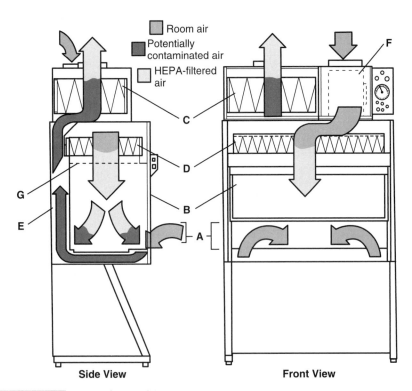

FIGURE 10-12 *Biosafety cabinet*

Redrawn from Centers for Disease Control and Prevention and National Institute of Health (1999). (Biosafety in Biomedical and Microbiological Laboratories—BMBL, 4th ed.)

REFERENCES

American Association of Occupational Health Nurses (AAOHN). (2001a). *Incident analysis* [AAOHN Advisory]. Atlanta, GA: AAOHN Publications.

American Association of Occupational Health Nurses. (2003a). *AAOHN worksite walkthrough program.* Foundation blocks: A guide to occupational & environmental health nursing. Atlanta, GA: AAOHN publications.

American Association of Occupational Health Nurses. (2003b). *AAOHN safety action plan template: General industry. Manufacturing setting. Worksite walkthrough program.* Foundation blocks: A guide to occupational & environmental health nursing. Atlanta, GA: AAOHN publications.

American Association of Occupational Health Nurses (AAOHN). (2004). Components of Ergonomics Programs. Available at http://www.ergore sources. org/components/ index.htm.

American Conference of Governmental Industrial Hygienists. (2004). *2004 Threshold limit values for chemical substances and physical agents and biological exposure indices.* Cincinnati, OH: American Conference of Governmental Industrial Hygienists Technical Affairs Office.

Bean, S. (2004). H&S strategy must be supported by training. *Occupational Health, 56*(6), 10.

Blackman, L., & Walkerdine, V. (2001). *Mass hysteria: critical psychology and media studies.* New York: Palgrave.

Breitenstein, B. D., Jr., & Spickard, J. H. (2002). Ionizing radiation. In P. H. Wald and G. M. Stave (Eds.). *Physical and biological hazards of the workplace.* New York: Van Nostrand Reinhold.

Centers for Disease Control and Prevention and National Institutes of Health. (1999). *Biosafety in microbiological and biomedical laboratories (BMBL)* 4th Edition. Available at http://www.cdc.gov/od/ohs/pdf files/4th BMBL.pdf

DiNardi, S. R. (Ed.). (2002). *The occupational environment: Its evaluation, control, and management* (2nd ed.). Fairfax, VA: American Industrial Hygiene Association.

Dobie, R. A. (2000). Noise. In P. H. Wald & G. M. Stave (Eds.). *Physical and biological hazards of the workplace.* New York: Van Nostrand Reinhold.

Eichenberger, J. (1995). How to achieve results through employee committees. *AAOHN Journal, 42*(7), 344-348.

Emery, A., & Malcolm, S. (1995) *An introduction to recombinant DNA in medicine* (2nd ed.). New York: John Wiley & Sons.

Fleming, L. E., Herzstein, J., & Bunn, W. B. (1997). International control of occupational and environmental health hazards, *International occupational and environmental medicine,* Boston: OEM Press, 47-62.

Friend, M. A., & Kohn, J. P. (2003). *Fundamentals of occupational safety and health* (3rd ed.). Rockville, MD: Government Institutes.

Garg, A. (1995). Revised NIOSH equation for manual lifting: A method for job evaluation. *AAOHN Journal, 43*, 211-216.

Grenyer, B., et al. (2004). Safer at work: development and evaluation of an aggression and violence minimization program. *Australian & New Zealand Journal of Psychiatry, 38*(10), 804-811.

Hau, M. L., & Dierwechter, D. W. (2000). Incident response. In D. B. Cox (Ed.), *Hazardous materials management.* New York: McGraw-Hill Inc.

Heimlich, J. E. (2004). Extension Fact Sheet: *Multiple Chemical Sensitivity, CDFS-192-96,* Ohio State University. Available at http://ohioline.osu.edu/ cd-fact/0192.html.

Klane, J. (2004). Really effective training. *Occupational Health & Safety, 73*(9), 179-184.

Levy, B. S., & Wegman, D. M. (2000). *Occupational health: Recognizing and preventing work-related disease* (4th ed.). Boston: Little, Brown and Company.

McDermott, H. J., (2004). *Air monitoring for toxic exposures* (2nd ed.). New York: JohnWiley & Sons.

Manuele, F. A. (2003a). *On the practice of safety* (3rd ed.). Itasca, IL: National Safety Council.

Manuele, F.A. (2003b) Severe injury potential: Addressing an often-overlooked safety management element. *Professional Safety, 48*(2), 26-32.

National Safety Council. (2001). *Accident prevention manual for business & industry:*

Administration & programs (12th ed.). Itasca, IL: National Safety Council.

National Safety Council. (2001). *Accident prevention manual for business & industry: Engineering & technology* (12th ed.). Itasca, IL: National Safety Council.

Occupational Safety and Health Administration (OSHA). (1992). *Concepts and techniques of machine safeguarding*. (OSHA 3067). Washington DC: U.S. Department of Labor.

Occupational Safety and Health Administration (OSHA). (1999). *OSHA technical manual*. Available at http://www.osha.gov/dts/osta/otm/otm_toc.html.

Perkins, J. L. (2003). *Modern industrial hygiene: Biological Aspects* (Vol. II). New York: Van Nostrand Reinhold.

Plog, B. A., Benjamin, G. S., & Kerwin, M. A. (2002). *Fundamentals of industrial hygiene* (5th ed.). Itasca, IL: National Safety Council.

Sparks, P. J., Daniell, W., Black, D. W., Kipen, H. M., Altman, L. C., Simon, G. E., & Terr, A. I. (1994). Multiple chemical sensitivity syndrome: A clinical perspective. I. Case definition, theories of pathogenesis, and research needs. *Journal of Occupational Medicine, 36*(7), 718-730.

Spear, J. (2002). Incident investigation, a problem-solving process. *Professional Safety, 47*(4), 25-29.

Stern, M B., & Mansdorf, S. Z. (1999). *Applications and computational elements of industrial hygiene*. New York: Lewis Publishers.

Sterns, M. (2004). Respirator fit testing requirement and procedures. *Occupational Health & Safety, 73*(5), 108-112.

Sullivan, T. (Ed.). (2003). *Environmental law handbook* (17th ed.). Rockville, MD: Government Institutes.

Swartz, G. (2002) Job hazard analysis. *Professional Safety, 47*(11), 27-33.

Swartz, G. (2001). *Job hazard analysis: Guide to identifying risks in the workplace*. Rockville, MD: Government Institutes.

United States Department of Justice, Federal Bureau of Investigation. (2004). *Workplace violence – issues in response*. Available at http://www.fbi.gov/publications/violence.pdf.

Weeks, J. L., Levy, B. S., & Wagner, G. R. (2004). *Preventing occupational disease and injury* (2nd ed.). Washington DC: American Public Health Association.

CHAPTER

11

Direct Care in the Occupational Setting

BARBARA BURGEL

Direct care consists of activities involved in the delivery of clinical care to individual clients. These activities include the steps necessary for appropriate clinical decision making, such as taking a health history, conducting a physical examination, and ordering diagnostic or screening studies as well as actually providing clinical services. This chapter provides an overview of the processes involved in planning and delivering direct care services in the occupational setting; it concludes with a description of outcomes that can be used to evaluate the effectiveness of services.

I Direct Care Professional Practice Concepts

A *Direct care* is defined as hands-on, clinical care delivery to individual clients. The range, scope, and depth of these activities vary with the educational preparation, knowledge, skills, and abilities of the occupational and environmental health nurse.

B *Advanced practice nursing* is an umbrella term for a licensed registered nurse prepared at the graduate degree level as a clinical specialist, nurse anesthetist, nurse midwife, or nurse practitioner (American Association of Colleges of Nursing [AACN], 1998).

C *Primary care* is the provision of integrated, accessible, and coordinated health-care service, which is:
1. Person-centered and holistic, involving all levels of prevention
2. Provided in a partnership with clients, within the context of family and community
3. Provided by a multidisciplinary health-care team with the goal to improve client health care outcomes (Bodenheimer et al, 2002; Grumbach & Bodenheimer, 2004)
4. "Health-care providers" and "clinicians" are additional terms used to describe those who provide primary care services within their scope of licensure

D There are several *professional and regulatory* parameters of practice.
1. The standards of occupational and environmental health nursing include several applicable standards for direct care, including Standard I: Assessment, and Standard II: Diagnosis (AAOHN, 2004a).
2. AAOHN competencies in occupational and environmental health nursing include Category I: Clinical and Primary Care. Performance criteria for

competent, proficient and expert practice in clinical and primary care can be found at http://www.aaohn.org./.

3. Licensure laws in each state outline the scope of practice for registered nurses and for advanced practice nursing (AAOHN, 2004b).

4. AAOHN supports the Nurse Licensure Compact, which is a mutual recognition model of nurse licensure that allows a nurse to have one license (in his or her state of residency) and to practice (both physical and electronic) in other states, subject to each state's practice law and regulation. Under mutual recognition, a nurse may practice across state lines unless otherwise restricted (National Council of State Boards of Nursing, 2005).

II Overview of Direct Care

A **Careful planning will determine the range of direct care services needed for a specific industry, and will help meet the goals for a healthy work force.**

1. The range and scope of direct care services may include the following:
   a. Care for occupational and/or nonoccupational conditions
   b. First aid, emergency care, minor acute care, chronic illness management, full-service primary care, and 24-hour call
   c. Prevention-based services, including health promotion and screening programs and services such as preplacement programs, immunizations, and health surveillance
   d. Case management of occupational and/or nonoccupational health problems
   e. Home care and telehealth services; *telehealth* refers to the use of electronic information to support long distance health service delivery, health education, and health administration

2. Direct care services can be offered to all workers, dependents, and retirees.

3. Health-care providers may be employees of the company or independent contractors; contractual arrangements with a health maintenance organization or other organizations for on-site providers may also be developed.

4. Depending on the types of conditions commonly treated, their medical complexity, and the number of anticipated visits, service providers on-site may include the following:
   a. Occupational and environmental health nurses, clinical nurse specialists in occupational health, and adult or family nurse practitioners who specialize in occupational and environmental health (AAOHN, 2004b)
   b. Family or primary care physicians or doctors of osteopathy who specialize in preventive medicine/occupational medicine
   c. Physical therapists, occupational therapists, and massage therapists
   d. Mental health professionals
   e. Other providers based on needs assessment

5. The rationale for providing on-site direct care services includes the following benefits:
   a. Greater convenience for workers, with less down-time resulting from absence due to sickness and visits to off-site health care providers
   b. Greater opportunity for case management to monitor quality, outcomes, and cost of care
   c. Fast and accurate determination of work-related etiology or aggravation of the symptom or disease, with the opportunity for timely prevention/loss control activities at the worksite

d. Accommodations, if needed, that are made by on-site providers who are knowledgeable about the work site

e. Opportunity to reinforce safe work practices with each worker encounter

f. Ability to tailor direct care services to the risk profile of the company and to complement/maximize the health benefit plan

g. Cost savings, which are realized by controlling duplicate health-care services and reducing absence resulting from sickness

h. Opportunity to reinforce a self-care approach to health

6. Determine the need for direct care on-site by evaluating the following factors:

a. Hazard profile of company

b. Geographic proximity of the nearest emergency facility

c. Injury and illness statistics (both occupational and nonoccupational)

d. Demographics of the work force (number of workers, age, gender, length of employment with firm)

e. Health benefit coverage (number of workers with coverage; inclusion or exclusion of preventive and mental health services)

f. Company philosophy about direct care activities for workers

g. Financial and personnel resources

7. There are multiple ethical, legal, and professional considerations for direct care activities in the occupational setting (Burgel, 1996).

a. Ethical considerations include the following:

1) Confidentiality of personal health information of workers and their dependents must be safeguarded ethically and legally according to professional codes of conduct and state and federal laws (i.e., Health Information Protection and Accountability Act, Privacy Rule; See Chapter 3) (AAOHN, 2004c).

2) The direct care provider must balance the "duty to warn" against the right to privacy of the worker or dependent.

3) Resources dedicated to occupational health and safety are often limited; it is therefore important to prioritize direct care activities to preventable work-related exposures, and not duplicate direct care services that may be funded through personal health insurance coverage.

4) Workers have a right to know about the hazards in their work settings and a right to be notified of an exposure or abnormal physical findings.

b. Legal considerations include the following:

1) Documentation must be done according to professional codes of conduct and AAOHN Standards of Occupational and Environmental Health Nursing (AAOHN, 2004d). (Chapter 3, Section IX.)

2) Advanced practice nurses can prescribe medications in many states. If medications will be dispensed or prescribed, state pharmacy laws must be followed.

3) Activities related to the care of clients must comply with OSHA standards, and compliance is needed with state laws for ensuring that direct care providers are free from infectious diseases (rubella, varicella, tuberculosis, and others).

4) Potential liability arises if there is malpractice by the direct care provider. In this case, is workers' compensation the exclusive remedy, or can the injured worker sue the direct care provider for malpractice?

Legal advice is needed to clarify the professional malpractice issues for on-site direct care.

c. Professional considerations include the following:
   1) Direct care providers must be competent to perform the direct care activities and must practice within the state's business and professions code and scope of practice.
   2) AAOHN's Standards of Occupational and Environmental Health Nursing guide professional practice.
   3) Outcomes of clinical care must be measured, and clinical care evaluated using a continuous quality improvement model.
   4) A standardized language for occupational and environmental health nursing, with a minimal data set (Toth, 2003), must be adopted for widespread use, to document direct care processes and outcomes as well as occupational and environmental health nurses' roles and functions.
   5) Secure data management systems must be created not only for individual care, but also for population-based disease management activities.
   6) Policies and procedures outlining practice understandings and consultation/referral mechanisms must be clearly delineated.
   7) Direct care activities must be linked to prevention activities at the worksite.

B **The primary emphasis of direct care activities is on health promotion and protection.**
1. Health promotion:
   a. Begins with people who are basically healthy
   b. Uses strategies related to personal lifestyle—those personal choices made in a social context—that can have a powerful influence over one's health status (U.S. Preventive Services Task Force, 2004; U.S. Department of Health and Human Services [USDHHS], 2000)
   c. Includes such activities as the promotion of physical exercise, weight control, nutrition, and the reduction of the use of alcohol and tobacco
2. Health protection strategies:
   a. Are related to environmental or regulatory measures that confer protection on large population groups
   b. Include food and drug safety and environmental health initiatives (U.S. Preventive Services Task Force, 2004; USDHHS, 2000)
3. The three levels of prevention include primary, secondary, and tertiary measures to protect and promote health and prevent disease (Chapter 14).

C **There are unique knowledge needs for direct care in occupational health.**
1. Providing direct care in the occupational setting requires:
   a. Knowledge of the physical and mental requirements of the worker's job, including an understanding of essential job criteria and reasonable accommodations, in compliance with the Americans with Disabilities Act.
   b. Knowledge of the work processes, potential hazards, and any personal protective equipment requirements.
   c. Recognition of the link between work-site exposure and adverse health effects, and between worker health status and a safe work environment.
   d. Familiarity with clinical practice guidelines and evidence-based practice for treatment and disability management unique to occupational health (Glass, 2004; Reed, 2001).

    e. A clinical care philosophy that promotes safe work as therapeutic, and uses the worksite as a critical component of the treatment/rehabilitation plan.

    f. An ability to counsel, educate, and coach effectively about risk communication, self-care, and return to work.

    g. Excellent communication skills to coordinate care, share rationale for treatment, and advocate for injured workers and their families through the workers' compensation/disability systems.

    h. Ability to manage multiple health and illness conditions, and interface with nurse case managers employed by insurance carriers, health plans, and/or employers.

    i. Awareness of the connection between the physical and psychosocial aspects of illness, and recognition of the red flags for delayed recovery.

    j. Medical record documentation that safeguards personal health information in employment settings.

    k. Legal standards that may specify care components for screening and surveillance; for example, the OSHA standard for asbestos, or the Department of Transportation requirements.

2. There are several operational requirements for direct care activities in an occupational health setting, including:

    a. Facility/equipment requirements

        1) Private space to maintain confidentiality

        2) Client gowns and sheets

        3) Handwashing facilities

        4) Locked file cabinet for medical records

        5) Small refrigerators for medications (clean) and specimens (dirty). Two refrigerators are desirable but not always possible.

        6) Emergency response equipment, capabilities, and facilities (e.g., oxygen, automatic external defibrillator, electrocardiogram, intravenous lines, allergic response, eyewash, decontamination area)

        7) Equipment to conduct examinations (e.g., clinic table, light source, blood pressure equipment, oto-ophthalmoscope, stethoscope, reflex hammer, tuning forks [256 and 512 Hz], cotton swabs, tongue depressors, peak flow meters, goniometer to measure range of motion, Jamar to measure grip strength, tape measure, gloves)

        8) Screening equipment (e.g., audiometer and sound booth, spirometer)

    b. Supplies

        1) Medications (e.g., vaccinations, epinephrine, prescribed medications, and over-the-counter medications.)

        2) Safe needle devices and needle disposal units

        3) Miscellaneous supplies (e.g., splints, ice packs, eye patches, suture kits, urine drug testing)

    c. Administrative needs

        1) Systems and supplies for recordkeeping (e.g., intake form, informed consent form for treatment, operations, procedures, billing [if applicable], health history questionnaire for initial visit and follow-up, physical examination form for initial visit and follow-up, encounter form, referral form, lab/x-ray forms, prescription pad, physical therapy order forms, reappointment process, release of medical information forms, workers' compensation forms, other mandatory reporting, and recording in OSHA-300 log). These systems are either paper or electronic.

2) Educational materials (e.g., culturally sensitive materials, with simple text and liberal use of diagrams, to manage literacy and language range; selected consumer-oriented health web sites for self-care education)
3) List of referrals (e.g., community resources, providers, organizations)

III Health History

A health history provides a database of subjective data that encompasses all aspects of the individual's health, including current and past occupational and environmental exposures.

A Purposes of a health history are:
1. To establish a health-care relationship
2. To identify active and potential physical and mental health problems
3. To determine a risk profile for preventable health concerns

B Components of a comprehensive health history include:
1. Client profile: demographic data, including age, sex, nationality, and job title
2. Chief complaint: reason for visit—illness, injury, or prevention focused
3. History of present illness (HPI): includes questions about the seven symptom descriptors and supportive positive and negative data from other sections of the database
   a. Seven symptom descriptors are:
      1) Location/radiation: Where exactly is the pain/symptom located? Trace where it radiates.
      2) Setting: What were you doing when you noticed the symptom?
      3) Quality: What is the pain/symptom like? (sharp/dull/cramping/throbbing)
      4) Quantity/severity: How bad is it? On a 1-10 scale, with 10 being the worst, how would you rate your symptom? What is the functional impact of symptom?
      5) Chronology: When did this start? Is it getting better, worse? How long does each episode last?
      6) Aggravating/alleviating factors: What makes it worse? What makes it better? (Describe specific work activities that may have caused or aggravated symptom)
      7) Associated manifestations: Are there any other symptoms associated with it?
   b. Supportive positive/negative data related to the symptom include:
      1) Past medical history (PMH) (e.g., Any prior workup of the same symptom? Any significant prior injury/illness that might contribute to current complaint?)
      2) Family history: Any significant family history of an illness that might contribute to current complaint?
      3) Personal/social history: Are there any contributing factors from diet, alcohol, smoking, drug use, exercise? Any new stressors?
      4) Occupational/environmental history: Is there anything in your work or home environment that could contribute to this symptom? Any coworker or family member with similar complaints?
      5) Review of systems: Are there any related symptoms not previously mentioned?

4. Past medical history: prior illnesses, hospitalizations, surgeries, obstetrical history, and current immunization status

5. Medications and allergies: over-the-counter, prescribed and illicit drug use; for allergies, note response to determine if true allergy or a sensitivity

6. Family history: genetic/hereditary risk factors, chronic disease in family, and any significant family problems

7. Personal and social history: status of current relationships; satisfactions, future goals, stressors, and coping style; housing, education, literacy levels, and any financial concerns; violence potential (e.g., is there a gun kept at the home?)

8. Health habits: exercise, alcohol, diet, smoking, illicit drugs, sleep, seat belt use

9. Occupational and environmental health history (Section III.D): a complete listing of past and current paid and unpaid positions, including military experience, and any exposures, injuries, impairments

10. Review of systems: a checklist of symptoms, by body system, that may prompt recall of an important symptom within the past 6 months

C **Components of a problem-specific history include:**
1. Client profile
2. Chief complaint
3. History of present illness
4. Key occupational health questions to help determine work-relatedness:
   a. Is the symptom temporally related to work?
   b. Is the symptom temporally related to a change in a work process?
   c. Does the symptom improve/go away when away from work (i.e., on weekends, on vacation, or when the work is modified and the worker is removed from the exposure)?
   d. Do co-workers have similar complaints?
   e. Is the worker exposed to an agent that is known to cause the symptoms? Does the symptom cause any difficulty with work?

D **The goals of the occupational and environmental exposure history are to identify current or past exposures, reduce or eliminate current exposures, and reduce adverse health effects (ATSDR, 2000).**
1. The purposes of the occupational and environmental exposure history are to:
   a. Identify asymptomatic occupational/environmental illness
   b. Provide epidemiologic correlation between symptoms and activities or exposures
   c. Help to correctly diagnose occupational or environmental health problems, and stimulate prevention activities at the work site so others are not similarly exposed
   d. Help prevent aggravation of existing injury/illness
   e. Allow assessment of synergistic risks; for example, whether worker smokes or lives in an urban area with air pollution, and is also exposed to a known pulmonary irritant
   f. Aid in teaching and counseling about health and safety rights and responsibilities, self-care strategies, and risk reduction activities at work

2. A screening occupational/environmental health tool is described by Blue and colleagues (2000):
   a. It is a focused screening tool for use in the primary care setting, to identify high risk job or home exposures
   b. It is based on the mnemonic "WHACS":
      1) **W**hat do you do?
      2) **H**ow do you do it?
      3) **A**re you concerned about any exposures on or off the job?
      4) **C**oworkers or others exposed?
      5) **S**atisfied with your job?
3. A comprehensive occupational and environmental exposure history includes the following (ATSDR, 2000) (Figure 11-1 presents a suggested format.):
   a. *Exposure survey*
      • Selected questions for an exposure survey include current exposure to metals, dust, loud noise; the use of protective equipment; and any recent job changes.
   b. *Work history*, including an occupational profile and occupational exposure inventory
      • Selected questions for an occupational profile include job title, type of industry, and dates of employment.
      • Selected questions for an occupational exposure inventory address missing more than one day of work because of an illness related to the job, and a job change because of any health problems or injuries.
   c. *Environmental history*
      • Selected questions for an environmental history include living next to an industrial plant or dump site; source of drinking water; year home was built.
4. Critical aspects of the exposure history require (ATSDR, 2000):
   a. Quantifying the amount, duration and frequency of exposure (dose)
   b. Detailing route of exposure (inhalation, dermal, ingestion, mucous membrane)
   c. Separating acute versus chronic exposures
   d. Separating acute versus chronic health effects
   e. Taking an environmental exposure history (See Box 11-1, p. 307, for a tool.)

E **Limitations of the health history include the following:**
1. Reliability of informant may be compromised because of language and communication barriers
2. Family and social history may be emotionally charged for the individual
3. Provider may fail to collect and/or pursue significant data from occupational and environmental history
4. Workers may lack knowledge about exposures
   a. Workers may lack understanding of the health implications of certain activities
   b. There may have been inadequate time during clinic encounter to gather data
   c. Providers may not know what to do with the information, if collected

IV The Physical Examination

A **Purposes of the physical examination in the occupational setting are to:**
1. Identify disease
2. Detect disease process in presymptomatic stage

EXPOSURE HISTORY FORM

Part 1. Exposure Survey   **Name:**_____**Date:**_____

Please circle the appropriate answer.   **Birth date:**_____**Sex (circle one):** Male   Female

---

1. Are you currently exposed to any of the following?
   metals   no   yes
   dust or fibers   no   yes
   chemicals   no   yes
   fumes   no   yes
   radiation   no   yes
   biologic agents   no   yes
   loud noise, vibration, extreme heat or cold   no   yes

2. Have you been exposed to any of the above in the past?   no   yes

3. Do any household members have contact with metals,
   dust, fibers, chemicals, fumes, radiation, or biologic agents?   no   yes

---

If you answered *yes* to any of the items above, describe your exposure in detail—how you were exposed, to what you were exposed. If you need more space, please use a separate sheet of paper.

---

4. Do you know the names of the metals,
   dusts fibers, chemicals, fumes, or radiation
   that you are/were exposed to?   no   yes ➔

5. Do you get the material on your skin or
   clothing?   no   yes

6. Are your work clothes laundered at home?   no   yes

7. Do you shower at work?   no   yes

If yes, list them below

8. Can you smell the chemical or material you
   are working with?   no   yes

9. Do you use protective equipment such as
   gloves, masks, respirator, or hearing protectors?   no   yes ➔

10. Have you been advised to use protective
    equipment?   no   yes

11. Have you been instructed in the use of protective
    equipment?   no   yes

12. Do you wash your hands with solvents?   no   yes

13. Do you smoke at the workplace?   no   yes
    at home?   no   yes

14. Are you exposed to secondhand tobacco smoke no   yes
    at the workplace?
    at home?   no   yes

If yes, list the protective equipment used

Continued

FIGURE 11-1 *Example of a format for occupational and environmental health history* (http://www.atsdr.cdc.gov/HEC/ CSEM/ exphistory/exphist_form.html)

Sources: From U.S Department of Health and Human Services Agency for Toxic Substances and Disease Registry, 2000.

15. Do you eat at the workplace?	no	yes
16. Do you know of any co-workers experiencing similar or unusual symptoms?	no	yes
17. Are family members experiencing similar or unusual symptoms?	no	yes
18. Has there been a change in the health or behavior of family pets?	no	yes
19. Do your symptoms seem to be aggravated by a specific activity?	no	yes
20. Do your symptoms get worse or better at work?	no	yes
at home?	no	yes
on weekends?	no	yes
on vacation?	no	yes
21. Has anything about your job changed in recent months (such as duties, procedures, overtime)?	no	yes
22. Do you use any traditional or alternative medicines?	no	yes

If you answered *yes* to any of the questions, please explain.

FIGURE 11-1 —*cont'd Example of a format for occupational and environmental health history*

3. Determine biologic markers/target organ measures at baseline; compare measures at time of surveillance
4. Determine any impairment that may impact the ability to do the job or may necessitate an accommodation
5. Document baseline objective findings, if there is prior impairment and potential future apportionment

B **Several things must be considered when conducting a physical examination.**
1. The primary purpose of the examination and use of the data will determine the scope of the physical examination. For example, it may be necessary to specify what is mandatory and what is voluntary in a preplacement evaluation.
2. Examination findings, or absence of findings, should be charted in an objective and nonjudgmental fashion.
3. The ethical principle of nonmaleficence (do no harm) is of primary concern.
4. Findings should be summarized and recorded consistently, so that any abnormalities from baseline can be clearly detected over time.

C **Techniques for physical examination are as follows:**
1. *Inspection* uses sight to look at the individual and to observe variations from the norm or from previously observed state.
2. *Palpation* uses light and deep touch to feel with hands and fingers to check temperature, moisture, texture, size, pulsation, vibrations, presence of joint swelling, nodules, masses, joint mobility, and organ size and location.
3. *Percussion* is the direct striking of a finger against skin or the indirect striking of a finger against a finger lying against an individual's skin. This technique is used to assess tenderness and/or to determine the density, size, and

EXPOSURE HISTORY FORM

Part 2. Work History   Name:_____ Date:_____
A. Occupational Profile   Birth date:_____ Sex: Male   Female

The following questions refer to your current or most recent job:

Job title:_____ Describe this job:_____

Type of industry:_____ _____

Name of employer:_____ _____

Date job began:_____ _____

Are you still working in this job? yes   no   _____

If *no*, when did this job end?_____ _____

Fill in the table below listing all jobs you have worked including short-term, seasonal, part-time employment, and military service. Begin with your most recent job. Use additional paper if necessary.

Dates of Employment	Job Title and Description of Work	Exposures*	Protective Equipment

*List the chemicals, dusts, fibers, fumes, radiation, biologic agents (i.e., molds or viruses) and physical agents (i.e., extreme heat, cold, vibration, or noise) that you were exposed to at this job.

Have you ever worked at a job or hobby in which you came in contact with any of the following by breathing, touching, or ingesting (swallowing)? If *yes*, please check the box beside the name.

☐ Acids	☐ Chloroprene	☐ Methylene chloride	☐ Styrene
☐ Alcohols (industrial)	☐ Chromates	☐ Nickel	☐ Talc
☐ Alkalies	☐ Coal dust	☐ PBBs	☐ Toluene
☐ Ammonia	☐ Dichlorobenzene	☐ PCBs	☐ TDI or MDI
☐ Arsenic	☐ Ethylene dibromide	☐ Perchloroethylene	☐ Trichloroethylene
☐ Asbestos	☐ Ethylene dichloride	☐ Pesticides	☐ Trinitrotoluene
☐ Benzene	☐ Fiberglass	☐ Phenol	☐ Vinyl chloride
☐ Beryllium	☐ Halothane	☐ Phosgene	☐ Welding fumes
☐ Cadmium	☐ Isocyanates	☐ Radiation	☐ X-rays
☐ Carbon tetrachloride	☐ Ketones	☐ Rock dust	☐ Other (specify)
☐ Chlorinated naphthalenes	☐ Lead	☐ Silica powder	
☐ Chloroform	☐ Mercury	☐ Solvents	

FIGURE 11-1 —*cont'd*

location of underlying organs; sounds range from tympanic to resonant, hyperresonant, dull, or flat.

4. *Auscultation* is the process of listening directly with the bell (for lower pitched sounds) or the diaphragm (for higher pitched sounds) of the stethoscope to assess sounds produced by the various organs and tissues.

D **Methods used to conduct the physical examination consider the following:**

1. The examination should be performed systematically; its scope and depth depend on its purpose and the proficiency of the direct care provider.

B. Occupational Exposure Inventory   *Please circle the appropriate answer.*

1. Have you ever been off work more than 1 day because of an illness related to work?	no	yes
2. Have you ever been advised to change jobs or work assignments because of any health problems or injuries?	no	yes
3. Has you work routine changed recently?	no	yes
4. Is there poor ventilation in your workplace?	no	yes

Part 3. Environmental History   *Please circle the appropriate answer.*

1. Do you live next to or near an industrial plant, commercial business, dump site, or nonresidential property?   no   yes

2. Which of the following do you have in your home?
   Please circle those that apply.

Air conditioner	Air purifier	Central heating (gas or oil?)	Gas stove
Fireplace	Wood stove	Humidifier	Electric stove

3. Have you recently aquired new furniture or carpet, refinished furniture, or remodeled you home?   no   yes

4. Have you weatherized your home recently?   no   yes

5. Are pesticides or herbicides (bug or weed killers; flea and tick sprays, collars, powders, or shampoos) used in your home or garden, or on pets?   no   yes

6. Do you (or any household member) have a hobby or craft?   no   yes

7. Do you work on your car?   no   yes

8. Have you ever changed your residence because of health problem?   no   yes

9. Does your drinking water come from a private well, city water supply, or grocery store?

10. Approximately what year was your home built? _____

If you answered *yes* to any of the questions, please explain.

FIGURE 11-1 —*cont'd Example of a format for occupational and environmental health history*

2. If the person reports a specific symptom—for example, sensory changes in a specific location—more in-depth sensory testing is indicated.
3. Abnormal physical examination findings should be matched with symptoms through a clinical decision-making process, with the goal to determine a working diagnosis; or the client can be referred for validation and follow-up to an appropriate health care provider.
4. Laboratory/diagnostic studies: Often, objective laboratory data are obtained at the time of the client encounter (e.g., urinalysis, pulse oximetry reading, or peak flow).
5. For a review of health assessment/physical examination skills, see Rasmor and Brown, 2001 and 2003.

BOX 11-1

Taking an environmental exposure history: questions to consider

Use the mnemonic **I-PREPARE**.

I Investigate potential exposures: Have you ever been sick after coming in contact with a chemical? Do you have symptoms that improve away from work or home?

P Present Work: Are you exposed to solvents, dusts, fumes? Do you know where to find material safety data sheets? Do you wear work clothes home?

R Residence: When was your residence built? What type of heating do you have?

E Environmental concerns: Are there environmental concerns in your neighborhood?

P Past work: What are your past work experiences?

A Activities: What activities or hobbies do you have? Do you garden, fish or hunt?

R Referrals and resources: Use these key resources:
Agency for Toxic Substances and Disease Registry
http://www.atsdr.cdc.gov/
Association of Occupational and Environmental Clinics
http://www.aoec.org/
Environmental Protection Agency
http://www.epa.gov/
Material Safety Data Sheets
http://www.hazard.com/msds
Occupational Health and Safety Administration
http://www.osha.gov/
Local Health Department, Environmental Agency, Poison Control Center

E Educate: Are materials available to educate the patient? Have prevention strategies been discussed? What is the plan for follow-up?

Source: U.S. Department of Health and Human Services Agency for Toxic Substances and Disease Registry, 2001.

V Clinical Decision Making

A *Clinical decision making* is the process of analyzing subjective and objective data and establishing a working definition of the health problem. This process includes the following steps (Bickley & Szilagyi, 2003):

1. Identify the abnormal findings: symptoms, physical signs, laboratory results, and any recent work-site sampling or surveillance results.

2. Cluster these findings into logical groups; for example, "numbness into the first and second digits, with atrophy of the thenar muscle in the same hand, with known awkward postures and repetitive motion of the upper extremity at work."

3. Localize the findings anatomically; for example, "the location of the above symptoms is in the distribution of the median peripheral nerve, but also could be the C6 cervical nerve root."

4. Interpret the findings in terms of probable process:
   a. Pathologic—involving an abnormality in a body structure
   b. Pathophysiologic—involving an abnormality in a body function
   c. Psychopathologic—involving a disorder of mood or thinking

5. In occupational health, probable process includes the toxicology of the substance, specifically determining the dose-response and known target-organ

effect. The material safety data sheet (MSDS) for hazardous chemicals provides additional objective data.

6. Make one or more hypotheses about the nature of the client's problem.
   a. Select the most specific and central findings around which to construct your hypothesis.
   b. Match your findings against all conditions you know can produce them.
   c. Eliminate the hypotheses that fail to explain the findings.
   d. Weigh the probabilities, based on the client's risk profile, extent of exposure, epidemiology of the condition, temporal issues, and toxicology of the exposure.
   e. Consider life-threatening, "do not miss" conditions and conditions that are treatable.
7. Test the hypothesis. In occupational health, this often includes removal from exposure or modification of work duties, with monitoring for changes in symptoms.
8. Establish a working definition of the problem, the "assessment," and share rationale of how the subjective and objective data and laboratory findings link to support the working diagnosis.
   a. It is important to include the client's response to the working diagnosis, and how he or she is coping with this diagnosis.
   b. Other questions to consider include the following:
      1) Is it a work-related condition, caused by work?
      2) Is it a pre-existing condition aggravated by work?
      3) Is it related to environmental health concerns?
      4) Is it not related to work or the environment?
      5) Does work pose any additional risks for injury/or any difficulties?
      6) Is the person physically and emotionally capable of meeting the essential criteria of the job, with or without accommodation?
9. Outline a plan:
   a. Diagnostic interventions: What additional laboratory tests or x-ray examinations need to be ordered? Is any environmental sampling data needed?
   b. Therapeutic interventions: What will be prescribed today? Include medications, exercise, modified work duties, ice, and splints.
   c. Client education: Describe the education and counseling provided at this visit.
   d. Record the date of the follow-up visit, and advise the worker to return sooner to the clinic if condition worsens in any way or if there are questions. Advise the worker regarding urgent care or emergency settings to access, if needed.
   e. Recordable-reportable conditions: Is it OSHA recordable on the OSHA 300 log? According to state workers' compensation law, is the condition reportable? Are there other mandatory reporting requirements, for example, loss of consciousness, suspected pesticide exposure?
   f. Temporary work restrictions/accommodations: direct communication with the supervisor is often needed to ensure a successful return to work. The diagnosis is kept confidential and not released to the supervisor unless the worker has signed a release of medical information consent, and there is a "need to know" by the employer.

10. The decision-making process then repeats itself with follow-up appointments, and the collection of new subjective, objective, and laboratory data. The working diagnoses may be revised and refined over time and the clinical management plan altered, if needed.

11. There is misdiagnosis and underdiagnosis of occupational health concerns by primary care and urgent care settings because of health care provider time and knowledge factors (Harber & Merz, 2001; Harber et al., 2003). Recognition and prevention of work-related illness and injury is highly dependent on the provider's taking an occupational and environmental health history, and pursuing knowledge of workplace hazards.

B **Another approach to clinical decision making includes the above steps, but is augmented by using a cognitive tool to prompt a complete list of possible diagnoses. This adapted cognitive tool is OVINDICATES. See Box 11-2 for an example of using the OVINDICATES mnemonic to stimulate possible diagnoses.**

C **Examples of prevention opportunities that can result from direct care and clinical decision making in the occupational setting include:**

1. When a worker presents with a work-related injury, it may signify a breakdown in a control measure. It is therefore critical to do an accident investigation to correct this problem at the root cause, so coworkers are not similarly exposed.

2. When a worker presents with a work-related injury or illness, it may be viewed as a sentinel event. Case-finding screening activities can seek other workers who may have been similarly exposed but are still asymptomatic.

VI Practice Guidelines

Practice guidelines are clinical practice recommendations based on a critical review of research/evidence; their primary aim is to standardize care.

A **There are numerous practice guidelines focusing on different aspects of care, including the following:**

1. The diagnosis of a specific health condition
2. The clinical management of a health condition
3. Client educational materials for a health condition

BOX 11-2

Clinical decision-making and reaching a diagnosis

Application of **OVINDICATES** to a presenting symptom: Headache
Occupational: Carbon monoxide exposure at work
Vascular: Vascular migraine headache
Inflammatory: Cervical sprain
Neoplastic: Brain cancer
Degenerative or Drug: DJD of neck or caffeine withdrawal

Infectious: Sinusitis or meningitis
Congenital: Aneurysm
Autoimmune: Temporal arteritis
Trauma: Subarachnoid bleed
Endocrine: Pituitary adenoma
Social/Psychologic: Stress/ somatoform disorder/ malingering

B Other purposes of clinical practice guidelines include:
1. Reduce variation in practice across geographic regions and across providers
2. Improve the quality of health care and ensure use of tools and interventions that are based on current research/evidence
3. Promote best practices and cost consciousness
4. Use as a quality assurance/audit tool
5. Assist in the insurance authorization process
6. Facilitate the disability management process

C Sources of practice guidelines include:
1. The Agency for Healthcare Research and Quality, in association with the American Association of Health Plans and the American Medical Association, has established a National Clearinghouse for Guidelines (http://www.guideline.gov/).
2. The Agency for Healthcare Research and Quality produced three practice guidelines relevant to occupational health: Acute Low Back Pain, Smoking Cessation, and Depression in Primary Care, available through their web site (http://www.ahcpr.gov/).
3. The American College of Occupational and Environmental Medicine guidelines, 2nd edition (Glass, 2004).
4. The Centers for Disease Control and Prevention (CDC) has many guidelines for occupational infectious disease. (http://www.cdc.gov/)
5. The occupational and environmental health nurse may also wish to develop or modify selected clinical guidelines; see the AAOHN's Advisory called *Developing Clinical Guidelines or Protocols for Practice* (2004).
6. Disability management guidelines include, for example, *The Medical Disability Advisor* (Reed, 2001).

D Direct care in occupational health is unique because of regulatory standards that require specific health-related examinations or screening tests based on airborne concentrations of a substance and years of exposure (Papp & Miller, 2000). The types of examinations that may be required are as follows:
1. Preplacement examination (e.g., asbestos)
2. Periodic examination (e.g., ethylene oxide)
3. Emergency/exposure examination and tests (e.g., selected carcinogens)
4. Termination examination (e.g., coke oven emissions)
5. Specific screening tests (e.g., spirometry for respiratory protection)

VII Application of Levels of Prevention to Direct Care Activities

A Primary prevention—Immunizations are widely underutilized as a primary prevention strategy.
1. The worksite is an ideal location for immunizing workers (CDC, 2000). CDC has specific standards for the safe delivery of vaccination programs and services.
2. Other resources related to immunization are available through the CDC; many are listed on their web page found at http://www.cdc.gov/nip/publications/ACIP-list.htm.

B Primary prevention—The preplacement physical follows a job offer.
1. The preplacement physical examination:
   a. Focuses on ability to perform the essential functions of the job

   b. Ensures protection of the worker from known risk factors
   c. Provides information so the worker can be placed in a job that does not compromise the worker's current health status
   d. Assesses the worker's need for accommodation
   e. Identifies any previously undiagnosed health problems
   f. Establishes baseline data such as impairment status, which is important in the event of future apportionment
   g. Ensures compliance with federal OSHA standards, the ADA, and other mandated programs and services such as DOT-required preplacement programs
   h. Introduces the worker to a health care system that is focused on prevention and early detection of disease
2. Components of the preplacement examination include:
   a. Job-specific health history (mandatory) and health maintenance questions that may not be relevant to performance of the job (voluntary)
   b. Physical examination of organ systems that are involved in job performance or may be affected by job performance
   c. Appropriate laboratory tests or screenings, based on job requirements (e.g., functional capacity testing, vision testing, spirometry, or selected blood chemistry)
   d. An offer of a vaccine (e.g., hepatitis B vaccination, if exposed to bloodborne pathogens in the course of employment) (Rogers, 2003; Nachreiner et al., 1999)
3. In order to conduct an effective preplacement examination program:
   a. The examiner must have the necessary skills to perform the examination.
   b. The examiner must have knowledge of the job requirements and be provided a copy of the job analysis that specifies specific requirements, such as climbing ladders, lifting 30 pounds on a continuous basis, reaching 70 inches to push a button to start a machine.
   c. The examiner must have knowledge of Americans with Disabilities Act (ADA) issues regarding pre-employment inquiries about drug and alcohol use, the use of drug testing, and how to interpret direct threat.
   d. The examiner must have knowledge of how the ADA interacts with workers' compensation.
   e. The examiner must have knowledge of the processes of accommodation, including the interactive process, the concept of undue hardship, and the legal issues regarding hiring decisions.
   f. The examiner must have knowledge of patient confidentiality laws.

C Secondary prevention—*Screening* is a secondary prevention measure to identify or treat individuals who have a disease or risk factors for a disease but who are not yet experiencing symptoms of the disease (USDHHS, 2000).
1. Criteria for health screening (U.S. Preventive Services Task Force, 2004) include:
   a. The disease must be one where early diagnosis and intervention has a positive effect on morbidity and mortality (e.g., blood sugar levels to detect diabetes mellitus).
   b. The method of administering the test must be acceptable to both the person administering the test and the worker receiving the test.
   c. Efficacy: the test must be able to detect the target condition earlier than it could be detected without screening and with sufficient accuracy to

avoid a large number of false negative results (sensitivity) and false positive results (specificity).

d. The occupational and environmental health nurse should be properly educated to perform the test, recognize abnormal results, and counsel, refer, and provide care for the worker.

2. Box 11-3 outlines the interventions recommended for the periodic health examination for normal-risk adults (U.S. Preventive Services Task Force, 2004).

a. The Task Force reviews evidence for screening tests and their frequency, including chemoprevention, and makes recommendations. Topical areas include cancer, heart disease, infectious disease, and musculoskeletal conditions. For low-back-pain prevention, for example, the evidence to support the efficacy of back strengthening programs and services/other

---

BOX 11-3

Clinical preventive services for normal-risk adults

Screening

Blood pressure, height and weight: Periodically, 18 years and older.

Total blood cholesterol: Men 35 years and older every 5 years; women 45 years and older every 5 years.

Pap smear: Women 18-65 years every 1-3 years.

Chlamydia recommendation is asymptomatic in pregnant women <25 years and others at increased risk for infection.

Colorectal cancer: Periodically, depends on test, 50 years and older.

Osteoporosis: Women, routinely, ≥65 years or ≥60 years if at increased risk for fractures.

Alcohol use: Periodically, 18 years and older.

Vision, hearing: Periodically, 65 years and older.

Immunization

Tetanus-diphtheria (Td): Every 10 years, 18 years and older.

Varicella (VZV): Susceptibles only—two doses, 18 years and older.

Measles, mumps, rubella (MMR):

Women of childbearing age—one dose, 18-50 years.

Pneumococcal pneumonia: One dose, 65 years and older.

Influenza: Yearly, 50 years and older.

Chemoprevention

Discuss aspirin to prevent cardiovascular events: men, periodically, 40 years and older; women, periodically, 50 years and older.

Discuss breast cancer chemoprevention with women at high risk.

Counseling

Calcium Intake: Women, periodically, 18 years and older.

Folic acid: Women of childbearing age, 18-50 years.

Breastfeeding: Women, after childbirth, 18-50 years.

Tobacco cessation, drug and alcohol use, STDs and HIV, nutrition, physical activity, sun exposure, oral health, injury prevention, and polypharmacy: Periodically, 18 years and older.

NOTE: Upper age limits should be individualized for each client.
Source: U.S. Preventive Services Task Force, 2004
STDs, Sexually transmitted diseases.

risk factor reduction, used in primary care settings for the prevention of back pain, is insufficient. However, there is limited evidence to support back education programs and services in occupational settings, with short-term modest benefits for those with chronic back pain (US Preventive Task Force, 2004).

b. Although the recommended interventions are for the general population, special attention should be paid to the needs of high-risk populations with unique health risks (e.g., for food handlers, consider hepatitis A vaccination). Note that there are additional screening guidelines that may differ, for instance, the American Cancer Society guidelines for cancer screening.

c. See screening summaries and sample flow sheets for "Putting Prevention into Practice" in Figure 11-2 (http://www.ahrq.gov/clinic/ppipix.htm).

D Secondary prevention—Surveillance is described as *health surveillance* and/or *medical surveillance*.

1. The term *medical surveillance* is used by OSHA to describe the process of determining whether workers are experiencing adverse health effects from exposure to hazards (Papp & Miller, 2000).

2. Medical surveillance refers to the requirements in the OSHA standards for specific clinical activities, including preplacement examinations, periodic examinations, emergency/exposure examinations, termination examinations, biologic monitoring, and other laboratory or screening tests (Papp & Miller, 2000). (Although the OSHA term is *medical* surveillance, the preferred terminology in occupational and environmental health nursing practice is *health* surveillance to better reflect the purpose and scope of practice.)

3. Occupational health surveillance is the process of monitoring the health status of worker populations to gather data about the effects of workplace exposures and to use the data to prevent illness or injury (AAOHN, 2004e).

4. Purposes of a surveillance examination are as follows:
   a. Protect the worker from exposures that might cause adverse health effects
   b. Ensure the worker's ability to perform the job activity
   c. Fulfill governmental surveillance requirements, such as those outlined in the standards for asbestos and lead exposure
   d. Ensure that environmental controls are working

5. Five goals of aggregate surveillance activities in occupational health are as follows:
   a. Identify illness, injury, or hazards that represent new opportunities for prevention
   b. Define the magnitude and distribution of the problem in the work force
   c. Track trends in the problem's magnitude and assess the effectiveness of prevention efforts
   d. Target educational and consultation efforts to specific work sites
   e. Publicly disseminate information to facilitate personal and societal policy making (Levy &Wegman, 2000)

6. Surveillance requires familiarity with the relevant standards, the routes of exposure, and toxic doses of chemicals. The primary activities involved in surveillance include the following:
   a. Collection of specific exposure data

Text continued on p. 322

Adult Preventive Care Flow Sheet

Name: _____   Date of Birth/Age: _____   Male: _____   Female: _____   MR# or SS#: _____

Ethnicity: _____   Medications: _____   Old Records: _____

Allergies: _____   Smoker: _____   ETS: _____   Date: _____

1. Immunizations	Population/Frequency	I.D.	Date/Site/Sig.	Date/Site/Sig.	Date/Site/Sig.	Date/Site/Sig.
Tetanus—diphtheria	q 10 yr					
Hepatitis B	Adults at increased risk—3-dose series					
Varicella	Nonimmune adults 2 doses delivered 4-8 wk apart					
Rubella	Women of chidlbearing age and health care workers without evidence of immunity or prior immunization—1 dose					
Hepatitis A	At high risk					
Influenza vaccine	q 1 yr ≥50 yr or at increased risk					
Pneumococcal vaccine	Once ≥65 yr or at increased risk					

Adult Preventive Care Flow Sheet (cont.)

Screening Test/Exam	Population/Frequency	Date	Age	N, Results Normal			A, Results Abnormal			R, Refused			P, Pending		
2. Blood pressure															
3. Height/weight															
4. Total cholesterol, HDL	≥35 yr males ≥45 yr females														
5. Diabetes	Adults with hyperlipidemia or hypertension														
6. Pap smear	q 3 yr														
7. Mammogram	q 1-2 yr ≥40 yr														
8. Colorectal cancer screening	Depends on screening test selected*														
9. Osteoporosis	≥65 yr females ≥60 yr females at increased risk for fractures														
10. Problem drinking															
11. Vision	>65 yr														
12. Hearing	≥65 yr														
13. Chlamydial infection	Sexually active women age ≤25														

* See www.preventiveservices.ahrq.gov for U.S. Preventive Services Task Force recommendation on colorectal cancer screening

FIGURE 11-2   *Putting prevention into practice. A, Adult prevention guidelines and sample flow sheets.*

Continued

Adult Preventive Care Flow Sheet (cont.)

	Population/Frequency	Date	N, Results Normal	A, Results Abnormal	R, Refused	P, Pending
		Age				
High Risk						
14. STD/HIV						
15. TB infection/PPD						
Chemoprevention						
16. Discuss aspirin to prevent CHD	High risk					
17. Discuss breast cancer chemoprevention	Women of older age Breast cancer in first-degree relative Atypical hyperplasia or breast biopsy					
Counseling						
18. Tobacco use						
19. Alcohol/drug use						
20. Nutrition						
21. Physical activity						
22. Oral health						
23. Sun exposure						
24. Injury prevention						
Sexuality/Reproduction						
25. STD/HIV						

Adult Preventive Care Flow Sheet (cont.)

Sexuality/Reproduction	Population/Frequency	Date	N, Results Normal	A, Results Abnormal	R, Refused	P, Pending
		Age				
26. Unintended pregnancy						
27. Multivitamin with folic acid	Females capable of pregnancy					
28. Osteoporosis/calcium						

Referrals (As indicated)	Date	Result
Diabetes education		
Nutrition education		
Tobacco cessation program		
Dental examination		
Eye exam/glaucoma		

Note: Screening tests/exams and counseling based on U.S. Preventive Services Task Force recommendations.

ETS = environmental tobacco smoke; HDL = high-density lipoprotein; STD = sexually transmitted disease; HIV = human immunodeficiency virus; TB = tuberculosis; PPD = tuberculin purified protein derivative; CHD = coronary heart disease.

First published in *A Step-by-Step Guide to Delivering Clinical Preventive Services: A Systems Approach.* U.S. Department of Health and Human Services, Agency for Healthcare Research and Quality. Rockville, MD, 20001. AHRQ Pub. No. APPIP01-0001.

Revised January 2003.

FIGURE 11-2—cont'd *Putting Prevention into practice. A, Adult prevention guidelines and sample flow sheets.*

Adult Health Risk Profile

Name: _____   Date of Birth/Age: _____   Male: _____   Female: _____   MR# or SS#: _____

Ethnicity: _____   Medications: _____   Old Records: _____

Allergies: _____   Smoker: _____   ETS: _____   Date: _____

Screening	Annual Assessment of Risk Factors	Counseling Provided
1. Vaccine-preventable diseases	Needs the following immunizations: ___ Td booster—≥10 yr since last booster ___ Date of last Td ___ Hepatitis B—at increased risk ___ Varicella—nonimmune adults ___ Rubella—nonimmune females of childbearing age and health care workers without evidence of immunity or prior immunization ___ Hepatitis A—at high risk ___ Influenza—≥50 yr or high risk ___ Pneumococcal—≥65 yr or high risk	
2. Blood Pressure (BP)	___ Weight ___ BP ___ Does not exercise 30 minutes most days of week ___ First-degree family history of high blood pressure or personal history of hypertension ___ Diabetes mellitus	
3. Height/weight	___ Above healthy weight range for height **OR** ___ BMI >25. Formula for calculating BMI is $\dfrac{\text{Weight (kg)}}{\text{Height (m)}^2}$	
4. Cholesterol	___ In males ≥35 yr and females ≥45 yr ___ >1 yr since previous abnormal test ___ Diabetes mellitus ___ Family history of cardiovascular disease <50 yr in male relatives, <60 yr in female relatives ___ Family history suggestive of familial hyperlipidemia ___ Multiple coronary heart disease risk factors (e.g., tobacco use, hypertension)	

Adult Health Risk Profile (cont.)

Screening	Annual Assessment of Risk Factors	Counseling Provided
5. Diabetes	____ Adults with hypertension or hyperlipidemia	
6. Pap smear	____ Is or has been sexually active ____ >3 yr since last Pap smear ____ Abnormal ____ Date	
7. Mammogram	____ ≥40 yr and has not had a mammogram within the past 1–2 yr ____ Family history of breast cancer	
8. Colorectal cancer screening	____ ≥50 yr ____ Family members who have a positive history of cancer of colon, intestine, breast, ovaries, or uterus ____ History of polyps	
9. Osteoporosis	____ Women ≥65 ____ Women ≥60 at increased risk for fractures	
10. Problem drinking	____ Drinks >2 drinks/day (men) OR >1 drink/day (women)	
11. Vision	____ If >65 yr, does not see an eye doctor for regular eye exams ____ Glaucoma ____ Diabetes mellitus ____ Wears glasses ____ Family history of glaucoma	
12. Hearing	____ >65 yr strains to hear a normal conversation ____ Turns up volume on TV and radio so loud that others complain	
13. Chlamydial infection	____ Is sexually active and ≤25 yr ____ Prior history of STD ____ New or multiple sex partners ____ Had cervical ectopy ____ Uses barrier contraceptives inconsistently	

Continued

FIGURE 11-2—*cont'd Putting prevention into practice. B, Adult health risk profile.* (http://www.ahrq.gov/clinic/ppipix.htm)

Adult Health Risk Profile (cont.)

For Persons at High Risk	Annual Assessment of Risk Factors	Counseling Provided
14. STD/HIV	____ Contraception ____ Has or has had any one of the following risk factors: ____ Previous STD, multiple sex partners, or shared needles	
15. Tuberculosis (TB) infection	____ Close contact with a person who has active TB ____ Occupational high risk (health care, correctional, residential, etc.) ____ Lived in endemic area in the past year (SE Asia, Africa, Latin America) ____ Medical risk factors (e.g., diabetes, HIV, alcoholism) ____ PPD status ____ INH	
Chemoprevention	**Annual Assessment of Risk Factors**	**Counseling Provided**
16. Discuss aspirin to prevent coronary heart disease	____ At risk for coronary heart disease	
17. Discuss breast cancer chemoprevention	____ Women of older age ____ Breast cancer in first degree relative ____ Atypical hyperplasia or breast biopsy	
Counseling	**Annual Assessment of Risk Factors**	**Counseling Provided**
18. Tobacco use	____ Currently smokes cigarettes, cigars, or pipes or uses smokeless tobacco ____ Is exposed to tobacco smoke regularly ____ Number of packs per day ____ Carcinoma ____ Coronary artery disease	
19. Alcohol/drug use	____ Long-term use of certain prescription drugs ____ Has had medical/social problems related to alcohol or drug use ____ Uses or has used "street drugs"	
20. Nutrition	____ Does not limit intake of fat and cholesterol, maintain caloric balance in diet, or eat foods containing fiber	
21. Physical activity	____ Does not exercise 30 minutes most days	

Adult Health Risk Profile (cont.)		
Counseling	**Annual Assessment of Risk Factors**	**Counseling Provided**
22. Oral health	___ Poor dental hygiene (e.g., does not brush with a flouride toothpaste and floss daily) ___ Does not see a dentist regularly ___ Smokes or chews tobacco and/or drinks alcohol	
23. Sun exposure	___ Immunosuppression ___ Family history of skin cancer ___ Freckles and poor tanning ability ___ Light skin, hair, and eye color	
24. Injury prevention	___ Does not use seatbelts when in a motor vehicle ___ Does not use a helmet when on a bike/motorcycle ___ Drinks alcohol and drives, or rides with someone who does ___ Medicines, chemicals/poisons, or firearms are accessible to children ___ Does not have working smoke detectors in the home ___ At risk for battering or abuse (emotional, verbal, or physical)	
25. STD/HIV	___ Contraception ___ Previous STD, multiple sex partners, or shared needles	
26. Unintended pregnancy	___ Sexually active male or sexually active female of childbearing age ___ Does not desire a pregnancy/is not using a reliable birth control method	
27. Multivitamin with folic acid	___ Sexually active female of child bearing age	
28. Osteoporosis	___ Does not do weight-bearing exercises ___ Does not get adequate calcium ___ Low body weight ___ Caucasian female ___ Hormone replacement therapy (HRT) ___ Menopause at <40 yr	

Notes/Instructions: _____

Completed by: _____ Date: _____

Reviewed by clinician: _____ Date: _____

Note: Information is based on U.S. Preventive Services Task Force recommendations

ETS = environmental tobacco smoke; Td = tetanus-diphtheria; BMI = body mass index; STD = sexually transmitted disease; HIV = human immunodeficiency virus; PPD = tuberculin purified protein derivative; INH = isoniazid.

First published in *A Step-by-Step Guide to Delivering Clinical Preventive Services: A Systems Approach*. U.S. Department of Health and Human Services, Agency for Healthcare Research and Quality. Rockville, MD, 20001. AHRQ Pub. No. APPIP01-0001. **Revised January 2003.**.

FIGURE 11-2—*cont'd Putting prevention into practice.* B, *Adult health risk profile.* (http://www.ahrq.gov/clinic/ppipix.htm)

b. Selection and application of appropriate medical examinations (OSHA, 2004)

7. Occupational and environmental health nurse responsibilities are as follows (Rogers & Livsey, 2000):
   a. Collaboration in the development of surveillance and screening policies (who to test; selection of testing methods based on hazard profile, toxicology, environmental sampling data, and legal requirements; frequency of testing; on-site versus vendor selection for analysis of results; storage of data; reporting of abnormal values; referral plan in response to abnormal values; ethical considerations; policy impact for the worksite)
   b. Development of health history questionnaire and physical examination forms
   c. Performance of test examination
   d. Interpretation of test, referral, follow-up, and care plans
   e. Maintenance of confidentiality, record retention, and storage
   f. Health education—recommending changes in personal and work habits
   g. Instruction in self-care techniques for prevention and early detection
   h. Counseling or referral for conditions unrelated to exposure

8. Recognized methods of surveillance include chest x-ray, urinalysis, liver function testing, kidney function studies, complete bloodwork, audiometric, spirometry, and other tests needed for specific indicators of organ system status. The frequency of testing depends on the incidence of disease in a specific target population. A written opinion is required from the person who conducts the examination.

9. OSHA publishes an *Appendix of Screening and Surveillance: A guide to OSHA Standards,* which augments the standards. This can be accessed through the web site found at http://www.osha.gov/ (Papp & Miller, 2000).

E **Secondary prevention involves early diagnosis and treatment of injury and illness (emergency response/first aid, urgent care, chronic care, occupational and nonoccupational).**

1. Anticipate the type of health problems that may present urgently or in event of a disaster.
   a. Disaster preparedness requires a policy and procedure to manage large groups in the event of a fire, earthquake, explosion, biologic or bomb threat, or act of violence
   b. Determine extent of direct care provided on site in event of a disaster
   c. Consider establishing Medical Emergency Response teams

2. Occupational and environmental health nurses must be prepared to provide first aid.
   a. Eight federal OSHA standards require the provision of first aid (OSHA, 1991). State OSHA programs and services may have additional requirements.
   b. Consider the scope of first-aid training, the contents of a first-aid kit, and how to respond to shock, bleeding, burns, etc.

3. Occupational and environmental health nurses provide urgent and chronic care to workers.
   a. Evaluate each health complaint to determine the following:
      1) Acuity of the condition and need for triage to outside referral
      2) Work causation or aggravation

3) Ability of the worker to safely do the job with his or her health complaint, and the need for accommodation
4) Reinforce individual prevention activities
5) Act on work-site hazard control measures

b. Go through each step of the clinical decision-making process.
   1) Collect and analyze subjective data (health history, including a thorough occupational and environmental history).
   2) Collect and analyze objective data (physical examination, laboratory findings, environmental sampling data).
   3) Formulate assessments (determine whether condition is occupational or nonoccupational, and establish risk profile).
   4) Outline plans (diagnostic, therapeutic, and client-education interventions, with reporting/recording if needed).
   5) Evaluate and follow up on both the individual and the work site to ensure that preventive measures are implemented and reinforced.

c. Box 11-4 presents a protocol for the diagnosis and treatment of tendinitis (Burgel, 1998).

4. Many direct care activities require use of over-the-counter or prescribed medications. (Refer to the AAOHN Advisory [AAOHN, 2004f] for a summary of over-the counter considerations.)

F **Tertiary prevention relates to disability and case management**

1. *Case management* is "a process of coordinating an individual client's total health care services to achieve optimal, quality care delivered in a cost-effective manner" (AAOHN, 2004g).

2. *Disability management* uses case management strategies to manage medical care, return to work, and needed accommodations for ill and injured workers with lost time; the goal is to prevent a protracted delay in returning to work.

3. *Modified/transitional work* is an important strategy in disability/case management. Studies examining the impact of modified work found that ill or injured workers who were offered modified work return to work about twice as often as those who are not (Krause, et al., 1998; Wassel, 2002).

4. *Clinical evaluation* for substance use and depression/anxiety disorders is important in disability and case management.

VIII Evaluating Outcomes

A **Health outcomes are the results or consequences of a process of care. Health outcomes may include the following:**

1. Satisfaction with care

2. Use of health care resources

3. Clinical outcomes, such as changes in health status and in the length and quality of life as a result of detecting or treating disease (USDHHS, 2000).

B **Examples of health outcome indicators for occupational health are as follows (Rudolph, 1996; Rudolph, 1998):**

1. Access to care: Initial treatment for nonemergency work-related conditions will be delivered within 24 hours after the injury is reported.

Text continued on p. 328

BOX 11-4

Protocol for the diagnosis and treatment of tendinitis (Burgel, 1998)

I. Definition: Tendinitis is an acute or chronic inflammatory pain response after an acute or cumulative trauma to the tendon structures.

II. Database

   A. Subjective information

      1. Age, hand dominance

      2. Pain diagram, with rating of pain on 1 to 10 scale

      3. Antecedent events, including nonoccupational risk factors such as trauma, sports, and repetitive activities at home. Describe work activities, detailing frequency of fine manipulations, grasps, lifts, reaches, or keystrokes per minute, presence or absence of awkward postures, degree of force used, amount of weight lifted, and whether extremity is resting against sharp edges. Describe tool use, presence of vibration (e.g., jackhammer). Describe use of any protective equipment (e.g., antivibration gloves).

      4. Describe environment: Automation versus manual operations, presence or absence of an adjustable workstation (e.g., height of work surface, adjustable chair), distance and height of required lift/reach.

      5. Note symptom course with time off work or vacation.

      6. Note presence of symptoms in coworkers with similar job tasks.

      7. Upper extremity symptoms: Erythema, swelling, locking of digits, numbness, tingling, weakness, nighttime awakening with paresthesias, neck pain

      8. Past treatments used: Nonsteroidal anti-inflammatory drugs, local injections of cortisone, physical therapy modalities, acupuncture, massage, chiropractic treatment, splint use (detail number of hours and for which tasks), assistive devices

      9. Impact on activities of daily living: Family responsibilities assumed by others; modification of repetitive household tasks such as shopping, cooking, vacuuming, and grooming; self-care strategies, including use of lightweight backpacks, "smart-grip" tools, and "quick fixes" to maintain neutral positions

     10. Past health history: Arthritis, diabetes, thyroid disorder, pregnancy, medications, allergies to medications, peptic ulcer disease, gastric distress with use of nonsteroidal antiinflammatory agents

     11. Family history: Arthritis, diabetes, thyroid disorder

     12. Personal/social history: Exercise (overall conditioning, overtraining, postural awareness), smoking and alcohol (vasoconstriction and impact on healing)

     13. Past occupational/hobby history: musical instrument, needlework, keyboard/mouse use, hand tool use/vibration

   B. Objective information

      1. General appearance, noting pain, posture

      2. Height and weight

      3. Skin: Erythema, bogginess, swelling, crepitus

      4. Musculoskeletal: Bony or soft tissue deformity, muscle atrophy, localized pain to palpation, anatomic distribution of pain/

Source: Burgel, B.J. (1998). Tendinitis. In Collins-Bride, G., Saxe, J. (editors): *Nurse Care*, San Francisco, UCSF Nursing Press.

BOX 11-4

Protocol for the diagnosis and treatment of tendinitis—cont'd

      paresthesias, range of motion, special maneuvers (see the table at the end of this box for selected special maneuvers)

    5. Neurologic: Sensory loss mapping, motor strength, deep tendon reflexes, special maneuvers (Phalen's and Tinel's maneuvers for nerve entrapment)

III. Assessment
  A. Determine exact location of tendinitis, its etiology, and whether acute or chronic. If work-related, notify workers' compensation carrier according to state labor code.
  B. Rule out nerve entrapment, distal versus spinal cord.
  C. Rule out arthritis presentation.

IV. Plan
  A. Diagnosis
    1. Laboratory, as indicated by the history and physical examination, possibly including the following:
      a. Antinuclear antibody, erythrocyte sedimentation rate, and rheumatoid factor (if you suspect a rheumatologic disorder)
      b. Blood urea nitrogen, creatinine, and liver function tests, if there is a history of prior renal disease, and with prolonged use of nonsteroidal antiinflammatory agents
      c. Thyroid function tests and fasting blood glucose (if you suspect carpal tunnel syndrome)
    2. Other diagnostics: Nerve conduction studies with electromyelogram, x-ray, magnetic resonance imaging
  B. Treatment
    1. Nonsteroidal antiinflammatory agents (e.g., ibuprofen 600 mg TID [three times a day] orally with food)
    2. Cortisone injection if tendinitis is severe, and if one isolated site of pain; the recommendation is not to inject more than three times per year in the same location.
    3. Splint or brace the affected extremity (do not immobilize shoulders for tendinitis). Wean the splint use, as symptoms decrease, to avoid muscle atrophy.
    4. Apply ice after any repetitive activity and at least 2 to 3 times per day for 15 to 20 minutes.
    5. Relative rest based on etiology: Omit, decrease by 50%, or modify the offending activity.
    6. After the acute phase, recommend gentle stretching and strengthening exercises to affected area; warm shower before repetitious activity.
  C. Client education (Refer to client education supplement on tendonitis.)
  D. Expected client outcomes
    1. Decrease in pain
    2. Increase in function
    3. Increase knowledge about avoidance of repetitious activities and need for overall conditioning

Continued

BOX 11-4

Protocol for the diagnosis and treatment of tendinitis—cont'd

E. Consultation
   1. Consult with or refer to an orthopedist or neurologist if there is muscle atrophy or grossly abnormal nerve conduction studies.
   2. Consult with specialist if symptoms persist beyond 3 to 6 months despite conservative treatment and modification of repetitious activity.

Client Education Supplement: Treatment for Tendinitis
Description
Tendinitis is a painful disorder caused by partial tearing or overstretching of the tendon sheath. Tendons are the fibrous "ropes" that connect muscle to bone. Inflammation is usually caused by a sudden movement that overstretches the tendon, or by small, micro tears to the tendon sheath that result from repetitive movements over time. Numbness and tingling may also occur with tendinitis, and are usually from localized swelling with pressure on a nearby nerve. Known risk factors for tendinitis are awkward postures, frequency of repetitions, amount of weight being lifted, sharp surfaces, and vibration. Treatment is aimed at eliminating these risk factors at home and at work.

Treatments
Rest, ice, compression, and elevation (RICE) are the treatment for tendinitis, in addition to using medications such as ibuprofen, which reduce the inflammation. Consider yourself an athlete as you prepare to do a repetitious activity at home or at work, and do appropriate warm-up and cool-down exercises every day. Other treatments aimed at prevention of these injuries include:
Re-choreographing your work and home tasks by doing the following:
- Slow the speed of your task.
- Keep your head, neck, wrists, elbows, and lumbar spine all in neutral position when doing a task.
- Divide the task into smaller parts, and scramble the job tasks, so your body is not using one set of muscles and tendons for a long period of time.
- Use long muscles to do the job (e.g., lift your whole arm to shift to a different position on a keyboard, instead of bending at the wrist; turn toward the task, instead of rotating your neck).
- For every one to two hours of repetitious work, get up and stretch, deep breathe, and change positions.
- Choose your home exercise to counter your work postures; for example, do the backstroke in swimming if you spend your workday leaning forward over a work surface.
- Alternate arms and feet, and do not overuse your dominant extremity.
- Brisk walking with deep breathing is a good exercise for overall conditioning.
If your work is causing your tendinitis:
- Notify your supervisor that you have a work-related complaint.
- Discuss your work tasks in detail with your health care provider.
- If you have photos of your work station, show them to your health care provider.

BOX 11-4

Protocol for the diagnosis and treatment of tendinits—cont'd

- A work station or work process can be analyzed by an ergonomic specialist, with recommendations to correct any design flaws that could cause a repetitive strain injury.
- Quick fixes can also be tried; for example, raise a computer screen into a better visual field by using old phone books, divide your lifting load in half, or shift more-frequent work tasks closer to your body.

Selected physical assessment maneuvers for workup of tendinitis

Maneuver	Technique	Possible diagnosis
Tinel's at the carpal tunnel	Strike two fingers over carpal tunnel region of wrist; if pain, numbness, or tingling occurs into the 1st, 2nd, or 3rd digits, this is a positive Tinel's sign.	Carpal tunnel syndrome (entrapment of the median nerve)
Phalen's	Flexion of both wrists to 90 degrees for 60 seconds; if pain, numbness, or tingling occurs into the 1st, 2nd, or 3rd digits, this is a positive Phalen's sign.	Carpal tunnel syndrome
Tinel's at the Guyon's canal	Strike two fingers over the hook of hamate above ulnar styloid; if pain, numbness, or tingling occurs into the 4th or 5th digits, this is a positive Tinel's at the Guyon's canal.	Ulnar nerve entrapment or neuritis at the Guyon's canal
Tinel's at the cubital tunnel	Strike two fingers between the medial epicondyle and the olecranon; if pain, numbness, or tingling occurs into the 4th or 5th digits, this is a positive Tinel's at the cubital tunnel.	Ulnar nerve entrapment or neuritis at the cubital tunnel
Finkelstein's test	Client makes fist over flexed thumb and gently ulnar deviates wrist; if pain occurs outside the first extensor compartment (located just above the radial styloid, on the flexor side of the anatomic snuff box), this is a positive Finkelstein's test.	DeQuervain's tendinitis
Resisted wrist extension	Client makes a fist and extends at wrist while resistance is applied downward; if pain occurs in the lateral epicondyle area, this is a positive tennis elbow test.	Lateral epicondylitis
Resisted wrist flexion	Client makes a fist and flexes at wrist while resistance is applied upward; if pain occurs in the medial epicondyle area, this is a positive test.	Medial epicondylitis
Palpation of insertion of biceps tendon into shoulder	Client, with elbow flexed at 90 degrees at side, externally rotates shoulder; if pain is palpated at the groove between the greater and lesser tubercles, this is a positive test.	Bicipital shoulder tendinitis

2. Client satisfaction: x percent of injured workers identified the occupational and environmental health nurse as very to extremely helpful in answering questions about the workers' compensation system on satisfaction survey.
3. Primary prevention: High-risk health care workers will have documentation in their preplacement record of hepatitis B immunity or the offer of vaccination.
4. Secondary prevention: Occupational health history is documented in x percent of medical records of workers with occupational injury; or, chart documentation of ergonomic evaluation is completed within one week of diagnosis of a work-related upper extremity complaint.
5. Tertiary prevention: Sustained return to work, without reinjury, for 90 days after release to return to work; or, litigated cases decreased to x percent after occupational and environmental health nurse case management intervention.

C **Continuous Quality Improvement includes self-assessment of direct care activities to improve health care outcomes (Lukes & Schiavone, 2001).**
1. Identify values: Define vision, mission, and goals/priorities of direct care.
2. Identify work: Detail current programs and services, including most common direct care activities.
3. Identify standards: List relevant standards, for example, OSHA standards and practice guidelines, against which all results will be measured.
4. Secure measurements/develop evaluation tools.
   a. Structure evaluation; for example, safe needle devices being available for immunization programs
   b. Process evaluation; for example, a work injury report was filed correctly and within a specified timeframe
   c. Outcome evaluation, for example, improved client satisfaction scores after treatment of a work related injury.
5. Make interpretations and apply results:
   a. Identify areas of program strength and any areas of noncompliance.
   b. Involve entire staff in feedback discussion of process and outcomes, and need for remediation.
   c. Set goals for improvement.

REFERENCES

Agency for Toxic Substances and Disease Registry. (2000). Taking an exposure history. *Case studies in environmental medicine.* ATSDR Pub. ATSDR-HE-CS-2001-0002. Atlanta, GA: U.S. Department of Health and Human Services, Division of Health Education and Promotion.

American Association of Colleges of Nursing. (1998). *Position statement: Certification and regulation of advanced practice nurses.* Washington, DC: AACN.

American Association of Occupational Health Nurses. (2003). Competencies of occupational and environmental health nursing. Available at http://www.aaohn.org/.

American Association of Occupational Health Nurses. (2004a). Standards of occupational and environmental health nursing. Available at http://www.aaohn.org/

American Association of Occupational Health Nurses. (2004b). *Nurse practitioners in occupational and environmental health.* AAOHN advisory. Atlanta, GA: AAOHN Publications.

American Association of Occupational Health Nurses. (2004c). *Confidentiality of employee health information: clarifying legal and ethical obligations of the occupational and environmental health nurse.* AAOHN advisory. Atlanta, GA: AAOHN Publications.

American Association of Occupational Health Nurses. (2004d). *Developing clinical guidelines or protocols for practice*. AAOHN advisory. Atlanta, GA: AAOHN Publications.

American Association of Occupational Health Nurses. (2004e). *Occupational health surveillance*. AAOHN position statement. Atlanta, GA: AAOHN Publications.

American Association of Occupational Health Nurses. (2004f). *Over-the-counter medications*. AAOHN advisory. Atlanta, GA: AAOHN Publications.

American Association of Occupational Health Nurses. (2004g). *The occupational health nurse as a case manager*. AAOHN position statement. Atlanta, GA: AAOHN Publications.

Bickley, L. S. & Szilagyi, P. G. (2003). *Bates' Guide to Physical Examination and History Taking* (8th ed.). Philadelphia: Lippincott Williams & Wilkins.

Blue, A. V., Chessman, A.W., Gilbert, G. E., Schuman, S. H., & Mainous, A. G. (2000). Medical students abilities to take an occupational history: Use of the WHACS mnemonic. *JOEM, 42*(11), 1050-1053.

Bodenheimer, T., Wagner, E. H., & Grumbach, K. (2002). Improving primary care for patients with chronic illness. *JAMA, 288*(14), 1775-1779.

Burgel, B. J. (1996). Primary care at the worksite: Policy issues. *AAOHN Journal, 44*(5), 238-243.

Burgel, B. J. (1998). Tendinitis. In G. Collins-Bride & J. M. Saxe (Eds.), *Nurse practitioner/physician collaborative practice: Clinical guidelines for ambulatory care*. San Francisco: UCSF Nursing Press.

Centers for Disease Control and Prevention. (2000). Adult Immunization Programs in Nontraditional Settings: Quality Standards and Guidance for Program Evaluation, *Morbidity and Mortality Weekly Reports, 49(RR01);* March 24, 2000, 1-13. Available at http://www.cdc.gov/epo/mmwr/ preview/mmwrhtml/rr4901a1.htm.

Glass, L.S (Ed.). (2004). *Occupational medicine practice guidelines*, 2nd edition. American College of Occupational and Environmental Medicine. Beverly, MA: OEM Press

Grumbach, K., & Bodenheimer, T. (2004). Can health care teams improve primary care? *JAMA, 291*(10), 1246-1251.

Harber, P., Bublik, M., Steimberg, C., Wallace, J., & Merz, B. (2003). Occupational Issues in Episodic Care Populations. *American Journal of Industrial Medicine, 43*, 221-226.

Harber, P., & Merz, B. (2001). Time and knowledge barriers to recognizing occupational disease. *Journal of Occupational and Environmental Medicine, 43*, 483-490.

Krause, N., Dasinger, L. K., & Neuhauser, F. (1998). Modified work and return to work: A review of the literature. *Journal of Occupational Rehabilitation, 8*(2), 113-139.

Levy, B. S., Wegman, D. H. (Eds.). (2000). Occupational Health: *Recognizing and preventing work-related disease and injury* (4th. ed.), Philadelphia: Lippincott Williams and Wilkins.

Lukes, E. N., & Schiavone, G. A. (2001). Self Assessment for Quality and Assurance: An Essential Component of Effective Health Care Delivery at the Worksite. *AAOHN Journal, 49*(1), 44-54.

National Council of State Boards of Nursing (n.d.). *Nurse Licensure Compact.* Retrieved February 28, 2005 from http://www.ncsbn.org/nlc/index.asp.

Nachreiner, N., McGovern, P., Kochevar, L. K., Lohman, W. H., Cato, C., & Ayers, E. (1999). Preplacement assessments: Impact on injury outcomes. *AAOHN Journal, 47*(6), 245-253.

OSHA. (1991) *Guidelines for First Aid Programs. Directive CPL 02-02-053.* Washington DC: Department of Labor.

OSHA. (2004). *Medical Screening and Surveillance*. Washington DC: Department of Labor. Available at http://www.osha-slc.gov/SLTC/medicalsurveillance/index.html.

Papp, E. M. & Miller, A. S. (2000). Screening and surveillance: OSHA's medical surveillance provisions. *AAOHN Journal 48*(2), 59-72.

Rasmor, M. & Brown, C. M. (2001). Health assessment for the occupational and environmental health nurse: Skills Update. *AAOHN Journal, 49*(7), 347-358.

Rasmor, M., & Brown, C. M. (2003). Physical examination for the occupational health nurse. *AAOHN Journal, 51*(9), 390-402.

Reed, P. (Ed.). (2001). *The medical disability advisor* (4th ed.). Westminister, CO: The Reed Group.

Rogers, B. (2003). *Occupational health nursing: Concepts and practice* (2nd ed.). Philadelphia: W.B. Saunders Co.

Rogers, B. & Livsey, K. (2000). Occupational health surveillance, screening and prevention activities in occupational health nursing practice. *AAOHN Journal 48*(2), 92-99.

Rudolph, L. (1996). A call for quality. *Journal of Occupational and Environmental Medicine 38*(4), 343-344.

Rudolph, L. (1998). Performance measures in occupational medicine: A tool to manage quality. *Occupational Medicine: State of the Art Reviews 13*(4), 747-753.

Toth, D. (2003). A standardized language for occupational health nursing—the minimum data set. *AAOHN Journal, 51*(7), 283-286.

U.S. Department of Health and Human Services. (2000). *Healthy people 2010: Conference edition*, Vols. I and II. Washington, DC: U.S. Government Printing Office. Available at http://www.health.gov/healthypeople.

U.S. Preventive Services Task Force. (2004). *Guide to clinical preventive services* (3rd ed.). AHRQ Publication No. 04-IP003. Rockville, MD: Agency for Health Care Quality and Research. Available at http://www.ahrq.gov/clinic/periodorder.htm.

Wassel, M. L. (2002). Improving return to work outcomes: Formalizing the process. *AAOHN Journal, 50*(6), 275-286.

CHAPTER

12

Disability Case Management

Mary Lou Wassel, Jean Randolph, and Lori K. Rieth

Occupational and environmental health nurses routinely coordinate and manage the care of ill and injured workers. Their role as case managers has grown more sophisticated with managed care as a primary cost-containment strategy in response to rising health care expenses. This chapter presents an overview of historical and recent trends in disability case management and discusses important issues and challenges that occupational and environmental health nurses must consider in fulfilling this practice function.

I Case Management

Case Management is a process of coordinating a worker's health care services to deliver optimal, quality care in a cost-effective manner (AAOHN, 2004a).

A *Disability case management* **is the coordination and management of work-related and nonwork-related injury and illness and includes aspects related to group health, workers' compensation, short-term disability, Family and Medical Leave Act (FMLA), and long-term disability benefits.**

B **Case management is designed to prevent fragmented care and delayed recovery, to manage the associated benefits, and to facilitate a worker's return to work to an appropriate transitional or full duty assignment or to an optimal alternative.**

C **A primary goal of case management is to justify the health care provided with a clear measurement of outcomes; cost savings often result, but the major emphasis should be on optimizing health care outcomes.**

II Important Case Management Terms

A *Benefits*—Services owed an individual, as defined by law (e.g., employment benefits or workers' compensation benefits) or based on criteria established in a policy or summary plan description (e.g., rehabilitation, retraining).

B *Cash Benefits*—Cash that is paid either as part of workers' compensation benefits or according to an employer's defined disability plan or negotiated in a union contract to replace a worker's loss of income or earning capacity due to disability resulting from an occupational or nonoccupational injury or illness.

1. The following four classifications describe monetary worker's compensation disability benefits. (These categories are described in terms of their effects on worker's employment in Chapter 3):
   a. *Temporary total disability (TTD)*—tax-free reimbursement for partial wages when a worker is temporarily totally disabled
   b. *Temporary partial disability (TPD)*—tax-free reimbursement for partial wages when a worker is temporarily partially disabled
   c. *Permanent total disability (PTD)*—tax-free reimbursement for partial wages when a worker is permanently totally disabled
   d. *Permanent partial disability (PPD)*—tax-free reimbursement for partial wages when a worker is permanently partially disabled
2. Worker's compensation benefits are determined and allocated according to state jurisdictional rules.
3. Other disability benefits (short term disability [STD] and long term disability [LTD]) can be either tax-free when the worker pays for these plans or after-tax in employer paid or employer self-funded programs.
4. These disability benefits are determined and allocated according to language in the employer's disability plan descriptions or policy statement.

C *Deductible*—**The amount that a member of the health care plan must pay for covered services per specified period (usually the policy year) before the insurer will pay benefits (e.g., health care, prescriptions).**

D *Earning capacity*—**The *potential* wages a worker *could achieve*, given his or her education, training, skill level, previous experience, medical condition, proximity to available work, and other factors.**

E *Exclusive remedy*—**The legal concept that receipt of workers' compensation benefits is the sole benefit (remedy) for the occupational condition incurred and leaves the worker without an additional course of action against the employer.**

F *Functional capacity evaluation* (FCE)—**A professional assessment to specifically determine a disabled person's residual physical abilities.**

G *Gatekeeper*—**The term commonly used to refer to a primary care provider (PCP) who is responsible for coordinating all of a member's medical care. Also may refer to a type of managed care plan that requires that the member have a formal referral from a PCP in order for other care to be covered by the plan (e.g., hospitalization, precertification).**

H *Indemnity* – **In worker's compensation language, generally refers to payments made for lost wages.**

I *Indemnity plan*—**A traditional health insurance program in which the insured person is reimbursed for covered expenses after a deductible is met.**

J *Independent medical examination (IME)*—**A second medical opinion related to a worker's health condition that can be legally binding in some jurisdictions and according to some plan designs.**

K *Job analysis*—**A detailed description of a worker's job duties and physical and mental activities that identifies the essential functions of the job.**

L *Managed care*—**A system of health care delivery that influences utilization of services, costs of services, channeling for services, and measures of performance.**

M *Maximum medical improve*ment—**Used in worker's compensation to indicate the final level to which a person improves/recovers after sustaining a**

disabling medical condition (may or may not equate to pre-disability level).

N *Rehabilitation*—Treatment or formal plan provided by multidisciplinary specialists intended to return the worker to optimal function.

O *Reserves*—Money set aside by a self-insured organization or an insurance carrier to pay the ultimate monetary cost of claims/losses.

P *Residual functional capacity* (RFC)—The final determination of a person's physical capabilities or restrictions at the conclusion of recovery from an illness or injury, usually determined from a physical evaluation and review of an FCE test. The RFC determination is compared with the physical demands of the job activity to determine the appropriateness of vocational options or limitations in daily living.

Q *Risk management*—The process of making and implementing decisions that will minimize the adverse effects of accidental and business losses on an organization.

R *Return to work* (RTW)—The desired goal for all workers after an injury or illness (occupational and nonoccupational).

S *Transitional work*—A temporary job that accommodates the worker's restrictions for a limited period during recovery from an illness or illness. Options for transitional work assignments include the following:
1. *Modified duty*, in which a worker's original job is adjusted to accommodate restrictions
2. *Alternative duty*, in which the worker performs a different job because restrictions rule out continued performance of original job duties

T *Third-party administrator* (TPA)—a company that handles all the administrative tasks involved in managing claims for self-insured employers who fund their own benefit plans (Mullahy, 2004).

U *Utilization review*—A process that measures use and consumption of available resources (including professional staff, facilities, and services) to determine medical necessity, cost effectiveness, and conformity to criteria for optimal use (Shrey & Lacerte, 1995).

V *Wage loss*—The actual *amount* of monetary losses sustained by a worker due to the inability to work.

III Historical Perspective

A *Case management* has been used to describe a variety of strategies for managing health and social services for individuals, families, and work-force populations.
1. Community service coordination, a forerunner of case management, began at the turn of the 20th century in public health programs (American Nurses' Association, 1988).
2. Case management is not a new process, but its scope has expanded and become more sophisticated.
3. The current trend in formalized case management began with Medicaid and Medicare demonstration projects in the early 1970s (Case Management Society of America, 2002).
   a. Managed care programs emerged as a strategy to contain health care costs.

b. As a result, the dual priorities of case management became meeting the worker's needs and making good use of community resources.

4. There have been several major shifts in the approach for disability case management, from orientation to work adjustment services in the 1970s, to work hardening in the 1980s, and to rehabilitation at the workplace in the 1990s (Shrey & Lacerte, 1995).

5. In 2003, there were 4.4 million reported injuries and illnesses in private industry; of these, 2.3 million were cases with days away from work, job transfer, or restriction (Bureau of Labor Statistics, 2004).

6. On any given day, approximately 3.9% of the workers in the U.S. workforce are absent from work, and more than half of employers are unaware of how their absence rates compare with competitors (Watson Wyatt Worldwide, 2001).

7. Keeping more workers at work more of the time is one "best practice" for responding to economic and productivity problems (Wassel, 2002).

B **Occupational and environmental health nurse case managers have historically been the ideal professionals to coordinate workers' health care services from the onset of illness or injury to the safe return to work or an optimal alternative.**

1. Focuses of occupational health case management are as follows:
   a. Providing a safe and healthful workplace
   b. Ensuring that ill or injured workers receive prompt, quality healthcare
   c. Facilitating ill and injured workers' return to work as soon as it is medically safe (Wassel, 2002)
   d. Coordinating total absence management programs (see Figure 12-1: Total Absence Management: Ideal Coordinated State, Watson Wyatt, 2004; and see AAOHN's Foundation block: Absence Management Program, 2004b for more information about these programs)

2. Occupational and environmental health nurses help injured workers achieve optimal outcomes by using the following (AAOHN 2003):
   a. Expertise in health care delivery
   b. Knowledge of the multitude of service options
   c. Expertise in managing return-to-work programs
   d. Understanding of workers' relationships with their environments

C **History has influenced the development and implementation of today's more sophisticated case management services.**

1. Today case management requires an understanding of how the health care delivery system is affected by various medical insurance, government, and corporate mechanisms.

2. In the practice setting, case management demands critical thinking skills, clinical knowledge, experience within the health care delivery systems, ability to access quality, professional resources (Mullahy, 2004), knowledge of the workplace, and knowledge of benefit plan designs and statutory requirements.

D **Changes in the payment for health care services have historically had the greatest effect on access and delivery.**

1. Before World War II, technology was simple and health care dollars were directed primarily toward the treatment of acute illnesses or injuries.

2. After World War II, technology became more complex, and health care expenses for the treatment of chronic, long-term, expensive-to-treat illness and injuries increased dramatically (Rooney, 1990).

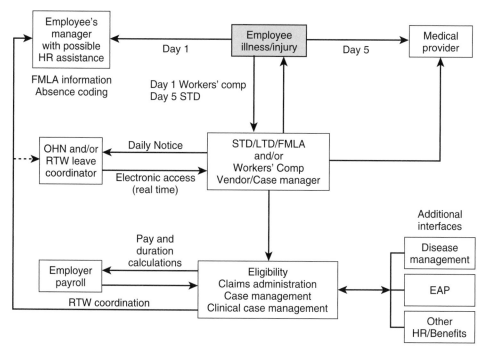

a. The health insurance industry and third-party payment systems emerged.

b. During postwar economic challenges, it was very common for employers to offer benefits such as pensions, disability benefits, and insurance plans instead of salary increases.

c. Health insurance payments rose as the insurance industry expanded from covering less than 20% of Americans before WWII to greater than 60% by the early 1960s.

d. It became generally expected that policyholders were entitled to whatever care or treatment licensed health care providers prescribed.

3. Third-party payments rose from covering about 33% of all personal health care costs in 1950 to almost 75% in the 1990s.

4. By the 1990s, most American workers expected their employer-funded health insurance benefits to cover the majority of their individual and their family members' health care expenses.

a. Direct costs for workers' health care expenses and lost wages resulting from occupational illnesses and injuries are generally paid under a variety of employer workers' compensation insurance arrangements at no cost to workers.

b. Costs for nonwork-related health care expenses are generally paid under a variety of employer group health insurance arrangements that include copayment costs for workers.

E The critical need for effective case management has grown largely as a result of uncontrolled and rising health care costs.

1. By the 1980s, employers were paying for a larger portion of the nation's health care and could no longer tolerate uncontrolled increases in both private and

public health care costs that had resulted in double-digit annual increases for their group health and workers' compensation insurance premiums.

2. Corporations found themselves challenged to make a profit in a climate where health care expenses were consuming approximately 15% of the gross domestic product.

F **Managed care as a cost-containment strategy emerged first in the group health insurance arena and later in the workers' compensation arena.**

1. Managed care incorporates use of preferred provider networks, health maintenance organizations (HMOs), direct contracting, bill audits, utilization review, preadmission authorization, concurrent and retrospective review, second surgical opinions, independent medical exams, and targeted case management (e.g., disease management, catastrophic cases).

2. In 1997, nearly 75% of workers who received health benefits from their employers were covered by some type of managed care plan, up from 51% in 1995 (Mullahy, 2004).

3. It has been estimated that more than 110 million Americans are enrolled in formal managed care plans, including a significant number of Medicare and Medicaid recipients as new enrollees.

4. Although managed care programs strive to reach all potential users of health care service, case management is a personalized process that focuses on certain high-risk or high-cost individuals; some of the greatest cost savings are achieved when case management efforts are focused on the 3% to 5% of the worker population responsible for 60% to 70% of the expenditures in any health plan (Mullahy, 2004).

5. Decision factors or triggers for case management are often developed based on the goals of the individual program.

G **Disability management utilizes services, people, and materials to minimize the impact and cost of disability to employers and workers and encourages return to work for employees with disabilities (Mobley, 2000).**

1. Disability management has a business side and a financial side that include designing return-to-work policies that are consistent with a company's operations and promote a return-to-work culture (Gilpin, 2000).

2. Using an effective disability management process, workers get the treatment they need with a goal of returning them to work as soon as medically feasible (Gilpin, 2000).

3. Corporations can realize significant cost benefit from effectively integrating workers' compensation, Family and Medical Leave Act (FMLA), short-term disability (STD), and long-term disability (LTD) programs with occupational health and safety and worksite disease management programs (Burton, 2000).

4. Supervisors must be shown how they can benefit from programs to keep valued workers on the job and from developing program evaluation strategies that link disability management with the corporate bottom line (Gilpin, 2000).

5. Employers should be prompted to incorporate integrated disability management into strategic planning as part of creating a healthy organization (Curtis, 2004).

6. Once disability management is included in the strategic plan, key success strategies in the disability management field must be incorporated into the design of the program (Curtis, 2004).

H Case managers are in a unique position to define, prevent, create, or reinforce disability by the following means (Mashburn, 2001):
  1. Understanding the relationship among impairment, work, and disability
  2. Promoting return to work solutions for individuals and employers
  3. Coordinating administration of the claim in a timely fashion
  4. Partnering with the employer and the worker to ensure positive return-to-work outcomes
  5. Utilizing basic return-to-work principles in disability management programming

I Competency in occupational and environmental nursing requires change over time as factors reshape the scope of practice.
  1. In 1999, the American Association of Occupational Health Nurses, Inc. (AAOHN) identified competency categories by an external consensus validation process and established performance criteria for each competency.
  2. These competencies were updated in 2003. Case management is one of the categories.
  3. The competent level of practice in the case management category includes (AAOHN, 2003):
      a. Identifying the need for case management.
      b. Conducting a thorough and objective assessment of the client's current status and case management needs.
      c. Using and evaluating available health care resources to achieve an optimal health care outcome.
      d. Collaborating with the client and others to use a multidisciplinary approach to achieve the desired outcome(s).
      e. Using and maintaining an accurate, complete recordkeeping system while maintaining confidentiality.
      f. Identifying changes in case management practice to bring about appropriate care and cost effective outcomes.
  4. Practice at the proficient and expert levels includes developing and managing case management programs and functioning as an expert to internal and external audiences (AAOHN, 2003).

IV Case Management Services: Practice Settings and Providers

Practice settings and providers for case management services are as follows:

A Workplaces/corporations

B Health care delivery systems (e.g., hospitals, clinics, rehabilitation facilities)

C Provider agencies/facilities (e.g., mental health, home health)

D Managed care organizations, including HMOs

E Public insurance providers (e.g., Medicaid, Medicare, Social Security Administration)

F Private insurance providers (e.g., workers' compensation, health, long-term care, disability, liability, casualty, auto, and accident)

G Independent case management companies and providers (e.g., nurses, vocational rehabilitation counselors)

V Team Roles and Responsibilities

A The *worker*, who is the central player in the case management process, has the following main responsibilities:

1. Communicating promptly with the employer about an occupational or non-occupational injury or illness.
2. Participating in the accident investigation process as appropriate.
3. Maintaining contact with the occupational and environmental health nurse regarding medical care, treatment, prognosis, follow-up appointments, and issues regarding return to work.
4. Keeping appointments with all health care providers.
5. Complying with treatment and medical protocols for recovery.

B The *occupational and environmental health nurse* is involved in all stages of the case management process. The nurse's responsibilities include the following (AAOHN, 2004c; AAOHN & CMSA, 2003):

1. Serving as first line contact with the ill or injured worker; this may include assessment, evaluation, treatment, and referral to or coordination with other health care providers.
2. Providing case management, with an emphasis on return to pre-injury function (AAOHN, 2004c).
3. Acting as a liaison with the worker, other health care professionals, insurers, TPAs, the employer, and the workers' compensation board, if applicable, on the worker's behalf (AAOHN, 2004c).
4. Establishing a target return-to-work date based on disability guidelines.
5. Working with the worker to establish recovery and rehabilitation goals and objectives.
6. Jointly setting a date for return to work; working with the physician to coordinate return to work in a transitional job or to establish a timely and individualized rehabilitation program.
7. Communicating with other health care professionals to negotiate care (e.g., home care, durable medical equipment, rehabilitation, hospice) and to assess social support resources.
8. Working with the employer to determine if transitional work is available and monitoring worker's progress upon return to work.
9. Researching sources of valuable information for developing specific job restrictions (i.e., Job Accommodation Network, where health care professionals can speak directly with trained consultants about specific needs and modification solutions). See Appendix I for contact information; http://www.jan.wvu.edu/ (Wassel, 2002).
10. Educating the worker about the benefits of the workers' compensation or disability system and answering or referring further questions to the claims manager or human resources, as appropriate.
11. Maintaining confidentiality of the worker's protected health information in accordance with professional codes, laws, and regulations.

C The *physician* is usually the primary care provider for the seriously injured or ill worker. The physician's responsibilities include the following:

1. Providing timely information regarding diagnosis, treatment, prognosis, and expected return-to-work date
2. Clarifying any work limitations that may apply upon return to work; approving transitional duty work
3. Being aware of workplace issues, including types of work available and transitional work options

4. Conducting a workplace walk-through assessment as needed in coordination with the employer
5. Communicating with members of the Return to Work Team, including the occupational and environmental health nurse or claims manager, before making referrals to other specialists for persistent symptoms

D The *employer's* **support is critical in an effective case management program, especially in identifying possible transitional duty to expedite return to work. The employer's responsibilities include the following:**
1. Investigating the accident or issues impacting illness and injury and reviewing workplace factors, which may need to be changed or modified (e.g., machine modifications, ergonomic improvements).
2. Maintaining contact between supervisor and worker during the disability to promote good will and help maintain the link between the ill and injured worker and the workplace.
3. Helping the occupational and environmental health nurse, human resources professionals, and the supervisor identify suitable transitional work.
4. Establishing and supporting a return-to-work program for both occupational and nonoccupational injuries and illnesses.
5. Facilitating the worker's return to work as soon as is medically safe.

E The *insurer or third party administrator (TPA)* **(whether internal or external), represented by the claims manager, acts as a consultant with all parties during all stages of the claim. Responsibilities of the insurer include the following:**
1. Determining compensability and/or eligibility of the claim.
2. Authorizing medical care and payment of bills to providers.
3. Ensuring the payment of appropriate wages specified in workers' compensation statutes and/or disability plans.
4. Communicating regularly and responding promptly and accurately to employer's and worker's questions regarding the claim, including referrals, entitlements (e.g., permanent partial disability [PPD], temporary total disability [TTD], settlements, and coordination of benefits).
5. Coordinating the flow of information by requesting periodic health and medical information from health care providers when necessary.
6. Consulting with attorneys, when necessary, regarding specific questions about workers' rights under state workers' compensation law (e.g., controverting or settling a claim).

F *Rehabilitation specialists* **(rehabilitation nurses, physical therapists, occupational specialists, and vocational counselors) work with the injured worker during the rehabilitation phases of recovery (AAOHN, 1999). Their major responsibilities include the following:**
1. Working with the injured worker so function and strength are regained to meet the goal of return to work as soon as medically possible
2. Communicating with the team regarding the worker's progress; be aware of "red flags" and issues affecting return to work (Box 12-1 lists several indicators of delayed recovery.)
3. Providing specialized programs to facilitate the worker's return to work, using such techniques as functional capacity assessments, ergonomic evaluations, labor market surveys, and work hardening programs
4. Providing realistic expectations regarding recovery
5. Helping the injured worker manage chronic pain

BOX 12-1

Indicators of delayed recovery (red flags)

- Poor job satisfaction
- A change in the story of injury occurrence
- Unresolved anger at employer about the injury
- Unwillingness to discuss or negotiate an RTW plan
- Multiple failures to return to work
- Perceived lack of support from supervisor
- History of job performance problems
- Time off without any change in symptoms
- Income on temporary disability equal to or greater than regular wage scale
- Double dipping between workers' compensation, STD, LTD, or SSDI

- Other secondary gain issues: disabled partner at home, multiple demands, and entitlement issues
- Limited job offerings in the area
- "Doctor shopping"
- Involvement of an attorney
- Requests for narcotics renewals
- Close to retirement age
- Undiagnosed or untreated depression (either preceding or concurrent with injury)
- Time off from the date of injury exceeds 6 months
- Continued subjective complaints without objective findings
- Unavailable when case manager calls

G The *union* (bargaining representative) is important in its support of the case management process and the injured or ill worker. Main responsibilities include the following:

1. Working with the employer and the occupational and environmental health nurse to understand and support objectives for the ill or injured worker.
2. Helping the ill or injured worker understand his or her responsibilities for return to transitional work.
3. Helping the ill or injured worker understand his or her benefits while disabled.

VI Steps in Program Development

Establishing an effective case management program requires several important steps: assessment, data analyses and diagnoses, planning, implementation, and evaluation.

A Assessment is the first step of the process.

1. Gather benefit cost and utilization data for nonwork-related health problems (health care and disability) for workers, specifically for the following (Rieth, 2000):
   a. High-cost cases
   b. Repetitive hospitalizations or extensions of hospital stays
   c. Selected diagnoses (e.g., spinal cord injuries, premature births, cancer, organ transplants, psychiatric diagnoses)
   d. Short-term disability/long-term disability coverage and plan designs for workers

  e. Numerous providers involved in a case
  f. Pharmacy-related expenses
2. Collect the following workers' compensation data by geographic region, department, and job class:
  a. Numbers and costs of first-aid, medical-only, and lost-time cases, and the range of diagnoses
  b. The type of permanent disability awarded and vocational rehabilitation costs
  c. High-reserve cases
  d. Workers' compensation experience rating
  e. Litigation costs (Box 12-2 presents strategies for avoiding litigation)
  f. Referral data on the number and types of specialty referrals, wait time before seeing specialist, length of physical therapy prescription, etc.
  g. Selected diagnoses (e.g., soft-tissue injury, upper-extremity musculoskeletal disorders, low back pain, and stress claims)
3. Review health benefit coverage for workers and dependents for the following:
  a. Pre-existing condition exclusions
  b. Mental health benefits (inpatient, outpatient, partial stays)
  c. Home-care coverage
  d. Pre-authorization procedures
  e. Second-opinion requirements
  f. Out-of-pocket costs
  g. Disease management programs
  h. Health promotion programs
  i. Prescription drug coverage
  j. Percentage of workers and dependents not covered by an employer-sponsored health plan

---

BOX 12-2

Strategies for avoiding litigation

- Be aware that miscommunication among the parties is one of the largest barriers to efficient case management (AAOHN, 1999).
- Treat injured workers with respect and dignity.
- Respect the worker's right to confidentiality of medical information whenever possible.
- Coach the employer regarding the benefits of instituting a transitional return-to-work program.
- Maintain regular contact among all parties on the health care team to address concerns, treatment, special needs, referrals, etc.

- Maintain contact with the worker to avoid misunderstandings and maintain the bond with the employer.
- Consider a home visit to the worker in cases that have medically complex diagnoses, are deemed catastrophic, or warrant assessment of rehabilitation needs.
- When the worker is hospitalized, consider a visit to the hospital to show support, answer questions, and establish a bond with the worker.
- Advocate and assist the worker with the multitude of potential issues with the health care system.

4. Review medical leave-of-absence, short-term disability (STD), and long-term disability (LTD) policies and communication between human resources and the occupational health services.
5. Assess success of transitional duty program.
   a. Number of successful return-to-work cases
   b. Supervisor cooperation
   c. Number of reinjuries
   d. Overall cost of accommodations
6. Determine workplace areas where employer cooperation could be improved.
7. Benchmark with other corporate case or absence management programs (Denniston et al., 2005).

B **Once the assessment has been completed, the data are analyzed and diagnoses formulated.**
1. Determine regional and programmatic "hot spots" where outcomes and costs have not been well monitored or may be a potential problem.
2. Conduct a brief, retrospective, cost-effectiveness analysis to determine whether case management could have made a positive impact on a sample of interest.
   a. Select two or three high-cost lost-time cases.
   b. Look at group aggregate data to determine opportunities for program development.
   c. Trend numbers against benchmark data and incidence rates
   d. Detail health costs and temporary/permanent disability costs.
   e. Determine the important outcome criteria, based on the natural history of the injury or illness and on published clinical disability duration guidelines (e.g., The American College of Occupational and Environmental Medicine's *Occupational Medicine Practice Guidelines* [2004]; *The Work Loss Data Institutes Official Disability Guidelines* [2005]; *Presley Reed's Medical Disability Advisor* [2005]).
3. Document a range of anticipated cost savings based on the cases identified for case management (e.g., in-house utilization review, pre-certification services, or return to work).
4. If a positive impact of case management can be demonstrated, proceed with formal planning for a pilot project; examples of positive impacts include the following:
   a. Cost savings cover the program's expenses
   b. Less invasive diagnostic procedures are ordered
   c. An improved quality of life results

C **Planning will be based on the diagnoses.**
1. Use the following criteria to identify one or two units within the organization to pilot a case management program:
   a. Size of the worker population and pattern of injury and illness statistics
   b. Opportunity to demonstrate a positive impact within a defined time frame
   c. Management and union support
   d. Willingness to provide transitional return to work options
   e. Strong occupational and environmental health nursing involvement
   f. Strong commitment to primary prevention of work-related hazards and health education for nonoccupational health hazards.

2. Develop a policy statement with program goals, objectives, and timetable.
3. Determine necessary resources (e.g., telephone, computer, fax, car, database management software, and staff) to provide the appropriate level of case management.
4. Network with other disability management professionals in the community.
5. Develop a marketing plan for workers, including communication with human resources, union, supervisor, workers' compensation, STD or LTD carriers and administrator, community referrals, etc.
6. Consider establishing a task force that will develop strategies to ensure the successful "buy-in" by workers.
7. Establish evaluation criteria.

D **The plan then needs to be implemented.**
1. Initiate a trigger system to notify the occupational health services of cases to be included in case management pilot programs.
2. Link the worker to the needed services and communicate the rationale for treatment choices.
3. Throughout the case management process, use primary, secondary, and tertiary preventive nursing interventions to prevent delayed recovery.
4. Document time spent with worker, nature of interactions, anticipated outcome, and cost savings in a computerized database management system.
5. Focus on a realistic return-to-work date and appropriate job accommodations
6. Verify that transitional work options are appropriate for any temporary work restrictions.
7. Establish an ongoing internal process to assist with return to work and transitional duty.

E **Evaluation using a structure, process, and outcomes approach is the last step in this process. (Figure 12-2 presents a case management evaluation model).**
1. Determine the effects of relevant structural elements on the resolution of cases. Structural elements include the following:

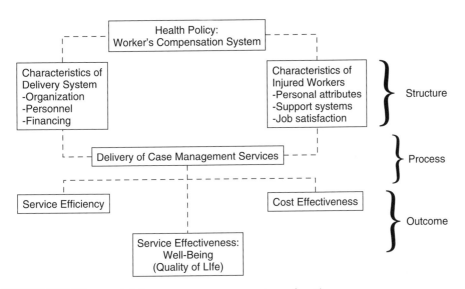

FIGURE 12-2 *Model for case management evaluation*

Source: Salazar, MK, Graham, L & Lantz, B 1999.

a. Policies, procedures, and regulations (e.g., workers' compensation, Department of Labor, Employee Retirement Income Security Act (ERISA)
b. The characteristics of the delivery system, including the organization of services, personnel involved in service delivery, and financing of services
c. The characteristics of the injured or ill workers, including their personal attributes, support systems, and attitudes about work
d. The characteristics of the workplace, including support and attitudes

2. Develop methods to ensure that appropriate processes, including the following, are used in the delivery of service:
   a. The interactions among case manager, other service providers, and the ill and injured worker are adequate and appropriate.
   b. Workers are informed and knowledgeable about the structures and processes affecting their cases.
   c. The cause of the injury or illness is analyzed, with the goal being to prevent similar occurrences in the future.

3. Assess the outcomes that are affected by case management services; outcomes include service efficiency (timeliness of services), service effectiveness (quality outcomes), and cost effectiveness (dollar outcomes) [Dyck, 2000].
   a. Measures of *service efficiency* include:
      1) A notification system that captures all the cases and triages them to meet the predefined case management criteria
      2) Appropriate and accurate entry of data by case managers
      3) Delivery of services within the anticipated time frame, with limited wait time, if referred
      4) Documentation of steady improvement in the worker's condition
      5) An active plan for return to work in a transitional capacity until able to resume full duty of the original job
   b. Measures of *service effectiveness* include the facts that:
      1) The worker is satisfied with care coordination and communication.
      2) The case manager is satisfied with the implementation of the case management program, including the integration of any suggestions to improve the program.
      3) Providers and management are satisfied with their collaboration with the case manager to improve care outcomes.
      4) The supervisor is satisfied with the implementation of the transitional duty component of the case management program.
      5) Union leadership is satisfied with a fair and equitable application of benefits for workers.
   c. *Cost effectiveness* is measured by evaluating direct and indirect costs.
      1) The *direct costs* of illnesses and injuries include the measurable medical expenses and payment for lost wages. These costs are fairly easy to quantify, but represent only a fraction of the total cost of illnesses and injuries when compared with the indirect or hidden costs of illnesses and injuries. Measuring direct cost savings necessitates the following:
         a) Placing a cost value on every intervention
         b) Selecting data for a particular work site and comparing several claims that included case management with other claims that were not case managed, trying to control for types of work demands and severity of workers' conditions

    c) Evaluating the frequency and costs of office visits, types of diagnostic interventions, numbers and costs of prescriptions, number of inpatient days, mean length of stay, etc.

    d) Measuring temporary disability, STD, sick leave, and LTD payments

    e) Determining the date of injury, date of permanent and stationary status, and amount and percent of any permanent disability award

    f) Detailing any vocational rehabilitation costs and resultant savings

    g) Listing legal costs (health evaluations, attorney representation, and settlements)

    h) Determining direct cost savings in insurance premiums (e.g., quantify savings from transitional work versus lost workdays on lowering experience modification rates)

    i) If work related and the worker did not return to work, evaluating the date of termination and continued costs in the social security/disability system if workers' compensation benefits are depleted or settled

    j) Determining the expenses of the case management program, including a percentage of overhead costs and the number of hours of case management time

2) The *indirect* or hidden costs of accidents are more difficult to measure and represent much greater costs. Measuring indirect cost savings necessitates the following:

    a) Determining time lost by supervisors and other workers (e.g., time needed to investigate the accident, time lost if work is suspended due to accident)

    b) Identifying replacement costs for hiring temporary workers or new staff

    c) Estimating decreased production levels, lost profits, potential loss of customers, and decreased worker morale

    d) Determining whether savings were realized with the cases analyzed

    e) Repeating the cost analysis for a group of claims with similar diagnoses and from a specific department, site, or region

    f) Communicating "added value" (quality and outcomes) of case management program to management, union, human resources, and case management staff

VII Return to Work (RTW)

A **Specific steps must be taken to formalize the RTW program.**

1. Companies should have an established RTW program with a *written* RTW policy statement.

    a. Having a written RTW policy statement will usually require the approval and commitment of upper management.

    b. A written RTW policy clarifies management expectations and reinforces a corporate culture in which all workers are valued, will receive prompt, quality health care, and will be returned to either full duty or temporary/transitional duty as soon as is medically safe.

    c. Companies usually have written policies for sick leave, short-term disability, and long-term disability referencing return to work and transitional work expectations.

    d. The corporate RTW policy and procedures should also be included in the worker policy and procedure manual.

BOX 12-3

Sample transitional work program policy

Purpose

The purpose of this program is to provide a process for assisting employees who are temporarily unable to perform some or all of their regular job functions because of injury or illness to return to productive work in a safe and timely manner. Employees who require permanent job accommodations are included in the company's Americans With Disabilities Act (ADA) policy.

Policy

- XYZ Company will make reasonable efforts to provide suitable alternative productive work to employees who are temporarily unable to perform all of their regular job functions. Transitional work assignments will be based on the physical limitations of the individual, the expected duration of the limitations, and the availability of suitable temporary work. Transitional work may include any of the following: reduced work hours, reduced production requirements, job modification, and assignment to alternative work within individuals' own or other departments.

- The company is under no obligation to create transitional work positions. The company reserves the right to discontinue an employee's transitional work assignment at any time. Employee refusal to accept transitional work assignments may result in a loss of disability benefits; however, participation in the transitional duty program is considered voluntary under the Family and Medical Leave Act guidelines.

Program Guidelines

- The program applies to any hourly or salaried employee with a medical condition, whether work related or non-work related, who is temporarily unable to perform his or her full job duties, as documented by work restrictions issued by a health care professional.

- Each case will be considered on an individual basis.

- Management may limit the number of employees working in the transitional work program (TWP).

- Every attempt will be made to keep employees working in their own department. If suitable work is not available in the home department, employees may be assigned to other departments or to temporary special projects (e.g., new employee training/shadowing, data collection for xxx program).

- Employees in the TWP may be limited to working a maximum number of hours on a daily or weekly basis.

- Time frame: transitional work assignments are considered temporary and will not exceed 8 total work weeks within any 12-month period, unless the employee is progressing satisfactorily and it is determined by the health care provider that an extension of no longer than 4 weeks should be sufficient to allow the employee to return to his or her regular job.

- Salary: employees in the program will be paid at the same rate of pay as their regular job.

Continued

BOX 12-3

Sample transitional work program policy—cont'd

Roles and Responsibilities
Occupational Health Nurse
- Responsible for overall management of the TWP.
- Determines which employees are eligible for inclusion in the program based on medical documentation and availability of suitable transitional job(s).
- Responsible for complying with established TWP procedures.

Injured or Ill Employee
- Must communicate any actual or anticipated medical absences in accordance with the attendance policy.
- Cooperate fully with the TWP.
- Provide appropriate medical information as requested by the occupational health nurse.
- Advise the supervisor and occupational health nurse immediately of any change in health status or other circumstances that affect the transitional work plan.

Department Management and Supervisors
- Fully support the program objectives.
- Refer potential program candidates to the occupational health nurse.
- Collaborate with the occupational health nurse to develop individual transitional work plans.
- Identify job opportunities within their department.
- Ensure that employees in the program work within the confines of the approved transitional work plan.

Human Resources
- Assist with administration of the TWP as requested by the occupational health nurse.
- Work to resolve any conflicts that may arise as the result of a transitional work assignment.
- Notify the occupational health nurse of potential program candidates.

e. Having a written RTW policy helps ensure equitable treatment and avoid potentially discriminatory situations where it may be tempting to have one policy for good performers and another policy for challenging performers.

f. A sample Transitional Work Program Policy is included in Box 12-3.

2. The corporate RTW policy and procedures should be communicated to all workers.

3. Labor representatives should be consulted and included when developing or modifying the company's RTW policy and program.

4. Labor representatives can often serve as the occupational and environmental health nurse's advocate in RTW efforts.

B **A goal of occupational health and safety programs and services is to prevent lost-time injuries.**

1. Even in workplaces with proactive health and safety programs and services, accidents and injuries still occur.

2. Accident/incident procedures should require prompt notification of supervisors, transportation of the worker to health care treatment, a requirement for accident investigation, and reporting the incident to the insurance carrier or TPA.

3. To ensure a safe and healthy workplace, loss prevention and safety programs should address the exposures for the class of business, and focus on loss sources revealed in a thorough analysis of recent, historical loss data obtained from OSHA logs and insurance loss/claims information.

4. Prompt, thorough investigation must be enforced as the primary strategy for learning from accidents and near misses, directing corrective efforts for faulty processes, and preventing future accidents.

5. Holding supervisors and department managers accountable for safety as a performance measure is one recommended method of ensuring compliance.

C **When injuries and illnesses occur, they should be addressed immediately.**

1. Workers are responsible for promptly notifying their supervisor of any injuries or prolonged illnesses.

2. Employers are responsible for immediately reporting any workplace injuries or illnesses necessitating time away from work to their workers' compensation insurance carrier or TPA.

3. In work sites where on-site occupational health services are provided, the occupational health professionals should also be notified promptly.

4. Case management ideally begins from the onset of the injury or illness and continues through the safe return to work or an optimal alternative (AAOHN, 2004c).

D **A program goal is to provide timely and quality health care to workers (see Case Study 1).**

1. In situations where the injury or illness occurs "in the course of employment" (compensable under workers' compensation laws), employers in most states can direct workers to a panel of pre-selected health care providers.

2. In an effort to ensure the best health care outcomes, employers or their occupational health professional representatives should preselect a panel of health care professionals who share their commitment to provide prompt, high-quality health care and treatment and returning injured workers to work as soon as is medically safe.

Text continued on p. 356

Case Study 1: Return to Work for Occupational Injury – Low Back Pain

Presentation: A 40-year-old airline baggage handler felt something "go out" in his back after lifting a particularly heavy suitcase onto a conveyor belt. After finishing his shift, he reported the incident to his supervisor, stating that he initially didn't think anything of it, but as his shift wore on he was feeling pain and stiffness increase. The incident was noted and:

"Best-Practice" Treatment Protocol*

The employee went home, took ibuprofen as directed and rested for the night.

The next morning, the employee reported to work reporting stiffness and pain in the lumber region and expressed anxiety about returning to his regular job.

His supervisor understood and concurred with his employee's reluctance to assume his normal duties until a medical professional checked his condition. The supervisor advised the injured worker to report to Employee Health to assess his condition and ability to return to work.

Note: Assessments of this nature may be made by Primary Care Physicians MD/DO (50%), Orthopedists (33%), or Chiropractors (17%).

Worst-Case

The employee went home, took ibuprofen as directed and rested for the night.

The next morning the employee felt pain and stiffness and decided to spend the next few days in bed. He left a message that he would not be in to work for the remainder of the week.

There was no direct communication with his supervisor or co-workers.

Commentary

Good communication between the employee and employer is key. Making the employee feel valued as a part of the team through support, reassurance, and early intervention has both physiologic and psychologic benefits.

Clinical findings:

No radiculopathy
No "red flags"
No history of back pain

Radiculopathy questionable
No "red flags"
No history of back pain

NOTE: Radiculopathy is often over-diagnosed. For unequivocal evidence of radiculopathy, refer to the AMA Guides to

Continued

Case Study 1: Return to Work for Occupational Injury – Low Back Pain—cont'd

	"Best-Practice" Treatment Protocol* Healthy patient Non-smoker	Worst-Case Healthy patient Non-smoker Abnormalities found in images. Indications of disc bulges or herniated disc.	Commentary *the Evaluation of Permanent Impairment,* 5th Edition, page 382-383.
Diagnosis:	Lumbar Sprain/Strain (847.2) Severity: Mild	Displacement of intevertebral disc, site unspecified, without myelopathy (722.2)	Indiscriminant imaging will result in false positive findings, such as disc bulges, that are not the source of painful symptoms and do not warrant surgery.
Treatment:	• Decreased activity, if necessary, based on severity and difficulty of job; passive therapy with heat/ice (3-4 times/day), stretching; appropriate analgesia (i.e., acetaminophen) and/or anti-inflammatory (i.e., ibuprofen) [*Benchmark cost: $14*]; back to work except for severe cases in 72 hours, possibly modified duty.* • Avoid prolonged bed rest • No x-rays unless significant trauma (e.g., a fall) • If muscle spasms, then consider muscle relaxant with limited sedative side effects [*Benchmark cost: $44*] (Note: The purpose of muscle relaxants is to facilitate return to activity, but muscle relaxants have not been shown to be more effective than NSAIDs.)	Rest. Avoid strenuous activity. May not return to his regular duties.	Anti-inflammatories are the traditional first line of treatment, to reduce pain so activity and functional restoration can resume. A comprehensive review of clinical trials on the efficacy and safety of drugs for the treatment of low back pain concludes that available evidence supports the effectiveness of non-selective nonsteroidal anti-inflammatory drugs (NSAIDs) in acute and chronic LBP, of muscle relaxants in acute LBP, and of antidepressants in chronic LBP.

Case Study 1: *Return to Work for Occupational Injury – Low Back Pain—cont'd*

Return to work:	• REASSURE PATIENT: common problem (90% of patients recover spontaneously in 4 weeks) Immediate. The physician conferred with the employer to determine availability of transitional work options. The employee was able to report right back to work after his initial examination for transitional duty, working a concession in the airport, with breaks as indicated. Transitional duty Clerical/Modified Work 0 days for a mild lumbar sprain or strain or 3 days for a severe lumbar strain (with transitional duty following the capabilities and activities modifications outlined below: **Capabilities and Activities Modifications:** Lifting with knees (with a straight back, no stooping) not more than 5 lbs up to 3 times/hr; squatting up to 4 times/hr; standing or walking with a 5-minute break at least every 20 minutes; sitting with a 5-minute break every 30 minutes; no extremes of extension or flexion; no extremes of twisting; no climbing ladders; driving car only up to 2 hrs/day.	Expected return: approximately 12 weeks Initial conservative medical treatment, regular work if cause of disability: 84 days Within this diagnosis, 84 lost workdays would be the case if there was either: • No communication between the physician and the employer indicating what the patient can or cannot do, or, • Unwillingness on the part of the employer to accommodate transitional work options.	The strongest medical evidence regarding potential therapies for low back pain indicates that having the patient return to normal activities has the best long-term outcome. There are many therapies, both invasive and noninvasive, whose purpose is to cure the pain, but there is no strong evidence that they accomplish this as successfully as therapies that focus on restoring functional ability, without focusing on the pain. However, transitional duty may be necessary, since there is evidence for a dose-response relationship between physical workload and LBP of longer duration, and unavailability of transitional work options for return to work plus a job requirement of lifting for three fourths of the day or more. All were significant, independent determinants of LBP chronicity.

Continued

Case Study 1:   Return to Work for Occupational Injury – Low Back Pain—cont'd

	"Best-Practice" Treatment Protocol*	Worst-Case	Commentary
Second visit	• Second visit (day 7 – about 1 week after first visit) –Document progress (flexibility, areas of tenderness, motor strength, straight leg raise – sitting & supine) –If still 50% disabled then prescribe manual therapy [Benchmark cost: $250]: Refer to massage therapist, chiropractor, physical therapist, or occupational therapist (3 visits in first week), or by treating DO/MD –Discontinue muscle relaxant	Magnetic resonance imaging (MRI) of the lumbar (or lumbosacral spine) requested to verify diagnosis. [Benchmark cost: $1,600] Electromyography and nerve conduction velocity testing (EMG/NCV) performed to ascertain radiculopathy. [Benchmark cost: $750]	There is strong evidence that physical methods, including exercise and return to normal activities, have the best long-term outcome in employees with low back pain. Direction from physical and occupational therapists can play a role in this. Medical evidence shows good outcomes from the use of manipulation in acute low back pain without radiculopathy. If manipulation has not resulted in functional improvement in three to four weeks, it should be stopped and the patient reevaluated.
Return to work: 10 days for a mild lumbar insecurity, sprain or strain or 14-17 days for a severe strain (with manual work following the capabilities and activities modifications outlined)	• Employee is now ready to assume increased duties/manual work with the following restrictions: Lifting with knees (with a straight back) not more than 25 lbs up to 15 times/hr; squatting up to 16 times/hr; standing or walking with a 10-minute break at least every 1-2 hours; sitting with a 10-minute break every 1-2 hours; extremes of flexion or extension allowed up to 12 times/hr; extremes of twisting allowed up to 16 times/hr; climbing ladders allowed up to 25 rungs 6 times/hr; driving car or light truck up to a full work day; driving heavy truck up to 4 hrs/day.	Employee still unable to return to work.	In this "worst case" scenario, there are two additional forms of disability in play. First, iatrogenic disability that is medically caused, in this case through misdiagnosis. The second type of disability is system-induced. From the start, the lack of initiative on the employer's part to communicate with the employee or try to get him back to work right away, suggests to the employee that his injury may be worse than he thought. Further, the unwillingness of the employer to provide transitional work options compounds the disability, adding to his feeling of dependency, inadequacy, depression, anxiety, job dissatisfaction, or insecurity.

Case Study 1: Return to Work for Occupational Injury – Low Back Pain—cont'd

Third visit	• Third visit (day 14 – about 1 week after second visit) -Document progress -Prescribe muscle-conditioning exercises -At this point 66%–75% should be back to regular work -If still disabled, then first imaging study (AP/Lateral 2-view X-Ray of lumbar) [*Benchmark cost: $150*] to rule out spondylosis, degenerative disc disease, tumor, fracture, osteoporosis, or joint narrowing/spinal stenosis (age related, not caused by recent trauma – will not change treatment) [ICD9 721.3, 721.4, 724.02] -Continue therapist, change from passive to active modality, 2 visits in next week, teach home exercises -End manual therapy at 4 weeks Patient is released to full duty four weeks after the injury.	Third Visit (after 4 weeks): Employee shows signs of weakening and atrophy of the muscles. Referral to a Chiropractor for manipulation. (18 visits over 6 weeks) [*Benchmark cost: $1,030*]	Patient should show signs of improvement in 3-4 weeks or manipulation should be stopped and the patient re-evaluated.
Return to work:		Fourth visit: (3 months after injury) No reported improvement by patient. Evidence of noncompliance with self-directed care. Patient exhibits signs of depression and still complains of pain.	Malingering, albeit unintentional, can foster other difficulties, like family and financial problems or alcohol or chemical dependencies, as well as depression. A recent clinical trial concluded that patients with chronic low back pain who followed cognitive intervention and exercise programs improved significantly in muscle

Continued

Case Study 1:   Return to Work for Occupational Injury – Low Back Pain—cont'd

"Best-Practice" Treatment Protocol*	**Worst-Case**	**Commentary**
	Referral to psychiatrist. [*Benchmark cost: $120/session/week for 4 months*] Medications for anxiety and depression are prescribed. [*Benchmark cost: $168*]	strength compared with patients who underwent lumbar fusion. Presurgical predictors of poor outcomes from fusion are number of prior low back operations, low household income at time of injury, older age, lawyer involvement, and the presence of depression.
	Patient consults with an attorney. [*Benchmark cost: Initial Consultation–no charge*] Physician referral to spine surgeon who recommends spinal fusion [*Benchmark cost: $45,000*] Fusion performed. Post-surgical physical therapy (34 visits over 16 weeks): [*Benchmark cost: $1,890*]	
Outcome: Four weeks after the employee's initial presentation to Employee Health, the employee was back to full duty in his original job. There were no lost workdays, due to transitional work opportunities.	7 months after injury, employee states that his pain is worse and he is unable to return to his original job. His depression continues and he has become chemically dependent on pain killers.	Most patients reported that their back pain was worse (67.7%) and their overall quality of life was worse or no better (55.8%) than before surgery, as measured at a 2-year follow-up assessment.
	No return to work	Approximately $15 billion was spent on spinal fusion in the U.S. last year, an estimated 90% of which were not supported by the results of high-quality medical studies. In addition to wasting money, many patients are having to suffer through an unnecessary surgery, which is highly invasive and even life threatening, when there are other therapies that would be more likely to help them return to functionality.
	Employee's attorney filing a total disability claim. [*Benchmark cost: $5,000 to prepare and file claim*]	

Case Study 1: Return to Work for Occupational Injury – Low Back Pain—cont'd

Direct costs to 7 months after injury:	Lost wages: $ 0 Medical: $ 723 Legal: $ 0	Lost wages to date: (7 mos.): $9800 Medical: $57, 763 Legal: $ 5,000 (to date) Note: Potential lost wages: $ 455,000* (25 years to age 65 times 52 weeks @ $350/week) *Possible lifetime benefits because of catastrophic claim
Total direct costs to date:	There was no permanent impairment. $773 $773	Open case $72,563 $480,700
Potential total direct costs:		Estimated ongoing medical care ($3,500); ongoing psychiatric care for an additional 15 months ($7,200); ongoing legal fees till resolution of case ($15,000); lost wages till age 65 ($455,000).
Savings to date:	$71,790 Savings over first 7 months	
Potential total savings:	$479,927	

Of utmost significance is that prolonged unnecessary treatment in and of itself, along with delayed return to activity, is not only costly (as illustrated by this case study), but most importantly, has been proven to be harmful to injured workers, their families, their quality of life and consequently, to society in general.

"Best practice" Treatment Protocol, and Return-to-Work Durations and Capabilities & Activity Modifications from *Official Disability Guidelines 2005 (ODG)*, tenth edition, and *ODG Treatment in Worker's Comp* (ODG/TWC), third edition, published by Work Loss Data Institute: <u>www.worklossdata.com</u>.

Case Study prepared by Patricia Whelan, Publisher, Work Loss Data Institute, Encinitas, CA 92024.

3. Jurisdictional rules dictate how workers access medical care.
    a. Some require channeling within networks
    b. Some require posted panels of providers
    c. Some allow employers to direct all referrals to health care providers
    d. Some allow employers to direct referrals to health care providers under certain provisions or time frames
    e. Some states are designated as worker choice states, and employers are restricted from directing or referring workers to providers
4. Case managers must maintain current knowledge of changes in workers' compensation laws in their jurisdictional areas.
    a. There are only a few states/jurisdictions that do not assert "exclusive remedy" protection for employers.
    b. Case managers need to know the jurisdictions in which they work to know those situations in which exclusive remedy does not apply and determine if an additional claim or suit may be active in conjunction with the workers' compensation claim.
5. Many managed care programs include brokered fee arrangements with a network of health care professional and treatment facilities.
    a. These fee arrangements are among the cost-control strategies for managing benefit costs and insurance premiums/fees.
    b. In addition to providing prompt access to cost-effective care for workers, it is imperative that there also be a process for monitoring and ensuring quality treatment outcomes for workers treated by network or panel health care providers.
6. Developing and fostering trusting relationships with quality health care providers is key to the success of case management and an effective RTW program.

E An additional goal of case management is to promote proactive transitional work programs.
1. The most important principle of disability case management is *early intervention* (Mullahy, 2004); early intervention is likely to result in cost savings to employers, disabled workers, and insurance carriers; and to important psychosocial benefits experienced by workers and their families (Shrey & Lacerte, 1995).
2. When injuries or illnesses result in actual or potential lost work days, a target return-to-work date should be established, using recognized disability guidelines (e.g., The American College of Occupational and Environmental Medicine's *Occupational Medicine Practice Guidelines* [2004]; *The Work Loss Data Institutes Guidelines* [2005]; *or Pressley Reed's Medical Disability Advisor* [2005]).
3. Ill or injured workers should be released to return to work as soon as is medically safe.
4. The preferred site for injured workers to rehabilitate in preparation for returning to their original job is in their own workplace.
5. This workplace rehabilitation/return to work model reduces or eliminates most of the disincentives that result from the worker's potentially lengthy separation from the work site and yields more cost.
6. The shift in the 1990s toward employers becoming more active participants in rehabilitation and return-to-work efforts is attributed to a reduced labor pool, efforts to minimize costs of ill and injured workers compensation or

disability, and the implementation of the ADA, which mandates job modification and accommodation for persons with qualifying disabilities (Shrey & Lacerte, 1995).

7. The functional match of an injured or ill worker to the job is the fundamental principle for transitional work programs.

8. Employers can expedite the RTW process by accurately completing a job analysis for each job category.
   a. *Job analysis* is a process that involves a formal analysis of the tasks associated with a specific job or group of jobs; a job analysis specifically identifies the essential functions of the job.
   b. The job analysis should paint an accurate picture of the essential physical, mental, and environmental requirements of the job and be made available to treating health care professionals to help determine work return dates and job modification requirements.
   c. The treating health care provider is responsible for identifying any job restrictions.
   d. Employers and case managers should use the job analysis to determine transitional duty options (modified or alternative work) for workers released to work with medical restrictions.
   e. The terminology *light duty* has developed a negative connotation; the preferred terminology is *transitional work*.
   f. Transitional work is intended to be temporary and progressive, not a permanent job accommodation.
   g. A time benchmark must be established for limiting and re-evaluating the continuation of transitional effective service results.

9. After 60 to 90 days of temporary transitional work, the RTW team, including the case manager, must evaluate the injured worker's progress, the reality of returning to the original job, and options for a permanent modified position or an alternative position.

10. Six months should be a sufficient time to determine permanence of a worker's recovery unless there are valid contributing variables or extenuating circumstances.

F **There are several considerations when occupational illnesses and injuries occur.**

1. Workers who become ill or injured in circumstances that "arise out of and in the course of employment" are eligible for workers' compensation benefits.

2. In addition, preexisting conditions aggravated by employment are compensable in many jurisdictions.

3. The majority of workers who become ill or injured in most workplaces receive medical treatment and return to work before absences result in payment for lost wages.

4. Generally most lost-time workers' compensation claims result in injured workers returning to full duty in their original position before completing 60 days of transitional work.

G **Employer disability benefits for nonoccupational illnesses and injuries may include the following (see Case Study 2).**

1. Salary continuance
2. Accumulated sick pay
3. Short-term disability

Case Study 2:   *Return to Work for Non-Occupational Disability—Stroke*

Presentation: A 56-year-old male with a job as a warehouse associate at a large manufacturing plant in the Midwest experienced a sudden onset of headache, weakness, and blurred vision, at work. He was transported by ambulance to the local emergency room for evaluation. After a series of diagnostic tests, he was diagnosed with a mild cerebrovascular accident (CVA).

Treatment: The employee was subsequently admitted and aggressively treated as an inpatient for 4 days. Upon his discharge, he was not experiencing any expressive or receptive aphasia or motor deficiencies. Medications included Plavix, 50 mg daily and ASA, 81 mg, daily.

Restrictions: Upon discharge from the hospital, the worker's treating physician restricted him to working half days for one week to be followed by resuming full time work after the initial week.

Initial Issues: The supervisor contacted the nurse case manager with concerns about the return to work and complying with the restrictions. The supervisor cited the potential concern for safety issues with the worker's ability to safely continue driving a forklift truck (safety-sensitive position) as part of his normal job duties.

Implementation: Initial concerns led to a team problem-solving session that resulted in the following:

1. The manager identified an open position for a customer service agent that did not require the worker to drive a forklift.
2. The worker was recognized as a knowledgeable employee, and it was determined that he could be an asset to this position.
3. The supervisor accommodated the week of part-time transitional duty. He agreed to monitoring the employee's condition and to call EMS if any signs and symptoms developed.

RTW Results: The employee was returned to work in one week's time (7 days). The Medical Disability Advisor guidelines for disability duration following a CVA to be 28 to 91 days, depending on the degree of symptoms and the job classification. This worker's new position is classified as light to moderate.

Cost Savings: Most importantly, the company was able to keep an experienced and valued employee. The financial savings include the following:

1. Wages—$17.50 per hour or $140 per day
2. Employee came back to work much earlier than standard guidelines (approximately 28-91 days). If he had been out for this entire time, he would have received 100% salary continuation benefits at $140/day.
3. Savings can be taken as a range from 21 days saved (28 days minus 7 days experienced) = $ 2940 to 84 days saved (91 days minus 7 days experienced) = $11,760. The majority of this was "saved" due to the nurse case management intervention and a proactive return to work that provided transitional work options.

Added Benefit: Management agreed to sponsor employee training in first aid /CPR to review the correct procedures for responding to illness and injury in the warehouse environment with all employees.

Case study prepared by Lori Rieth and Cathy Junor.

a. Conditions and benefit amounts vary per plan description.
b. The benefit is income replacement for a portion of regular earnings as defined by the employer's plan.
c. The length of benefit period can vary; it is generally 26 weeks.
d. This benefit may be statutory in some states (NY, NJ, CA, RI, PR, HI).
e. Workers receiving benefits may be required to provide appropriate documentation from treating medical providers as proof of continued need for benefits, as determined by plan.

    f. Short-term disability (SSD) can bridge to long-term disability or Social Security Disability Insurance (SSDI).

    g. Short-term disability may coordinate benefits with Family and Medical Leave Act (DiBenedetto & Haag, 2000).

4. Long-term disability
    a. Long-term disability is an income replacement plan; it does not cover any medical payments
    b. Plans vary but generally start after 26 weeks or after the STD elimination period.
    c. Plans generally move from STD to LTD
    d. It is desirable for benefits to coordinate with expiration of short-term disability, but it is not always possible to avoid coverage gaps.
    e. The emphasis of long-term disability is on return to work, retraining, or vocational rehabilitation; it is also directed at the advocacy of Social Security benefits.
    f. Long-term disability may coordinate with SSDI, pension, workers' compensation, and other income replacement.
    g. Long-term disability is an employer-sponsored or worker-paid group benefit, not required by statute in most jurisdictions.
    h. After the defined period of time (e.g., two years), a plan may require the worker to meet an "any occupation" provision in order to continue to receive LTD benefits.
       1) The "any occupation" provision is a common requirement of LTD plans, meaning that if the worker is qualified to perform *any* other comparable job or occupation, benefits will cease.
       2) Vocational rehabilitation specialists are often called on to assess the worker's earning capacity to help determine if the worker meets the "any occupation" provision and other criteria and is therefore eligible for continuation of long-term disability benefits.

5. Case managers play a pivotal role in the following:
    a. Coordinating communications with health care providers, ill and injured workers, and employers
    b. Facilitating the worker's timely return to work
    c. Helping the worker reintegrate into the original job as medical restrictions are lifted

VIII Integrated Disability Management Programs

A **Occupational and environmental health nurses recognize that workers' absence from work as a result of either occupational or nonoccupational injuries or illnesses affects the overall work environment and productivity.**
1. Profitable companies understand the value of keeping their employees healthy, safe, and productive at work (Wassel, 2002).
2. These companies consider it a priority to seek prompt, quality health care for ill or injured workers and return them to work as soon as it is medically safe (Wassel, 2002).

B **Payments for medical costs and lost wages may be generated from different sources, but all have a common goal of timely, effective return to work.**
1. Employers purchase workers' compensation insurance as mandated by law, and provide health care and disability benefits to be competitive, and to attract and retain workers.

2. Managed care arrangements are present in both the health care and workers' compensation delivery models.
3. Often medical costs are lower for nonoccupational injuries than for the same conditions treated under workers' compensation benefits under separate programs (Reese, 1998).

C Integrated disability management programs are being developed with efforts to include the following characteristics:
1. Coordinated workers' compensation, short-term disability, FMLA, and long-term disability claims administration
2. Single intake and claims-reporting process
3. Coordinated case management of occupational and nonoccupational disability
4. Coordinated return to work efforts for occupational and nonoccupational disability
5. Integrated information management systems
6. Streamlined administrative processes
7. Disability definitions and regulatory compliance issues consistently defined and managed across all programs that meet the organization's needs and objectives (DiBenedetto & Haag, 2000)
8. Coordinated with other benefit programs (i.e., Employee Assistance Programs [EAP] and disease management)

D Case managers need to help educate medical providers accustomed to working in a non-occupational/managed care environment to understand and embrace the more aggressive return-to-work approach of the workers' compensation system (Reese, 1998).

IX Federal Acts

A There are many regulations that may affect RTW and case management services. These include:
1. Family and Medical Leave Act
2. Americans with Disabilities Act
3. Department of Transportation Drug and Alcohol Testing
4. Employee Retirement Income Security Act
5. Consolidated Omnibus Budget Reconciliation Act

B Case managers must understand the impact of regulations on their workers' particular situations and craft their case management plans accordingly.

X Delivery Models

A *On-site (in-person) case management* refers to services provided in-person with the disabled worker at various locations (home, treatment facilities, workplaces, etc.).
1. Advantages of on-site case management include:
   a. Provides opportunities to establish a firmer, more trusting professional relationship with the worker (Donofrio, 1997)
   b. Allows first-hand observation of the worker's medical condition and his or her response to and compliance with treatment (Alliotta, 1999)
   c. Allows more opportunities to identify personal, familial, environmental, and other factors that may impede the worker's progress in recovery (Donofrio, 1997)

    d. Once a more comprehensive evaluation of all impacting factors is done, more appropriate interventions can be developed for the case management plan (Donofrio, 1997)

  2. Disadvantages of on-site case management include:

    a. Services are costlier because of the travel and time involved to meet parties involved in the case (Donofrio, 1997).

    b. On-site case managers must always justify the benefit of their services in relation to the cost to overcome skepticism of some consumers (Mullahy, 2004).

B *Telephonic case management (TCM)* **refers to services provided by telephone by employer representatives or vendor representatives hired to perform the services (Donofrio, 1997).**

  1. Advantages of TCM include:

    a. Allows more immediate assessment of case management needs

    b. Establishes at least some level of rapport with the worker and family immediately upon identification of an injury or disabling diagnosis

    c. Communicates concern for the worker's well being, helping to avoid misunderstandings and feelings of abandonment by the worker

    d. Allows early opportunity to ease the workers' fears and anxieties by educating them regarding policies, procedures, and jurisdictional requirements, which they need to understand and navigate in the course of their treatment and recovery (Aron, 1997; Bechtel, 1998; Donofrio, 1997)

    e. Reduces anxiety, which in turn reduces the need to seek education from outside sources, such as legal counsel or poorly informed family and friends (Reese, 1998)

    f. Facilitates communication between worker and supervisor to reduce anxiety and resolve concerns the worker may have about job security, relationship with their supervisor, etc. (Aron, 1997)

    g. Allows immediate communication with health care providers to facilitate appropriate treatment, overall case management planning, and interventions (Aron, 1997; Donofrio, 1997; Wright & Eggleston, 1997)

    h. Establishes the telephonic case manager as a coordinator and point of contact for the worker, health care providers, and employer

    i. Quickly identifies needs requiring on-site evaluation or additional medical interventions, that otherwise could have been delayed

    j. Reduces costs compared with on-site case management services, because of the travel and time involved to perform on-site services

    k. Because of reduced costs, allows employers and insurers to offer services to larger numbers of workers

    l. Because it allows earlier intervention, TCM facilitates earlier resolution of cases or identification of severe cases requiring more comprehensive on-site case management services (Donofrio, 1997)

  2. Disadvantages of TCM include:

    a. It is more challenging to form personal and trusting relationships telephonically than in person with workers, health care providers, and other parties.

    b. Dependence on verbal information from workers and others may limit the identification of issues that could have been identified with an on-site visit (Donofrio, 1997).

    c. Multiple state licenses may be required for nurses providing case management services over different jurisdictions.

    d. Because of its cost-effectiveness, TCM may be used even when factors indicate more-comprehensive on-site services (e.g., catastrophic cases) (Donofrio, 1997; Wright & Eggleston, 1997).

    e. Telephonic case managers need to be mindful of their liability when providing services in this manner; concerns about liabilities may limit the case manager's ability to provide comprehensive information.

    f. Frequently, the caseload for TCM nurses is higher than on-site caseloads, potentially limiting their effectiveness.

    g. A high-volume caseload can restrict services to a cursory level, perhaps leading to missed follow-up or confusion of cases.

3. Ethical considerations are as follows:

    a. Because on-site case managers have opportunities to develop more personal relationships with all parties of a case, they need to recognize their own and others' limitations.

    b. Programs limit or dictate the benefits available to the worker.

    c. Case managers need a clear understanding of when they may or may not go outside of a program for other available resources.

    d. If case managers do obtain resources outside a program, it is important to know under what circumstances and by what source their time and expenses will be compensated.

    e. Case managers must be diligent in their ethical conduct and avoid any coercion by referral sources to perform or authorize questionable services.

    f. On-site case management should not be used as a substitute for fraud investigation or surveillance on a case.

REFERENCES

Alliotta, S. (1999). Patient adherence outcome indicators and measurement in case management and health care. *Care Management.* 5(4), 24-81.

American Association of Occupational Health Nurses. (2003). Competencies in occupational and environmental health nursing. *AAOHN Journal, 51*(7), 290-302.

American Association of Occupational Health Nurses. (2004a). *Standards of occupational and environmental health nursing.* Atlanta, GA: AAOHN Publications.

American Association of Occupational Health Nurses. (2004b) *Foundation blocks: A guide to occupational & environmental health nursing. Absence Management Program.* Atlanta, GA: AAOHN Publications.

American Association of Occupational Health Nurses. (2004c). *Position statement: The occupational health nurse as a case manager.* Retrieved on January 3, 2005 at http://www.aaohn.org/.

American Association of Occupational Health Nurses and Case Management Society of America. (2003). *Joint position statement: Role of occupational and environmental health nurses and nurse case managers in protecting confidentiality of health information.* Atlanta, GA. AAOHN Publications.

American College of Occupational and Environmental Medicine. (2004). *Occupational medicine practice guidelines* (2nd ed). Beverly Farms, MA. OEM Press.

American Nurses Association. (1988). *Nursing case management.* Kansas City, MO: Task Force on Case Management.

Aron, L. J. (1997). What's up with workers' compensation? *Care Management, 3*(3), 16-20.

Bechtel, G., Newman-Giger, J., & Davidhizar, R. (1998). Case managing patients from other cultures. *Care Management, 4*(5), 87-91.

Bureau of Labor Statistics (2004). *Workplace injuries and illnesses in 2003.* Washington DC: US Department of Labor.

Burton, W. N. and Conti, D. J. (2000). Disability management: Corporate medical department management of Employee health and productivity. *Journal of Occupational and Environmental Medicine, 42*(10), 1006-1012.

Case Management Society of America. (2002). *Standards of practice for case management.* Little Rock, AR: Case Management Society of America.

Childre, F. (1997). Nurse managed occupational health services: A primary care model in practice. *AAOHN Journal, 45*(10), 484-490.

Consumers and managed care. (1997, February 9). *The New York Times,* p. 14.

Curtis, J., & Scott, L. R. (2004). Integrating disability management into strategic plans. *AAOHN Journal, 52*(7), 298-301.

DiBenedetto, D. V., & Haag, A. B. (2000). *Principles of workers' compensation and disability case management,* Vol. 1. Yonkers, NY: DVD & Associates.

Donofrio, J.M. (1997, Summer). Telephonic case management: Does it work and who really benefits? *Case Review,* 34-37.

Denniston, P. L., & Whelan, P. (2005). Benchmarking medical absence: Measuring the impact of occupational health nursing. *AAOHN Journal, 53*(2), 84-93.

Dyck, D. E. (2000). *Disability management: Theory, strategy and industry practice.* Markham, Ontario: Butterworths Canada Ltd.

Fireman's Fund Insurance Company. (1997). *SmartCARE return to work guide.* Novato, CA: Fireman's Fund Insurance Company.

Gilpin, S. (2000). Disability management: It takes a pro to solve the puzzle. *Business & Health, 18*(2), 37-39.

Gliniecki, C. M.., & Burgel, B. J. (1995). Temporary work restrictions: Guidelines for the primary care provider. *Nurse Practitioner Forum, 6*(2), 79-89.

Head, G. L. (1997). *Essentials of risk management* (3rd ed.), Vol. 1. Malvern, PA: Insurance Institute of America.

Hessellund, T. A., & Cox, R. (1996). Vocational case managers in early return-to-work agreements. *Care Management, 2(6),* 34-78.

Mashburn, K., & Mitchell, K. (2001). The role of the case manager in an impairment-based return-to-work process. *Case Manager, 12*(1), 58-61.

Mobley, E. M., Linz, D. H., Shukla, R., Breslin, R. E., & Deng, C. (2000). Disability case management: An impact assessment in an automotive manufacturing organization. *Journal of Occupational and Environmental Medicine, 42*(6), 597-602.

Mullahy, C. M. (2004). *The case manager's handbook* (3rd ed.). Gaithersburg, MD: Aspen Publishers, Inc.

Reed, P. (2005). *The medical disability advisor: Workplace guidelines for disability duration.* (5th ed.). Westminster, CO: The Reed Group.

Reese, S. (1998). Integration: The case for blended benefits. *Business and Health, 16*(4), 62-69.

Rieth, L. (2000). The occupational health service: Staffing, facilities and equipment. *AAOHN Journal, 48*(8), 395-404.

Rooney, E. (1990). Corporate attitudes and responses in rising health care costs. *AAOHN Journal, 38*(7), 304-311.

Salazar, M. K., Graham, K. Y., & Lantz, B. (1999). Evaluating case management services for injured workers: Use of a quality assessment model. *AAOHN Journal, 47*(8), 348-354.

Shrey, D. E., & Lacerte, M. (1995). *Principles and practices of disability management in industry.* Boca Raton, FL: CRC Press.

Strasser, P. (2004). Managing transitional work—Program foundation. *AAOHN Journal, 52*(8), 323-326.

U.S. Chamber of Commerce. (1999). *Analysis of workers' compensation laws.* Washington, DC: U.S. Chamber of Commerce. (NOTE: This document is prepared and published annually and is an excellent reference for details on workers' compensation laws. To order call toll free, 800-638-6582).

U.S. Department of Health and Human Services. (1994). *Acute low back problems in adults: Assessment and treatment* (AHCPR No. 95-0643). Rockville, MD: Public Health Service, Agency for Health Care, Policy and Research.

Washington State Department of Labor and Industries (1994). *Industrial insurance: glossary.* Olympia, WA: State of Washington Department of Labor and Industries.

Wassel, M. L. (1995). Occupational health nursing and the advent of managed care: Meeting the challenges of the current health care environment. *AAOHN Journal, 43*(1), 23-28.

Wassel, M. L. (2002). Improving return to work outcomes: Formalizing the process. *AAOHN Journal, 50*(6), 275-285.

Watson Wyatt Wordwide. (2001). *Staying @ work: Integrated disability management around the world—2000/2001*. Retrieved October 10, 2004, from http://www.watsonwyatt.com/homepage/images/database_uploads/w376global/Swwp2000.pdf.

Wolfe, G. S. (1998). Cost savings and case management. *Care Management, 4*(5), 5.

Work Loss Data Institute. (2005). *Official disability guidelines* 2005, (10th ed.). Encinitas, CA: Work Loss Data Institute.

Work Loss Data Institute. (2005). *Official disability guidelines treatment in worker's comp.* (3rd ed.). Encinitas, CA: Work Loss Data Institute.

Wright, L. & Eggleston, M. (1997) Catastrophic case management. *Case Review, 3*(3), 59-61.

CHAPTER

13

Disaster Planning and Management

MARILYN L. HAU

Disaster management poses challenges that are distinct from normal predictable emergencies. It requires a paradigm change from the application of unlimited resources for the greatest good of each individual client, to the allocation of limited resources for the greatest good to the greatest number of casualties. This is achieved most effectively by planning and training for disasters (Frykberg 2003). While no one wants to overreact, occupational and environmental health nurses must recognize their responsibilities to the employer and the employee population through disaster planning and management.

I Disaster Characteristics

A "Disasters are events that occur when significant numbers of people are exposed to hazards to which they are vulnerable, with resulting injury and loss of life, often combined with damage to property and livelihoods" (Wisner & Adams, 2002).

1. Disaster events can be caused by nature, technology, human conflict, or a combination of these (Table 13-1).
2. Disasters exceed the capacity of the affected community to respond effectively; thus they require outside assistance.

TABLE 13-1

Disaster potential hazards: a few examples

Natural	Technological	Conflict
Firestorms	Hazmat spills	Riots
Flood	Explosions	Strikes
Landshift	Utility failure	Suicide bombings
Tornado	Building collapse	Bomb threat
Epidemic	Transportation accident	Employee violence
Earthquake	Power outage	Mass shootings
Volcano	Nuclear accident	Equipment sabotage
Hurricane	Dam failure	Hostage events
High winds	Fire	Transportation disruption
Blizzard	Water loss	Weapons of mass destruction
Heat wave	Ruptured gas main	Computer viruses/worms

3. Disasters can be classified by several parameters, such as the number of fatalities, the number of ill and/or injured, the length of time for the impact, the rescue time, or the radius of the disaster area.
4. Measurement devices are used to determine the magnitude of natural events (Wisner & Adams, 2002).
   a. Richter scale is used to measure the magnitude of an earthquake.
   b. Modified Mercalli Intensity (MMI) is a subjective measurement used to describe the intensity, or nature and spatial extent of the damage from an earthquake.
   c. Saffir-Simpson scale is used to measure the strength of hurricanes.
   d. Fujita scale is used to measure the strength of tornadoes.
5. *Na-tech disasters* are technological emergencies that result from natural disasters (called *joint disasters*). Examples are an earthquake causing ruptured natural gas lines and fires, or a tornado causing a chemical tank breach and chemical spill (Wisner & Adams, 2002).
   a. Response will be required for both events simultaneously.
   b. There is likely to be more than one technologic event, since the natural disaster may affect several industrial facilities in the disaster zone.
   c. Major utilities (e.g., water, power, communications) may be disrupted.
   d. Mitigation efforts may not work as anticipated because of the upset from the natural disaster.
6. Disasters may cause mass-casualty incidents (MCI) that limit the ability of the occupational and environmental health nurse to provide definitive care to the victims due to the numbers, severity, and diversity of injuries.
7. Several factors contribute to the increased probability and the severity of the consequences of disasters.
   a. The risk of disasters is greater today as a result of a growing population, more technology, and increased political turbulence resulting in the threat of terrorism.
   b. Nature has not become more violent; rather, people have become more vulnerable due to mass migration, urbanization, building in high-risk areas such as earthquake faults and coastal hurricane areas, and war causing more people to live in exposed places with fewer resources to fall back on.
   c. Technologic disasters are more frequent and severe as a result of increased complexity and dependency in areas such as telecommunications, computer systems, high-rise buildings, widespread power-supply grids, and global marketing.
8. "Interest in disaster preparedness is proportional to the recency and magnitude of the last disaster" (Auf der Heide, 1989).
9. Disasters are never identical.
10. Disaster nursing is "the systematic and flexible utilization of knowledge and skills specific to disaster-related nursing, and the promotion of a wide range of activities to minimize the health hazards and life threatening damage caused by disasters in collaboration with other specialized fields" (Society of Disaster Nursing, 2002).

B **"Emergencies are any natural or manmade situations that result in severe injury, harm, or loss" of humans, property and/or environment (Wisner & Adams, 2002).**
1. Emergencies are individual situations that can arise out of disasters where rapid and effective action is required to prevent further loss of life and livelihood (Wisner & Adams, 2002).

2. Daily emergencies can be managed by mobilizing additional personnel and resources. Disasters cannot be managed this way (Veenema, 2003).

3. "The degree and effectiveness of preparedness often spell the difference between emergency and disaster" (Kelly 1989).

C **Various disaster models have been developed; several describe the sequence of events and activities that occur in the course of a disaster.**

1. The Disaster Life Cycle model consists of several general phases (Wisner & Adams, 2002) (Figure 13-1).
   a. The *prodromal* phase is the warning period when signs or public announcements occur. Evacuation or taking shelter may occur in this phase if there is sufficient time.
   b. The *impact* phase is when the disaster-causing event occurs. It may be short, as in a tornado, or more prolonged, as in a hurricane.
   c. The *rescue* or *emergency* phase is the period when immediate assistance is provided by bystanders and first responders.
   d. The *recovery* or *reconstruction* phase is the period when all the necessary services and resources are applied to return to predisaster conditions. This may last for days, months, or years.
   e. The *quiescent* or *interdisaster* phase is the period between disaster events.

2. Another model for disaster chronology is defined by the use of a timeline (Veenema, 2003).
   a. The *preimpact* phase includes planning/preparedness and disaster warning.
   b. The *impact* phase is divided into 0-24 hours and 24-72 hours. It includes response and emergency management.
   c. The *postimpact* phase begins after 72 hours with efforts aimed at recovery, rehabilitation, reconstruction, and evaluation.

3. The Jennings Disaster Nursing Management Model (Figure 13-2) was developed to assist educators to add disaster nursing to community health nursing courses. It enables community nurses to plan for and manage disasters in conjunction with other personnel in each of the segments of each phase of the model (Jennings-Saunders, 2004).

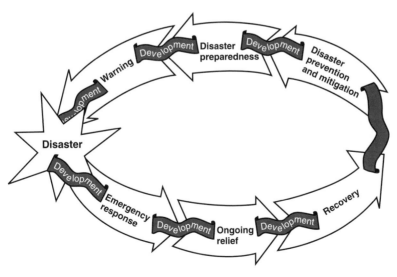

FIGURE 13-1 *The disaster cycle*

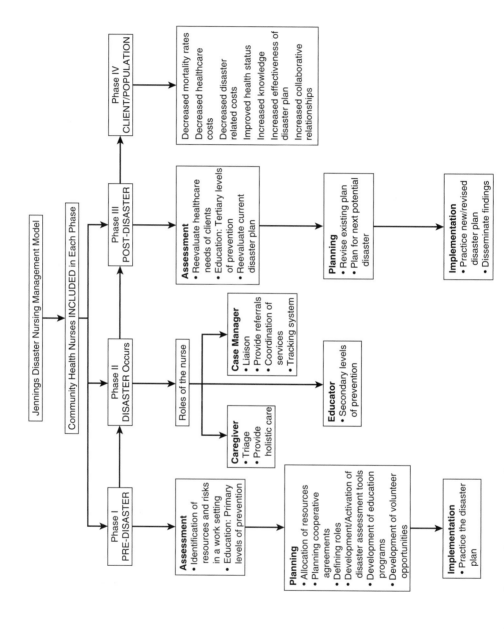

FIGURE 13-2 *Jennings Disaster Nursing Management Model*

Source: Jennings-Saunders, 2004.

a. Phase I (pre-disaster) includes assessment, planning, primary prevention education, and plan practice activities.

b. Phase II (disaster) includes direct nursing care provision, case management, and secondary prevention education activities.

c. Phase III (post-disaster) requires client needs reassessment, tertiary prevention level education, a reevaluation and revision of the disaster plan, and communication of the experiences and findings.

d. Phase IV (positive client/population outcomes) defines outcome expectations. Examples are decreased mortality rates and costs, improved knowledge and health status, and improvement in disaster plan effectiveness and collaboration. Phases I through III impact these outcomes.

II Disaster Planning and Preparedness

Disaster planning and preparedness occur during the pre-disaster phase. *Planning* includes the determinations made with others on how to respond and manage resources if a disaster event occurs; *preparedness* includes the measures taken and policies formed before an event occurs that allow for prevention, mitigation, and readiness. "A rededication to preparedness is perhaps the best way to honor the memories of those we lost that [September 11, 2001] day." (National Commission on Terrorist Attacks Upon the United States 2004).

A **Regardless of the cause or phase of a disaster, disaster planning and preparedness share common overall problems (Auf der Heide, 1989).**

1. "Conventional wisdom" and routine emergency response don't work. Disasters often pose unique problems rarely faced in daily emergencies, such as blocked access, inadequate resources, unfamiliar tasks and procedures, unfamiliar faces and roles, overload of communications, and the need for interorganizational coordination.

2. Disaster problems cross interdisciplinary boundaries, triggering the mobilization of resources not ordinarily used in local emergencies. The normal procedures for emergency response do not adapt as well to the disaster situation.

3. Actual human attitudes often differ from what one might expect.
   a. Some people have experienced the periphery of disaster events and, as a result, they mistakenly underestimate the risk and overestimate their ability to survive the event.
   b. Overestimation of an entity's capability to deal with a disaster is called the *Robinson Crusoe syndrome*. (We're the only ones on the island.) The result is neither collaboration nor a coherent overall strategy.
   c. Fatalism and denial are manifested in comments such as "There's nothing to worry about because nothing can be done about it anyhow," and "It can't happen here."
   d. People may be lulled by a false sense of security when precautionary measures are in place; for example, they may assume that flood control projects prevent all floods.
   e. Some responders have a need to be identified as heroes by their peers and others. They add to the problem—and often to the number of victims.

4. There are multiple organizational barriers to preparing for and responding to a disaster:

a. In some cases, no institution, person, or government agency is seen as responsible or accountable for disaster preparedness; persons or groups perceive that it is "not my [our] job."
b. Competing demands for resources needed to prepare for disasters may be at the bottom of the list of priorities.
c. Often disaster responses are plagued with over-response from untrained volunteers, miscommunication in resource allocations, lack of incident command, and sightseers.
d. Persons in authority at an agency or organization may assume command because they are the "boss;" however, they may not have the necessary expertise or training.
5. Groups and organizations can contribute in various ways to ineffective disaster response; for example, vested interest groups can create the setup for disasters, such as the rights of property owners to build in flood prone areas.
6. Because companies, local agencies, and organizations experience the fewest exposures to disaster loss compared to the state or nation, they are the least apt to perceive disaster planning and resources as important issues.

B **There are many actual and potential benefits to a workplace to plan and prepare for disaster events.**
1. Protection of workers, citizens, and the environment is a moral responsibility, as are Western values of goodness, truth, and justice (Schneider, 2000); planning and preparedness help companies meet these responsibilities.
2. Criminal charges are now appearing in the pursuit of legal responsibility in industrial disasters (Schneider, 2000); planning and preparedness help companies avoid these risks.
3. Planning and preparedness may reduce disaster impacts and, consequently, exposure to civil liability in the event of an incident.
4. Several different regulatory programs require planning under such names as emergency response plans, emergency action plans, contingency plans emergency and fire prevention plans, and risk management plans (Table 13-2).

TABLE 13-2

OSHA regulations requiring emergency plans

Standard	Type of Plan
29 CFR 1910.35 36, 37	Means of Egress
29 CFR 1910.38	Emergency Plans and Fire Prevention Plans
29 CFR 1910.119	Process Safety Management of Highly Hazardous Chemicals
29 CFR 1910.120	Hazardous Waste Operations and Emergency Response
29 CFR 1910.146	Permit-Required Confined Spaces for General Industry
29 CFR 1910.151	Medical Services and First Aid
29 CFR 1910.156	Fire Brigades
29 CFR 1910.158	Portable Fire Extinguishers
29 CFR 1910.159	Automatic Sprinkler System
29 CFR 1910.160	Fixed Extinguishing Systems
29 CFR 1910.165	Employee Alarm Systems

5. Costs of addressing the effects of a disaster only after it has happened will be much greater than they would be if preparations were taken in advance (Federal Emergency Management Agency [FEMA], 2004).

6. Local, state, and federal aid is usually insufficient to cover the extent of resulting damages.

7. Planning and preparedness can lessen the impact of a disaster and speed the response and recovery phases, enhancing a company's ability to recover from financial losses, regulatory fines, loss of market share, damages to equipment or products, or business interruption (Jones et al., 2000).

   a. 47% of businesses that experience a fire or major theft go out of business within two years.

   b. 44% of companies that lose records in a disaster never resume business.

   c. 93% of companies that experience a significant data loss are out of business within five years.

   d. The majority of businesses spend less then 3% of their total budget on business recovery planning.

8. Disaster preparedness and planning enhance a company's image and credibility with employees, customers, suppliers, and the community.

9. Disaster preparedness and planning may reduce insurance premiums or make the difference in whether or not an insurance carrier will contract to provide coverage.

10. All organizations are vulnerable to disaster events: it's not a matter of "if" it will happen, but "when."

11. Lessons learned from recent events suggest that integration of occupational and environmental health into public health should lead to an all-hazards approach, with better overall disaster preparedness (Sokas & Perrotta, 2003).

C **Disaster preparedness has reached a new level of urgency, mandating that nurses be able to function effectively in disaster situations (Jennings-Saunders, 2004).**

1. Because occupational and environmental nurses have regular interaction with workers, the workplace, and the community, they are likely to be aware of the strengths and needs of clients, enabling them to assess and respond holistically in disaster events.

2. Occupational health nurses have a long history of protecting workers from the adverse effects of a multitude of workplace exposures; they are well positioned to serve on the frontlines of the terrorist affront to workers (Salazar, 2002).

D **There are several different types of plans, some of which have specifically defined functions for particular agents, and others which are broader in scope to cover all potential hazards; the priority in all plans is life safety.**

1. The *Emergency Action Plan* is required by the Occupational Safety and Health Administration (OSHA) to ensure that worker evacuation plans and drills have been developed, particularly in response to facility fires.

2. The *Business Continuity Plan* focuses on policies, practices, and activities that reduce business losses and enhance actions to resume operations; it requires that all operations performed by a particular unit or component be listed, prioritized, and identified as to their importance to continued business operations.

   a. Critical operations are those operations a business cannot do without or that have a role that is vital to the operation and/or may pose a life-safety risk. For each critical business activity, mitigation strategies should be implemented and a recovery process developed.

b. Essential operations are not critical, but are difficult to operate without, although the facility could function for awhile without them.

c. For nonessential operations, interruption would merely be an inconvenience.

3. The *Risk Management Plan* evaluates potential off-site consequences of chemical releases.

   a. It requires the identification of "worst case scenarios" and how they will be managed.

   b. 40 CFR Part 68 Risk Management programs for Chemical Accidental Release Prevention is an Environmental Protection Agency (EPA)-mandated plan.

4. The *Emergency Response Plan (ERP)* governs the immediate response to a disaster to provide life safety, rescue, damage control, evacuation and/or sheltering-in-place; OSHA requires an ERP for hazardous waste sites and hazardous materials spill response (29 CFR 1910.120).

5. The *Contingency Plan* is a generalized emergency plan to handle unforeseen events not identified in a hazard and risk assessment.

6. The *Federal Response Plan* coordinates federal resources in any disaster or emergency situation in which there is need for federal assistance, as identified in the Robert T. Stafford Disaster Relief and Emergency Assistance Act (42 U.S.C. 5121 et seq.).

7. The *Spill Prevention, Control and Countermeasures Plan (SPCC)* describes measures to prevent, contain, and clean up oil spills; its intent is to protect waterways from oil contamination.

   a. A facility is required to have an SPCC plan if it meets the following criteria:

      1) It is non–transportation-related.

      2) It has above-ground capacity greater than 1,320 gallons or buried capacity greater than 42,000 gallons.

      3) There is a reasonable expectation that a spill could occur to navigable U.S. waters.

   b. SPCC plans are required by federal regulation 40 CFR 112, which is implemented by the Environmental Protection Agency.

   c. The plan includes procedures to be followed to prevent oil spills from occurring.

   d. It also provides procedures for responding to and controlling oil spills at the facility.

8. A *Mutual Aid Plan* calls for participating firms to share resources to help each other during an emergency.

   a. This is especially helpful for small facilities with limited resources and for larger facilities with significant hazards.

   b. Mutual aid agreements are also instituted among community first-responder agencies.

9. *Recovery Plans* govern the repair and rebuilding, including prioritization of facilities and communities after a disaster.

10. An *Emergency Management Plan* is required by the Joint Commission for Accreditation of Healthcare Organizations for hospital, ambulatory care, behavioral health, home care, and long-term care facilities (Joint Commission Resources, 2001).

    a. This plan is required under the following Environment of Care (EC) standards:

1) EC.1.4 to develop the plan using the four phases of mitigation, preparedness, response, and recovery
2) EC.2.4 to implement the plan
3) EC.2.9.1 to execute the plan by conducting drills

b. The plan must include emergencies that develop within the organization or facility and handling of patient care demands from emergencies occurring in the community.
c. The plan has extensive requirements, including the requirement for an incident command structure and a known Hospital Emergency Incident Command System (HEICS) that links to the community structure.

11. An *All-Hazard Disaster Management Plan (DMP)* is the most broad in scope.
   a. The DMP covers natural disasters and man-made disasters. Manmade disasters can be subdivided into technologic disasters and conflict-induced disasters.
   b. The plan incorporates all of the other more specific plans, including emergency response plans and business recovery/continuity plans.
   c. The ultimate goal of the DMP is to predict and prepare for the unpredictable (Hans, 1995).

E **The All-Hazard Disaster Management Plan serves as an excellent template for a disaster plan.**

1. The objectives for the all-hazard disaster plan are:
   a. To eliminate or reduce the chance of a disaster occurring
   b. To reduce the resulting impact, injury, illness, and/or damage
   c. To use emergency response to prevent additional harm
   d. To strengthen the ability to withstand disruption of infrastructure (e.g., vital building and community services such as water, sanitation, and transportation)
   e. To enable rapid recovery and restoration of production, services, and pre-disaster conditions

2. There are several key principles that determine the success or failure of the plan.
   a. Support of upper management is essential; if production considerations always supersede preparedness, planning efforts will be sabotaged by low prioritization.
   b. Disaster planning requires the expertise of many people; planners may include representatives of company management, occupational health and safety personnel, human resources, risk managers, accounting, security, and union representatives.
      1) More people will be participating and investing in the plan.
      2) The plan experiences increased visibility and importance.
      3) The plan receives a more broad perspective on key issues.
      4) Important networking and collaborative relationships can develop.
   c. Businesses must avoid the attitude that they can handle events by themselves; planning must be done in partnership with community resources (Archibald et al., 2002).
   d. The planning process takes time and proper project management; during this process, an interim plan should be developed to provide some initial guidance (Wallace & Webber, 2004).
   e. The occupational and environmental health nurse should be prepared to be the prime mover, or motivating force, for the plan.

F **A logical progression of activities can be followed to develop a disaster management plan.**

1. A first step is to establish a planning team.
   a. Some persons may be active members while others may serve as advisors.
   b. Input from personnel in all key functional areas should be obtained, including upper and line management, environmental health and safety, occupational and environmental health, human resources, maintenance, security, public relations, marketing, legal, financial, purchasing, telecommunications and other workers in accordance with the size and sophistication of the facility.
   c. Team appointments should be made in writing from upper management.
2. A clear line of authority between group members and the group chairperson should be defined.
   a. Senior management should give and announce the authority to the planning team to develop the plan.
   b. The authority may be provided through a mission statement.
3. There are several logistical preparations that need to be completed.
   a. Preliminary deadlines and timelines should be established.
   b. Progressive budgetary needs should also be outlined, such as consulting fees, travel fees, research costs, clerical costs, and other expenses.
4. All existing plans should be located and reviewed. These may include a site evacuation plan, fire protection plan, security procedures, bomb threat procedure, hazardous materials response plan, risk management plan, and others.

G **A logical progression of activities can be followed in analyzing potential disasters to include in the disaster management plan.**

1. Conduct a *hazards identification,* determining what adverse events are possible. (See Table 13-1.)
   a. *Hazard* is "the potential for harm or damage to people, property, or the environment" (Manuele, 2003).
   b. All hazards with a potential for a disaster that could occur within a facility, or that could occur within the community and would affect the facility, should be identified.
   c. Sources of information regarding hazards include knowledgeable company representatives, knowledgeable community agencies and representatives, health and safety professionals, professional publications and courses, area historical data, government agencies' data, and news media.
   d. Business functions should be identified according to their critical functions and the amount of time they can be inoperative.
2. Next, perform a *vulnerability assessment.*
   a. Vulnerability is the degree to which a population or an individual is unable to anticipate, cope with, resist, and recover from the impacts of disasters; it is a function of susceptibility, resistance, and resilience.
      1) *Susceptibility* is a product of social, political, economic, and cultural forces and activities that determine the proneness of individuals and groups to being adversely affected by disaster.
      2) *Resistance* is the ability of buildings and the infrastructure to resist the strain or force exerted by natural or human-induced agents.
      3) *Resilience* is the amount of coping capacity.
   b. Each identified hazard should be reviewed for potential human loss, property loss, economic impact, and environmental impact.

    c. Relevant questions include: What is the vulnerable location? What population exists within this location? What essential services, facilities, and environmental systems exist within this zone?

    d. Each business function, component, or department should conduct its own individual risk assessments (Jones et al, 2000).

        1) They should examine all the processes they perform and critical areas or activities that are necessary to avoid significant loss of revenue, customers, or business operation.

        2) When combined, these individual assessments compose the risk assessment for the entire business.

    e. The capabilities that exist and that would prevent or respond to the identified hazards and consequently reduce vulnerability should be determined.

        1) This may include existing response plans, available emergency response equipment, and plant security.

        2) The number of trained on-site responders, experience, site expertise, equipment, supplies, facilities, contract services, community response capabilities, detection and alarm devices, data backup resources, site security, and archive practices should be considered.

    f. Worst-case assumptions for each hazard should be used in the vulnerability analysis.

    g. When evaluating business interruption, the amount of time a business interruption can be tolerated without causing critical disruption should be considered (Jones et al, 2000).

        1) Immediate—0 to 24 hours. (May require immediate alternate or "hot" site)

        2) Delayed—24 hours to 7 days. (Prearranged site that would be needed for a short period)

        3) Deferred—Beyond 7 days. (No immediate need for an offsite location)

    h. Business functions can also be assessed by their degree of vulnerability to each potential threat or hazard (Jones et al, 2000):

        1) Highly vulnerable—Those business functions that have a great risk of experiencing a threat or hazard.

        2) Vulnerable—May experience a threat or hazard.

        3) Not Vulnerable—Threat or hazard not likely to occur

3. The next step is to set priorities by performing a risk analysis.

    a. *A risk analysis* evaluates and compares different hazards by assigning a measure to the hazards and ranking them.

    b. *Risk* is a possibility of suffering harm from a hazard, while a hazard is a substance or action than can cause harm.

    c. Determine how probable it is that the hazard could occur.

    d. Determine how severe this hazard could be in consequences compared to others identified and analyzed.

    e. Determine how vulnerable the affected location and persons are to the hazard and its severity; in other words, how great is the risk with one hazard compared to the others.

4. The final product of these analyses is a list of potential disasters identified by priority for the purposes of mitigation, preparedness, response, and recovery. (Refer to Chapter 6 for further information on quantifying risks.)

H **After organizing resources for plan development and prioritizing hazards based on a risk analysis, the next critical activity to perform is *mitigation*.**

    1. *Mitigation* is the effort to eliminate hazards or lessen the impact of an event should it occur.

2. Examples are storing critical data off site, substituting less-hazardous raw materials in a process, or reinforcing storage tanks in an earthquake-prone area.
3. Mitigation efforts should be initiated according to the priorities set by the risk analysis.

I **Basic response preparedness is the next step in the disaster planning process.**

1. *Response* consists of efforts that are made during and immediately after a disaster to assist victims and reduce the likelihood of secondary harm.
2. The response period begins with the notification or warning and lasts until the critical incident is resolved.
3. Detailed response plans must cover several key elements.
   a. An alarm system must be established with distinctive signals utilized if it is a multipurpose alarm system.
   b. The preferred means of reporting fires and other emergencies must be identified.
   c. The evacuation of personnel must be planned.
      1) The type of evacuation must be designated, such as total or partial evacuation of certain areas of a plant, based on the nature and extent of the emergency.
      2) Emergency escape procedures and emergency escape route assignments must be included.
      3) Procedures to be followed by employees who remain to operate critical plant operations before they evacuate must be identified.
      4) Procedures to account for all employees after emergency evacuation has been completed need to be established.
   d. Sheltering-in-place may need to be considered as an alternative to evacuation; sheltering-in-place is accomplished by selecting a location with no or few windows and taking refuge there (American Red Cross, 2004).
      1) Chemical, biological, or radiologic contaminants released into the environment can make evacuation unsafe; staying inside where exposure is less could be preferable.
      2) In some circumstances, it is recommended that the location air intakes be closed off.
      3) Human behaviors should be kept in mind; having workers remain at a facility sheltered-in-place versus evacuating to their cars and going home can be difficult to enforce if the employees do not have an understanding of sheltering-in-place concepts and how, in certain situations, they are safer than by evacuating.
   e. Plans must include procedures for persons with disabilities.
      1) The hearing impaired will need direct notification or visual warnings.
      2) The visually impaired may need audible or vibratory notification.
      3) Nonambulatory personnel may need special rescue services by trained responders, or may need to have an area of rescue assistance with fire code compliance and two-way communications established.
   f. Rescues and medical duties for employees who are to perform them should be outlined.
   g. The person in charge can vary according to the nature of the emergency, such as medical versus hazardous materials release; it is essential to determine who this person is.
   h. A list of the company personnel who should be notified in the various cases of emergencies should be developed.

1) The means to summon and communicate with them throughout the emergency should be determined.
2) Names or regular job titles of persons or departments who can be contacted for further information or explanation of duties should also be identified.
3) A list of community agencies to be called should be available; methods of communication should be determined.

CAUTION: Do not assume that community response agencies are able to handle any facility emergency. For instance, many emergency medical services will not accept for treatment or transport a chemically contaminated patient. Company-trained personnel must decontaminate the patient first.

J **The final activity in planning is implementing the plan.**
1. The plan should be reviewed with all personnel when it is completed, on initial assignment of a new employee, when employee responsibilities change or the plan changes, and annually or more often as needed.
2. Training to meet plan requirements should be implemented; training needs may include fire equipment and response, use of personal protective equipment, first aid and cardiopulmonary resuscitation (CPR), decontamination procedures, bomb threat procedures, and others.
3. An emergency response team should be trained, if this is needed and feasible.
4. The plan should be tested through practice evacuations, sheltering-in-place, documented tests of alarm systems, communications systems tests, fire response equipment inspections, and other plan elements.
5. One or more of the various practice drills of the plan should be conducted when more advanced response is planned. The types of drills are as follows:
   a. Orientation—Briefing or low-stress training to familiarize participants with team roles, responsibilities, and expectations; this provides a good overview of the emergency response plan.
   b. Tabletop—Limited simulation or scenario of an emergency situation to evaluate plans, procedures, coordination, and assignment of resources.
   c. Functional—Limited involvement or simulation by field operations to test communication, preparedness, and availability/deployment of operational resources.
   d. Full-scale—Conducted in an environment created to simulate a real-life situation.
6. Review and update the plan frequently, at least once a year.

III Disaster Response

The response phase is the point at which emergency actions are started to save lives, property, and the environment, and to prevent secondary harm. "Emergency response is a product of preparedness." (National Commission on Terrorist Attacks Upon the United States, 2004). There are five basic stages of response to an emergency or disaster: recognition, notification/warning, immediate employee safety, community/public safety, property protection, and environmental protection.

A **The length of each stage depends on the emergency situation; for example, the notification/warning stage for a hurricane may be several hours, whereas the notification stage for an explosion may be minutes or only seconds.**
1. The priority ranking in emergency response is persons, then property, then environment.

2. Each stage depends on effort in earlier stages; for example, the extent to which evacuation assures immediate employee safety greatly influences whether response can be refocused to property.
3. Property protection deals with property at the emergency scene as well as protecting property on which the event may impinge.
4. Environmental protection involves reduction and elimination of emergency incidents affecting air, waterways and groundwater, soil, and wildlife.

B **A strategic decision that must be made during response is whether to respond in a defensive or an offensive mode.**
1. A defensive response mode is undertaken to prevent exposure or damage with no intentional entry or contact with the incident scene, for example, going to a distant valve to shut off a leaking pipeline.
2. An offensive mode response requires proper personal protective equipment and personnel who have been trained to this level of response, for example, entering a chemical release area to plug and patch a leaking tank.
3. Persons responding to disasters must know their own capabilities and not exceed them; for instance, rescue may not be possible without involving too much risk to the rescue personnel.
4. The following basic measures should be taken, according to the specific disaster event.
   a. Approach any scene cautiously from upwind, uphill, and upstream. Resist the urge to rush in.
   b. Secure the scene by keeping people away from the site, outside a safety perimeter.
   c. Identify the hazards, using all available information and reevaluating as more information becomes available.
   d. Assess the situation by considering whether there is fire, chemical spill, weather-related hazard, and/or terrain/location hazard.
   e. Determine who or what is at risk: people, property, or the environment.
   f. Determine what actions should be taken, such as evacuation versus shelter-in-place.
   g. Determine what resources are required and whether they are readily available.
   h. Decide what can be done immediately.
   i. Obtain the help of responsible agencies and qualified personnel.
   j. Respond using the scene's safest entry route, if response is possible.
   k. Set up decontamination, if these measures are needed.
   l. Establish first aid and medical treatment arrangements.

C **When a disaster occurs, the first response will be the local emergency medical system (EMS), police, fire, and other identified responders.**
1. Upon notification of a disaster, hospitals, medical facilities, and public health agencies will activate their disaster plans. If these agencies are also affected by the disaster, the response will be modified accordingly.
2. County or city emergency organizations will become activated and responsive.
   a. In the event of a hazardous materials disaster, the Local Emergency Planning Committee (LEPC), an agency mandated by the US EPA, will be activated.
   b. The American Red Cross and other voluntary agencies will respond.
3. "On the morning of September 11, 2001, the last best hope for the community rested not with national policymakers but with private firms and local public servants, especially the first responders: fire, police, emergency med-

ical service, and building safety professionals." (National Commission on Terrorist Attacks Upon the United States, 2004).

D **Local activities may be mirrored at the state level and possibly the federal level, depending on the magnitude of the event.**

1. The Federal Emergency Management Agency (FEMA) may respond with activation of the Federal Response Plan.
2. The National Disaster Medical System (NDMS) provides for the establishment of Disaster Field Offices (DFOs) in the disaster region.
   a. Emergency Response Teams (ERTs) are located in the DFOs.
      1) An Operations Section coordinates federal, state, and voluntary efforts.
      2) The ERT Operations Section has a Human Services Branch that is responsible for:
         a) Needs assessment
         b) Establishment of disaster recovery centers
         c) Initiation, coordination, and delivery of recovery programs authorized by the Stafford Act
         d) Managing the Department of Homeland Security (DHS) and state grant programs
   b. An Infrastructure Support Branch deals with restoration of public utilities and other infrastructure services.
   c. A Deputy Field Coordinating Officer for Mitigation coordinates with the Infrastructure Support Branch and otherwise promotes mitigation and preparedness activities.

E **In March 2004, the Department of Homeland Security developed the National Incident Management System (NIMS).**

1. A goal of NIMS is to enable responders at all jurisdictional levels and across all disciplines to work together more effectively and efficiently.
2. Beginning in 2006, federal funding for state, local, and tribal preparedness will be tied to compliance with NIMS.

F **One of the "best practices" incorporated in the National Incident Management system is the Incident Command System (ICS), a standard, on-scene, all-hazards incident management system already in use by firefighters, hazardous materials teams, rescuers, and emergency medical teams.**

1. The ICS is based on basic business management practices in which leaders perform the basic tasks of planning, directing, organizing, coordinating, communicating, delegating, and evaluating; these functional areas are under the overall direction of an Incident Commander.
2. The system can be implemented on a company, community, state and/or national basis and under a variety of conditions.
3. Utilization of the ICS is mandatory under certain circumstances.
   a. The Superfund Amendments and Reauthorization Act requires that organizations that deal with hazardous material incidents respond under an ICS.
   b. Most fire and EMS departments implement the ICS at fire scenes and in mass casualty incidents.
   c. Certain insurance companies and local regulations require implementation of an ICS.
4. The ICS is designed to organize the response so that the maximum amount of resources is provided to the greatest areas of need. Features that enable this are:

a. *Integrated communications*—Communications procedures and protocols; frequency allocations and uses; and procedures to receive, record, and acknowledge incoming and outgoing communication are integrated and coordinated. Plain language is used in all communications exchanges.

b. *Span of control*—A desirable range of from three to seven subordinates is assigned to any one supervisor for effective management.

c. *Unified command*—When multiple agencies are involved, responsibility for the overall management of an incident is shared with all agencies contributing to the command process.

d. *Action plan*—The plan addresses strategic goals, tactical objectives, and all support activities and actions that are required for all responders and response agencies.

e. *Comprehensive resource management*—Resources are identified, recorded, and given status monitoring throughout all phases of the incident in order to maximize resource utilization, consolidate large numbers of individual resources, and reduce communications loading of radio channels.

f. *Modular format*—A top-down organizational structure is used for any incident. Top down means "that the command function is established by the first arriving officer." (http://training.fema.gov/EMIWeb/downloads/ISI95untl.pdf

5. The ICS contains five areas of function, that is, key elements that must be present to respond effectively.

a. The command function involves directing, ordering, and controlling resources by virtue of explicit legal, agency, or delegated authority.

b. Operations is responsible for management of all tactical activities at the event, including medical response, rescue, fire suppression, hazmat response etc.

c. Planning is the function for collection, evaluation, dissemination, and use of information about the progress of the incident and the status of resources; it plays a key role in the creation of a disaster/emergency-specific action plan.

d. Logistics is responsible for locating, organizing, and providing facilities, services, and materials for the response.

e. Finance carefully records and justifies cost and financial operations and reimbursement of costs.

6. Several critical officer positions are found in the system.

a. The *incident commander* is the one person in overall charge of the operations; this position is mandatory in all responses.

b. The *safety officer* reports directly to Command and can shut down operations if anything poses a threat to personnel safety; this position is mandatory in all responses.

c. Agency representatives work within the command function and decision-making process with the incident commander through the *liaison officer*.

d. The *operations section officer* or *chief* has primary responsibility for tactical operations taking place at any specific phase of the emergency's event.

e. The *planning officer,* responsible for the planning function, reports to the incident commander.

f. The *logistics office* oversees the logistics function and reports to the incident commander.

    g. The staging area is controlled by the *staging area manager*, who dispatches resources when called for at the scene.

7. The staging area is a resource-marshalling area, where units such as ambulances report while waiting for specific assignments and direction.
    a. There may be one or more staging areas established.
    b. Only those resources that can be readily employed and utilized at the scene of the emergency should be on the immediate site. The rest should be held in the staging area.

G A *command post*, **which serves as the command center, must contain the necessary communications equipment to allow direction of units out in the field.**

1. Trying to run an emergency response without a command post would be like trying to drive a car without a steering wheel. The command post has several functions.
    a. It serves as an operations center for command staff and community agency command staff away from the disaster scene to enable smooth operations at both the command post and the scene.
    b. It must serve as a center for incoming information from the scene and other site units and for outgoing information to the media and community.
    c. It can be a planned site at a fixed facility or a specially designed vehicle.
    d. Only one command post is used per incident.
2. A command post must have certain features to become operational quickly; these include:
    a. A designated command post location
    b. An alternative if the primary site is unusable
    c. Backup heat and/or power/battery-operated equipment
    d. The necessary communications equipment: telephones (cellular?), radios, fax machine, weather radio, and megaphone/PA system
    e. Adequate protection against potential hazards
    f. Access to restroom facilities, water, garbage/sanitation supplies, food and utensils, etc
    g. A separate area for media briefings
    h. The Disaster Plan, Emergency Action Plan, other plans, resources lists, plot plans, and other essential documents
    i. Documentation capability, which may include tape recorders, forms, copy machine, clip boards, computer diskettes, office supplies
    j. Controlled and secure access
    k. Necessary information resources, such as material safety data sheets (MSDSs), DOT Emergency Response Guidebook, NIOSH Pocket Guide, chemical compatibility charts, etc.

H Key persons, such as department heads, government officers and officials, and volunteer agency members gather at an Emergency Operations Center (EOC) to coordinate their response to an emergency event.

1. Most jurisdictions maintain an EOC as part of their community's emergency preparedness program.
2. The proper interface between the EOC and the on-scene management should be worked out in advance, if possible.
3. The EOC does not compete with the command post but operates in conjunction with it.

I **Important measures must be taken in the response phase to reduce legal liability.**

1. Reasoned actions, decisions, and responses, including telephone, radio, and traffic activities must be documented.
2. Photographs and videos should be taken.
3. All documents, such as shipping papers or notes that have been collected should be retained.
4. Work should be conducted within defined responsibilities and levels of authority.
5. Records and reports should be filed promptly.
6. Legal counsel may need to be consulted.
7. If response deficiencies are noted, they should be corrected.
8. Any new hazards identified during the response should be noted, and arrangements should be made to mitigate them when the crisis is over.

J **The news media represents the public's First Amendment right-to-know at a news incident.**

1. The press is committed to finding out what has occurred and to providing objective and responsible reporting on the best available information that can be obtained.
2. Different media outlets have different needs; thus a single statement issued by a public information officer may not meet the needs of everyone.
   a. The television reporter is looking for a good shot; radio reporters want good sound bites.
   b. Newspaper reporters want details and background information.
   c. Specialty services may want to cover "the story behind the story."
3. The media will be present at several locations, including:
   a. The incident site, which is the first place the press will go; it provides the best source of information for the first-in journalist.
   b. Command and control centers (i.e., command posts, emergency operations centers)
   c. Fire and police stations
   d. Offices of public officials
4. Media must make preparations related to the preparations and distribution of information.
   a. A site should be preselected for media operations and interviews.
   b. A packaged press kit can be prepared with generic information months in advance; sample information contained in package press kits can include:
      1) Telephone numbers for press lines at the emergency operations center
      2) Background information on emergency service units
      3) Background information on emergency response teams
      4) Glossary of terms used
      5) Diagrams of specialized equipment
      6) Training photographs
      7) Explanation of procedures, for example, use of a chlorine B kit
      8) Safety information
      9) Interview procedures and policies
      10) Information on past incidents/disasters

K **Resources are all personnel and major items of equipment (including crews) that are available or potentially available, for assignment to incidents;** *resources are a major response need* **(Emergency Management Institute, FEMA, 2004).**

1. Resources are described by several predetermined definitions:
   a. Kind or function (e.g., a patrol car or bulldozer)
   b. Type or performance capability (e.g., capacity or pressure factor)
   c. Single resources are individual pieces of equipment and their personnel complement—or a crew of individuals with an identified supervisor—that can be used in a tactical application at an incident
2. Resources are defined in various combinations.
   a. A combination of single resources assembled for a particular operational need, with common communications and a leader, is a *task force*.
   b. A group of resources of the same kind and type (e.g., three drug K-9 teams, six patrol units, etc.) is a *strike team*, managed by a *strike team leader*.
3. All resources will be in one of three category conditions.
   a. *Assigned* resources are performing active responses.
   b. *Available* resources are ready for immediate assignment and are usually in the staging area.
   c. *Out-of-service* resources are not ready for response, because of such factors as mechanical problems, rest periods, or weather conditions.
4. A major problem that can occur when resources are being assembled is that there are too many untrained personnel.
   a. *Convergent volunteerism* is "the arrival of unexpected or uninvited personnel wishing to render aid at the scene of a large-scale emergency incident" (Cone et al, 2003).
   b. Volunteers may freelance without the knowledge and direction of incident command.
   c. Untrained personnel may include medical, fire, law enforcement, and civilian personnel showing up at natural, technological, and conflict-origin disasters.
   d. These untrained persons must be kept out of the scene and provided a response outlet, such as availability at a staging area.

L **Communications are needed to report initial and secondary emergencies, to warn personnel of hazards as they appear, to keep families and the community informed about what is happening at the facility, to coordinate evacuation and response actions, and to keep in contact with emergency response agencies and command centers;** *communication is a major response need.*
1. Communications can be disrupted on a short-term basis or by a total communications failure.
2. Facility communications should be prioritized to identify those that should be restored first.
3. Options include messengers, telephones, cell phones, portable microwave, amateur radios, point-to-point private lines, satellite, high-frequency radio, two-way radio, FAX machine, dial-up modems, local area networks, bull horn, whistles/bells, pagers, and hand signals.
4. Battery-operated communications systems such as National Oceanic and Atmospheric Administration (NOAA) weather radios and AM radios to keep informed of the disaster impacts and responses should be considered.

M **Evacuation of the facility or area may be a necessary response.**
1. An accounting for all personnel, using post-evacuation assembly areas, is needed.
2. Employees' transportation needs for community-wide evacuations must be considered.

3. Persons with disabilities and those who do not speak English may need special assistance.
4. Posted evacuation procedures and routes must be followed.
5. Critical operations must be continued or shut down while an evacuation is underway. Persons assigned to these responsibilities must be capable of recognizing when to abandon the operation and evacuate themselves.
6. Primary and secondary evacuation routes and exits that have emergency lighting in case a power outage occurs must be identified.
7. Evacuation routes and emergency exits must be wide enough to accommodate the number of evacuating personnel, clear and unobstructed, unlikely to expose evacuating personnel to additional hazards.
8. The names and last known locations of personnel not accounted for should be determined and given to the Emergency Operations Center.
9. An accounting of nonemployees, such as suppliers and customers, is needed.
10. Additional evacuation in case the incident worsens should be considered; for example, employees may be sent home by normal means or they may be provided with transportation to an off-site location.
11. Shelter may be provided within the facility or away from the facility in a public building in certain events, such as chemical releases, tornado warnings and parking lot shootings.
12. The need for emergency supplies such as water, food, sanitation, and medical supplies must be determined if long-term sheltering is anticipated.
13. Coordination with local authorities needs to occur.
14. Search and rescue should be conducted only by properly trained and equipped professionals.
15. Untrained employees should not be allowed to reenter a damaged or contaminated facility until professional responders have declared the all clear.

N **Protecting facilities, equipment, and vital records is essential.**
1. Vital records can be protected by labeling them and securing them in insulated containers.
2. Computer systems should be backed up and then data should be stored off-site, where they would not likely be damaged.
3. When an event affects the facility, vital records and computer facilities may need additional security.
4. Arrangements should be made for the evacuation of critical original records, such as patents, to backup facilities.
5. Arrangements should be made for backup power.

O **Response efforts may need to include environmental protection considerations such as:**
1. Waterways may need to be protected from oil or chemical runoff.
2. Soil may need to be collected and disposed of as hazardous waste.
3. Air may need to be protected by preventing evaporation of volatile materials.
4. The National Response Center (NRC) must be notified immediately when dangerous goods or hazardous substances at or above reportable quantities are spilled. (1-800-424-8802)
5. The Department of Defense military shipments incidents must be reported to the US Army Operations Center for incidents involving explosives and

ammunition, and the Defense Logistics Agency for incidents involving non-explosive and non-ammunition military shipments.

6. The Federal Bureau of Investigation (FBI) field office, along with local authorities, must be notified of a credible terrorist threat or of a suspected incident involving weapons of mass destruction (WMDs).

IV Disaster Recovery

Recovery, the last phase of the cycle, continues until return to normal operation is accomplished. This may be short term, medium term, or long term, depending on the size and circumstances of the emergency or disaster.

A **Recovery activities should always include evaluation of ways to avoid future similar emergencies.**

1. Accurate damage assessment is important to the recovery process.
2. Recovery should not conflict with "crime scene" preservation and examination.
3. Fast recovery is desirable, but the cause of the incident must be established.
4. Accurate projections of recovery times should be estimated and communicated.

B **Recovery efforts can last from days to weeks or even months.**

1. Often responders do not recognize the need to take care of themselves and to monitor their own emotional and physical health.
2. Rescue and recovery operations take place in extremely dangerous work environments. Mental fatigue over long shifts can place emergency workers at greatly increased risk for injury.
3. Co-workers may be intently focused on a particular task and may not notice a hazard nearby or behind, placing themselves and others at risk.
4. The paths to recovery appear to be determined by the physical characteristics of the disaster agent, the types and quantities of community resources that survive the disaster, the external aid that the community can obtain, and the reconstruction strategies that these communities adopt and implement.

C **The disaster recovery phase can be divided into particular periods of activity.**

1. The *restoration* period is the period when security of the damage area is established; repairs to utilities are made; debris is removed; evacuees return; continuing care is provided to victims; and commercial, industrial, and residential structures are repaired or prefabricated housing or other temporary structures go up and temporary bracing is installed for buildings and bridges.
2. The *reconstruction/replacement* period involves rebuilding capital stocks and getting the economy back to pre-disaster levels. This period can take some years.
3. Public information should flow constantly to disaster victims, and be monitored for effectiveness.

D **A critical responsibility during recovery is to ensure that mandatory reports are made to various authorities.**

1. A fatality or multiple hospitalizations must be reported to the nearest OSHA office within eight hours.
2. A recordable occupational injury or illness must be entered on the OSHA 300 log within six days.

3. Release of a listed carcinogen must be reported to OSHA within 24 hours.
4. Release of hazardous air pollutants must be reported to the EPA Regional Administrator at a time varying with the specific pollutant.
5. In some cases, "less than reportable quantities" of a release must be reported to local, state, and regional authorities.
6. There are federal reporting requirements (as many as 40 citations in the CFR), state requirements, regional requirements, and local requirements. The responsible person at the facility must know and meet these reporting requirements.

V Natural Hazard–Specific Considerations (FEMA, 2004)

A Hurricanes bring torrential rains, high winds, and ocean storm surges, causing floods and other damage; floods are the most common natural disaster.

1. Floods can also be caused by spring rain, heavy thunderstorms, winter snow thaws, and failed dikes or dams, but also from technologic events such as ruptured water mains or leaking water tanks.
2. Planning includes inspecting areas in the facility that could be subject to flooding or wind damage.
   a. Identify vulnerable records and equipment that can be moved to a higher location.
   b. Consider storing backup and data media in watertight containers.
   c. Plan to protect outside equipment and structures.
   d. For all natural disasters, consider obtaining a NOAA Weather Radio with a warning alarm tone and battery backup for early natural-event warnings.
3. Mitigation measures can also be taken.
   a. Have the means and personnel available and trained to move equipment and other critical items to a safe location if a flood watch or warning is announced.
   b. In flood-prone areas, consider flood proofing the facility by blocking off doors and windows, reinforcing and sealing walls, installing check valves at utility and sewer line entrances, and constructing floodwalls and levees outside.
   c. New construction can be elevated on walls, columns, or compacted fill.
   d. Careful assessment for floodplain locations is an important mitigation factor when new facility locations are being contemplated.
   e. Have backups systems ready for hurricane events; these include emergency lighting, alternative power sources, and portable pumps.
   f. To protect from high winds, install window storm shutters. A second option is to cover windows with 5/8-inch marine plywood.
   g. Identify alternate storm shelters, particularly underground shelters, for protection against high winds.

B Hurricanes can also spawn tornadoes, which are often accompanied by thunderstorms and heavy rains.

1. Tornadoes can occur with little or no warning but can also be identified by the National Oceanic and Atmospheric Administration (NOAA) through storm watches and reports.
2. Should a tornado watch be announced, be ready to take shelter. Listen for radio announcements and community sirens.

3. Should a tornado warning be issued, take shelter immediately. A tornado has been sighted or is showing on radar.

4. In addition to the natural hazard considerations listed in Section A, identify designated tornado shelters in your area or have a shelter identified at your facility by a structural engineer or architect. *Auditoriums, cafeterias, and gymnasiums with flat wide-span roofs are not safe.*

5. Have worker notification procedures established.

6. Consider the need for spotters to watch for approaching storms and funnel clouds.

7. Train and practice on tornado notification and shelter responses frequently.

C **Earthquakes can occur anywhere in the United States, suddenly and without warning.**

1. Earthquakes can trigger other disaster events, such as fires, explosions, landslides, tidal waves (tsunamis), and floods.

2. Often the greatest danger to people occurs when equipment and nonstructural elements such as ceilings, lighting fixtures, and windows shake loose.

3. Planning for earthquakes includes assessment of the facility for vulnerability.

4. Mitigation requires developing and prioritizing facility-strengthening measures, such as adding steel bracing and sheer walls to frames, reinforcing columns and building foundations, and replacing unreinforced brick and façade.

5. Interior mitigation includes moving large and heavy objects to floor level; securing shelves, furniture, computers and cabinets; securing fixed machinery to the floor; anchoring large utility and process piping; and installing safety glass.

6. Hazardous materials must be properly stored and in a manner that incompatible chemicals are not kept adjacent to each other.

7. Training and drills should be provided to workers on building evacuation procedures and on designated safe areas should evacuation be unnecessary. Be prepared for aftershocks.

8. Local government agencies and insurance carriers can provide comprehensive area assessments, planning and mitigation guidance, and response and restoration support.

D **The guidelines provided above for selected natural disasters can be applied to other events as well.**

1. The keys to each of these disasters are thorough hazard identification, vulnerability analysis, planning, and mitigation measures.

2. A well-conceived plan with proper training and drills is essential.

VI Technologic Hazard-Specific Considerations

A **Fires are the most common hazards, causing deaths, injuries, and extensive property damage (FEMA, 2004).**

1. Prevention of fires is the key element to planning.
   a. Inspect the facility regularly for fire hazards.
   b. Install and maintain fire notification and suppression systems in accordance with local and consensus fire codes.
   c. Install smoke detectors and change batteries annually. Test them monthly.

2. Properly trained employees can reduce the risk of fire and the extent of injuries and damage.
    a. Train employees on fire prevention, fire containment, fire alarms and reporting, and evacuation.
    b. Conduct evacuation drills regularly.
    c. Ensure proper functional emergency lighting and evacuation maps.
    d. Provide fire extinguisher training if employees are expected to use these devices.

B *Hazardous materials* **are substances that are explosive, flammable, combustible, toxic, corrosive, oxidizable, radioactive, or an irritant.**
1. Many regulations define hazardous materials according to the intent of the requirements, including the Superfund Amendments and Reauthorization Act of 1986 (SARA), the Resource Conservation and Recovery Act of 1976 (RCRA), the Toxic Substances Control Act (TSCA), and the Hazardous Materials Transportation Act (HMTA).
2. OSHA has standards that address hazardous materials in general, such as 29 CFR 1910.1200 Hazard Communication standard and 29 CFR 1910.1450 Chemical Hazards in Laboratories.
3. Other standards address specific materials or applications, such as OSHA standards for asbestos, carcinogens, and others, or the Hazardous Waste Operations and Emergency Response standard.
4. These standards define training requirements, handling and transportation restrictions, written plans, emergency spill and release response, and reporting requirements.
5. Preparedness and emergency planning include several essential steps.
    a. Ensure that all hazardous materials are properly labeled and stored.
    b. Have Material Safety Data Sheets (MSDSs) readily available for workers to consult for proper use and personal protection measures as well as spill cleanup precautions and PPE.
    c. Include the fire department in site walk-throughs and response training.
    d. Ensure that only properly trained and equipped employees are permitted to work with hazardous materials and to respond to spills or releases.
6. Identify neighboring facilities and transportation routes that could impact the facility with a hazardous materials incident.
7. Be prepared to conduct a safe evacuation if required, or to shelter-in-place if this is the more appropriate option.

C **High-rise buildings (4 stories or higher) pose unique problems in emergency events; mitigating the effects of a disaster in such buildings is a critical concern.**
1. Evacuation plans should be reviewed to ensure the presence of redundant power and lighting systems, evacuation chairs for the disabled, and reflective paint on evacuation routes.
2. In order to be realistic, evacuation practice should include staff; early responders, such as firefighters, police officers; and utility company emergency personnel.
3. Information about hazards and risk analyses should be updated regularly.
4. Emergency plans should be developed jointly with early responders.
5. Security should be improved with low-tech options, such as landscaping with cactus and bougainvillea, and high-tech options, such as surveillance cameras.

6. Care should be taken to avoid locked stairwell doors that would prevent evacuees from returning to a floor if their egress is blocked. Automatic unlocking doors are an option.

D **Other technologic emergencies include loss of a utility, a power outage, and interruption of critical business elements such as information systems or equipment.**

1. Planning requires that all critical needs be identified, followed by determination of the impact should a service disruption occur.
2. Mitigation is a critical element to reducing the impact of these events.
   a. It includes the installation of back-up systems, such as emergency power generators.
   b. Data back-up, retrieval, and recovery methods should be defined for critical operations.
   c. Vital records, such as patents and software licenses, should be identified and secured in disaster-resistant/exposure-resistant containers with copies kept offsite.
   d. Establish preventative maintenance programs for equipment and operations.
3. Should an event occur, have only properly trained personnel or contractors restore system operations to avoid further damage and provide a more rapid recovery.
4. Have essential service-provider contact information available, such as telephone numbers, account numbers, and facility service addresses.
5. Be prepared to notify regulatory agencies should critical equipment such as pollution prevention units fail.

VII Conflict-Related Hazard-Specific Considerations

A **Workplace violence can occur in several forms, such as robberies and assaults perpetrated by criminals, domestic dispute that has spilled over into the workplace, and a disgruntled worker. (See Chapter 15.)**

1. Planning for workplace violence should be included in the emergency action/disaster management plan (Parker, 2004).
   a. Engineering controls can be implemented as mitigation measures.
      1) Crime Prevention Through Environmental Design (CPTED) includes measures to keep the perpetrator out of the workplace, such as placing counters near the front door for visibility, reducing hiding places by limiting the height of landscaping, or providing weapons-proof barriers in high-risk locations such as emergency department entrances.
      2) Prevent access to rooftops and air intakes.
      3) Prevent access to mechanical rooms and units.
      4) Use see-through fencing that will not obscure visual detection of potential violence.
      5) Install closed-circuit TVs, security lighting, or intrusion detection sensors in restricted areas.
      6) Install emergency phones in the facility and on the grounds.
      7) Install panic alarms in high-risk locations.
      8) Maintain escape routes by preventing obstructing furniture.
      9) Provide staff-only locked areas such as restrooms.
   b. Administrative controls should also be instituted (Parker, 2004).

1) Educate employees to understand that when a coworker threatens with a violent act, he or she should be taken seriously and reported to the employer.
2) Perform preplacement background checks.
3) Have a sound workplace violence policy that is communicated to all employees and new hires.
4) Consider establishing a multidisciplinary team to evaluate reports of threatened violence.
5) If domestic issues are a problem, assist the employee with counseling, such as through employee assistance programs and with protection through restraining-order enforcement.
6) Avoid employees' working alone by providing buddy systems and increased staffing.
7) Utilize easily recognized employee ID tags, but minimize information contained on them.

2. Planning should also include measures to take should an incident occur, including getting the work environment back to normal as soon as possible and networking with trained professionals to aid employee coping.
   a. Identify safe places to escape inside and outside the facility.
   b. Train on defusing violent situations and in self-defense.
   c. Have clear procedures for calling for help and for notifying the essential authorities.
   d. Ensure that the involved work area is secured for further investigation.

B **Mass shootings are similar to workplace violence events, with most of these events occurring either in the workplace or in schools (Wisner & Adams, 2002).**

1. Many perpetrators carry more than one weapon, including fragmentation devices such as those used at the Columbine High School in 1999.
2. None of the shooters have been found to wear body armor; in one survey 40% took their own lives (Wisner & Adams, 2002).
3. Planning, response, and recovery should follow the guidelines provided for workplace violence.
4. Should the shooter be outside the facility, sheltering-in-place should receive the greatest emphasis to avoid workers' evacuating into harm's way.
5. Workers should be trained to understand that they cannot "talk down" the shooter or persuade him or her to surrender.
6. Workers should learn how to take cover away from hazardous materials containers and away from reflective surfaces.
7. Noise-producing devices, such as wristwatch alarms, pagers, and cell phones, should be deactivated or silenced.

VIII Terrorism

A *Terrorism* **is the calculated use of violence or threat of violence to inculcate fear; it is intended to coerce or to intimidate governments or societies in the pursuit of goals that are generally political, religious, or ideologic (Wallace, 2004).**

1. A legal definition from the FBI is "the unlawful use of force against persons or property to intimidate or coerce a government, the civilian population, or any segment thereof, in the furtherance of political or social objectives (Code of Federal Regulations, 2001).
2. Areas with high population densities, such as the workplace, make them desirable terrorist targets.

3. The terrorist attacks of September 11, 2001, and the anthrax attacks of 2001 targeted people in workplaces, making them the frontline in the United States in a new "21st-century battlefield" (Secretary of Defense Donald Rumsfeld in Krames, 2002).

4. During the response phase of an event, first-responders, rescue and recovery workers, and healthcare workers must face these hazards in the course of their work.

5. Some of the risk factors for attracting terrorism are aggregations of more than 100 employees at a facility, high-rise buildings, government sites, defense contractors, symbolic and historical structures, international business operations, and critical infrastructure services (Hudson & Roberts, 2003).

6. Key factors need to be added to disaster plans to address terrorism preparedness.
   a. Identify ways to reduce the risk of an attack, such as reducing aggregation, enhancing building security, and preventing access to building air intakes.
   b. Collaborate, plan, and train with local response agencies, public health agencies, and law enforcement and intelligence agencies.
   c. Keep current with plans, security programs, clinical advances, and training tools through colleagues, government agency web sites, and key infrastructure organizations.
   d. Protocols must include reducing risks to first responders (Deitchman, 2003).
      1) Administrative controls include written, well-practiced plans, appropriate immunizations, and post-exposure prophylaxis.
      2) Engineering controls include use of self-sheathing needles, improved rescue/ambulance ventilation systems, and use of rapidly deployed decontamination units.
      3) Personal protective equipment controls include provision of properly fitted N-95 respirators in response vehicles and heavy gloves for protection from sharps during extrications and rescues.

B *Weapons of mass destruction* **(WMDs) are any destructive device or weapon that is designed or intended to cause death or serious bodily injury through the release, dissemination, or impact of toxic or poisonous chemicals, disease organisms, or radiation or radioactivity at a level dangerous to human life (United States Code 2004).**

1. Terrorists prefer mass destruction because of the harm, injury, and possible economic systems paralysis it generates.

2. WMDs increase the psychologic impact of the event, using fear, outrage, and a sense of helplessness as a force multiplier.

3. WMDs are described with an acronym B-NICE: *b*iologic agents, *n*uclear agents, *i*ncendiary devices, *c*hemical agents, and *e*xplosive devices (Cangemi, 2002).

C *Biologic agents* **are bacteria, viruses, rickettsiae, and toxins that are adaptable, easy to conceal, cheap, and impact significant population sizes rapidly (Sullivan et al, 2003). (See Table 13-3.)**

1. The infrastructure of agriculture and livestock, food products, and water sources can be targets as well as human targets.

2. For a biologic weapon to succeed, it must have a payload containing the agent, a container that keeps the agent intact, a delivery system, and a dispersal mechanism.

TABLE 13-3

Potential biologic weapons

Biotoxins	Infectious Agents
Botulinus toxin	Viral hemorrhagic fever (VHF)
Ricin	Ebola virus
Staphylococcal enterotoxin B	Plaque
Trichothecene mycototoxin	Q fever – rickettsia Coxiella burnetii
Aflatoxin	Venezuelan equine encephalitis (VEE)
Saxitoxin	Anthrax
Tetrodotoxin	Cholera
	Pneumonic plague
	Smallpox
	Tularemia
	Brucellosis
	Yellow fever
	Multidrug-resistant tuberculosis

Source: Centers for Disease Control and Prevention, 2004.

    a. Dissemination can be accomplished with aerosol sprays, through contaminated food and water, through direct skin contact, and by injection (Cangemi, 2002).

    b. The perpetration of a hoax, such as the anthrax hoaxes that occurred after the anthrax incidents in 2001, impedes the ability of first responders to identify the actual biologic weapon.

3. Infectious agents require an incubation period after exposure is accomplished, resulting in an often insidious onset; biotoxins do not require an incubation period.

4. Occupational and environmental health nurses, primary health care providers, and first responders have the potential for being the first health care providers to observe and report unusual illness or injuries (Salazar, 2002).

5. A disaster management plan must include specific procedures for bioterrorist events.

    a. Occupational and environmental health nurses must become familiar with the toxins and infectious agents subject to terrorist attacks. Refer to Table 13-3 for a significant agent list.

    b. Occupational and environmental health nurses must be able to recognize early signs and symptoms.

    c. Occupational and environmental health nurses must be ready to implement transmission precautions and infection control measures, treatments, health education requirements, and prevention measures such as vaccinations when available.

    d. Occupational and environmental health nurses must know public health reporting requirements and how to access community resources.

6. The onset of a biologic attack may be detected through identification of clusters, dead insects, animals or fish, and unexplained illnesses.

7. The CDC and the U.S. Department of Agriculture have mandated the implementation of provisions of the Public Health Security and Bioterrorism Preparedness and Response Act of 2002 to provide protection against

misuse of select agents and toxins whether inadvertent or the result of terrorist activity.

    a. The interim final rule from the CDC is 42 CFR Part 73, the Possession, Use, and Transfer of Select Agents and Toxins.

    b. Select agents are biologic agents and toxins that have the potential to pose a severe threat to public health and safety.

    c. Requirements for select agent program compliance include registration of government agencies, universities, research institutions, and commercial entities; security risk assessments; safety plans; a designated facility Responsible Official (RO); security plans; emergency response plans; training; transfers; record keeping; inspections; and notifications.

    d. Requirements include FBI background checks and fingerprinting by the FBI's bioterrorism unit of all persons requesting approval to access select agents and toxins.

    e. The regulations include severe criminal and civil penalties for possession or transfer of, or access to, select agents and toxins without FBI clearance and for noncompliance with CDC regulations.

D Several types of *nuclear and radiologic incidents* can be employed by terrorists (Louisiana State University, 2003).

    1. The dispersion of nuclear and radioactive agents can occur in multiple ways.

        a. A nuclear weapon can be detonated, creating a partial (e.g. suitcase bomb) or total yield of its nuclear contents (e.g., A-bomb).

        b. A radioactive source can be hidden in a location frequented by many people for extended periods of time (e.g., an unenclosed cobalt therapy source).

        c. Radioactive materials can be dispersed by an explosive device, known as a "dirty bomb" or radiation dispersal device (RDD) (e.g., radionuclides such as strontium 90).

        d. Radioactive materials can be deposited into food and water supplies (e.g., radionuclides such as H3 tritium).

        e. The use of radioactive materials in an RDD or to contaminate food and water are the most likely potentials.

            1) Nuclear fission devices are difficult to obtain and to launch.

            2) Nuclear sealed sources are risky to the perpetrator and bulky to handle.

            3) Radionuclides are in prevalent use in industry, medicine, research, etc., and thus easiest to obtain, particularly outside the United States.

    2. Radiation exposure exists in several forms (Breitenstein & Spickard, 2002).

        a. Alpha radiation consists of invisible particles with very little penetration power. A piece of paper or a layer of skin stops them.

        b. Beta particles have a greater penetration power and can require a thicker barrier.

        c. Gamma rays and X-rays are not particles but rather high-energy, short wavelengths at the end of the electromagnetic scale. Lead and concrete barriers are necessary for adequate shielding.

        d. Contrary to popular belief, a nuclear power plant will not explode when impacted. It may release various forms of radiation, however.

        e. Most radioactive materials have the capability of emitting more than one form of radiation.

3. Exposures can consist of external exposure, internal exposure, or both.
   a. Internal exposure occurs from inhaling, ingesting, or injecting radioactive materials. This is a serious exposure, because the internal organs are receiving a direct effect that cannot be decontaminated.
   b. External exposure occurs from radioactive particles on the skin, such as in nuclear fallout, and from an unprotected presence to gamma-emitting radioactive materials and x-ray generating equipment. Decontamination and/or removal of the source or generating unit stops the exposure.
4. The occupational and environmental health nurse must be able to recognize the possibility of radiation exposure and radiation sickness signs and symptoms, including acute radiation sickness.
   a. External exposure may appear as dermal desquamation or burns.
   b. A flu-like illness, followed by a latency period, and then an acute illness involving the gastrointestinal tract, blood-forming organs, and central nervous system may indicate a high-intensity exposure over a short period of time. Death or recovery depends on the type, location, and amount of exposure.
   c. Chronic exposure, less likely in a terrorist incident, would be manifested in blood dyscrasias and genetic effects.
5. The occupational and environmental health nurse must have or be able to summon resources with radiation detection equipment, decontamination capability, and treatment capabilities.
   a. Alpha and beta particles can be washed from the skin through victim decontamination.
   b. Gamma radiation can be detected and measured using a Geiger-Mueller counter. Beta and alpha radiation require different detection equipment.
   c. Internal radiation exposure treatment may consist of drugs that bind the agent and excrete it through the urine or feces.
   d. Potassium iodide is administered prior to or at the immediate occurrence of a release of radioactive iodine (I-125, I-131) in order to saturate the thyroid gland and prevent uptake of the radioactive form.

E An *incendiary device* **can be a container with flammable materials, an ignition source, and possibly a time-delay mechanism (Veenema, 2003).**
1. The device is intended to produce a violent ignition, intensely hot fire, and a fire duration for an extended period of time.
2. These devices can be very simple or quite complex and can be in any form or size.
3. The occupational and environmental health nurse should have a high level of suspicion when an out-of-place or unfamiliar container is found in a highly populated or vulnerable area.
4. Only trained "bomb squad" personnel with special personal protective equipment should handle and detonate the device.

F *Chemicals as weapons* **have been identified by their health effects (Sullivan et al, 2003).**
1. Samples of health effects are as follows:
   a. Nerve agents interfere with the central and peripheral nervous systems.
   b. Vesicants or blister agents cause severe burns to the skin, eyes, lungs, and mucous membranes.
   c. Blood agents interfere with the ability to absorb and transport oxygen to the cells.

    d. Choking agents disable the respiratory function.

    e. Irritants cause pain, tearing, and respiratory distress.

2. Chemical agents are likely to create casualties within an hour or less. Routes of exposure are inhalation, ingestion, skin or mucous membrane absorption, and rarely, injection.

3. The occupational and environmental health nurse must be prepared to suspect, identify, and treat these exposures without personal endangerment.

    a. Several levels of hazardous materials response training are identified by OSHA. (29 CFR 1910.120)

        1) The Awareness Level includes recognition and identification of the material, employing proper notification procedures, and following the employer's emergency action plan (no minimum number of hours training specified).

        2) The First Responder Operations Level includes Awareness training plus basic hazard and risk assessment of the scene, personal protective equipment (PPE) selection, confinement and containment procedures, and decontamination procedures. Response is only defensive, with no intentional contact with the material (minimum 8 hours of training).

        3) The Hazardous Materials Technician receives advanced training in hazardous materials behavior models and in offensive response, using specialized chemical protective clothing, self-contained breathing apparatus and control and resolution of the incident (minimum 24 hours of training).

        4) The Hazardous Materials Specialist has advanced knowledge of chemical agents to respond with and serve as a consultant to the Technicians (minimum 24 hours of training).

        5) The On-Site Incident Commander receives First Responder Operations training plus training in the Incident Command System and the Emergency Response Plan (minimum 24 hours of training).

        6) If the occupational and environmental health nurse plans to respond to an incident, or a chemically contaminated person seeks the occupational and environmental health nurse for care, the occupational and environmental health nurse should have a minimum of First Responder Operations training.

    b. It is imperative that health care providers wear the correct personal protective equipment while patient decontamination and/or treatment are underway.

    c. Terrorist events can consist of a combination of agents.

        1) Bomb devices have been loaded with rat poisons containing warfarin, which prevents blood clotting.

        2) Some chemicals are released as a liquid, and then volatilize to become an inhalation hazard.

        3) Some chemical agents may be dispersed high above the ground to create a vapor plume that can travel long distances, affecting a large population.

        4) Some chemical agents are also radioactive, creating both chemical and radiation health effects.

    d. Treatment protocols should be planned in advance to include site-specific chemical exposure risks as well as access to community resources for terrorist chemical agents.

1) Initial treatment includes airway establishment and maintenance, decontamination (simultaneously), standard infection control practices, and supportive care.
2) Pharmacotherapy may be available to treat the toxicity of some hazardous materials (Hurlbut et al, 2003) (Table 13-4).

G *Explosive devices* **are bombs that either detonate or deflagrate to produce a powerful release of intense heat and extremely high-pressure gas.**
1. Explosive devices are divided into two types.
   a. Primary explosives are used as fuses and detonators. They must be kept wet to avoid instability and explosion.
   b. Secondary explosives require a booster and include such compounds as nitrated organic mixtures.
2. Military and civilian explosive devices include grenades and antipersonnel devices.
3. Homemade explosives consist of a fuel plus an oxidizer, or mixtures of oil or gasoline with powdered metals, and come in a wide variety of devices.
4. Terrorist bombs are usually targeted for mass gatherings to create a large number of victims with multiple and complex injuries, disorganization, and chaos.
5. The *blast* is the detonation and conversion of an explosive material into a large quantity of pressure and heat energy. The *blast injury* comprises the soft-tissue and visceral injuries caused by the initial blast and its subsequent effects; four categories of blast injuries can occur (Carmona & Sullivan, 2003).
   a. The *primary blast injury* is the result of the sudden changes in pressure caused by the blast wave.
      1) Solid organs are less compressible and may sustain contusions.
      2) Hollow organs that are gas-filled are more compressible and experience more severe tissue damage.
      3) Primary blast injuries typically damage the middle ear, pulmonary alveoli, gastrointestinal tract organs, and the central nervous system.

TABLE 13-4

Examples of hazardous materials exposure treatments

Pharmacotherapy	Hazardous Material Exposure
Atropine	Organophosphates and carbamates
Pralidoxime (2-PAM)	Organophosphate poisoning
Methylene blue	Nitro compound–induced methemogobinemia
Calcium gluconate	Hydrofluoric acid
Dimercaprol (BAL)	Lewisite, heavy metals
Dimercaptosuccinic acid (DMSA)	Lewisite, heavy metals
2,3 Dimercapto-1-propanesulfonic acid (DMPS)	Mercury, heavy metals
Cyanide antidote kit: amyl nitrite, sodium nitrite, and sodium thiosulfate	Cyanide gas inhalation, hydrogen sulfide gas inhalation
DTPA	Plutonium, neptunium, americium, and rare earth radionuclide metals: cesium
Inhalation sodium bicarbonate	Chlorine gas inhalation

Source: Hurlbut et al, 2003.

      4) Symptoms include pulmonary manifestations of pneumothorax, respiratory failure, and air embolism; GI symptoms of hemorrhage and organ perforation; and central nervous system concussion and air embolism.

   b. *Secondary blast injuries* occur from the flying debris generated from the primary blast. Injuries can be superficial or serious including amputations.

   c. *Tertiary blast injuries* occur from the victim's body being hurled against other objects from the blast force.

   d. *Miscellaneous blast injuries* occur from inhalation of heated or toxic vapors, burns, and radiation exposures.

6. Blast injuries, particularly unseen internal injuries, can often be missed because of their insidious nature.

7. In addition to the explosive device, some of these devices are equipped with nails, bolts, ball bearings, and pesticides.

8. Suicide bombings are considered by terrorists as one of the best means for reaching a target.

   a. Devices have included belts, vests, jackets, backpacks, suitcases, bicycles, shoes, and other cases carried on the person.

   b. Victims and responders are at risk for exposure to HIV and hepatitis from infected suicide bombers.

IX Template Emergency Preparedness/Disaster Management Plan

An emergency preparedness/disaster management plan should be tailored to establish regulatory compliance for the applicable region or jurisdiction and to protect workers and the community against potential disaster conditions. The following basic outline can serve as a framework to use in the development of a site-specific all-hazard disaster management plan (DMP); the outline can be copied, modified, and expanded according to site-specific needs.

A **The purposes of an emergency preparedness/disaster management plan are as follows:**

1. Prevent—or at least control—harm to people (highest priority) and property (secondary priority) in the event of an emergency or disaster.

2. Contain the extent of property loss only when the safety of all staff and neighbors at risk has been clearly established.

3. Prevent harm to the environment and the surrounding community.

4. Facilitate automatic disaster response by avoiding delays caused by decision making.

5. Identify previously unrecognized hazardous conditions that would aggravate an emergency and take steps to eliminate them.

6. Identify deficiencies, such as lack of resource coordination to handle an emergency.

7. Raise safety awareness.

8. Demonstrate the company's commitment to the safety of its workers.

9. Establish regulatory compliance with OSHA's 29 CFR 1910.38 plans for emergency action and fire response; 29 CFR 1910.119 for process safety management; 29 CFR 1910.120 for hazardous waste operations; and 29 CFR 1910.151 for medical services and first aid.

10. Provide consistency with and support for local emergency plans and response agencies.

B **The emergency preparedness/disaster plan is site specific; it applies to all persons on site, including workers, contractors, and visitors.**
   1. The plan is governed by the following factors:
      a. Nature of work performed
      b. Number of workers and contractors at site
      c. Hours of operation
   2. A vulnerability assessment, which evaluates required responses and necessary resources, should be completed; this should include input from community agencies with responsibilities for emergency response.
   3. The plan should include regular planning meetings and drills.
   4. Because major emergencies are low-probability events, they compete with other company financial allocations.
   5. Hazard control, emergency response, legal requirements, and administrative concerns must be addressed in the plan.
   6. A written plan should be available for inspection and copying by workers, their representatives, community emergency-response agencies, and OSHA personnel.

C **The program will require the input of multiple groups and individuals within the organization.**
   1. A disaster planning committee can assist in the planning and oversight of the program; the number of people and their functions will depend on the size and complexity of the workplace.
   2. Personnel to carry out the activities of the plan include the following:
      a. The safety director, who performs the function of emergency-response team coordinator for planning and training; the safety director also:
         1) Provides and maintains the inventory of hazard monitoring equipment and personal protective clothing and equipment used for hazardous materials response
         2) In an emergency response, acts as the safety officer
         3) Conducts post-emergency investigations
      b. Management encourages and supports emergency-response plans, activities, and training by:
         1) Ensuring that workers are familiar with and follow the procedures of the plan
         2) Informing the disaster planning committee of any new conditions or potential problems that warrant planning for emergency responses
         3) Reviewing and approving revisions to the plan
         4) Ensuring adequate resources for implementation and maintenance of the plan
         5) Supporting coordination with local community emergency-response programs
      c. Supervisors encourage and support worker emergency-response activities and training, ensure that workers are familiar with and follow the plan's procedures, and inform the disaster planning committee of any new conditions or potential problems that warrant planning for emergency responses.
      d. The human resources director acts as public relations officer in an emergency by maintaining communication to the news media, providing communications between upper management (site and corporate) and the emergency-response team, and communicating with families that may be affected by the emergency.

e. The environmental protection manager ensures proper reporting of environmental contamination as required by law and corporate policy and ensures proper disposal of hazardous and medical waste in an emergency.

f. The health center manager acts as medical officer, as defined in the National Fire Academy Incident Command System, during an emergency. In the absence of a physician, an occupational and environmental health nurse should assume this role. The health care manager:

   1) Provides and maintains an inventory of emergency medical equipment and supplies

   2) Supervises on-site medical emergency-response team members in caring for victims during an emergency response

   3) Directs or provides emergency victim triage, treatment, and transportation

   4) Communicates with community rescue and medical emergency responders and with hospital emergency department staff

   5) Ensures that current emergency patient care protocols are signed by the appropriate health care professionals and updated regularly

   6) Ensures that the on-site training of the medical emergency-response team in first aid and cardiopulmonary resuscitation (CPR) is provided and kept current according to criteria of the certifying agency

   7) Schedules and arranges physical examinations for respirator users and emergency responders according to company protocol and regulatory requirements, such as for hazardous materials (hazmat) technicians outlined in OSHA 29 CFR 1910.120

g. Other personnel include emergency-response and first-aid team members, hazardous materials response team members, and fire brigade members; these workers:

   1) Provide rapid emergency services within the property boundaries in accordance with the assigned response team

   2) Maintain knowledge and skills through participation in on-site training programs and drill exercises

   3) Refrain from response activities that are beyond the level of their training and equipment

   4) Keep emergency-response routine activities from interfering with their normal job responsibilities

h. The information technology manager (ITM) ensures the creation and maintenance of computer data backup files; the ITM maintains off-site contingency data storage and ensures capability of reinstallation and restoration of computer hardware and software.

i. Workers need to know the facility evacuation plans and evacuate as instructed during actual and practice alarms; report all emergencies, including health, fire, chemical, and intrusion, by calling a designated phone number; and follow instructions of the evacuation team leaders, emergency-response team members, and community emergency-response personnel.

j. Security personnel rope off the pre-designated section of parking lot for emergency-response vehicles during an emergency; additional roles include:

   1) Preventing curiosity seekers from entering the site

   2) Preventing removal of company documents and property during the disruptions of a site emergency

3) Escorting arrivals to meet with the appropriate company representative (e.g., the news media to the human resources director) at a pre-designated meeting location

k. The switchboard operator properly handles emergency calls by determining the nature of the emergency and assessing the details outlined on the emergency call form; other roles include:

1) Notifying the on-site emergency-response personnel when an employee emergency call is received

2) Summoning community emergency-response agencies at the direction of the emergency-response manager in charge

3) Activating the site alarm system when directed by the emergency-response manager in charge

4) Receiving and documenting all bomb threats telephoned to the switchboard, and reporting them immediately to management

l. The maintenance supervisor provides, maintains, and ensures monthly inspections of all fire-response equipment and supplies, self-contained breathing apparatus equipment and tanks, and rescue hardware and tools stored for emergency response; he or she is responsible for:

1) Maintaining emergency power-generating capability

2) Directing shutdown, repair, and start-up of utilities involved in site emergencies

3) Providing post-incident assessment of hazards and damage to property and equipment

4) Making regular rounds, being alert to fire potentials, chemical leaks, and utility failures

m. Technical consultants respond to the incident command operations center, when requested, to interpret and advise on the status and potential escalation of a chemical incident and attend annual training on hazardous materials emergency response.

D **There are several emergency procedures that are part of a general plan; these include communication strategies, personnel responsiblities, evacuation plan, monitoring personnel, sheltering-in-place procedures, information dissemination, notification and reporting to proper authorities, and record keeping.**

1. Communication strategies include the following:

a. *Notification phone list:* a list of names, site phone extensions, home phone numbers, and pager numbers of everyone whose support your company might need

b. *Community-response phone list:* a list of agencies with names, phone numbers, and pager numbers of every agency whose support your company might need; possibly include security companies, insurance companies, photographers, attorneys, and public relations firms

c. Bright red, manual, *fire-alarm pull stations* that are linked to the local fire department alarm console throughout the facility

d. *Evacuation alarms,* located throughout the facility, that can be activated by the switchboard operator

e. An *internal communication system* consisting of a designated emergency telephone number and a pager system

f. *Family notification procedures,* to be conducted as necessary by the human resources director or other company official

g. *Contact with utility companies* by the maintenance supervisor as necessary

    h. *Notification of regulatory agencies* requiring reporting of hazardous materials release by the environmental protection manager; the local OSHA office will be notified by the safety director in accordance with OSHA requirements in the event of a work-related fatality or hospitalization of workers

2. Personnel in command will be established according to the nature of the emergency, as follows:

    a. Medical emergencies: the occupational health physician or the occupational and environmental health nurse is in command.

    b. Fire emergencies: the fire brigade captain is in command in incipient level fires; in major structural fires, the local fire department is in command.

    c. Hazardous materials releases: the HazMat team captain is in command; in major releases involving the community, the local fire department's HazMat technician team is in command.

    d. Natural disasters, intrusions, and bomb threats: the human resources and safety directors share command in coordination with security; in events of immediate threat involving bomb threats, violence, and intrusions, the local police authority is in command.

    e. Overall coordination of plan development and implementation is under the direction of the emergency-response team coordinator.

    f. Design and annual review of this plan are under the direction of the disaster planning committee chairman.

3. Evacuation and fire drills should be held at least annually to practice the documented plans; every drill or actual emergency incident should be followed by an in-depth evaluation to include all levels of responders.

    a. Individuals should be assigned to assist handicapped workers in emergencies.

    b. Evacuation routes and alternate means of escape should be identified; these need to be made known to all persons at site.

    c. Routes must be kept unobstructed through regular safety inspections.

    d. Evacuation routes should be clearly posted.

4. During an evacuation, methods to ensure that personnel are accounted for need to be in place.

    a. Safe locations for staff to gather for head-counts to ensure that everyone has left the danger zone must be specified.

    b. Each department must assume responsibility for its workers and its visitors.

    c. The building can be reentered only after staff have been advised to do so by the senior management.

    d. A designated and an alternate head-counter should be appointed, one for every 20 workers.

    e. The incident command needs to be notified of the results of the count and of any missing persons.

    f. Sufficient inside locations must be designated when sheltering-in-place (workers are moved to a designated safe location within the building) is preferred over evacuation, as in tornadoes, hurricanes, earthquakes, or hazardous materials vapor clouds.

5. Information is disseminated to:

    a. Insurers, who will be notified by the human resources department or site management.

b. Community and media contacts, who will be advised by the human resources director; a preselected site should be designated for media and press releases.

6. Authority notification and reporting will occur as follows:
   a. The local emergency planning committee will be notified by the local fire department as required by regulations.
   b. The national response center will be notified by the safety director when mandated by regulatory requirements.
   c. The local environmental protection agency will be notified, when mandated, by the environmental protection manager.
   d. Other notifications may be necessary for different regions; company policy may require certain company representative notifications.

7. Several people are responsible for recordkeeping functions.
   a. The occupational and environmental health nurse will establish and maintain all health records.
   b. The maintenance supervisor will maintain all fire maintenance and repair records.
   c. The maintenance supervisor will maintain boiler records and emergency generator testing records.
   d. An appropriate designee will establish and maintain incident response records.
   e. The environmental protection manager will establish and maintain hazardous materials release reports.
   f. The human resources director and the safety director will establish and maintain all other records, based on the nature of the record and the incident.

E **The emergency procedures outlined in this section can be applied to numerous emergency scenarios, including hurricane, flood, major blizzard, bomb threat, fire, medical emergency, and hostile events.**

1. A tornado is imminent.
   a. Description: A tornado is imminent, and you have no time to report to the designated tornado shelter.
   b. Action plan: Seek safety under a table, desk, or heavy piece of equipment that offers protection from falling debris; use a coat or similar item to protect your face and eyes; put on safety equipment such as safety glasses and hard hat.
   c. Post-threat plan: Call the designated numbers for help (if phones are operational); inspect your work area for damage; follow evacuation, cleanup, or other recovery activities as directed.

2. A tornado warning has been issued.
   a. Description: A tornado warning has been issued, and time permits additional preparation.
   b. Action plan: Seek shelter immediately in interior rooms without windows, such as bathrooms or closets; shut off utilities and processes that will not become hazardous when interrupted; wear any personal safety equipment.
   c. Post-threat plan: Call the designated numbers for help if needed (if phones are operational); inspect your work area for damage; follow evacuation, cleanup, or other recovery activities as directed.

3. Hazardous material—a small spill or release
   a Description: A small spill has occurred that poses no safety, environmental, or health danger and can be handled safely without additional assistance or equipment beyond standard personal safety equipment.

    b. Action plan: Close valves and right drums or bottles according to your training and the MSDS; prevent the chemical from entering a drain; add neutralizing agents, adsorbents, or pillow.

    c. Post-threat plan: Dispose of material according to site hazardous waste procedures. Fill out an accident form.

4. Hazardous material–a large spill or release has occurred!

    a. Description: A large spill or release has occurred; it poses a significant threat to health and safety from vapors or fume inhalation, skin contact, flammability, environmental contamination, rapid spill proliferation, and loss of site safety control.

    b. Action plan

      1) Get yourself and others out of the danger zone. Rope off the area to prevent entry, call the designated number immediately and advise on the nature of the spill, the chemicals involved, and the exact location; do not attempt to rescue co-workers.

      2) The on-site HazMat team will respond to the incident according to their training and equipment capabilities or will request help from the local fire department's HazMat technician team.

      3) Occupational health providers will respond to provide emergency victim care and monitor the HazMat team members.

      4) Exposure victims will be decontaminated as necessary by the HazMat team before being released to community emergency-response providers. The hospital will be notified.

    c. Post-threat plan: The size of the release may necessitate a report to governmental authorities. Cleanup operations will be arranged according to the nature of the spill, such as via commercial chemical cleanup companies.

F **Recovery procedures are multifaceted; they include stress debriefing, incident investigation, report development, damage assessment, and cleanup and restoration.**

1. Critical incident stress: "Reactions to trauma/crisis in the workplace may have far-reaching repercussions on the emotional and financial status of an organization. It is imperative to address these issues and situations as they occur" (Lewis, 1993).

    a. Psychologic assistance will be offered to all affected employees in the event of an emotionally traumatic emergency response, which can precipitate critical incident stress similar to post-traumatic stress disorder.

    b. This will be offered between 24 to 48 hours after the event.

    c. Trained psychologist services will be obtained.

2. Incident investigation: Its chief purpose is to prevent similar future losses by identifying and evaluating present losses, reporting to OSHA, and assessing insurance claim needs.

    a. The investigation should be conducted at the scene of the incident, keeping the site as undisturbed as possible.

    b. Photos should be taken, drawings developed, and measurements taken as appropriate.

    c. All witnesses should be interviewed, one at a time and privately.

    d. An effort should be made to determine the root causes.

3. Reports include regulatory reports as required, internal reports according to company policy, and press releases as needed.

4. Each worker is expected to evaluate the worksite for damages, make a report to supervisors, and complete a maintenance work order.

   a. The occupational health department will provide a report of injuries, fatalities, and hospitalizations to the safety and human resources departments and establish follow-up case-management procedures.
   b. Maintenance will evaluate utilities, building structure, and major processing equipment for damage and report to the safety department and upper management.
   c. Section supervisors will evaluate worker reports and departmental damages—including lost records, lost or damaged equipment, and any damages that pose a safety hazard or delay the return to normal operations—and will report these to the maintenance and safety departments and management.
5. Cleanup operations will be supervised by the maintenance department, which will use outside contractors as needed, after approval from management. Management will establish a priority list for restoration processes to return to normal operations.
   a. The company's employee assistance program (EAP) will be contacted for services if applicable.
   b. Accounting will quantify financial losses and restoration costs for management.
   c. Management will arrange professional services such as legal assistance as applicable.
   d. Information technology will provide smooth and rapid restoration of computer services.

G **In order to maintain the program, the plan will be reviewed and updated annually by the disaster planning committee, with changes being implemented by the chairman.**
1. The emergency plan document will be distributed to plant manager, shift supervisors, emergency-response team coordinator, safety, occupational health services, human resources, maintenance, switchboard, local fire department, and local emergency planning committee.
2. Testing and drills will occur on a regular basis:
   a. Evacuation drills will be conducted at least annually.
   b. Emergency-response team drills will be conducted monthly, using methods such as table-top drills, skills practice, and mock drills.
   c. A mock disaster drill will be conducted annually and should include community emergency-response agencies.
   d. Emergency responders will be required to pass annual performance tests of procedures such as CPR, according to their area of response.
   e. Follow-up assessment will include identifying processes that proceeded as planned, areas requiring improvement, and equipment and operating procedures that need to be added, deleted, or modified. Participants will be advised of the findings.
3. The type and nature of training will vary according to personnel's responsibilities.
   a. The HazMat team will be trained by a recognized, qualified training firm that is able to provide awareness, operations, and technician levels of training in accordance with the requirements of 29 CFR 1910.120. Training will be provided for appropriately designated workers, who will also receive annual refresher training.
   b. Fire brigade members will be trained to the level of incipient fire response in accordance with NFPA (National Fire Protection Association,

2005) 600 and OSHA Standard Subpart L by the local fire department, with refresher training annually.

  c. First-aid and CPR training will be provided by the occupational and environmental health nurse with monthly training sessions and annual refresher programs; training curriculum will be in accordance with the standards of the American Heart Association or National Red Cross and with the OSHA Compliance Guideline 2-2.53C, promulgated in October, 1990.

4. Multiple types of equipment must be maintained.

  a. Each emergency-response team will maintain its own equipment, with the exception of the fire and self-contained breathing apparatus equipment, which will be maintained by the maintenance department.

  b. Equipment inspections will be conducted and recorded monthly; deficiencies will be reported to the emergency-response coordinator.

  c. The emergency-response coordinator will provide annual updated lists of on-site equipment to the disaster planning committee chairman for inclusion in the appendices of this plan as labeled.

  d. Medical and first-aid equipment will be located at the occupational health service center, and additional first-aid kits, stocked by the occupational and environmental health nurse, will be located at the entrance of each department.

5. Workers need to be familiar with the facilities that will serve their needs in the event of an emergency.

  a. The occupational health service will be the site for client care, if it is not conducted at the scene.

  b. A designated meeting location will serve as the media center and will contain a site plot plan, photographs of emergency-response drills for reference, telephones, fax machine, podium, and extra tables and chairs.

  c. A predesignated location will serve as the incident command post to conduct centralized emergency operations management. This facility will contain two-way radios, site plot plans, telephone, fax machine, set of MSDSs, a copy of this plan, and emergency lanterns.

X Appendices to Include in a Written Plan

A **Appendix A: Hazardous Materials Inventory with Location. Provide a complete list of all the hazardous substances on site and the department and building where they are located.**

B **Appendix B: Facility/Site Plot Plan. Provide a current map of the entire site. If appropriate, provide building plans for each building on site, including locations of fire equipment, emergency exits, evacuation routes, alarm locations, first-aid equipment locations, and other sites as needed.**

C **List of Fire Protection Equipment. Provide a comprehensive list of all fire alarm and response equipment, including fire-fighting foam, fire coats and other protective equipment, fire hoses, etc.**

D **Appendix D: List of Plant Emergency Safety and Rescue Equipment. Provide a comprehensive list of all plant safety and rescue equipment, such as tripods and confined-space harnesses, chemical neutralizers, spill blankets, shovels, respirators, etc.**

E Appendix E: List of Plant Emergency Medical Equipment. Provide a list of all on-site first-aid and professional medical equipment, such as stethoscopes, antidotes, stretchers, splints, etc.

REFERENCES

American Public Health Association. (1990). *Control of communicable diseases in man* (15th ed.). Washington, DC: American Public Health Association.

American Red Cross. (2004). *Shelter-In-Place*. Available at http://www.red cross.org/services/disaster/beprepa red/shelterinplace.html.

Archibald, R.W., Medby, J. J., Rosen, B., & Schachter, J. (2002). *Protecting occupants of high-rise buildings*. Available at http://www.rand.org/publications/ran dreview/issues/rr.08.02/occupants.html

Auf der Heide, E. (1989). *Disaster response principles of preparation and coordination*. St. Louis: Mosby.

Bartosh, D. (2003). *Incident command management in the era of terrorism*, Washington, DC: Police Executive Research Forum.

Breitenstein., B. D., Jr., & Spickard, J. H. (2002). Ionizing radiation. In P. H. Wald & G. M. Stave (Eds.). *Physical and biological hazards of the workplace*. New York: Van Nostrand Reinhold.

Bush, President George W. (2004). at the Wisconsin Emergency Management's 37th Annual Governor's Conference on Emergency Management. Available at http://www.whitehouse.gov/news/re leases/2004/03/20040330-6.html

Cangemi, C. W. (2002). Occupational response to terrorism, *AAOHN Journal* 50(4), 190-196.

Carmona, R., and Sullivan, J.B. (2003). Explosives and antipersonnel agents. In Chase, K. (Cons. Ed.). *Clinics in occupational and environmental medicine, terrorism: Biological, chemical, and nuclear*, 2(2), 339-361.

Centers for Disease Control and Prevention. (2004). *Bioterrorism agents/diseases*. Available at http://www.bt.cdc.gov/agent/agentlist.asp

Centers for Disease Control and Prevention. (2002). *Guidance for protecting building environments from airborne chemical, biological or radiological attacks*. Cincinnati, OH: NIOSH Publications. Available at http://www.cdc.gov/ niosh.

Cone, D. C., Weir, S., & Bogucki, S. (2003). Convergent volunteerism. *Annals of Emergency Medicine*, 41(4), 457-462.

Deitchman, S. D. (2003). Managing infectious risks to first responders. In Chase, K. (Cons. Ed.). *Clinics in Occupational and Environmental Medicine, Terrorism: Biological, Chemical, and Nuclear*, 2(2), 427-443.

Federal Emergency Management Agency (FEMA). (2000). *Planning for sustainability: The link between hazard mitigation and livability*, Washington, DC.: FEMA

Federal Emergency Management Agency (FEMA), (2004). *Emergency management guide for business and industry*, Washington, D.C.: FEMA. Available at http://www.fema.gov/

Federal Emergency Management Agency (FEMA), Emergency Management Institute, (2004) *IS 195—Basic incident command system*. Available at http://training.fema.gov/EMIWeb/do wnloads/IS195unt4.pdf.

Frykberg, E. R. (2003). Disaster and mass casualty management: A commentary on the American College of Surgeons position statement. *Journal of the American College of Surgeons*, 197(5), 857-859.

Hans, M. (1995). Are you prepared for a crisis? *Safety + Health*, 151(6), 38.

Hau, M. (1995). Emergency action plans: Is yours just an illusion? *Safety + Health*, 151(9), 156.

Hudson, T. W. & Roberts, M. (2003). Corporate response to terrorism, In Chase, K. (Cons. Ed.). *Clinics in Occupational and Environmental Medicine, Terrorism: Biological, Chemical, and Nuclear*. 2(2), 389-404.

Hurlbut, K., Tong, R.G., & Sullivan, J.B. (2003). Pharmacotherapy for the toxicity of hazardous materials. In Chase, K. (Cons. Ed.). *Clinics in occupational and environmental medicine, terrorism: biological, chemical, and nuclear*, 2(2), 299-313.

Jennings-Saunders, A. (2004), Teaching disaster nursing by utilizing the Jennings Disaster Nursing Management Model, *Nurse Education in Practice*, 4, 69-76.

Joint Commission Resources. (2001), Using JACHO standards as a starting point to prepare for an emergency, *Joint Commission Perspectives,* 21(12), 2514.

Jones, R. W. , Kowalk, M. A., & Miller, P. P. (2000), Critical Incident Protocol—A Public and Private Partnership supported by Grant No. 98-LF-CX-0007 awarded by the Office for State and Local Domestic Preparedness Support, Office of Justice Programs, U.S. Department of Justice., Lansing, MI: Michigan State University.

Kelly, R. B. (1989). *Industrial emergency preparedness.* New York: Van Nostrand Reinhold.

Krames, J. A. (2002). *The Rumsfeld way.* New York: McGraw Hill.

Lewis, G. W. (1993). Managing crises and trauma in the workplace: How to respond and intervene. *AAOHN Journal,* 41(3), 124-130.

Lloyd, D. W. and Wilson, H. (2002) Interpretation of subjective ratings: some fundamental aspects, *Prevention and Management: An International Journal,* 11(4), 308-311.

Louisiana State University, National Center for Biomedical Research and Training, Academy of Counter-Terrorist Education (2003), *WMD Response Guide Book*

Manuele, F. A. (2003a). *On the practice of safety* (3rd ed.) Itasca, IL: National Safety Council.

National Commission on Terrorist Attacks Upon the United States. (2004). *The 9/11 Commission Report* (Authorized Edition), New York: W.W. Norton.

National Fire Protection Association. (2005a). *NFPA 1561, Standard on emergency services incident management System,* Quincy, MA: National Fire Protection Association.

National Fire Protection Association. (2005b). *NFPA 101, Life safety code,* Quincy, MA.: National Fire Protection Association.

Parker, J. G. (2004). Planning and communication crucial to preventing workplace violence. *Safety + Health* 170(3), 57-61.

Salazar, M. K. (2002). Preparing for crisis-occupational health nurses respond. *AAOHN Journal,* 50(4), 161.

Salazar, M. K., & Kelman, B. (2002). Planning for biological disasters—occupational health nurses as "First Responders," *AAOHN Journal,* 50(4), 174-181.

Schneider, R. O. (2000), Knowledge and ethical responsibility in industrial disasters, *Disaster Prevention and Management: An International Journal,* 9(2), 98-104.

Society of Disaster Nursing, (2002) *Disaster Nursing.* Available at http://www.jsdn.gr.jp/eng/disaster/_nhtml.

Sokas, R. K., and Perrotta, D. M. (2003). Preparedness: where is occupational and environmental health? *Journal of Occupational and Environmental Medicine,* 45(11), 1133-1135.

Sullivan, J. F., Steward, C., & Phillips, S. (2003). Weapons of mass destruction: biologic agents. In Chase, K. (Cons. Ed.). *Clinics in Occupational and Environmental Medicine, Terrorism: Biological, Chemical, and Nuclear,* 2(2), 191-207.

Sullivan, J.F., Steward, C., & Phillips, S. (2003). Weapons of mass destruction: chemical agents. In Chase, K. (Cons. Ed.). *Clinics in Occupational and Environmental Medicine, Terrorism: Biological, Chemical, and Nuclear,* 2(2), 263-279.

United States Code, (2004). Title 18 Part I, Chapter 113B, §2332. at http://assembler.law.cornell.edu/uscode/html/uscode18/usc_sup_01_18_10_I.html

Veenema, T. G. (2003). *Disaster nursing and emergency preparedness for chemical, biological and radiological terrorism and other hazards.* New York: Springer.

Wallace, M., & Webber, L. (2004). *The disaster recovery handbook: A step-by-step plan to ensure business continuity and protect vital operations, facilities, and assets.* New York: American Management Association.

Wisner B., & Adams, J. (2002). *Environmental health in emergencies and disasters.* Geneva: World Health Organization.

14

Health Promotion and Adult Education

KAY N. CAMPBELL

Health promotion and adult education are essential elements of today's occupational and environmental health practice. The basic principles of adult education provide tools that can be applied to health education and to workplace health promotion. By helping individuals assess their health needs and developing strategies to meet those needs, the occupational and environmental health nurse creates an environment that values and supports healthy workers, thereby contributing to the bottom line of the company. Healthy workers are creative, engaged, and productive workers.

I Overview of Health Promotion

Health promotion is a process that supports positive lifestyle changes through corporate policies, individual efforts to lower risk of disease and injury, and the creation of an environment that provides a sense of balance among work, family, personal, health, and social concerns.

A **The emphasis on health promotion began with the nineteenth-century epidemiologic revolution.**
  1. Nineteenth century: The focus was on hygiene, sanitation, housing, and working conditions.
  2. Twentieth century: The emphasis was on disease prevention and health.
     a. 1970s: There was recognition that more than half of premature deaths were preventable by lifestyle changes.
     b. Early 1980s: Comprehensive workplace health promotion programs were instituted to help people change their health behaviors.
     c. 1990s: The concept of workplace health promotion broadened to include not only behavioral and lifestyle change, but also organizational strategies that supported healthy work environments.
  3. Twenty-first century and beyond: As healthcare costs continue to soar, adding a significant burden to industry, the major thrust becomes one of cost containment.
     a. Companies struggle to introduce insurance benefits changes in the form of cost shifting and decreased healthcare coverage to contain these costs.
     b. Health promotion and disease management become a critical factor in the strategy to keep people healthy or complement their treatment regimens, thus reducing the healthcare cost burden.

B **Health promotion activities are conducted by and draw upon the expertise of health professionals from many fields.**
1. Examples of these fields are nursing, health education, medicine, psychology, nutrition, occupational and physical therapy, safety, and ergonomics.
2. Occupational and environmental health nurses are often responsible for developing health promotion programs in work settings (AAOHN, 2003).

C **Health promotion focuses on:**
1. Prevention of illness and injury with return to work strategies to prevent relapse
2. Promotion of personal health accountability while partnering with the employer for enhanced outcomes
   a. The term *consumerism* is used to describe the provision of education to consumers of health care so that they become more prudent users of healthcare services and can advocate for better care.
   b. *Self-care* refers to individuals, each taking responsibility for his or her own health. Lifestyle and psychosocial factors have a great impact on morbidity and mortality (see Figure 14-1 for a checklist of self-care actions).
3. Development of strategies for behavioral change
4. Movement to optimal health by balancing physical, emotional, social, spiritual, and intellectual health
5. Creation of a supportive work environment through policy, programs, and culture

D **The rationale for health promotion includes the following:**
1. Treating preventable illness and injury unnecessarily increases the cost of health care.
2. Health promotion strategies result in improved teamwork, innovation, and creativity within the work force.
3. Health promotion improves productivity, morale, and quality of life.

E **Costs and productivity are affected by health promotion programs and services.**
1. Mounting research supports health promotion as a prudent investment for business (O'Donnell & Harris, 2001).
2. Healthcare costs continue to rise, with costs for large employers totaling $1.8 trillion, or 15.5% of the gross domestic product (GDP), up from 11.1% fifteen years ago (CMS Health Accounts, 24 March 2004); it is expected to rise to 18.4% of GDP by 2013 (Heffler and al, 2004).
3. There are direct links between absenteeism and lifestyle behaviors. Employees not at work are not productive.
4. Factors related to productivity, such as engagement, morale, physical or emotional fatigue, and desire to work are more difficult to measure (O'Donnell & Harris, 2001).

F **When a workplace health promotion program is being established, a balance of organizational and personal health goals should be achieved through:**
1. Business goals, such as improved employee productivity and morale, reduced health care costs, and recruitment and retention of employees.
2. Health goals, such as identification and reduction of major health risks, maintenance and improvement of health and health conditions, improved energy and resilience, and balanced work and personal life.

SELF-CARE ACTIONS

Completed	Self-care action	Recommended guidelines
☐	Annual physical exam (one per calendar year)	Have an established relationship with a provider and schedule appropriate preventative care
☐	Tetanus-diphtheria	Vaccine every 10 years (booster may be needed following an injury)
☐	Annual influenza immunization for high risk individuals and others wanting to avoid the flu	High risk people with heart or lung problems, older than 65, chronic metabolic diseases such as diabetes, kidney dysfunction, lowered immunity, individuals providing care to high risk persons in the home setting
☐	Travel immunizations	Consult your personal provider as soon as you know you are going to travel. The sooner you consult your provider the better (some series take up to 6 months to complete).
☐	Suggested health goal: <120/80	Check annually
☐	Suggested health goal: Total cholesterol <200 mg/dL LDL <100 mg/dL DHL <40 mg/dL Triglycerides <150 mg/dL	Check every 5 years if within normal limits At risk, consult healthcare provider
☐		At age 40, start annual fecal occult blood testing
☐		After age 50, flexible sigmoidoscopy every 3-5 years or complete evaluation of the colon, colonoscopy, every 5-10 years
☐		Oral exam and cleaning every 6 months
☐		Ages 20 to 29 – one complete eye exam Ages 30 to 39 – at least 2 exams Ages 40 to 64 – exams every 2-3 years Age 65+ – exams every 1-2 years

FIGURE 14-1 *Self-care actions*

Continued

Women

Completed	Self-care action	Recommended guidelines	Resources
☐	PAP smear and pelvic exam	Every 1 to 3 years after age 18 to screen for cervical cancer	JAMA Woman's Health Care Network, www.ama-assn.org/special/womh/womh.htm
☐	Clinical breast exam	• Every 1 to 3 years • Annually after age 40	National Women Health Information Center www.4women.gov
☐	Mammography	• Age 40-49 every 1 to 2 years • Age 50+, annually • At risk women, consult healthcare provider for frequency	

Men

Completed	Self-care action	Recommended guidelines	Resources
☐	Prostate cancer screening	• At risk, personal or family history or African American age 40 – annual digital rectal exam • Age 50: annual digital rectal exam • Discuss PSA blood testing with your healthcare provider	Men's Health Network, www.menshealthnetwork.gov
☐	Testicular exam	Annual healthcare provider exam	

FIGURE 14-1 —*cont'd Self-care actions*

G Comprehensive health promotion programs use the following strategies to reduce unnecessary health care utilization (Lusk, 1999):
1. Encouraging appropriate use of health care delivery services
2. Preventing acute illness and injury and delaying development of chronic illness
3. Reducing symptom severity, discomfort, and disability

H Levels of health promotion programs may include:
1. Awareness and support programs and services that increase the level of interest in a health-related topic through newsletters, flyers, posters, seminars, and health fairs
2. Screening programs and services to help identify high-risk employees
3. Lifestyle behavior change programs and services designed to help individuals adopt healthy behaviors, such as regular exercise, good nutrition, stress management, and smoking cessation
4. Work-culture enhancement that supports and encourages work/life programs, organizational change efforts, and flexible work alternatives

I Occupational and environmental health nurses contribute to:
1. Keeping healthy people healthy

2. Identifying high-risk populations and developing targeted interventions to reduce employee health risks, thereby reducing healthcare costs and increasing productivity
3. Developing interventions for management of disease conditions
4. Evaluating outcomes on health, healthcare costs, productivity, and morale
5. Contributing to the development of a comprehensive healthcare strategy for the organization

II National Health Promotion Objectives

A **Healthy People 2010: Objectives for Improving Health (USDHHS, 2000): Describes 467 objectives in 28 focus areas by health behavior, disease, or setting; Healthy People objectives seek to increase life expectancy and quality of life, and to eliminate health disparities.**

B **To meet these goals, the implementation plan:**
1. Supports gains in knowledge, motivation, and opportunities for better decision making
2. Encourages local and state leaders to accomplish the following:
   a. Develop community and state efforts to promote healthy behaviors
   b. Create healthy environments
   c. Increase access to high-quality health care

C **Several areas of Healthy People 2010 are of interest to occupational and environmental professionals.**
1. Directly related to health promotion activities are the goals associated with increasing physical activity, obesity and weight loss, tobacco use, substance use, mental health, injury, violence, and immunizations.
2. Less directly related are goals associated with sexual behavior, environmental quality, and improved access to health care.

D **Occupational and environmental nurses use the objectives to:**
1. Benchmark with national norms
2. Justify program and service needs in discussions with management
3. Focus interventions
4. Develop site-specific population health goals and outcomes based on population data

See Table 14-1 for an example of health promotion goals for an organization.

III Health Models

Health models are developed as a means of explaining the concept of health and its relationship to people's health decisions.

A **The *Health Belief Model* was developed by Godfrey Hochbaum, Stephen Kegeles, Howard Leventhal, and Irwin Rosenstock in the 1950s (Rosenstock, 1990).**
1. Major components of the model include the following (Janz, Champion, Strecher, & Rosenstock 2002):
   a. *Perceived susceptibility* is an individual's subjective estimation of his or her own personal risk of developing a specific health problem.
   b. *Perceived severity* refers to an individual's own personal judgment of how serious a health condition may be; perceived susceptibility and perceived severity are often combined into *perceived threat*.

TABLE 14-1

Example of Healthy People 2010 Goals for a Company Population

2010 Goals	Business Strategies/ Business Impacts	2005 Baseline	2010 Targets
Increase proportion of workers who engage in regular exercise	*Strategy:* Employer will improve walking paths near the worksite and will allocate space for after hours exercise class. *Impact:* Workers will have more energy, better weight control, less mental stress and fewer disability claims.	Currently, 25% of workers engage in regular exercise	The proportion of workers who engage in planned activity at least three times per week or more will increase to 50%. Planned activities include walking (10,000 steps per day), swimming, jogging, sports strength training, or exercise classes such as aerobics that positively affect physical health, increase cardiovascular fitness, muscular strength and flexibility and assist in disease prevention.
Increase the proportion of workers (and their families) who are at their desired weight	*Strategy:* Company nurse will provide lunchtime nutrition courses. *Impact:* Workers will generally feel better; they will have more energy, less mental stress and fewer disability claims.	Currently, 53% of workers are overweight or obese based on their body mass index (BMI).	The proportion of workers who participate in weight control programs, attend nutrition courses, and engage in physical activity will increase so that by 2010, less than 25% of the worker population will be overweight or obese based on their BMI.
Increase the proportion of workers (and their families) who do not use tobacco.	*Strategy:* At least one smoke cessation lecture series will be offered each quarter. *Impact:* Workers will generally feel better; they will have more energy, less mental stress, and fewer disability claims	Currently, 24% of the workers smoke or use other tobacco products.	The proportion of workers who participate in smoke cessation programs or strategies will increase; and by 2010, less than 15% of workers will use tobacco products. Smoke cessation strategies include smoke cessation clinics and using patch or other devices to discourage tobacco use.

    c. *Perceived benefits* are an individual's estimation of how effective a health recommendation may be in removing the threat.

    d. *Perceived barriers* are an individual's estimation of the obstacles to the performance of a health-related behavior.

    e. *Cues to action* are strategies to activate one's readiness for action.

    f. *Self-efficacy* refers to one's confidence in one's own ability to take action.

  2. The likelihood of an action being taken is driven by the positive difference between the perceived barriers and the perceived benefits (O'Donnell & Harris, 2001).

  3. See Case Study 1 for application of the Health Belief Model.

B The *Health Promotion Model* by Pender (2002) is derived from social learning theory (Section IV.C) and is organized like the Health Belief Model. It is based on the following premises:

  1. Health promotion is directed at increasing the level of well being and self-actualization of an individual or group.

  2. Health-promoting behaviors are continuing activities that must be an integral part of an individual's lifestyle.

  3. Health-promoting behaviors are viewed as proactive rather than reactive.

C The *Health Promotion Planning Model* (known as the PRECEDE model) is used to help plan and evaluate health promotion activities (Green & Kreuter, 1999).

  1. The PRECEDE model consists of **p**redisposing (attitudes, knowledge), **r**einforcing (rewards, positive feedback), and **e**nabling factors (resources that facilitate or hinder performance of desired outcome).

  2. This model considers the multiple factors that shape health (e.g., behavior, lifestyle, and environment).

  3. Health promotion education and policy are viewed as important influences on the quality of life.

  4. Epidemiologic data provide information about behavior, lifestyle, and the environment.

  5. Quality of life is the expected outcome.

  6. Application of this model begins with the determination to work on controllable health behaviors; it addresses factors in the environment that influence behaviors, such as positive rewards or feedback by friends and family, and the attitudes and knowledge of the person modifying his or her behavior.

Case Study 1: Application of the Health Belief Model

Mary is the caregiver for her mother who is dying from breast cancer. She thinks the disease is really awful and is frightened that she might develop it (perceived susceptibility). She is motivated to get her annual health exam, mammography, and perform monthly breast checks, because she thinks it may provide a means for her to detect the disease early and thus get treated successfully (perceived benefits). On the other hand, she tells the occupational and environmental health nurse that she forgets to do her breast self-examination (BSE) because she is afraid she might find a lump (perceived barrier). The nurse reinforces the need and rationale for early detection (reinforcing perceived benefits); she then provides Mary with a chart, watches her do BSE in the office, and discusses her concerns about finding a lump. The nurse helps Mary establish a routine for the BSE (decreasing perceived barriers).

D The *Model of Health Promotion Behavior* proposes that self-efficacy beliefs play a central role regarding health beliefs and behavior (O'Donnell, 1989).
  1. The basic premises of this model are that:
     a. Optimal health represents a balance between physical, emotional, social, spiritual, and intellectual health.
     b. Programs and services are targeted at three levels: awareness, lifestyle and behavioral change, and supportive environments.
  2. An expanded version of this model, which includes a dimension labeled "Occupational/Environmental," has been developed (van der Merwe, 2005).
     a. A unique aspect of this more comprehensive model is the inclusion of the concept of work.
     b. It draws attention to the importance of work and how work is integrated into the fabric of our lives.

E The *Harm Reduction Model* assumes that health risks can be decreased by having clients ask, "What is healthier, safer, or less risky than what I am doing now?" and "What steps am I willing and able to take in order to be healthier, safer or less risky?" (Bradley-Springer, 1996; Caplan, 1995). Basic principles of this model are as follows:
  1. Most people are competent to make informed decisions about health behaviors.
  2. Needs are diverse, so it is better to offer numerous behaviors rather than one solution.
  3. Incremental changes in steps will work better than making large, difficult changes.
  4. People need social support, education, referrals, and assistance to make changes.

IV Behavior Change Theories and Models

As occupational and environmental health nurses work with clients to assist them in changing their lifestyle behaviors, it is critical to have an understanding of behavior change theories. With this knowledge, the nurse will be in a better position to help clients overcome their barriers and move toward successful outcomes.

A An analysis of psychotherapy theories for behavior change was performed to identify psychotherapeutic principles that relate to helping people change their behavior (Prochaska & Norcross, 2003).
  1. *Verbal* theories use language and emotions to guide changes in behaviors.
     a. *Consciousness raising* uses the individual's personal experience feedback to stimulate responses.
     b. *Catharsis* allows individuals to express emotions, which produces personal relief and improvement.
     c. *Choosing* gives alternative responses for individuals, and self-liberation occurs when they choose an alternative.
  2. *Action* or *behavioral* theories use stimuli outside the individual to evoke an action or behavior.
     a. *Conditional stimuli* refers to critical changes made in the stimuli that influence responses; *counter-conditioning* occurs when an individual changes his or her response to a stimulus, and *stimulus control* occurs when the environment is changed.

b. *Contingency control* refers to managing change by making changes in the environment to cause individuals to change. *Reevaluation* occurs when individuals change in response to consequences without contingency changes in the environment.

B *Transtheoretical Theory*—**Stages of Change Model (Prochaska & DiClemente, 1983), describes interventions tailored to individual responses at specific levels or stages.**

1. The theory was formulated by using numerous psychotherapy theories to develop the stages of change model to produce sustained behavioral change.
2. The content of the model varies from client to client, depending on the client's history of actions, present environment, and personality.
3. The stages of change include the following:
   a. Precontemplation: clients are not considering making a change.
   b. Contemplation: clients are beginning to explore or think about making a change.
   c. Planning: clients are determined to stop and begin to develop a plan.
   d. Action: clients modify their behavior, which may also mean they change their environment.
   e. Maintenance continues as the new behavior continues to be practiced.
   (Table 14-2 presents examples of processes to facilitate change.)
4. The central premise is that people progress through a series of stages when they attempt to change behaviors.
5. Ten different processes are used to enhance progression through the stages of change. These include:
   a. Consciousness raising (increasing awareness)
   b. Dramatic relief (experiencing and expressing feelings)
   c. Environmental reevaluation (assessing how environment affects the situation)
   d. Self-reevaluation (how person feels about the situation)
   e. Self-liberation (belief in ability to change)
   f. Relationships (support)
   g. Social liberation (assessing social changes that support changes)
   h. Counterconditioning (substituting healthier behaviors)
   i. Stimulus control (restructuring the environment)
   j. Reinforcement management (getting rewards)
6. Identifying and classifying the population into these stages should guide program planning and interventions.
7. Behavior change tools developed; using these stages, provide a comprehensive framework to move more behaviors towards maintenance.

C *Social Learning Theory* **proposes that people's thoughts have a strong effect on their behavior, and their behavior affects their thoughts (O'Donnell & Harris, 2001).**

1. Social Cognitive–Self-Efficacy Theory (Bandura, 1986) describes the factors involved in making decisions related to healthy behavior.
   a. These factors include one's personal efficacy (self-efficacy), social and environmental support, and behavioral experiences.
   b. Self-efficacy is an individual's confidence in his or her ability to perform.
   c. An individual's efficacy expectation determines his or her choice of activity, how much effort he or she will expend, and how persistent he or she will be.

TABLE 14-2

Stages of change model and examples of processes to facilitate change

Stages	Precontemplation	Contemplation	Planning	Action/maintenance
Psychotherapy theories		Consciousness raising	Choosing	Contingency control
		Feedback	Self-liberation Catharsis	Reevaluation Conditional stimuli Stimulus control
Health promotion activities	Posters Invitation classes Buddy system	Health Fairs	Health education classes	Follow-up contact
		Newsletter Brochures	Counseling	Environmental supports
		Pamphlets Health education classes Buddy system HRA	Health Planner	Health education

Source: Prochaska & DiClemente, 1982

    d. Supporting an individual's self-efficacy efforts may be the single most important factor in that person's success in changing personal health behaviors.

    e. See Case Study 2 for application of the social learning theory.

2. The Locus of Control Theory:

    a. An individual's belief (outcome expectation) that his or her own behavior determines reinforcements (outcomes) is called *internal locus of control*.

    b. An individual's belief that reinforcements are controlled by others is called *external locus of control*.

    c. Theoretically, individuals with internal locus of control are more likely to take control of their health and to engage in health promotion activities than are those with external locus of control.

Case Study 2: Application of Social Learning Theory

Joe is a supervisor. He has few friends, a problem he blames on being 30 pounds overweight. Joe sees that people he knows and admires seem to get job opportunities he does not. He believes it is because they are fit and slender. Joe is depressed. He confides his feelings to the nurse, who acknowledges his feelings, but then reminds Joe of his positive attributes; for example, she notes that he has good leadership skills which would help him get promoted. She reminds Joe of the successes he has had in the past with reducing his weight. Joe begins to gain confidence in his ability to lose weight and get into shape. He begins to eat nutritionally sound meals and goes to the company fitness center. The support he gets from the nurse helps to support his self image; this leads to him feeling better about himself. The nurse needs to continue to support his efforts and guide him into a maintenance plan when appropriate.

    d. The occupational and environmental health nurse should find ways to motivate individuals for improved internal locus of control, thus increasing their chances for success in changing health behaviors. (See XI, Motivating Adults to Learn.) These may include the following strategies:
        1) Increase the participants' perception of success (intrinsic motivation).
        2) Reinforce positive actions (external stimulus applied to intrinsic motivation).
        3) Provide incentive for participation and accomplishment of goals (extrinsic motivation).
        4) Involve family support (extrinsic motivation).
        5) Reinforce health messages in the environment, for example, vending machines, cafeteria, work spaces, and management communications (extrinsic motivation).

D *Transactional Theory* **is characterized by "reciprocal determinism," in which individuals change behavior then begin to actively participate with others in the new behavior.**
1. This experience strengthens the individual's desire to continue the new behavior or find the need to change the environment.
2. Efficacy and support can modify behavior, and direct experience with the new behavior increases the level of efficacy and support.
3. Occupational and environmental health nurses can establish recreational leagues, teams, buddy systems, and support groups that reinforce these principles.

E The *Theory of Reasoned Action* **proposes that behavioral intentions are the result of one's attitude and subjective norms (Fishbein & Ajzen, 1975).**
1. *Attitudes* are determined by beliefs regarding the consequences of a behavior and one's positive or negative evaluation of those consequences.
2. *Subjective norms* refer to a person's beliefs or perceptions about what others think he or she should do.
3. *Intentions* are the immediate determinant of behavior.
4. Occupational and environmental health nurses should gain management support and take measures that will result in a culture that reinforces healthy lifestyles and influences people in making better health decisions.

F The *Theory of Planned Behavior* **builds on the Theory of Reasoned Action; the element added to that theory is the belief that one has the resources to perform the behavior (Ajzen, 1988).**

G The *Theory of Goal Setting* **(Strecher et al., 1995) states that setting goals can help people change health-related behaviors by focusing effort, persistence, and concentration. The steps to setting goals include:**
1. Determination of commitment to change
2. Analysis of tasks required to make changes; breaking complex tasks into smaller tasks
3. Assessment of the client's self-efficacy for performing required behaviors
4. Establishment of reasonable goals
5. Feedback for continued success
6. Case study: John made his usual New Year's resolution to exercise daily for 20 minutes. After the first month, he had to make a business trip, which interrupted his routine. He began to miss days and found himself just not exercising. After talking with the company nurse, John decided to start out slowly by exercising three days a week and then work up to more frequent exercise.

H The *Theory of Social Behavior* states that the probability that an act will occur in a specific situation is equal to the sum of the person's habit and intention (Triandis, 1999).

I The *Protection Motivation Theory* combines features of the Health Belief Model with self-efficacy theory and other social psychologic constructs such as fear, arousal, appraisal, and coping (Prentice-Dunn & Rogers, 1986).

J The *Health Action Process Approach* states that health behavior change takes place over time (Schwarzer, 1992).

V Levels of Prevention

Comprehensive health promotion and health protection programs and services comprise three levels of prevention (Leavell & Clark, 1979):

A *Primary prevention* is aimed at eliminating or reducing the risk of disease through specific actions; examples include immunizations, stress management, smoking avoidance, risk factor appraisal, seat belt use, work-site walk-throughs, and use of personal protective equipment.

B *Secondary prevention* is directed at early case-finding and diagnosis of individuals with disease in order to institute prompt interventions; examples include screening programs, health surveillance, monitoring health and illness trend data, and preplacement and periodic examinations.

C *Tertiary prevention* is directed at rehabilitating and restoring individuals to their maximum health potential; examples include disability case management, early return to work, chronic illness monitoring, and substance abuse rehabilitation.

VI Framework for a Health Promotion Program (Figure 14-2)

A Health promotion program planning is a first step.
  1. Management should be involved in early stages of planning.
     a. Management personnel are more likely to support the program if they understand the value of health promotion and wellness. This can be achieved by:
        1) Providing management with an estimate of cost savings (including indirect cost savings such as increased productivity, reduced absenteeism, and health-care costs) that will be realized as a result of the program.
        2) Using supportive background, including case histories of successful programs, to generate management support.
        3) Using examples of success stories to garner support, for example describing previous participant "stories" of the positive impact of a program to their health, life, and/or productivity.
     b. Management should be kept informed of all program and service activities and invited to participate in planning as appropriate.
  2. Advisory committees, representative of the employee population, should be formed; representatives include management, line supervisors, union members, the benefits manager, and employee representatives.
     a. The advisory committee provides assistance and advice through all stages of the program, from planning to evaluation.

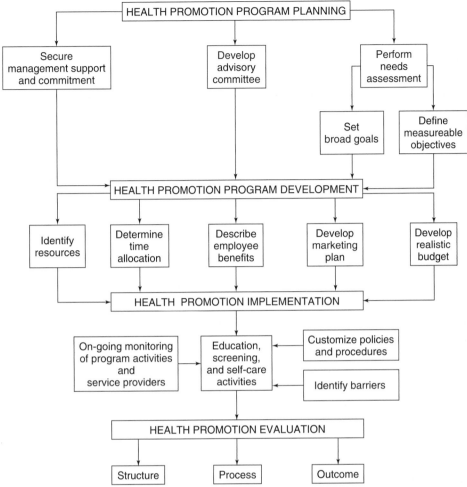

FIGURE 14-2 *Guiding framework for workplace health promotion programs*

Source: Rogers, B. (1994). Occupational health nursing: concepts and practice. Philadelphia: Saunders.

    b. Workers' involvement in and support of programs at this level are critical to a successful program.

3. To develop appropriate goals and objectives to guide program implementation and evaluation, a well-planned needs assessment should be conducted.

    a. A needs assessment can be used to collect information about the interests and health status of employees through written surveys, interviews, focus groups, or a combination of these methods.

    b. Workers' compensation data, insurance records, absenteeism reports, and other data that reflect health care costs within an organization are an important component of the needs assessment.

    c. A health risk appraisal is an efficient and relatively inexpensive tool that can identify a specific employee's health behavior and risks (Box 14-1).

    d. Development of targeted health risk interventions has proven to reduce healthcare costs and improve productivity.

BOX 14-1

Health risk appraisal

- A health risk appraisal (HRA) is a health education tool that is used to compare an individual's health-related behaviors and characteristics with those of the general population by comparing statistics and epidemiologic data. An HRA estimates an individual's life expectancy on the basis of current risk behaviors, and it calculates the amount of risk that could be eliminated by making appropriate behavioral changes.
- A health risk appraisal is easy to administer, confidential, provides information specific to the individual, and is easy to interpret. It includes a section that recommends corrective action, and provides positive feedback for results that demonstrate healthy behaviors.

- A health risk appraisal is used to assess nutrition/weight-management needs, fitness, stress levels, drug and alcohol problems, smoking behaviors, and cancer signs and risks.
- The benefits of a health risk appraisal include the following:
  - It provides the health-care counselor with a rational teaching aid that can be used as a point of focus during discussions about health and behavior.
  - It relies on a self-administered questionnaire, simple physiologic measurements, and computer-assisted calculations.
  - It can be used with large groups because it is efficient and relatively inexpensive.
  - It is science-based; it uses precise data based on appropriate studies.

B **Program planning is critical to the development of health promotion programs and services.**

1. Internal and external organizational resources should be identified when developing a health promotion program.
   a. The personnel needed to implement the program should be determined.
      1) Personnel from health services within the organization may implement programs, or they may be outsourced.
      2) Programs may require personnel with special skills and knowledge, such as an exercise physiologist to lead an exercise program.
      3) Personnel from various community agencies, such as the American Cancer Society or the American Red Cross, offer services or programs that can be provided at work sites.
   b. Audiovisual equipment may be essential, as well as other equipment specific to the programs and services (e.g., screening supplies, exercise devices).
   c. Paper, pencils, computer products, and other incidental supplies should be readily available.
   d. The availability of facilities and space appropriate for the purposes of the activity should be determined.
2. Negotiations must be carried out with the company for personal versus company time required to develop the program and for workers to use the program.

3. The program's existing and potential benefits should be determined.
   a. Existing benefits might include insurance incentives for employees who participate in certain activities.
   b. Potential benefits might be negotiated with management; for example, a "wellness" day could be traded for a certain number of sick days.
4. In order to be successful, marketing strategies should include participation of employees affected by the program.
5. A successful program depends on the inclusion of a realistic and a feasible budget; if costs exceed available resources, the occupational and environmental health nurse will be required to submit a revised budget to management or to adjust the programs to accommodate the available funds.

C **Health promotion program implementation involves many considerations.**
1. The primary strategy used in health promotion programs is education; screening and self-care activities are also important elements of a program. (Note: Referral and follow-up procedures must always be included as part of a screening program.)
2. Once a program is implemented, it is continually monitored to assess time frames, costs, and management interest and support; adjustments are made as needed.
3. The advantages and disadvantages of the health service providers (in-house or contracted) should be constantly monitored; in today's business climate, providers will need to prove how their services are cost beneficial and how they give a return on investment.
4. Policies and procedures that affect the provision of health promotion services should be customized to meet the needs of the organization.
5. Barriers to program implementation must be identified and considered in future planning.

D **Health promotion programs and services are evaluated by using a structure, process, and outcome framework.**
1. Examples of the structural elements to be considered in the evaluation include:
   a. Qualifications and adequacy of the staff involved in all phases of the program
   b. Appropriateness of the equipment and supplies used to carry out the program
   c. Demographics of workers who participated in the program
   d. Appropriateness of the facilities
   e. Match of the program with the mission and goals of the organization
   f. Management's commitment to wellness and support of the program
2. Examples of process elements to be considered in an evaluation include:
   a. The specific activities that characterize the program (e.g., if a diabetic screening program is in place, are the protocols and procedures state-of-the-art and appropriate for this employee population?)
   b. Evidence of collaboration and support among the various personnel involved in the program
   c. A monitoring system adequate to detect the need for changes
   d. Documentation and recordkeeping that meet legal requirements and effectively support communication
3. Examples of outcome elements to be considered in an evaluation include:
   a. Injury, illness, and absenteeism records

b. Surveys that evaluate knowledge about self-care (e.g., American Cancer Society screening guidelines) and attitudes about health (i.e., reflected in an expressed desire to participate in healthy behaviors)

c. Epidemiologic data that reflect behavioral choices related to health (e.g., decreased smoking rates)

d. Identification of health risks, participation in targeted interventions, lifestyle behavior change, and resulting impact to healthcare costs.

e. Observations of health activities (e.g., increased use of company exercise equipment)

4. Costs and benefits are a critical outcome measure that can determine whether a company will continue to support a program. (Chapter 9 describes steps in conducting cost-effectiveness/cost-benefit analyses.)

5. Outcomes should be communicated to management in order to ensure continuing support.

E **Incentives can be used to:**

1. Encourage employees to continue and maintain participation in health promotion programs and services.

2. Create a selling point for marketing health programs and services. (Program participation is competing for time and energy with other factors in the lives of employees.)

VII Lifestyle and Health Promotion

Modifiable lifestyles have been identified as a major cause of premature death in the United States.

A **Addiction behaviors are characterized by compulsion, loss of control, and continued involvement despite adverse consequences.**

1. Tobacco use causes nearly one in five deaths in the United States, making it the most preventable cause of death.

   a. About 8.6 million people in the United States have at least one serious illness caused by smoking (CDC web 2004).

   b. The latest trends indicate that 90% of the new smokers are children and teens.

   c. Figure 14-3 provides a test for measuring nicotine dependence.

2. Alcohol is the most misused drug.

   a. One out of every 13 adults in the United States abuses alcohol or is alcoholic.

   b. Moderate alcohol use—up to two drinks per day for men and one drink per day for women and older people—is not harmful for most adults.

   c. Box 14-2 presents a test for measuring alcohol dependence.

3. Drug misuse includes abuse of caffeine, alcohol, nicotine, cocaine, heroin, opiates, marijuana, designer drugs (drugs manufactured in an illegal laboratory that mimic a controlled substance), and prescription drugs.

B **Stress is a contributing risk factor to cardiovascular disease; more than half of the visits to health-care professionals are for stress-related disorders.**

1. Often, employee's absence from work is directly or indirectly related to stress and psychosocial factors. These issues are the most difficult to manage; they often affect the nurse's ability to get the employee back to work in a timely way.

The Fagerstrom Test

Questions		Points
1. How soon after you wake in the morning do you smoke your first cigarette?	Within 5 min.	3
	6-30 min.	2
	31-60 min.	1
	After 60 min.	0
2. Do you find it difficult to refrain from smoking in places where it is forbidden, e.g., church, library, cinema?	Yes	1
	No	0
3. Which cigarettes would you most hate to give up?	First one in the A.M.	1
	All others	0
4. How many cigarettes do you smoke per day?	10 or fewer	0
	11-20	1
	21-30	2
	31 or more	3
5. Do you smoke more frequently during the first hours after waking than during the rest of the day?	Yes	1
	No	0
6. Do you smoke even if you are so ill that you are in bed most of the day?	Yes	1
	No	0

Score: 1-6 = Low to moderate dependence
7-11 = High dependence

FIGURE 14-3 *The Fagerstrom test for nicotine dependence*

From Heatherton, T. F., et al. (1991). The Fagerstrom Test for Nicotine Dependence: A revision of the Fagerstrom Tolerance Questionnaire. *British Journal of Addictions, 86,* 1125.

BOX 14-2

Alcohol and other drug validation question set (CAGE questionnaire)

C Have you ever felt the need to *cut down* on your drinking?
A Have you ever felt *annoyed* by criticism of your drinking?
G Have you ever felt *guilty* about drinking?
E Have you ever used an *eye-opener* or taken a drink the first thing in the morning to steady your nerves or get rid of a hangover?

A positive response to two or more questions creates a high degree of suspicion regarding alcohol dependency.

---

2. Stress management education focuses on teaching people to manage their stress in a variety of ways, for example, progressive relaxation, meditation, cognitive restructuring, and physical activity.
3. The focus for today is to build skills for becoming more resilient, thus avoiding stress and remaining productive.
   a. Resilient people can be successful at work and in their personal lives even in a face-paced, ever-changing environment.

b. Resilient people make wise use of their energy, always ensuring that they eat well, are physically active, and manage themselves well.

C **Diet is associated with six of the top 10 causes of death: heart disease, stroke, atherosclerosis, non–insulin-dependent diabetes, cancer, and chronic liver disease.**

1. Eating foods low in fat and high in fiber reduces the risk of heart disease and cancer.

2. Low-fat, high-fiber diets also help to control body weight, which is a growing concern, according to the U.S. Public Health Service, because approximately 34% of Americans are overweight (USDHHS, 2000).

3. Obesity is currently an epidemic in the United States, with more than 64% of all adults overweight or obese (Office of the Surgeon General, n.d.).

   a. The annual cost of obesity in the United States is nearly $117 billion (CDC web 2004).

   b. Poor diet and physical inactivity lead to 300,000 deaths each year—second only to tobacco use (CDC web 2004).

   c. Body mass index (BMI) is a tool for estimating the weight status of individuals (Table 14-3).

      1) A person's BMI level is calculated by multiplying weight in pounds by 703; then dividing by height in inches twice (AAOHN, 2004a).

      2) Example: The formula for the BMI of a 5 foot 4 inch, 135-pound person is:

$$\frac{135 \times 703}{64 \times 64} \quad \frac{94,905}{4,096} \quad BMI = 23.2$$

      3) Normal scores range from 18.5-24.9; scores under 18.5 indicate underweight; between 25 and 29.9 overweight; over 30 indicates obesity.

   d. Effective weight-management programs can avoid substantial amounts of medical costs in addition to preventing overweight/obesity-related diseases.

   e. Workplace weight-management programs play a tremendous role in helping employees achieve weight loss. According to an AAOHN survey, nearly half of all respondents who claimed to participate in workplace weight-management programs reported success in reaching and maintaining their long-term goals (AAOHN, 2004b).

4. The food pyramid (Figure 14-4) encourages the following:

   a. Eating a variety of foods

   b. Choosing a diet with plenty of grain products, vegetables, and fruits

   c. Balancing food consumption with physical activity

   d. Choosing diet low in fat, saturated fat, and cholesterol

   e. Eating moderate quantities of sugars, salt, and sodium and drinking moderate amounts of alcohol.

D **Regular physical activity helps prevent coronary heart disease, high blood pressure, non–insulin-dependent diabetes mellitus, cancer, osteoporosis, obesity, mental health problems, and low-back problems.**

1. Physiologic evidence demonstrates that physical activity improves many biologic measures associated with health and physiologic functioning (USDHHS, 2000).

TABLE 14-3

Body mass index chart

Body mass index (BMI) is the measure of body fat based on height and weight.

How to calculate:

$$BMI = \left(\frac{Weight\ in\ Pounds}{(Height\ in\ Inches) \times (Height\ in\ Inches)} \right) \times 703$$

BMI	Normal						Overweight					Obese										Extreme Obesity						
	19	20	21	22	23	24	25	26	27	28	29	30	31	32	33	34	35	36	37	38	39	40	41	42	43	44	45
Height (inches)	Body Weight (pounds)																										
58	91	96	100	105	110	115	119	124	129	134	138	143	148	153	158	162	167	172	177	181	186	191	196	201	205	210	215
59	94	99	104	109	114	119	124	128	133	138	143	148	153	158	163	168	173	178	183	188	193	198	203	208	212	217	222
60	97	102	107	112	118	123	128	133	138	143	148	153	158	163	168	174	179	184	189	194	199	204	209	215	220	225	230
61	100	106	111	116	122	127	132	137	143	148	153	158	164	169	174	180	185	190	195	201	206	211	217	222	227	232	238
62	104	109	115	120	126	131	136	142	147	153	158	164	169	175	180	186	191	196	202	207	213	218	224	229	235	240	246
63	107	113	118	124	130	135	141	146	152	158	163	169	175	180	186	191	197	203	208	214	220	225	231	237	242	248	254
64	110	116	122	128	134	140	145	151	157	163	169	174	180	186	192	197	204	209	215	221	227	232	238	244	250	256	262
65	114	120	126	132	138	144	150	156	162	168	174	180	186	192	198	204	210	216	222	228	234	240	246	252	258	264	270
66	118	124	130	136	142	148	155	161	167	173	179	186	192	198	204	210	216	223	229	235	241	247	253	260	266	272	278
67	121	127	134	140	146	153	159	166	172	178	185	191	198	204	211	217	223	230	236	242	249	255	261	268	274	280	287
68	125	131	138	144	151	158	164	171	177	184	190	197	203	210	216	223	230	236	243	249	256	262	269	276	282	289	295
69	128	135	142	149	155	162	169	176	182	189	196	203	209	216	223	230	236	243	250	257	263	270	277	284	291	297	304
70	132	139	146	153	160	167	174	181	188	195	202	209	216	222	229	236	243	250	257	264	271	278	285	292	299	306	313
71	136	143	150	157	165	172	179	186	193	200	208	215	222	229	236	243	250	257	265	272	279	286	293	301	308	315	322
72	140	147	154	162	169	177	184	191	199	206	213	221	228	235	242	250	258	265	272	279	287	294	302	309	316	324	331
73	144	151	159	166	174	182	189	197	204	212	219	227	235	242	250	257	265	272	280	288	295	302	310	318	325	333	340
74	148	155	163	171	179	186	194	202	210	218	225	233	241	249	256	264	272	280	287	295	303	311	319	326	334	342	350
75	152	160	168	176	184	192	200	208	216	224	232	240	248	256	264	272	279	287	295	303	311	319	327	335	343	351	359
76	156	164	172	180	189	197	205	213	221	230	238	246	254	263	271	279	287	295	304	312	320	328	336	344	353	361	369

Source: Adapted from Clinical Guidelines on the Identification, Evaluation, and Treatment of Overweight and Obesity in Adults: The Evidence Report.

http://www.nhlbi.nih.gov/guidelines/obesity/bmi tbl.htm

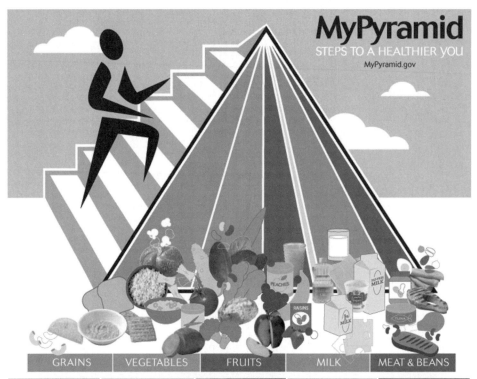

GRAINS	VEGETABLES	FRUITS	MILK	MEAT & BEANS

GRAINS Make half your grains whole	**VEGETABLES** Vary your veggies	**FRUITS** Focus on fruits	**MILK** Get your calcium-rich foods	**MEAT & BEANS** Go lean with protein
Eat at least 3 oz. of whole-grain cereals, breads, crackers, rice, or pasta every day 1 oz. is about 1 slice of bread, about 1 cup of breakfast cereal, or ½ cup of cooked rice, cereal, or pasta	Eat more dark-green veggies like broccoli, spinach, and other dark leafy greens Eat more orange vegetables like carrots and sweetpotatoes Eat more dry beans and peas like pinto beans, kidney beans, and lentils	Eat a variety of fruit Choose fresh, frozen, canned, or dried fruit Go easy on fruit juices	Go low-fat or fat-free when you choose milk, yogurt, and other milk products If you don't or can't consume milk, choose lactose-free products or other calcium sources such as fortified foods and beverages	Choose low-fat or lean meats and poultry Bake it, broil it, or grill it Vary your protein routine — choose more fish, beans, peas, nuts, and seeds

For a 2,000-calorie diet, you need the amounts below from each food group. To find the amounts that are right for you, go to MyPyramid.gov.

Eat 6 oz. every day	Eat 2½ cups every day	Eat 2 cups every day	Get 3 cups every day; for kids aged 2 to 8, it's 2	Eat 5½ oz. every day

Find your balance between food and physical activity
- Be sure to stay within your daily calorie needs.
- Be physically active for at least 30 minutes most days of the week.
- About 60 minutes a day of physical activity may be needed to prevent weight gain.
- For sustaining weight loss, at least 60 to 90 minutes a day of physical activity may be required.
- Children and teenagers should be physically active for 60 minutes every day, or most days.

Know the limits on fats, sugars, and salt (sodium)
- Make most of your fat sources from fish, nuts, and vegetable oils.
- Limit solid fats like butter, stick margarine, shortening, and lard, as well as foods that contain these.
- Check the Nutrition Facts label to keep saturated fats, trans fats, and sodium low.
- Choose food and beverages low in added sugars. Added sugars contribute calories with few, if any, nutrients.

MyPyramid.gov
STEPS TO A HEALTHIER YOU

FIGURE 14-4 *MyPyramid*

Source: U.S. Department of Agriculture Center for Nutrition and Promotion, April, 2005, CNPP_15.

2. Physical activity can build and maintain healthy bones, muscles, and joints; build endurance and muscular strength, and promote psychologic well being and self-esteem.
3. Moderate physical activity for at least 30 minutes a day for the majority of the week is recommended for adults.
4. Research has determined that walking is a good form of exercise.
   a. It is recommended to walk 10,000 steps per day, which is like walking 5 miles.
   b. A pedometer is a useful tool to count the number of steps a person takes; when the stride length is entered, the pedometer can calculate the distance one walks.

E **Cancer awareness can lead to early detection and prevention of this disease.**
1. Skin cancer is the most common type of cancer; lung cancer, however, causes the most deaths.
2. Breast cancer is the most common cancer among women in the United States, occurring in one out of nine women; some studies suggest it may be affected by a high-fat diet and excessive alcohol consumption.
3. The risk for uterine cancer increases with age (over 45), obesity, and levels of female hormones.
4. The incidence of prostate cancer increases with age; over 80% of all prostate cancers occur after age 65.

F **Accidents are a common cause of death and serious injury.**
1. Alcohol-related traffic accidents are the leading cause of death and spinal cord injuries in young Americans.
   a. Alcohol-related traffic deaths are the second leading cause of teen death.
   b. During a typical weekend, an average of one teenager dies each hour in a car crash and nearly 50% of these crashes involve alcohol. Box 14-3 presents safe-driving tips.
2. Safety also includes preventing falls, fires, and traffic accidents, both on and off the job.

G **The World Health Organization (WHO) recognizes infection with the human immunodeficiency (HIV) virus as a worldwide epidemic, for which prevention is the only control; currently there is no cure, although drug therapies have significantly impacted longevity of those infected with this virus.**

H **The occupational setting is an ideal location for the development of health-promotion programs and services.**
1. Health-promotion programs and services are an essential part of a comprehensive health and safety program in the occupational setting.
2. The timing and type of programs and services will be based on the needs of the worker population (Table 14-4).

BOX 14-3

Safe driving tips

- Do not drink alcohol and drive:
  - Use a designated driver
  - Use a taxicab
- Use seatbelts consistently
- Use infant/child car seats correctly and consistently

TABLE 14-4

Program development in the occupational setting

Health promotion activity	Type of program	When program is appropriate
A. Addictive behaviors:		

1. Tobacco use	Smoking cessation
	Nicotine gum/patches
	Individual behavioral
	  modification
		Smoker wants to quit:
		Assess dependency for
		  appropriate program and
		  support. (See Fig. 14.3.)

2. Alcohol and/or
  drug misuse
	Awareness
	Referral
	Employee assistance
	Community
		Job performance degenerates
		Absentee pattern appears
		  (see Cage Questionnaire in
		  Box 14.2.)

B. Stress reduction	Biofeedback Time management Visual imagery Exercise Humor Resilience training	Company experiences changes (e.g., downsizing) Increased client visits Increased EAP utilization

C. Nutrition	General nutrition
	Weight management
	Low fat/low cholesterol
	Cooking demonstrations
	Nutrition tables
	  interpretation
		Elevated cholesterol level HRA
		  results are out of the norm
		BMI > 25
		Reports of high blood pressure
		Concern about weight

D. Fitness	Recreational
	Flexibility
	Strengthening
	Aerobic
	Steps
		Anytime: everyone benefits
		  from exercise and activity
		  (recommended level assessed
		  at preplacement physical)
		Walking 10,000 steps/day

E. Cancer awareness		

1. Breast	Cancer awareness
	Breast self-exam instruction
	Clinical breast exams
	Mammography
		When worker population
		  includes female workers who
		  are age 20 and older

2. Uterine	Annual pap smears	

3. Prostate	PSA with digital exam	When worker population
		  includes male workers who
		  are age 20 and older

4. Testicular	Testicular self-exam instruction Clinical testicular exams	
5. Skin	Skin cancer awareness	
6. Colon	Fecal occult blood test Sigmoidoscopy	Anytime: All workers can benefit from this knowledge

TABLE 14-4

Program development in the occupational setting—cont'd

Health promotion activity	Type of program	When program is appropriate
F. Safety	Safety awareness education Driving safety Fire awareness safety Carbon monoxide safety	Anytime: Entire worker population can benefit from this information
G. HIV/AIDS	HIV/AIDS awareness World AIDS Day recognition	Anytime: All workers, particularly those at high risk, can benefit from these activities

3. Health Promotion is now heralded as one of the measures to curb the health-care cost epidemic.
4. See AAOHN Foundation Blocks that describe approaches for dealing with cardiovascular health (2004c) and diabetes management programs (2004d) in the workplace.

VIII Employee Assistance Programs (EAPs)

A An EAP is a work-based mental health program designed to provide support services to employees and, in some cases, employees' families who have personal issues that may affect their well-being and ability to perform their jobs.
  1. From the mid 1940s to 1950s, EAPs were designed to deal with alcohol and substance abuse problems.
  2. Currently, EAPs address an array of problems, including family, legal, financial, interpersonal, and organizational issues.
  3. The program may include referral, short-term counseling, crisis debriefing, and management coaching.
  4. Workplace mental health issues are steadily increasing. EAPs can develop programs to deal with depression, anxiety, and other mental health concerns.

B Standards for programs and professionals providing EAP services are developed by:
  1. The Employee Assistance Professional Association
  2. The Employee Assistance Society of North America

C Objectives of an EAP are:
  1. To effectively and efficiently provide services for ameliorating mental health problems, as well as alcoholism and other drug-related problems of the work force
  2. To identify employees with job performance problems and to respond to those seeking assistance by directing them toward the best assistance possible and providing continuing support and guidance throughout the problem-solving period

3. To serve as a resource for management and labor in intervening with employees whose personal problems affect their job performance

D **The core functions of EAPs include:**
1. Identification of employees' behavioral problems, based on job performance
2. Provision of expert consultation to employers and managers
3. Use of constructive confrontation appropriately
4. Creation and maintenance of links between the work organization and community resources
5. Evaluation of the success of employee assistance utilization, primarily on the basis of job performance

E **Criteria for successful programs include:**
1. Confidentiality as the cornerstone of the program
2. Accessibility of voluntary self-referral with an on-site or off-site counselor
3. Ability of supervisors to identify and refer employees with problems

F **EAP models may be external or internal**
1. Internal programs are staffed by employees of the organization or a sponsoring agency.
   a. The standard is one staff member for every 2,000 employees.
   b. The advantage is familiarity with the culture of the organization.
   c. The disadvantage is employee concern about confidentiality.
2. External programs are contracted by the organization.
   a. Services are provided by a variety of treatment centers, private companies, and other organizations.
   b. The advantage is that contracted programs are more accessible to small and medium-sized companies.
   c. The disadvantage is that the arrangement may not provide convenient access for employees.
3. Combinations of internal and external programs are sometimes possible.

G **The scope of services, which varies among organizations, may include:**
1. Assessment, short-term counseling, and diagnostic and referral services
2. Crisis counseling 7 days a week, 24 hours a day
3. Assistance in the development of a company's mental health policies and benefits program
4. Employee orientation, supervisory training, and union representation
5. Group education programs, such as stress management, conflict resolution, parenting, and organizational change
6. Prepaid alcohol and drug rehabilitation services
7. Management coaching for effective employee interactions

H **The role of the occupational and environmental health nurse in providing employee assistance services depends on the nature of services provided by the organization and on the nurse's knowledge and educational preparation. Occupational and environmental health nurses:**
1. Should be able to detect and recognize signs of potential psychologic or emotional distress among employees; stressed employees should be referred as appropriate
2. May provide counseling services related to lifestyle and health behaviors, personal issues, and work-related problems as part of routine care in the occupational setting; the provision of formal counseling sessions usually requires advanced preparation and credentialing in an appropriate field, such as clinical psychology

3. Should work with management to ensure that confidential and appropriate employee assistance services are part of a comprehensive occupational health and safety program
4. May provide crisis intervention to an employee (or department), who is then referred to an EAP counselor
5. May serve as liaison between company management and the EAP
6. May participate in the development of the program from assessment to evaluation

IX Introduction to Adult Education

Adult education principles enable occupational and environmental health nurses to effectively provide adult populations with preventive health information and help them modify lifestyle behaviors.

A **Characteristics of adult education are as follows:**
1. Adult education is the purposeful exploration by adults of a field of knowledge, attainment of skills, or a collective reflection upon common experiences.
   a. Explorations take place in group settings.
   b. An individual's personal experiences, skills, and knowledge influence how new ideas are received, new skills acquired, and experiences of others interpreted.
2. Settings for adult education programs include continuing education, training, networks, self-directed learning, distance education, and computer-based and community activity.
3. Participants in adult education are likely to have a variety of learning styles that affect their ability to acquire and retain information.
   a. Using multiple methods of presenting information will maximize the effectiveness of health education programs.
   b. Teaching styles should be adjusted to accommodate the needs of the learner; for example, older workers may require written material with large print and a setting that facilitates their ability to hear the speaker.

B **There are central principles that guide effective adult education.**
1. Participation is voluntary, with adults engaging in learning of their own volition.
2. Facilitation is characterized by a respect among participants for each other's self-worth.
3. Facilitators and learners are engaged in a cooperative group process involving a continuous renegotiation of activities and priorities.
4. Learners and facilitators are involved in a continual process of activity, reflection on activity, collaborative analysis of the activity, new activity, reflection, and so on.
5. Facilitation inspires adults to appreciate that values, beliefs, behaviors, and ideologies are culturally transmitted and to critically reflect on aspects of their professional, personal, and political lives.

C **Self-directed learning is the process in which individuals take the initiative in designing learning experiences, diagnosing needs, locating resources, and evaluating learning for themselves (Knowles, 1988).**
1. Contracts written by students are the chief mechanism used to enhance self-direction and allow students to diagnose their learning needs, plan activities, and identify and select relevant resources.

2. Techniques for self-directed learning involve the development of problem-solving skills to enhance students' ability to respond to typical problems and challenges.
3. Self-directed learners rely heavily on peer learning groups for support, information exchange, stimulus of new ideas, and locating relevant resources.
4. More time is required for extended exploration of curricular concerns, diagnosis and exploration of perceived needs (of learners) and prescribed needs (by educators), and negotiation of an agreed-upon learning plan.

D **Teaching involves presenting alternatives, questioning givens, and scrutinizing the self.**
1. Effective teaching:
   a. Sets an emotional atmosphere conducive to learning
   b. Uses learners' experiences as educational resources
   c. Gives constructive feedback to students
   d. Encourages collaboration and participation
2. The best teaching methods for self-directed learning involve:
   a. Leading discussions that present intellectual challenges in a nonthreatening setting
   b. Forming peer learning groups to experiment with ideas
   c. Encouraging the expression of opinions and alternative interpretations
   d. Providing lectures, demonstrations, independent study, and programmed computer learning

E **Adult educational programs are series of learning experiences designed to achieve, in a limited period of time, certain specific instructional objectives. Overall planning includes:**
1. Identifying the gaps between the learner's current and desired proficiencies
2. Assessing learning needs by the use of questionnaires, conducting individual interviews, observing participants, or consulting with experts
3. Using behavioral objectives to state the intended outcome or proficiency level the learner should obtain as a result of participating in the educational experience (Box 14-4).
4. Developing a plan that considers the objectives, outcomes, characteristics of the learner, size of the group, available times, equipment, facilities, and budget
5. Evaluating the program in terms of attainment of behaviors
   a. *Summative* evaluations are used to justify the program and focus on the program's worth and impact on the outcomes (e.g., a cost-benefit analysis).
   b. *Formative* evaluations focus on the program's procedures and are used for decision making to make improvements in the program (e.g., standardized tests and inventories).

X Philosophies of Adult Education

Adult educators' philosophies and systems of beliefs develop from values, principles, and experience.

A **Personal values affect adult educators' approaches to program development.**

B **Adult educators should develop and use a working philosophy of adult education to accomplish:**
1. Providing a point of reference on which to base activities
2. Helping avoid pitfalls in strategy development

BOX 14-4

*American Association of Occupational Health Nurses, Inc.
Behavioral Objectives*

A behavioral objective states what the learner will be able to do on completion of a continuing education activity. A behavioral objective identifies the terminal behavior or outcome of the program.

Objectives are critical to continuing education activity development, because they: (1) reflect input from learners relative to educational needs; (2) determine the selection of content and teaching methods; and (3) provide a guide to the evaluation phase.

Be sure that all written objectives:
- Use verbs that describe an ACTION that can be OBSERVED
- Are measurable within the teaching time frame
- Consist of only one action verb per objective
- Describe the learner outcome, not the instructor's process or approach
- Are appropriate for the designated teaching method(s)

Behavioral Terms to Use

apply*	define	distinguish	relate
analyze*	demonstrate*	explain	repeat
choose	describe	identify	revise*
compare	design*	list	select
compile*	develop*	outline	state
conduct*	differentiate	name	summarize
critique*	discuss	recall	synthesize*

* Use these action verbs with teaching methods that involve participants beyond a lecture/discussion approach (e.g., return skills demonstration, written/group exercises, etc).

Avoid using words that describe mental responses that cannot be measured, or terms that are broad, vague, difficult to measure, and permit a variety of interpretation.

Nonbehavioral Terms to Avoid

appreciate	enjoy	perceive
be acquainted with	gain a working knowledge of	recognize
be aware of	grasp the significance of	remember
be familiar with	have knowledge of	sympathize with
comprehend	increased interest in	think
develop an appreciation of	know	understand
develop conceptual thinking	learn	

C Recognized philosophies that can guide the adult educator are:
1. Liberalism—Knowledge is transmitted from expert to novice.
2. Humanism—Knowledge is acquired voluntarily based on individual needs and is self-directed, experimental, self-evaluated, and facilitative.
3. Progressivism—Knowledge is accumulated experimentally by use of one's senses and interaction with the world.

4. Behaviorism—Knowledge is gained by use of scientific method and through programmed learning.
5. Radicalism—Knowledge is gained through dialogue, dialectical process of reflection and action, problem posing, and critical thinking.
6. Deconstructionism: Knowledge is achieved through linguistic and literary analysis, by constructing individual reality, using dialectical process of reflection and action, problem posing, and critical thinking.

D **Approaches may be:**
1. Eclectic, developed by combining several elements of identified theories
2. Traditional, developed by adopting one particular theory and building on it

E **Adult education centers on the objectives of the program, needs of participants, curriculum, program content, analysis of the teaching/learning process, and the relationship of the education to the community in which the education takes place.**
1. The primary role of the occupational and environmental nurse as an educator is to help guide workers to accomplish their own goals, even when the nurse judges there are other goals that may be of more benefit to these individuals.
2. Designing the program around the worker will ensure successful completion for the worker and a willingness to continue the learning process.

XI Motivating Adults to Learn

Motivation is the concept that helps explain why people learn as they do. When adults are motivated to learn, they work harder, learn more, have a sense of enjoyment and achievement, and want to continue to learn. Occupational and environmental nurses will be of more assistance to clients if they are able to understand the motivational needs of health promotion program participants.

A **Motivational instructors function in the following ways:**
1. Present instructional material in a logical and orderly manner, thus providing clarity to difficult and new information, and are prepared to convey their knowledge through instruction.
2. Use motivation to arouse behavior, give direction or purpose to behavior, cause behavior to persist, and influence the learner to choose a particular behavior.
3. Have a realistic understanding of the needs and expectations of adults that influence their motivation to learn.
4. Teach in a manner that expresses care for the learner and knowledge of the subject, together with the intent to encourage similar feelings in the learner.

B **Several definitions are associated with motivating factors:**
1. An *attitude* is a combination of concepts, information, and emotions that result in a predisposition to respond favorably or unfavorably to particular people, groups, ideas, events, and objectives.
   a. Attitudes can be acquired through experience, direct instruction, or identification of role behavior.
   b. Attitudes can be modified by a new experience.
2. A *need* is a condition experienced by the individual as an internal (intrinsic) or external (extrinsic) force.
   a. A need leads the person to move in the direction of a goal.
   b. Identifying and addressing the learner's needs enhances motivation.
3. *Stimulation* is any change in perception or experience with the environment that makes people active.

a. Stimulation sustains adult learning behavior.

b. Attention, interest, and involvement are goals for learner participation.

4. An *affect* is the emotional experience of feelings, concerns, and passions that influences behaviors; when appropriate, the instructor should relate content and instructional procedures to learners' concerns.

5. *Competence* and *self-confidence* are motivating forces in learning; consistent feedback to learners regarding their mastery, progress, and responsibility will enhance their learning.

6. *Reinforcement* is a positive or negative response to an individual's behavior that affects the probability of the behavior's recurrence.

XII Teaching Methods and Techniques (Table 14-5)

A *Learning contract*—A formal agreement, written by the learner, detailing conditions of learning, including timelines and written evaluation

B *Lecture*—A planned oral discourse on a particular subject by a qualified person

C *Discussion*—An exchange of ideas between teacher and learner about subjects and issues

D *Mentorship*—An informal role in which the teaching function is primarily a means to advancement and secondarily a contribution to the learner

E *Case study*—An in-depth study of a representative problem or situation

F *Demonstration*—A presentation showing how something works and the procedures followed when using it

G *Simulation*—A method of obtaining skills, competence, or knowledge by participating in activities similar to a real-life activity of interest

H *Forum*—An open discussion with one or more resource persons and an entire group

I *Panel*—A small group of three to six persons who have a purposeful discussion of a topic about which they have specialized knowledge; discussion is in presence of an audience

J *Symposium*—A series of presentations by two to five persons of notable authority on different aspects of the same or closely related themes

K *Computer-enhanced education:* use of computers as an enhancement to teacher-learner interaction

L *Distance education:* communication between teacher and learner occurring through print, writing, telephone, or electronic media

M *Nominal group technique:* a type of group process that emphasizes the way people learn as contrasted to what they learn

N *Brainstorming:* a sharing of free-flowing ideas that is intended to stimulate creative thinking and the development of new ideas

XIII Effective Presentations

Presentations involve the preparation and delivery of critical subject matter in a logical and condensed form, leading to effective communication.

TABLE 14-5
Teaching methods and techniques

Method	Definition	Purpose	Specifics	Advantages	Limitations
Learning contracts	Formal agreement written by learner detailing what will be learned, how learning will be accomplished, timeline, and written evaluation	Individualizes the learning process	Components include objectives, resources and strategies, target dates for completion, evidence of accomplishment, and evaluation strategies	Flexible; learners control the process; preferred methods	Uncomfortable for learners and teacher if not used before; learners question quality of learning; teacher placed at risk for excess time pressures
Lecture	A planned oral discourse on a particular subject by a highly qualified individual	Cognitive transfer of information from teacher; framework for learning activities; identifies, explains, and clarifies different concepts, problems or ideas; challenges beliefs, attitudes, and behaviors; and stimulates the audience to further inquiry	Preparation includes preplanning, organization, compliance with time constraints, handouts, and practice	Precise and orderly format; popular; useful when no handouts; use for large groups; forum for one-on-one and enhances listening	Audience is exposed to one view; biased information may be given; discourages learners from the teaching/learning interaction; not able to determine impact on audience; speaker may not know audience level of knowledge or experience; evaluated on entertainment value rather than content
Discussion	Allows learners and teacher to talk about subjects and issues	Allows cognitive and affective exploration of issues	Prepare by setting discussion themes; providing resource materials; evoking consensual rules; personalizing discussion topics; and attending to group composition	Most favored, inclusive, and participatory	May uncover emotional issues which may need to be dealt with before further learning can take place

	Description	Purpose	Role/Types	Advantages	Disadvantages
Mentorship	Designates an informal role in which the teaching function is recognized primarily as a means to personal and institutional advancement and only secondarily as contribution to the overall well-being of the protégé	Promotes the development of the learner	Role of the mentor involves being supportive, challenging, and visionary	Promotes critical thinking; develops personal power and independence; provides a role model	Provides an environment where power may be misused, emotional dependence fostered and favoritism practiced. Hero worship, values conflicts, and feelings of abandonment may be experienced
Case study	An in-depth study of a problem or situation	Presents real life examples for study	Types include: case reports, analysis, and discussion. Design the study by focusing on the problem; developing supporting materials; reviewing; and field testing the case	Causes critical thinking; develops decision-making and problem-solving skills; and is participatory	Long preparation time; requires a facilitator to think on the spot
Demonstration	Presents how something works and the procedures followed in using it	Arouses interest and motivation; directs attention; supports verbal explanation; enables economical use of time and resources; and provides step-by-step guidelines in performing tasks or improving skills	Types include: instructional, participant volunteers, and full participation Roles Teachers must be technically expert; able to analyze process and break into small steps; and have all materials ready for use Learner must practice each step, communicate problems, and practice deficiencies	Illustrates point to enable learners to comprehend complex and difficult materials in a short time; reduces gaps between the learner and practice; and provides variety to facilitate different learning styles	Discourages some learners; difficult to isolate tasks, skills, and procedures into step-by-step manuals; time consuming; uses only small groups; limited individualized feedback

(Continued)

TABLE 14-5

Teaching methods and techniques—cont'd

Method	Definition	Purpose	Specifics	Advantages	Limitations
Simulation	A technique that enables learners to obtain skills, competence, or knowledge by becoming involved in activities that are similar to those in real life	An attempt to address real problems under real-life conditions and discuss them; develops complex cognitive skills such as decision making, evaluating, and synthesizing; impacts the learners' values, beliefs, and attitudes; induces empathy; sharpens interpersonal communication skills; and helps learners unlearn negative attitudes or behaviors	Types include: role play, case study, and critical incident. Steps are experience, sharing, processing, generalizing, and application. Roles. Facilitator should explain the purpose; give short, clear, and understandable instructions; provide relevant, real-life situations; involve problem solving appropriate to the level of the learner; have adequate interaction with learners; and give appropriate feedback. Learners should participate in all activities; develop an attitude of sharing and support; have open feedback with facilitators, and apply knowledge, skills, or attitudes to personal life situations	An opportunity to apply teaming to a new situation; participatory; no consequences of wrong decisions; immediate feedback; generates new ideas and changed attitudes; and is cost effective	Negative learning may occur if situation too complex; teacher must be proficient; expensive to design and conduct; time consuming

A **Elements of a presentation**

1. The goal of any presentation is effective communication, which means getting the message across in a manner that accomplishes the stated objectives.

2. Audience needs must be identified in order to reach the goals; audience needs are the determining factor in the selection of appropriate resource materials.

3. Meaningful content is supported by presentation aids, presentation techniques, and logistical details.

B **Types of presentations**

1. *Persuasive* or selling presentations pique the interest of potential participants, convince management to approve programs, or sell existing customers on the benefits of making changes.

2. *Explanatory* presentations make new information available or refresh an audience's understanding of a given topic by providing a general overview or description of a new development.

3. *Instructional* presentations teach how to use something, such as a new procedure or piece of equipment.

4. *An oral report* brings the audience members up to date on a subject they already know something about, by providing details suited to the needs and interest of the audience.

C **Preparing the presentation**

1. Establish written behavioral objectives, stating specific expected results and measurable accomplishments (see Box 14-4).

2. Audience analysis:
   a. Identify the objectives for the audience.
   b. Develop an overall approach to achieve objectives.
   c. Describe the social and demographic characteristics of the audience.
   d. Select appropriate information and techniques.

3. Prepare a preliminary plan consisting of no more than five main ideas or concepts, and discuss it with the officials who are planning the event.
   a. The plan is a guide for the presenter, keeping ideas channeled, focusing on points to be emphasized, and preventing the omission of information.
   b. Know the audience. If possible, determine the number of participants, where they work, what type of work they do, and their attitudes toward the subject.
   c. Make modifications as necessary before the presentation.

4. When selecting resource information, determine the purpose of the presentation material to be covered and the level of detail needed to meet the audience's needs.
   a. Questions to be answered:
      1) What is the purpose of this presentation?
      2) What do the participants expect and need from this presentation?
      3) What should be covered? What should be eliminated?
      4) What amount of detail is necessary?
      5) Will members of the audience have limitations (e.g., physical disabilities, language limitations, illiteracy, or other barriers to learning) that require adjustments?
      6) What can be withheld from the presentation but offered as a resource?

5. Organize the materials into the introduction, body, and conclusion of the presentation.

    a. The introduction should include:
      1) A direct statement concerning the subject of the presentation and its importance
      2) Some audience interest linked to the subject
      3) Examples leading directly to the subject
      4) Strong quotations related to the subject
      5) Important statistics that emphasize a point
      6) Strong or anecdotal information illustrating the subject
    b. The body of the presentation should consider:
      1) Visual illustrations as important aids to support the content
      2) Reiteration, statistics, comparisons, analogies, and expert testimony to present the main ideas
    c. The conclusion should consist of:
      1) A summary of the main ideas
      2) A review of the purpose of the presentation
      3) An appeal for audience action

6. Practice the presentation aloud to yourself, videotape or audiotape the practice session, or give a pilot presentation.
7. Conduct an evaluation.
    a. Evaluation is a critical component in assessing the effectiveness and efficiency of a program intervention in achieving a predetermined objective.
    b. Evaluations cannot be accomplished without taking into account people and their environments.
    c. By using the planning process data, measurable objectives, and program participants, a meaningful evaluation can be undertaken.

D **Development and use of audiovisuals can vary for different presentations.**
1. People retain about 30% of what they hear; about 20% of what they see; and about 50% of what they both hear and see; visual aids are used in a presentation to facilitate learning.
2. Characteristics of effective visual aids include:
    a. Each aid represents one key concept.
    b. They are appropriate to the audience.
    c. Text is restricted to a maximum of six words per line and 10 lines per visual, consisting of short phrases and key words rather than complete sentences.
    d. They use color or contrast to highlight important points.
    e. They represent facts accurately.
    f. They should be checked for spelling and accuracy; they can be unconvincing if inaccurate or misspelled.
3. To maintain quality, the presentation should contain no more than one visual for every 2 minutes of presentation time; the presentation, not the visuals, should be the center of attention.
4. Guidelines for using media include visibility and audibility, ease of operation, and accessibility.
    a. Consider room size, number of people, any distracting noises, seating arrangement, visual obstacles, and lighting.
    b. Organize the equipment before the presentation; arrange presentation components in sequence, and designate someone to help with lighting, if needed.
    c. Select aids based on availability, cost, and convenience.

5. Specific tools used in teaching include an overhead projector, slides, video, flip charts, handouts, audio recorder, chalkboards, computer visuals (e.g., Internet, PowerPoint), and models. Table 14-6 lists advantages and disadvantages of each.

6. Aids to further understanding (Note: When using any of the aids listed in this section, it is important to consider that all nonoriginal material may be subject to copyright.)

   a. The purpose of a chart is to direct thinking, clarify points, summarize information, and show trends, relationships, and comparisons. There are numerous types of charts (Box 14-5, p. 446).

   b. Illustrations, diagrams, and maps clarify points, emphasize trends, get attention, or show relationships or differences.

   c. Exhibits show finished products, demonstrate the results of good and bad practices, attract attention, arouse and hold interest, and adequately illustrate an idea.

   d. Manuals, pamphlets, outlines, and bulletins provide standard information and guidelines as well as reference and background material.

   e. Cartoons, posters, and signs attract attention, arouse interest, and often promote critical thinking.

   f. Photographs and illustrations from textbooks or magazines tie the discussion to actual situations and people, illustrate the immediate relevance of a topic, or show local activities.

   g. Examples and stories relieve tension, fix an idea, get attention, illustrate a point, clarify a situation, or break away from a delicate subject.

   h. Field trips present a subject in its natural setting, stimulate interest, blend theory with practical application, and provide additional material for study (Morrisey & Sechrest, 1997).

E **Several logistical steps are required when preparing for a presentation.**

1. Invite the audience to the presentation by letter, memo, phone call, formal announcement, electronic mail, or word of mouth.

2. Room set-up options depend on the size and shape of the meeting room, size and nature of the audience, type of presentation, delivery method, and kind of participation wanted from the audience.

   a. *Auditorium* style is used for large groups when there is no need for the audience to write or consult reference materials and when audience participation is limited to a question-and-answer period; generally, no tables or writing areas are available for participants.

   b. *Classroom* style is useful for relatively formal situations where participants need to write or actively use reference materials; tables or desks are provided.

   c. *Horseshoe,* or U-shaped, style is useful when eye contact with the audience and relatively informal discussions are desirable and participants may write or use materials easily; this is most desirable for small groups.

   d. *Buzz* style is useful when small-group discussions are conducted as part of the presentation; these discussions can be held easily at small tables distributed around in the room.

   e. *Chevron* or herringbone style is useful for group discussions, creating a more formal climate than buzz style and a less formal climate than classroom style; rectangular tables are preferred.

TABLE 14-6
Specific media tools

	Definition	Advantages	Disadvantages
Laptop computer with LCD projector	Use of laptop computer, PowerPoint presentations (slide show). Use of an electric device to project the presentation to a large screen	Predominately used. Convenient, easily modifiable, high quality, and inexpensive	Technical set-up. Make sure the laptop is compatible and working prior to the presentation. Have back-up CD, disc, or local hard drive with presentation in case the network is not accessible
Overhead projector	An electric device designed to project transparent materials as large as 10 by 10 inches and as small as 2 by 2 inches	The projected image is visible in a lighted room and transparencies are made inexpensively	Teachers must be able to talk and use transparencies simultaneously; machines require electric outlet and bulb
Slides	A small piece of film on which a single pictorial graphic image has been placed for still projection	Convenient to use, easy to obtain in high quality, relatively inexpensive, easy to use with no more than 5 to 6 lines per slide, and can be made from anything that is drawn, painted, written, typewritten, printed, or photographed	Slides must be viewed in a darkened room; each presentation requires filing, storing, and organizing slides
Video	Motion on tape shown on a television monitor with sound	Provides a common stimulus for students, with specific examples which achieve identification and involvement of the viewer with characters and situations presented	Expensive; not all information being presented may be consistent with what is being presented; must be shown in a darkened room and equipment often fails

	Description	Advantages	Limitations
Flip charts	A series of bound sheets of paper or poster board that can be flipped over, one at a time, to show a series of thoughts, pictures, outline points, questions, cartoons, or symbols	Portable, economical, and versatile; can be prepared ahead of time and used repeatedly	Not useful with large audiences; do not store easily; good handwriting skills are needed to develop
Handouts	Printed or duplicated material given to learners, such as outlines, job descriptions, bulletins, cartoons, charts, and problems	Allows learners to receive the same information and to be able to review or reference after presentation	A supplement, not a substitute for presentation; may distract from the main point or confuse the learner
Audio recorder	Recorded sound on a magnetic tape	Flexible timing and interruption of instruction; inexpensive, reusable, and easy to use; and tape is useful in large and small groups	Poorly prepared or used materials may distract or discourage learners
Chalkboard	A board whose writing surface is specially treated for use with chalk	Minimal cost; allows for spontaneity, audience involvement, and on-the-spot revisions	Not a permanent record; it has limited use in a large group
Models	Scaled representation, which may be equal in size, smaller, or larger than original	A model shows clearly and quickly "how" and "why" something works and permits close up observation, investigation, and analysis	Commercial models are costly to purchase; require large storage space, special atmospheric conditions, or extreme care in handling

Source: Adapted from Morrisey & Sechrest, 1987.

BOX 14-5

Types of charts

- *Highlight charts* present a direct copy or emphasize a point.
- *Time sequence charts* show relationships over time.
- *Organizational charts* indicate the relationships among individuals, departments, and jobs.
- *Cause-and-effect* charts illustrate causal relationships.
- *Flow charts* show the relation of parts to the finished whole or to the direction of movement of a process (e.g., PERT [Program Evaluation and Review Technique] charts).
- *Inventory charts* show a picture of an object with its parts labeled off to the side.
- *Dissection charts* present enlarged, transparent, or cut-away views of an object.

- *Diagrammatic or schematic* charts provide a simple portrayal of a complex subject by means of symbols.
- *Multibar graphs* represent comparable data using horizontal or vertical bars.
- *Divided-bar graphs* show the relation of parts to the whole by using a single bar divided into parts by lines.
- *Line graphs* display information using a horizontal scale and a vertical scale.
- *Pie graphs* show relations of parts to the whole, like a divided-bar graph.
- *Pictographs* represent comparable quantities in a given time by use of symbols such as a stack of coins representing comparable costs.

---

3. Equipment that may be needed includes a table, laptop computers, projection equipment, extension cords, spare bulbs, flip chart, and markers.
4. Download the presentation onto a compact disk (CD) or minicruzer (USB memory) if using from the network or hard drive in case there is a problem with connections.
5. Always check equipment, room temperature, and lighting; put slides, transparencies, and handouts in order; hide displays that should be out of sight before presentation; number transparencies or slides in order in case they become mixed up.
6. Coordinate arrangements at the presentation site by giving clear instructions regarding the specific needs; arrange for shipping materials in advance; arrive early to prepare the room; and always know how to operate equipment personally.
7. Announce "housekeeping" details before the presentation begins: rules regarding smoking, eating, or drinking; rest room locations; time and location of breaks; and registration requirements.

F Deliver the presentation.
1. Effective communication is a two-way process, involving both the speaker and the listener, that leads to some form of action or response.
2. In the communication process, the listener is the more important of the two members.

3. Platform techniques, such as eye contact with the audience, appropriate dress, confidence, and relaxed hand movements are important behaviors to exhibit.
    a. Gestures can be effective if they are properly synchronized with certain words or phrases and are not overused.
    b. Body movements are effective in releasing some of the speakers' tension, drawing attention back to the speaker from the visual aid, and changing the pace of the presentation.
    c. Facial expressions should be lively, varied, and appropriate to the mood of the audience.
    d. Concentrate on reducing distracting mannerisms such as lip licking, nose patting, ear tugging, stretching, or playing with pens, rubber bands, or paper clips.
4. Develop good voice quality: a natural, conversational pitch and injection; a level of volume that can be heard by all; a rate and tempo that varies enough to maintain the audience's interest; and deliberate pauses, used as needed.
    a. "Uh" results when the thought process interrupts the speech process; the problem is eliminated with increased familiarity with the subject.
    b. Trailing sentences or loss of voice at the end of sentences lose the audience.
    c. Faulty pronunciation and poor enunciation can be corrected by checking the dictionary for correct pronunciations and by adopting a manner of speaking that is clear, precise, and easy to listen to.
5. Tools facilitate the delivery of a speaker's message.
    a. A lectern provides a surface on which notes may be placed; provides an out-of-sight storage space for aids and handouts; gives a resting place for hands; establishes a type of relationship with the audience.
       1) Remaining behind the lectern establishes a formal relation with the audience.
       2) Moving to the side or front of the lectern removes the barriers and is less formal.
    b. The pointer draws attention to specific items on a visual aid and should be put down when not in use.
    c. The podium or lavaliere microphones should be used in practice until the presenter is speaking comfortably in a natural voice and with equipment at the proper height or on the lapel close to the mouth.
6. Learning to deal with audiences' questions is a vital skill for presenters.
    a. Conducting question-and-answer sessions involves accepting the question as a compliment from the participant, being prepared for possible questions, paraphrasing the question to ensure that everyone understands it, making the question relevant to the discussion, and trying to give a correct answer.
    b. Dealing with some difficult situations requires experience.
       1) Arguments should be postponed until after the session because they limit the participation of the rest of the audience.
       2) "Curves" or "loaded" questions may be intended to put the speaker on the spot, so end the discussion quickly and move on.
       3) Long-winded questioners should be handled by picking out a word or an idea that is being expressed and show its relationship to the presentation; or, as a last resort only, cut the questioner off in the interest of time.

4) The audience grows tired very quickly of a questioner who takes over to make a speech; the presenter should take control of the situation by asking the questioner to ask the question and then move on.

5) A question may come up for which the speaker has no answer; in that case, the speaker should admit it and ask the group if they have an answer.

G Always finish the presentation or program by evaluating the process and content.

1. Allow participants to rate the instructor.
2. Participants should evaluate whether the program addressed the stated goals and objectives and their own personal objectives.
3. Participants should be evaluated to determine the knowledge they gained during the presentation; this could be done using a pretest/posttest format.

REFERENCES

Ajzen, I. (1988). Attitudes, personality, and behavior. Chicago: Dorsey Press.

American Association of Occupational Health Nurses. (AAOHN) (2003). Competencies in occupational and environmental health nursing. *AAOHN Journal, 51* (7), 290-302.

American Association of Occupational Health Nurses.(2003c). *AAOHN cardiovascular health programs in the workplace.* Foundation blocks: A guide to occupational & environmental health nursing. Atlanta: AAOHN publications.

American Association of Occupational Health Nurses. (2003d) *AAOHN diabetes management programs in the workplace.* Foundation blocks: A guide to occupational & environmental health nursing. Atlanta: AAOHN publications.

American Association of Occupational Health Nurses. (AAOHN) (2004a). *Obesity management programs in the workplace.* Foundation Blocks. A guide to occupational & environmental health nursing. Atlanta: AAOHN publications.

American Association of Occupational Health Nurses. (AAOHN) (2004b). *AAOHN Survey: Employees tip scales of weight loss success.* Atlanta: AAOHN, Inc.

Bandura, A. (1986). *Social foundations of thought and action: A social cognitive theory.* Englewood Cliffs, NJ: Prentice-Hall.

Bradley-Springer L. (1996). Patient education for behavior change: help from the transtheoretical and harm reduction models. *Journal of Association of Nurses AIDS Care. 7* Suppl 1, 23-33; discussion 34-40.

Caplan D. (1995). Smoking: issues and interventions for occupational health nurses. *AAOHN Journal, 43*(12), 633-643.

Centers for Disease Control and Prevention (2004). *Cessation: Fact sheet.* From http://www.cdc.gov/tobacco/factsheets/cessation_factsheet.htm

Centers for Disease Control and Prevention (2004). *Key Stats.* From http://www.cdc.gov/obesity/keystats.htm

Centers for Disease Control and Prevention (2004). *Key Stats.* From http://www.cdc.gov/smoking/keystats.htm

CMS Health Accounts, 24 March 2004—cited by Thorpe, HA, 2004.

Corbridge, S.J., & Wilken, L: (2005). Smoking cessation-Part I, *AAOHN Journal 53*(2), 63-64.

Fishbein, M., & Ajzen, I. (1975). *Belief, attitude, intention and behavior: An introduction to theory and research.* California: Addison-Wesley, Publishing Company.

Galbraith, M. W. (Ed.). (2004). *Adult learning methods.* Malabar, FL: Krieger Publishing.

Green, L., & Kreuter, M. (1999). *Health promotion planning: An educational and environmental approach.* Mountain View, CA: Mayfield Publishing.

Heatherton, T. F., Kozlowski, L. T., Frecker, R. C., & Fagerstrom, K. O. (1991). The Fagerstrom Test for Nicotine Dependence: A revision of the Fagerstrom Tolerance Questionnaire. *British Journal of Addictions*, 86, 1119-1127.

Heffler, S., Smith, S., Keehan, S., Clemans, M. K., Zezza, M., & Truffer, C. (2004).

Health spending projections through 2013. *Health Affairs,* 11 February, pp. 79-93. Available at http://www.healthaffairs. org/cgi/content/abstract/hlthaff.w4.79, Retrieved 12 February 2004.

Janz, N. K., Champion, V. L., Strecher, V. J., & Rosenstock, I. M. (2002). The health belief model: Explaining health behavior through expectancies. In K. Glanz, F. M. Lewis, & B. K. Rimer (Eds.). *Health behavior and health education: Theory, research, and practice.* San Francisco: Jossey-Bass.

Knowles, M. S. (1988). *Self-directed learning: A guide for learners and teachers.* New York: Cambridge Books.

Leavell, H., & Clark, E. (1979). *Preventive medicine for the doctor in the community.* New York: McGraw Hill.

Lundy, K S., & Janes, S. (2001). *Community health nursing caring for the public's health.* Sudbury, MA: Jones and Bartlett.

Lusk, S. L. (1999). Demand management programs. *AAOHN Journal, 47*(6), 277-279.

Morrisey, G. L., & Sechrest, T. L. (1997). *Effective business and technical presentations* (3rd ed.). Reading, MA: Delmar Publishers.

O'Donnell, M. D. (1989). Definition of health promotion: Part III: Expanding the definition. *American Journal of Health Promotion, 3* (3), 5.

O'Donnell, M. D., & Harris, J. S. (2001). *Health promotion in the workplace* (3rd ed.). New York: Delmar Publishers.

Office of the Surgeon General. (n.d.). The surgeon general's call to action to prevent and decrease overweight and obesity. Retrieved March 2005 at http://www.surgeongeneral.gov/topics obesity/calltoaction/fact_glance.htm

Pender, N. (2002). *Health promotion in nursing practice* (4th ed.). Indianapolis, IN: Prentice Hall.

Prentice-Dunn, S., & Rogers, R.W. (1986). Protection motivation theory and preventive health: Beyond the health belief model. *Health education research: Theory and practice, 1*(3), 153-161.

Prochaska, J. O., & Norcross, J. C. (2003). *Systems of psychotherapy: A transtheoretical analysis.* Pacific Grove, CA: Brooks/Cole Publications.

Prochaska, J. O., & DiClemente, C. C. (1982). Transtheoretical theory: Toward a more integrative model of change. *Psychotherapy, 19*(3), 276-288.

Prochaska, J. O., & DiClemente, C. C. (1983). Stages and processes of self-change of smoking: Towards an integrative model of change. *Journal of Consulting and Clinical Psychology 51*(3), 390–395.

Rosenstock, I. M. (1990). Theory, research and practice. The health belief model: Explaining health behavior through expectancies. In K. Glanz, F. M. Lewis, & B. K. Rimer (Eds.), *Health behavior and health education: Theory, Research and Practice* (pp. 39-62). San Francisco, CA: Jossey-Bass.

Schwarzer, R. (1992). Adaptation and maintenance of health behaviors: A critical review of theoretical approaches. In R. Schwarzer (Ed.), *Self-efficacy: Thought control of action.* New York: Hemisphere.

Sitzman, K. (2004). Expanding food portions contribute to overweight and obesity. *AAOHN Journal, 52*(8) 356.

Strecher, V. J., Seijts, G. H., Kok, G. J., Latham, G. P., Glasgow, R., DeVellis, B., Meertens, R. M., & Bulger, D. W. (1995). Goal setting as a strategy for health behavior change. *Health Education Quarterly, 22*(2):190-200.

Triandis, H. C. (1999). Values, attitudes, and interpersonal behavior. In M.N. Page (Ed.), *Nebraska Symposium on Motivation, 1979.* (pp. 195-259), Lincoln, NE: University of Nebraska Press.

United States Department of Health and Human Services. (2000). *Healthy people 2010:* Volume I and Volume II (DHHS Publication No. 2000-0152). Washington, DC: U.S. Government Printing Office.

Van der Merwe, A. (2005). What are the different dimensions of wellness?, www.health24.com/mind/A healthy mind

CHAPTER

15

Managing Psychosocial Factors in the Occupational Setting

Mary K. Salazar and Randal D. Beaton

The quality of one's work life is related to a multitude of psychosocial factors in the workplace. Knowledge and recognition of these factors are essential to the development of effective and efficient occupational health and safety programs and services. This chapter provides an overview of the various dimensions of psychosocial factors; it describes methods to assess and respond to them, and it concludes with a discussion of things to consider when evaluating stress reduction programs and services.

I Overview of Psychosocial Factors

Psychosocial factors are directly related to the organization of work, organizational characteristics, interpersonal relationships at work, the meaning of work, and the characteristics of the workers themselves.

A Organization of work

1. The organization of work refers to how work is structured; it includes the work processes and organizational practices that affect the job design (NIOSH, 2002).
   a. The structure of work has changed in recent years as organizations have downsized, restructured, and increased their reliance on non-traditional work practices.
   b. Changing work practices may result in more stressful and hazardous working conditions such as reduced job stability and increased workloads.
   c. The number of hours Americans work each year has increased dramatically in the last two decades.
   d. Despite these negatives, the modern-day workplace offers workers more flexibility, responsibility, and learning opportunities than was available in the past; this can result in career growth, self-development, and greater job satisfaction.
2. NIOSH (2002) has developed a conceptual model to illustrate the multilevels of context inherent in the work environment (Figure 15-1).
   a. The *work context* refers to characteristics of the job; these include the job demands and conditions in the workplace.
   b. The *organizational context* refers to the structures and processes at the organizational level; they include management styles, production methods, and human resource policies.

External Context

Economic, legal, political technological and demographic forces at the national/international level

- Economic developments (e.g., globalization of economy)
- Regulatory, trade, and economic policies (e.g., deregulation)
- Technological innovations (e.g., information/computer technology)
- Changing worker demographics and labor supply (e.g., aging population)

↓

Organizational Context

Management structures, supervisory practices, production methods, and human resource policies

- Organizational restructuring (e.g., downsizing)
- New quality and process management initiatives (e.g., high performance work systems)
- Alternative employment arrangments (e.g., contingent labor)
- Work/life/family programs and flexible work arrangements (e.g., telecommuting)
- Changes in benefits and compensation systems (e.g., gainsharing)

↓

Work Context

Job characteristics

- Climate and culture
- Task attributes: temporal aspects, complexity, autonomy, physical, and psychological demands, etc.
- Social-relational aspects of work
- Worker roles
- Career development

FIGURE 15-1   *Organization of work*

Source: National Institute for Occupational Safety and Health.

    c. The *external context* refers to the multitude of forces at the national and international level that affect the work environment; these include such things as demographic trends, economic conditions, policy and regulations, and social and cultural norms.

  3. The organization of work will determine whether the workers' talents, knowledge, and other personal resources are properly used.

B **Organizational characteristics**

  1. Organizational culture and climate set the tone for worker communication patterns, prioritization of tasks, worker behavior, and the nature of worker interactions. (Chapter 7 provides more information about climate and culture.)

  2. The various work environments (physical, biologic, chemical, mechanical, and psychosocial) affect workers' perceptions of health, safety, and security within their organizations.

  3. Other organizational structures include organizational mission and philosophy, the size of the organization, its physical arrangement, and its service or product.

C **Interpersonal relationships and work**

  1. Relationships with managers and supervisors are determined by the management styles that prevail in an organization (Chapter 7); management styles determine the level of communication, decision-making power, and level of control experienced by the worker.

2. Co-worker relationships can be supportive, nonsupportive, or conflictual (Beaton et al., 1997).

a. When co-worker social support exists, workers are less likely to experience fatigue and exhaustion (Bultmann, et al., 2002; Schnorpfeil, et al., 2002).

b. Strong co-worker support has been associated with better employee retention rates and higher levels of job satisfaction (Landon, et al., 2004; Ndiwane, 2000)

c. Workers who perceive low co-worker support are at higher risk for occupational injury and widespread chronic pain (Haahr & Andersen, 2003; Harkness, et al., 2004; Hoogendoorn, et al., 2001).

3. New styles of labor, such as computerized recordkeeping, electronic communication, and computer and video monitoring have threatened workers' ability to have interpersonal relationships with co-workers and supervisors.

D **The meaning of work**

1. Work is a central part of most people's lives.

a. According to Sigmund Freud, work is an essential ingredient to a happy and well-adjusted personality.

b. Studs Terkel (1984) describes work as a search "for daily meaning as well as daily bread, for recognition as well as cash, for astonishment as well as torpor."

2. Work is basic to one's sense of his or her own social or personal identity; it is a symbol of personal achievement and values.

3. Work is often viewed as an important responsibility, and a means to "not be a burden" on others.

E **Characteristics of workers**

1. *Personal attributes* include the demographic attributes of workers, their personality traits, feelings about work, spirituality, and levels of motivation.

2. *Social networks,* especially family support, can affect workers' attitudes about work, their response to occupational illness and injury, and their ability to return to work when an injury or illness occurs.

3. A worker's level of job satisfaction is related to the structure of work, the organizational culture and climate, and interpersonal relationships at work.

II   Psychosocial Hazards

Although psychosocial hazards tend to be more nebulous and less tangible than other categories of hazards, they nevertheless exert a pervasive influence on health and safety.

A **Workplace violence in the modern day workplace**

1. Workplace violence is an act of aggression that causes physical or psychologic harm to a worker in the course of his or her work day; workplace violence is a serious and potentially deadly workplace hazard.

a. While mass murder by disgruntled workers is a serious concern, these incidents constitute only a small portion of violent events.

b. Threats, harassment, bullying, physical and emotional abuse, intimidation, stalking, and other assaults constitute the majority of violent incidents in the workplace.

    c. The 2,886 workplace deaths that occurred as a result of terrorist acts on September 11, 2001 were a tragic reminder of the threats to worker safety posed by international terrorism (US Department of Justice [USDOJ], 2002; US Department of Labor, 2004).

2. Most workplace violence falls into one of four categories (AAOHN, 2004; USDOJ, 2002; University of Iowa, 2001):

    a. Type 1, the most common category of violence, describes incidents in which the violence is associated with the commitment of a crime.

        1) In most cases, the perpetrator has no legitimate relationship with the employees or the worksite.

        2) This type of violence is most likely to occur among vulnerable work groups such as taxi drivers, workers in late night establishments, and others who work in isolated or dangerous areas or who handle money.

        3) About 80% of violent incidents are in this category.

    b. Type II involves a worker-client relationship; the "client" can be a customer, patient, student, inmate, or other recipient of services.

        1) These incidents occur in the course of doing business, for example, while a client is receiving a service.

        2) Workers in health care professions are the most likely to experience type II violence; the most common settings are psychiatric facilities, emergency rooms, admitting areas, intensive or critical care units, and medical response units.

    c. Type III includes worker-worker incidents; the perpetrators in this category are current or past employees who threaten or attack other current or past employees.

        1) Type III incidents may result from personality conflict, mishandled termination or disciplinary action, drug or alcohol abuse, or a grudge over a real or imagined grievance.

        2) In this type of violence, the perpetrator often provides warning signs; these include belligerence, hypersensitivity to criticism, preoccupation with violent themes, outbursts of anger, and other noticeable changes in behavior.

        3) Workplace factors that may contribute to Type III violence are listed in Box 15-1.

        4) A high injury rate and frequent employee grievances may serve as clues to problem situations in the workplace

    d. Type IV, called *personal relationship*, involves persons who have a personal relationship with a worker; type IV incidents are oftentimes spill-overs of domestic violence.

        1) Events in this category include stalking, threats, and harassment; 5% of workplace homicides are related to domestic violence.

        2) Because it is difficult to determine the boundaries between private and personal affairs, employers are reluctant to involve themselves in this category; however, once an event comes through the workplace door, it becomes the employer's concern.

        3) Types III and IV are the most preventable categories of workplace violence.

3. Homicide is the third leading cause of job-related death among all workers in the United States, and the second leading cause of workplace fatalities among women (USDL, Bureau of Labor Statistics [BLS], 2004).

> **BOX 15-1**
>
> *Workplace factors that contribute to workplace violence*
>
> - Understaffing that leads to job overload and compulsory overtime
> - Frustrations arising from poorly defined tasks and responsibilities
> - Downsizing and reorganization
> - Labor disputes and poor labor-management relations
> - Poor management styles (e.g., arbitrary or unexplained orders;
> over-monitoring, corrections or reprimands in front of other employees, inconsistent discipline)
> - Inadequate security or poorly trained, poorly motivated security force
> - A lack of employee counseling

Source: US Department of Justice, 2002.

    a. An average of 13 workers are murdered each week, accounting for 11.3% of all fatal work injuries, and for 31% of occupational deaths among women (compared to 9% among men).

    b. Robbery is the primary motive for job-related homicide, accounting for 75% of deaths.

    c. Disputes among co-workers and with customers account for about 10% of the total number of deaths.

    d. Sales workers experience the highest number of homicides, followed by taxi drivers, chauffeurs, and law enforcement officers; although they do not have the highest number of deaths, taxi drivers have the highest risk at 41.4 per 100,000 persons.

4. There are approximately 1.7 million assaults and threats of violence against American workers each year (USDOJ, 2001).

    a. Unlike homicides, nonfatal workplace assaults are slightly more likely to occur among women (56%) than among men (44%).

    b. Although fatal events are most often associated with robberies, nonfatal violence is more likely to result from anger or frustration of customers, clients, or co-workers.

    c. Most nonfatal workplace assaults occur in service settings such as hospitals, nursing homes, and social service agencies. Health care patients commit 48% of nonfatal assaults in the workplace (USDL, OSHA, 2004).

5. According to OSHA (USDL, OSHA, 2004), risk factors for workplace violence include the following:

    a. Contact with the public

    b. Exchange of money

    c. Delivery of passengers, goods, or services

    d. Having a mobile workplace, such as a taxicab or a police cruiser

    e. Working with unstable or volatile persons in health care, social services, or criminal justice settings

    f. Working alone or in small numbers

    g. Working late at night or during early morning hours

    h. Working in high crime areas

    i. Guarding valuable property or possessions

    j. Working in community-based settings

6. In order to prevent workplace violence, OSHA recommends that companies establish clear goals and objectives that are consistent with the size and complexity of the organization; at a minimum, workplace violence programs and services should do the following (USDL, OSHA, 2004):
   a. Establish and widely disseminate a clear zero tolerance for any form of workplace violence, including verbal or nonverbal threats, and related actions
   b. Ensure that workers who report any threats do not receive any type of reprisal
   c. Encourage workers to promptly report incidents and suggest ways to eliminate risks; require records of incidents to assess risk and monitor progress
   d. Outline a comprehensive plan for maintaining security in the workplace; possibly including having a liaison with law enforcement representatives and others who can help to identify ways to prevent and mitigate violence

---

BOX 15-2

Examples of violence prevention and control measures

Engineering Controls and Workplace Adaptations

- Security systems for use by staff: panic buttons, handheld noise devices, cellular phones
- Metal detectors at high-risk doorways
- Closed-circuit video recording in high-risk areas
- Curved mirrors in hallway intersections and secluded areas
- Bullet-resistant, shatterproof glass in reception, triage, and admitting areas
- Furniture arrangement to avoid entrapment of staff
- Limitation or elimination of items that can be used as weapons
- Two exits provided whenever possible
- Bright lighting indoors, outdoors, and in parking areas
- Lockable, secure rest rooms for staff, separate from visitor facilities
- Locks on rarely used doors, in accordance with local fire codes
- Vehicles used in the field maintained in good working condition

Administrative and Work Practice Controls

- Conduct periodic workplace safety and security analyses
- Establish a zero-tolerance violence policy
- Establish a trained response team to respond to emergencies
- Ensure adequate and qualified staffing at all times
- Provide management and administrative support during emergencies
- Control access to areas other than waiting rooms or lobbies
- Prohibit employees from working alone in high-risk areas
- Use adequate numbers of properly trained security personnel
- Provide security escort to parking lots
- Develop specific policies and procedures for off-site workers' safety
- Train workers in de-escalation and personal protection techniques

Source: USDL, OSHA, 1996.

e. Assign responsibility and authority to persons and teams with appropriate training and skill; ensure that adequate resources are available for this effort

f. Affirm management commitment to a work environment that places much importance on worker health and safety

g. Set up a company briefing to address such issues as preserving safety, supporting affected employees, and facilitating recovery

7. OSHA has developed recommendations for engineering and administrative controls that can be used to prevent workplace violence (Box 15-2).

8. Behavioral controls include training workers to (AAOHN, 2004):

a. Recognize and manage assaults when they occur

b. Use nonviolent response and conflict resolution

c. Maintain hazard awareness within the workplace

B Mistreatment and harassment

1. Workplace mistreatment or harassment is any act against an employee that creates a hostile work environment and negatively affects the employee, either physically or psychologically (Spratlen, 1994).

a. These acts of workplace mistreatment include hostile verbal and nonverbal behaviors directed at obtaining compliance from others (Keashly, 1998).

b. Examples of workplace mistreatment include yelling, use of derogatory names, shunning, and ridiculing someone in front of others.

c. Spratlen (1994) reported that most of the perpetrators of workplace mistreatment in an academic setting were males.

2. Sexual harassment consists of any "unwanted verbal or physical sexual advance"; this can range from "sexual comments and suggestions, to pressure for sexual favors, accompanied by threats concerning one's job, to physical assault, including rape" (Levy & Wegman, 2000).

a. "Studies indicate that 40 to 60 percent of women have experienced some form of sexual harassment at work" (Levy & Wegman, 2000).

b. Sexual harassment of nurses in the workplace undoubtedly increases their anxiety and can impair their ability to provide safe and competent patient care (Valente & Bullough, 2004).

c. Working in an organizational context perceived as hostile towards women can affect employees' well-being, even without personal hostility experiences (Miner-Rubino & Cortina, 2004).

C Unemployment and underemployment

1. "Unemployment is more destructive to physical and mental health than all but the most dangerous jobs" (Levenstein et al., 2000).

a. Studies have found a link between unemployment and increased rates of smoking, depression, drug use, and subsequent stroke (Gallo et al, 2004; Khlat et al. 2004).

b. The adverse effects of unemployment have been documented in a number of industrialized countries.

2. The underemployed include contingent, temporary, or part-time workers; an increasing percentage of employers are employing temporary and part-time workers.

a. The rate of job growth in the "temp" (temporary) help industry continues to outstrip the rate of overall job growth (US DHHS, 2001).

b. Temporary or contingent workers are less likely than permanent workers to have health insurance or employer-provided pensions.

3. Downsizing is an intentional reduction of a work force as a means of improving efficiency and effectiveness within an organization (Moore, 1999).
   a. Studies suggest that "survivors" of downsizing (those individuals who were not laid off when the reduction occurred) experience increased workloads, lowered trust in management, diminishing job security, and decreased morale.
   b. One study found the stress of hospital downsizing and restructuring led to burnout/emotional exhaustion in hospital nurses (Greenglass & Burke, 2002).
   c. Job insecurity is no longer a mere temporary break in an otherwise predictable work-life pattern, but instead, it may be a structural feature of the New Economy (Scott, 2004).
   d. Multiple health effects related to threats to employment security have been reported, including sleep disorders, increased blood pressure, and increases in cholesterol levels (Ferrie et al., 1998).

D Shift work
1. In 2000, approximately 20% of the American work force were shift workers working evening, night, or rotating shifts (Rajaratnam & Arendt, 2001).
2. Research suggests that a forward rotation of shifts (from day to evening to nights) is better than a backward rotation in terms of helping workers adjust to changes in sleep patterns (Box 15-3).
3. Short-term effects of shift work include sleep deprivation and disturbances of circadian rhythms, which result in decreased work performance and increased risk of accidents.
4. Long-term effects of shift work include gastrointestinal disturbances, coronary heart disease, and adverse pregnancy outcomes (Knutsson, 2003).

BOX 15-3

Suggestions for improving shift work schedules

- Avoid permanent (fixed and non-rotating) night shifts; most workers never really get used to nights.
- Keep consecutive night shifts to a minimum (2 to 4 days in a row before a couple of days off).
- Avoid quick shift changes (less than 10 hours between shifts).
- Allow some free weekends, at least two each month.
- Avoid several days of work followed by minivacations; this can be very fatiguing.
- Keep long work shifts and overtime to a minimum; if working 12-hour shifts, two or three in a row should be the maximum.
- Consider different lengths for shifts, possibly shorter shifts when there are lighter workloads.
- Examine start-end times; flextime may help workers cover their child-care needs.
- Keep the schedule regular and predictable; this assists in planning.
- Examine rest breaks; shift workers may need more than the standard coffee and lunch breaks.

Source: NIOSH, 1997.

5. "Poor working conditions add to the strain of shiftwork. Adequate lighting, clean air, proper heat and air conditioning, and reduced noise will avoid adding to the shiftworker's burden" (NIOSH, 1997).
6. Shift workers may be more sensitive to toxic substances because of changes in circadian rhythms.

E **Characteristics of work**
1. *Workload* refers to the total information load that a worker is required to perceive and interpret while performing tasks (Baker & Karasek, 2000).
   a. *Overload* occurs when the information processing load is greater than the worker's information processing capability
   b. *Underload* occurs when the information processing is not challenging enough for the worker; underload results in monotonous, boring work.
2. *Role stress* results from an interpretation of one's role within an organization (Kahn & Boulding, 1964; Baker & Karasek, 2000).
   a. *Role conflict* occurs when a worker experiences conflicting demands or is required to perform a task that is outside of the perceived requirements; as many as 48% of workers are affected by role conflict at some time in their work life.
   b *Role ambiguity* results from lack of clarity about the scope and responsibilities of the job; about 35% to 60% of U.S. workers are affected by role ambiguity.

F **Stresses in the modern workplace**
1. Electronic performance monitoring, which has become increasingly common in the modern workplace, has been related to increased anxiety, depression, anger, and fatigue among monitored workers (Stiles, 1994).
2. Organizational practices in the United States and abroad have changed dramatically in the New Economy (US DHHS, 2001).
   a. Companies have restructured and outsourced many functions.
   b. Organizations are adopting new and flatter management structures and implementing more flexible and lean production technologies
3. Automated machinery and robots have eliminated or threatened some jobs; some workers' jobs have become de-skilled as a result of new high-tech equipment and machinery.
4. Increased globalization of workplaces has led to the development of multinational companies, increased competition, and decreased profitability.
   a. As a result of globalization, occupational health and safety problems have become ubiquitous, affecting workers nationally and internationally.
   b. Because of decreased profitability, management is no longer willing to honor its "social contract" with workers. (*Social contract* is "management's commitment to maintain decent wages and working conditions in return for some job security and a rising standard of living." [Levenstein et al., 2000]).
   c. For a sizable portion of U. S. workers, international competition has resulted in lower wages, compulsory overtime, and an increased pace of work accompanied by decreased attention to occupational health and safety (Levenstein et al., 2000).
5. Technostress, defined as stress stemming from new and multiple technologies, may be the price we pay for adopting almost any technology that improves worker productivity (Ookita & Tokuda, 2001).

6. Home-based telework (telecommuting) has become an increasingly attractive option to employers and workers (Standen, Daniels, & Lamond, 1999).
   a. The number of telecommuters increased by 40% between 2001 and 2003. By 2003 it was estimated that approximately 40 million US employees engaged in some form of telecommuting at least one day per month (ITAC, 2003).
   b. The effects of telework and telecommuting on the psychologic well being of workers are complex and significant.
   c. It has been hypothesized that employers' expectations of greater performance and accountability of teleworkers has the potential to increase job pressures (Harpaz, 2002).
   d. There is a need for further research to identify and manage the potential psychologic effects of working at home (Hill et al, 2003).

III Occupational Stress

A Definitions

1. *Occupational stress* is "the harmful physical and emotional responses that occur when the requirements of the job do not match the capabilities, resources, or needs of the worker" (NIOSH, 1999).
   a. Stress can be either a positive (eustress) or a negative (distress) influence on one's sense of well being (Selye, 1974).
   b. *Stressors* refer to the physical or psychologic demands or stimuli to which an individual or worker group must adjust.
2. A *stress reaction* occurs when there is a mismatch between the work conditions and the individual worker (Levy & Wegman, 2000).
   a. *Acute stress reaction* refers to the initial and relatively brief biobehavioral and neuroendocrine fight-or-flight reaction to a stressor.
   b. *Chronic stress reactions* are long-term stress reactions or strains that involve the mobilization of the neuroendocrine and neurotransmitter systems affecting every organ system; they may be manifested as physiologic, psychological, or behavioral chronic stress responses.

B Facts about occupational stress

1. A Northwest National Life survey in 1991 found that 40% of U. S. employees surveyed viewed their jobs as "very or extremely stressful."
2. According to AAOHN (2005), "Nearly 20 percent of the American workforce claim that an episode of violence against an employee occurred within their workplace."
3. About two thirds of occupational stress that results in days away from work is experienced by white collar workers; in contrast, over half of *all* occupational injuries and illnesses occur to blue collar workers (USDL, BLS, 1999).
4. St. Paul Fire and Marine Insurance Company (1992, cited in NIOSH, 1999) concluded that ". . . problems at work are more strongly associated with health complaints than any other life stressor."
5. Nearly 50% of states in the United States allow workers' compensation claims for emotional disorders and stress-related disability.

C Job conditions that can lead to stress

NIOSH (1999) has identified several types of work conditions that can result in a stressful work environment. These include:

1. Excessive workload, lack of rest breaks, long work hours, shift work, and monotonous and boring tasks
2. Management style that precludes worker's participation in decision-making and results in poor communication between workers and supervisors or workers and co-workers
3. Interpersonal relationships that result in "poor social environment and lack of support from co-workers and supervisors"
4. Work roles with "conflicting and uncertain job expectations, too much responsibility, and too `many hats to wear'"
5. Career concerns, which result in "job insecurity and lack of opportunity for growth, advancement, or promotion"
6. Environmental conditions, such as "unpleasant and dangerous physical conditions"

IV Effects of Stress on Workers

Stress is manifested by an array of physiologic, psychological, and behavioral disorders.

A Psychologic disorders among workers

1. Depression is one of the most prevalent psychologic conditions observed in the occupational setting (Sears et al., 2000); one study found that depressed workers had between 1.5 and 3.2 more short-term work-disability days in a 30-day period than other workers (Kessler et al., 1999).
2. The prevalence of posttraumatic stress disorder in urban U. S. firefighters and paramedics has been documented to exceed 20% (Corneil et al, 1999).
3. "Burnout is a psychological syndrome of emotional exhaustion, depersonalization, and reduced personal accomplishment" (Maslach, 1993).
   a. *Emotional exhaustion* refers to feelings of being emotionally overextended and depleted of one's emotional resources.
   b. *Depersonalization* refers to a negative, callous, or excessively detached response to other people.
   c. *Reduced personal accomplishment* refers to a decline in one's feelings of competence and successful achievement in one's work.
4. Substance abuse has been directly correlated with the amount of stress experienced by workers; for example, one study demonstrated a direct relationship between job complexity and increased use of substances (Oldham & Gordon, 1999).

B Physiologic responses to stress

Epidemiologic research has documented a relationship between job conditions and certain types of physiologic responses, including the following:

1. Cardiovascular disease, such as hypertension and myocardial infarctions
2. Musculoskeletal disorders, such as headaches, myofascial back pain, and upper extremity cumulative trauma disorders
   a. Studies have found a relationship between dissatisfaction with work status and the risk of low-back pain (Bigos et al, 1992).
   b. Psychosocial factors have been identified as the "best predictor of chronicity" of musculoskeletal pain; pain-related disability has its genesis in the first few days or weeks after a problem (injury) occurs (Kendall, 1999).
3. Gastrointestinal conditions, such as peptic ulcers, gastritis, and other digestive disorders

    4. Impaired immune functioning; for example, one study found that even a month of high levels of job stress dramatically increased an individual's susceptibility to common cold viral infections (Cohen et al, 1998)

C **Behavioral responses**

    1. Inordinate workplace stress can lead to work performance decrements, decreased attention/concentration, increased distractibility, increased muscle tension, and poor judgment.

    2. Other behavioral responses include irritation, self-neglect (e.g., poor nutrition, lack of exercise), and interpersonal conflict.

    3. In more extreme cases, homicide or suicide may be a behavioral response.

V Effects of Stress on Organizations

Organizations experience both tangible (i.e., workers' compensation costs, lost work days) and intangible effects (i.e., lowered worker morale, increased interpersonal conflict) from stress.

A **Measuring work performance**

    1. Work performance is measured by productivity and the quality of work.

    2. Research suggests that policies benefiting worker health also benefit the bottom line because of better productivity and fewer performance errors.

    3. Healthy organizations are those organizations that have low rates of illness, injuries, and disabilities and that are competitive in the marketplace.

    4. Examples of characteristics that are associated with low-stress work and high levels of productivity include (NIOSH, 1999):

        a. Recognition of employees for good work performance

        b. Opportunities for career development

        c. An organizational culture that values the individual worker

        d. Management actions that are consistent with organizational values

B **Economic consequences of stress**

    1. Claims for stress-related conditions are the most costly claims in the workers' compensation system.

    2. Stressful working conditions are associated with increased absenteeism, tardiness, increased insurance costs, and worker turnover.

    3. Estimates of losses to the U. S. economy because of stress-related illnesses, injuries, worker's compensation claims, and decreased productivity range between $200 and $300 billion annually.

VI Occupational Stress Models

Multiple conceptualizations of occupational stress have resulted in the development of many occupational stress models over the years. These models help us to understand the interrelationships between the work environment and the worker that result in occupational stress.

A **The Person-Environment Fit (P-E) Model**

    1. The person-environment (P-E) fit postulates that stress occurs because of a poor fit between the subjective person and the subjective environment (French et al., 1982).

    2. According to the P-E model, a mismatch is present in one of two forms:

a. Between the demands of the job and a person's ability to meet those demands

b. Between the motives of the person (e.g., income, self-actualization) and the environmental supplies to satisfy those motives

3. A deficiency of this model is that it has limited ability to predict what objective conditions result in stress.

B The Demand-Control (D-C) Model

1. The demand-control (D-C) model categorizes occupations on the basis of psychologic demands and job control (also called *decision latitude*) (Karasek & Theorell, 1990).

2. The D-C model proposes that strain occurs when there is an imbalance between the demands of the job and the worker's decision latitude.

3. The amount of control that a worker has is now recognized as a decisive factor in the development of occupational stress.

C Effort-Reward Imbalance (E-RI) Model

1. Effort-reward imbalance (E-RI) models emphasize the effort and reward dimensions of the work environment (van Vegchel, Jonge, Bosma & Schaufeli, 2005).

a. Efforts include the job demands and obligations that are imposed on a worker.

b. Rewards include money, esteem, job security, career opportunities, and other benefits associated with employment.

2. The E-RI model postulates that work contracts provide for a reciprocal relationship between the efforts spent and the rewards received by a worker.

a. Jobs that are characterized by an imbalance between high efforts and low rewards are stressful and lead to adverse health outcomes (Siegrist, 1996).

b. When an effort-reward imbalance exists, a worker may experience "active distress," which leads to physiologic responses, which leads to the development of adverse health effects.

c. The original model (Siegrist, 1986) focused on cardiovascular outcomes; more recently, the model has been extended to apply to other psychologic and behavioral disorders.

D Systems models

1. Systems models view occupational stress from an organizational systems perspective.

2. The NIOSH systems model uses comprehensive schemata to examine the interaction of work and nonwork stressors (Hurrell & McLaney, 1988).

a. A combination of job stressors, nonwork factors, individual factors, and buffer factors predict acute reactions.

b. Acute reactions are categorized as physiologic, psychologic, and behavioral effects.

c. Outcomes include work-related disabilities and other diagnosed problems.

3. The ecologic model (Salazar & Beaton, 2000) offers a method of examining stress in the context in which the stress occurs (Section VII).

4. These system approaches are consistent with the position that dealing with occupational stress requires looking beyond the individual worker or worker groups to the conditions of work.

VII An Ecologic Approach to Occupational Stress

A **Ecologic theory**

1. Ecologic theory is a type of systems theory that describes multiple layers of influence; ecologic theory evolved from the biologic and social sciences.
    a. Its biologic origins date back to 1859, when Darwin described the complex interrelationships between organisms and their environments.
    b. The term *human ecology* was coined in the 1920s in a sociologic context in an attempt to systematically apply the basic theoretic scheme of plant and animal ecology to the study of human communities (Hawley, 1950).
2. In the 1970s, Bronfenbrenner generated a new wave of interest in using an ecologic approach to examine human problems.
    a. Bronfenbrenner (1977) felt that the study of humans requires the "examination of multiperson systems not limited to a single setting and must take into account aspects of the environment beyond the immediate situation containing the subject."
    b. Bronfenbrenner believed that human relationships and interactions could be best understood when they were viewed in context, and that the context could be viewed at various levels of organizational complexity.
3. The basic premises of ecologic theory are as follows:
    a. Systems are complex and interrelated.
    b. Everything is connected to everything else.
    c. Change is constant.
    d. Systems are dynamic.

B **The ecologic model**

1. The ecologic model offers a method of examining stress that goes beyond the individual worker to the context in which the stress occurs.
2. This approach is consistent with the position that dealing with occupational stress requires a workplace approach.
3. The model goes one step further, proposing that the broader context in which the organization is embedded may also influence the occurrence of stress in the workplace.

C **Components of the ecologic stress model**

1. The ecologic model of occupational stress (Figure 15-2) includes four nested levels of occupational stressors: the microsystems, the organizational system, the peri-organizational system, and the extra-organizational system (Salazar & Beaton, 2000).
    a. The *microsystem* consists of the environment immediately surrounding the worker or group of workers. It includes the physical features of the environment, the interactions that a worker experiences, and the activities that occur there.
    b. The *organizational system* is made up of the multiple structures and functions that constitute a work organization. Examples of organizational structures are labor unions, the size of the organization, its physical arrangement, and its service or product; examples of functions include communication, work processes, and worker training.
    c. The *peri-organizational system* refers to the forces within the societal system in which the individual and organization are imbedded that have an immediate effect on the work organization. These include regional economic conditions, the political climate, prevailing social conditions, and the general health of the community, which relate directly to the organization.

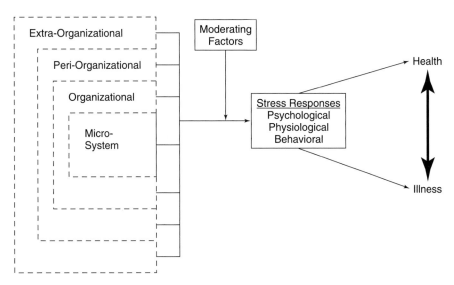

FIGURE 15-2 *An ecologic model of occupational stress*

Source: Salazar and Beaton, 2000.

     d. The *extra-organizational system* includes the cultures, societal norms, traditions, and government and economic policies that directly or indirectly affect workers. Direct effects are related to government policies, regulations, and standards.

2. Moderating factors serve as a means to ameliorate or intercept the effects of the identified stressors. They include the personal attributes, coping strategies, and social support systems of the worker.

3. A multitude of physiologic, psychologic, and behavioral stress responses can result from the interaction of multiple stressors (Section IV).

D **Health and illness outcomes**

1. The health-illness continuum describes the outcomes that result from the interaction of the ecosystems, moderating factors, and stress responses.

2. These outcomes can be positive (health) or negative (illness), or anywhere between.

     a. The health end of the continuum might be related to the sense of esteem and personal satisfaction that one derives from work.

     b. The illness end of the continuum includes ulcers, hypertension, angina, chronic headaches, cardiovascular diseases (e.g., myocardial infarction), and a multitude of mental health disorders.

3. Occupational and environmental health nurses are in a prime position to determine where workers are on the health-illness continuum; the ecologic model can then serve as a useful tool to identify and assess stress-related problems.

VIII Managing Psychosocial Factors in the Occupational Setting

Managing occupational stress is a cyclic process; it includes multiple steps between identifying the sources of stress and evaluating the intervention.

A **Principles underlying programs and services**

1. There are two prevailing approaches to workplace stress: the worker approach and the workplace approach.

    a. *Worker approach* includes stress management, employee assistance programs, and counseling strategies that are designed to improve workers' ability to cope with their occupational stressors.

    b. In contrast to the worker approach, the organizational *workplace approach* is based on the principle of improving working conditions (and decreasing occupational stressor exposures) for all workers (Box 15-4).

        1) This approach addresses the root causes of identified stress in the workplace by designing strategies that reduce or eliminate identified stressors.

        2) As a result of years of research and experience, NIOSH favors this approach.

2. Comprehensive stress-prevention programs and services involve a combination of organizational change (workplace approaches) and individual stress management (worker approaches) to prevent or ameliorate job stress to create a healthier workplace.

BOX 15-4

Approaches to organizational change to prevent job stress

Workload
- Ensure that the workload is in line with the worker's capabilities and resources.
- Avoid underload as well as overload.
- Increase control over the pace of work.

Work Schedule
- Establish work schedules that are compatible with workers' demands and responsibilities outside the job.
- Use flex time, job sharing, or a compressed work week to allow flexibility.

Work Roles
- Clearly define workers' roles and responsibilities.
- Avoid conflicts related to expectations of workers.

Content
- Design jobs to provide meaning, stimulation, and opportunities for workers to use their skills.

- Rotate jobs to increase stimulation and challenge.

Participation/Control
- Give workers opportunities to participate in decisions and actions affecting their jobs.
- Develop strategies to encourage positive interpersonal relations with co-workers and supervisors.

Job Future
- Improve communications; reduce uncertainty about career development and future employment prospects.
- Keep workers informed about decisions that will affect their positions, including the potential for promotions and mechanisms for professional growth.

Social Environment
- Provide opportunities for social interaction among workers.

Source: Sauter, Murphy, & Hurrell, 1990.

B **Assessing psychosocial factors**

1. A first step in managing psychosocial factors in the workplace is to identify the job conditions that can lead to stress (Section III.C. provides a list of job conditions).

   a. The sources of occupational stress in a given workplace can be assessed by using a variety of approaches, including interviews of the major stakeholders of a workplace organization, an employee survey, and observations at the workplace.

   b. Group discussions with management, labor representatives, and employees can provide valuable and rich information about the problem.

2. The second step in the management of psychosocial factors is to measure the stress reactions; both subjective and objective indices of occupational strain should be assessed.

   a. Subjective indices include self-reports of stress-related symptoms, job satisfaction, and perceptions of workplace morale, including the following (Baker & Karasek, 2000):

      1) Symptoms and motivations related to work conditions
      2) Anxiety, depression, and other emotional reactions
      3) Cognitive functioning and work performance
      4) Behavioral changes, such as sleep disturbances and substance abuse
      5) Physiologic measures, such as blood pressure monitoring, measuring the metabolites of catecholamines, and galvanic skin responses
      6) Other symptoms or diseases that are related to stress

   b. Objective indices include turnover rates, health care costs, absenteeism, and rates of on-the-job injury.

C **Strategies for preventing and controlling adverse effects of psychosocial factors**

1. On the basis of the assessment, the specific sources of occupational stress for a worker group and work organization can be targeted for organizational change.

   a. The identified source of stress can guide the intervention; for example, upper extremity pain and dysfunction might require an ergonomic improvement.

   b. If the stress is related to organizational dysfunction (e.g., ineffective communication), managers and workers should be involved in the design of the intervention.

2. The levels of prevention can be applied to stress control strategies (Baker & Karasek, 2000).

   a. Primary prevention focuses on the reduction of job stressors; for example, making changes within the organization.

   b. Secondary prevention focuses on the development of strategies to deal with stressful conditions; for example, improving the workers' ability to cope with the stressors.

   c. Tertiary prevention focuses on programs and services that provide treatment and rehabilitation for stress-related conditions; it includes employee assistance programs (EAPs) and counseling services.

3. Preparation for a stress prevention program should include the following (NIOSH, 1999):

   a. Building awareness about job stresses

   b. Securing top management commitment and support

c. Involving employees in all phases of the program

d. Obtaining the resources needed to develop an effective program

IX Evaluating Interventions That Promote Psychosocial Health in the Occupational Setting

A Using the Quality Assessment Model (structure, process, outcome) as an evaluation framework. (See Chapter 9 for description of this model.)

1. Certain *structural characteristics* of a workplace are essential to assuring psychosocial health; examples of these characteristics include an organizational mission and goals that address worker health and safety, management that is committed to a safe and healthy work environment, availability of employee assistance services, an emergency response plan, and an organizational climate and culture that values the individual worker.

2. *Processes* that protect the psychosocial health of workers include health and safety training for workers, strategies to resolve conflicts, workers' active participation in the development and implementation of health and safety programs and services, recordkeeping, and other stress-monitoring techniques.

3. *Outcomes* can be measured through an examination of job satisfaction, absenteeism and turnover rates, injury rates, workers' compensation costs, particularly for stress related claims, and rates of reported worker conflict.

B Characteristics of evaluation

1. Evaluations of interventions designed to prevent and control the adverse effect of psychosocial factors should include both short-term and longer-term measures as well as objective and subjective measures.

2. The evaluation of job stress prevention and control techniques is a continuous process.

C Benefits of evaluation

1. Evaluation serves to inform the occupational and environmental health nurse regarding needed changes in stress reduction programs and services.

2. Evaluation serves to appropriately guide the development of intervention strategies.

REFERENCES

American Association for Occupational Health Nurses (2004). Workplace violence program. *Foundation blocks: A guide to occupational & environmental health nursing. Absence Management Program.* Atlanta, GA: AAOHN publications.

Baker, D. B., & Karasek, R. A. (2000). Stress. In B. S. Levy & D. H. Wegman (Eds.), *Occupational health: Recognizing and preventing work-related disease and injury* (4th ed., pp. 419-436). Philadelphia: Lippincott Williams & Wilkins.

Beaton, R., Murphy, S., Pike, K., & Corneil, W. (1997). Social support & network conflict in firefighters and paramedics. *Western Journal of Nursing Research, 19,* 297-313.

Bigos, S. J., Battie, M. C., Spengler, D. M., Fisher, l. D., Fordyce, W. E., Hansson, T., Nachemson, A., & Zeh, J. (1992). A longitudinal, prospective study of industrial back injury reporting. *Clinical Orthopedics, 279,* 21-34.

Bronfenbrenner, U. (1977). Toward an experimental ecology in human development. *American Psychologist, 32*(7), 513-531.

Bultmann U., Kant I. J., Van den Brandt, P. A., & Kasl, S. V. (2002). Psychosocial work characteristics as risk factors for the onset of fatigue and psychological distress: prospective results from the Maastricht Cohort Study. *Psychological Medicine, 32*(2), 333-345.

Cohen, S., Frank, E., Doyle, W., Skoner, D., Rabin, B., & Gwaltney, J. (1998). Types of stressors that increase susceptibility to the common cold in healthy adults. *Health Psychology, 17,* 214-223.

Corneil, W., Beaton, R., Murphy, S., Johnson, C., & Pike, K. (1999). Exposure to traumatic incidents and prevalence of posttraumatic stress symptomatology in urban fire fighters in two countries. *Journal of Occupational Health Psychology, 4,* 131-141.

Ferrie, J. E., Shipley, M. J., Marmot, M. G., Stansfield, S. A., & Smith, G. D. (1998). An uncertain future: The effects of threats to employment security in white-collar men and women. *American Journal of Public Health, 88*(7), 1030-1036.

French, J. R., Caplan, R. D., & Van Harrison, R. (1982). *The mechanisms of job stress and strain.* Chichester, United Kingdom: John Wiley & Sons.

Gallo, W. T., Bradley, E. H., Falba, T. A., Dubin, J. A., Cramer, L. D., Bogardus, S. T., Jr., & Kasl, S. V. (2004). Involuntary job loss as a risk factor for subsequent myocardial infarction and stroke: findings from the Health and Retirement Survey. *American Journal of Industrial Medicine, 45*(5), 408-416.

Greenglass, E. R., & Burke, R. J. (2002). Hospital restructuring and burnout. *Journal of Health and Human Services Administration, 25* (1), 89-114.

Haahr J. P., & Andersen, J.H. (2003) Physical and psychosocial risk factors for lateral epicondylitis: a population based case-referent study. *Occupational and Environmental Medicine, 60*(5), 322-329.

Harkness E. F., Macfarlane, G. J., Nahit, E., Silman, A. J., & McBeth, J. (2004). Mechanical injury and psychosocial factors in the work place predict the onset of widespread body pain: a two-year prospective study among cohorts of newly employed workers. *Arthritis Rheumatology, 50*(5), 1655-1664.

Harpaz (2002) Advantages and disadvantages of telecommuting for the individual, organization and society. *Work Study, 51* (2).

Hawley, A. H., (1950). *Human ecology: A theory of community structure.* New York: Plume Press.

Hoogendoorn, W. E., Bongers, P. M., de Vet, H. C., Houtman, I. L., Ariens, G.A., van Mechelen, W., & Bouter, L.M. (2001). Psychosocial work characteristics and psychological strain in relation to low-back pain. *Scandinavian Journal of Work Environment and Health, 27*(4), 258-67.

Hill, J. E., Ferris, M., and Martinson V. (2003). Does it matter where you work? A comparison of how three work venues (traditional office, virtual office and home office) influence aspects of work and the personal/family life). *Journal of Vocational Behavior, 63*(2), 220-241.

Hurrell, J. J., & McLaney, M. A. (1988). Exposure to job stress—a new psychometric instrument. *Scandinavian Journal of Environmental Health, 14* (suppl.1), 27-28.

International Telework Association and Council. (2003) Results from the Dieringer research group's interactive consumer survey. Press Release August 18, 2003 Available at http://www.telecommute.org

Kahn, R. L., & Boulding, E. (1964). *Power and conflict in organizations.* New York: Basic Books.

Karasek, R., & Theorell, T. (1990*). Healthy work: stress, productivity, and the reconstruction of working life.* New York: Basic Books.

Keashly, L. (1998). Emotional abuse in the workplace: Conceptual and empirical issues. *Journal of Emotional Abuse, 1*(1), 85-117.

Kendall, N. A. (1999). Psychosocial approaches to the prevention of chronic pain: the low back paradigm. *Baillieres Best Practice Research in Clinical Rheumatology, 13*(3), 545-554.

Kessler, R. C., Barber, C., Birnbaum, H. G., Frank, R. G., Greenberg, P. E., Rose, R. M., Simon, G. E., & Wang, P. (1999). Depression in the workplace: effects on short-term disability. *Health Affairs, 18*(5), 163-71.

Khlat, M., Sermet, C., & Annick, L. P. (2004). Increased prevalence of depression, smoking, heavy drinking and use of psycho-active drugs among unemployed men in France. *European Journal of Epidemiology, 19,* 445-451.

Knutsson, A. (2003) Health disorders of shift workers. *Occupational Medicine, 53,* 103-108.

Landon B, Loudon J, Selle M, & Doucette S., (2004). Factors influencing the retention and attrition of community health aides/practitioner in Alaska. *Journal of Rural Health, 20*(3), 221-230.

Levenstein, C., Wooding, J., & Rosenberg, B. (2000). Occupational health: A social perspective. In B. S. Levy & D. H. Wegman (Eds.), *Occupational health: Recognizing and preventing work-related disease and injury* (4th ed., pp. 27-50). Philadelphia: Lippincott Williams & Wilkins.

Levy, B. S. & Wegman, D. H. (2000). *Occupational health: Recognizing and preventing work-related disease and injury* (4th ed.). Philadelphia: Lippincott Williams & Wilkins.

Maslach, C. (1993). Burnout: A multidimensional perspective. In W. B. Schaufeli, - C. C. Maslach, & T. Marek (Eds.). *Professional burnout: recent developments in theory and research.* New York: Taylor & Francis.

Miner-Rubino, K., & Cortina, L. (2004). Working in a context of hostility toward women: implications for employees' well-being. *Journal of Occupational Health Psychology*, 9, (2), 107-122.

Moore, S. Y. (1999). The effect of layoff threat and personal mastery on work performance over a three year period. Paper presented at APSA/NIOSH conference, Washington, DC.

National Institutes of Health. (1988). *Proposed national strategies for the prevention of leading work-related diseases and injuries*, Part 2. Cincinnati, OH: U.S. Department of Health and Human Services.

National Institute for Occupational Safety and Health (NIOSH). (1997). *Plain language about shiftwork.* Cincinnati, OH: U.S. Department of Health and Human Services.

National Institute for Occupational Safety and Health (NIOSH). (1999). *Stress at work.* Cincinnati, OH: U.S. Department of Health and Human Services.

National Institute for Occupational Safety and Health (NIOSH). (2002). *The changing organization of work and safety and health of working people.* Cincinnati, OH: U.S. Department of Health and Human Services.

Ndiwane A., (2000). The effects of community, coworker and organizational support to job satisfaction of nurses in Cameroon. *ABNF Journal, 11*(6), 145-9.

Oldham, G. R., & Gordon, B. I. (1999). Job complexity and employee substance use: the moderating effects of cognitive ability. *Journal of Health and Social Behavior, 40*(3), 290-306.

Ookita, S. & Tokuda, H. (2001). A virtual therapeutic environment with user projective agents. *Cyberpsychological Behavior, 4* (1), 155-167.

Rajaratnam, S., & Arendt, J. (2001). Health in a 24-hour society, *Lancet, 358*, 999-1005.

Salazar, M. K. & Beaton, R. (2000). Ecological model of occupational stress: Application to urban firefighters. *AAOHN Journal, 48*(10), 470-479.

Schnorpfeil, P., Noll, A., Wirtz, P., Schulze, R., Ehlert, U., Fre, K., & Fischer, J. E. (2002). Assessment of exhaustion and related risk factors in employees in the manufacturing industry—a cross-sectional study. *International Archives of Occupational and Environmental Health, 75*(8), 535-540.

Scott, H. K. (2004). Reconceptualizing the nature and health consequences of work-related insecurity for the new economy: the decline of workers' power in the flexibility regime. *International Journal of Health Services, 34* (1), 143-153.

Sears, S., Urizar, D., & Evans, G. (2000). Examining a stress-coping model of burnout and depression in extension agents. *Journal of Occupational Health Psychology, 5*, 56-62.

Selye, H. (1974). Stress and distress. *Comprehensive Therapeutics, 1*(8), 9-13.

Siegrist, J., Siegrist, K., & Weber, I. (1986). Sociological concepts in the etiology of chronic disease the case of ischemic heart disease, *Social Science & Medicine, 22*, 247–253

Siegrist, J. (1996) Adverse health effect of high-effort/low-reward conditions. *Occupational Health, 1*, 27-41.

Spratlen, L.P. (1994). Perceived workplace mistreatment in higher education: characteristics and consequences. *AAOHN Journal, 42*(11), 548-54.

Standen, P., Daniels, K., & Lamond, D. (1999). The home is a workplace: Work-family interaction and psychological well-being in telework. *Journal of Occupational Health Psychology, 4*(4), 368-381.

Stiles, D. (1994). Video display terminal operators: Technology's biophysical stressors. *AAOHN Journal, 42*(11), 541-547.

Terkel, S. (1984). *Working: people talk about what they do all day and how they feel about what they do.* New York: Ballantine.

U.S. Department of Health and Human Services (US DHHS). (2001). *Low-income and low-skilled workers' involvement in nonstandard employment*. Retrieved March 2, 2005, from http://aspe.hhs.gov/hsp/temp-workers01/index.htm

U.S. Department of Justice (US DOJ). (2001). *Violence in the workplace 1993-1999*. Bureau of Justice Statistics, Office of Justice Programs. Retrieved January 6, 2005 from http://www.ojp.usdoj.gov/bjs/pub/pdf/vw99.pdf

U.S. Department of Justice (US DOJ). (2002). *Workplace violence: Issues in response*. Critical Incident Response Group, National Center for the Analysis of Violent Crime, FBI Academy, Quantico, VA.

U.S. Department of Labor, Bureau of Labor Statistics. (1999). White-collar workers account for most cases of occupational stress, MLR: The Editor's Desk Retrieved March 2, 2005 from http://www.bls.gov/opub/ted/1999/oct/wk2/art03.htm

U.S. Department of Labor, Bureau of Labor Statistics. (2004). *National census of fatal occupational injuries in 2003*. News: US Department of Labor USDL 04-1830, Bureau of Labor Statistics, Washington DC.

U.S. Department of Labor. (1998). *Dealing with workplace violence: A guide for agency planners*. Available at http://;-20/www.opm.gov/ehg/workplace/index.htm

U.S. Department of Labor, Occupational Safety and Health Administration. (2004). *Guidelines for preventing workplace violence for health care & social service workers*. Publication OSHA 3148 01R. Washington DC: US Department of Labor.

University of Iowa (2001). *Workplace violence: A report to the nation*. Injury Prevention Research Center. University of Iowa: Iowa City, Iowa.

Valente, S., & Bullough, V. (2004) Sexual harassment of nurses in the workplace. *Journal of Nursing Care Qualifications*, 19(3), 234-241.

van Vegchel, N., de Jonge, J., Bosma, H., & Schaufeli, W. (2005). Reviewing the effort-reward imbalance model: drawing up the balance of 45 empirical studies. *Social Science Medicine*, 60(5), 1117-1131.

OTHER RESOURCES

Giga, S., Faragher, B., & Cooper, C., (2003). Part 1: Identification of good practice in stress prevention/management. In J. Jordan, E. Gorr, G. Tinline, S. Giga, B. Faragher, & C. Cooper (Eds.), *Beacons of excellence in stress prevention* (Health and Safety Executive Contract Research Report No. 133, pp. 1-45). Sudbury, England: HSE Books.

Lindstrom, M. (2004). Psychosocial work conditions, social capital, and daily smoking: a population based study. *Tobacco Control*, 13(3), 289-295.

16

Examples of Occupational Health and Safety Programs

MICHELLE KOM GOCHNOUR, ANNIE BRUCK, AND DENISE SOUZA

This chapter describes selected examples of occupational health and safety programs and services that can be used as models in a variety of work settings. Some of these programs are mandated by law (e.g., hearing loss prevention program, hazard communication, drug and alcohol testing); others may be of interest or importance to specific industries or businesses (international travel health and safety, ergonomic programs). The basic template used to describe these programs and services can be applied to other kinds of work-site programs.

Hearing-loss prevention programs and services

The passage of the Hearing Conservation Amendment to the OSH Act in 1983 provided the thrust for the development of hearing-loss prevention programs in industry. Hearing-loss prevention programs and services can either be conducted within the work site or contracted to a certified audiology testing service. It is recommended, and in some cases required by law, that individuals performing as audiometric technicians become certified through the Council for Accreditation in Occupational Hearing Conservation. The program outlined in this section can serve as a guide to developing a hearing-loss prevention program. It is advised that the program coordinator review and follow requirements established by the Occupational Safety and Health Administration (OSHA) or by states with OSHA-approved state plans.

I Noise-Induced Hearing Loss

Noise-induced hearing loss (NIHL) caused by occupational exposure has been a compensable occupational disease since the 1950s.

A **Noise-induced hearing loss has been identified as "one of the most common occupational diseases and the second most self-reported occupational illness or injury" (NIOSH, Fact Sheet, 2001).**

1. Estimates suggest approximately 30 million workers are exposed to hazardous noise levels (NIOSH, 2001).
2. Key industries with high numbers of workers exposed to hazardous noise include agriculture, mining, construction, manufacturing and utilities, transportation, and the military (NIOSH, 2001; NIOSH 1996).

B NIHL is preventable; however, once present it is permanent. The impacts of hearing impairment are far reaching.

1. Hearing loss affects an individual's quality of life in multiple ways (Lusk et al. 2003; 2004; May, 2000).
2. NIHL adds millions of dollars annually to the costs of workers' compensation systems (American Academy of Audiology, 2003; Lipscomb, 2003; NIOSH 2001).
3. In addition to hearing loss, noise exposure has been associated with multiple other psychologic and physical health effects, including anxiety, depression, blood pressure and heart rate changes, and myocardial infarction (Davies, 2005; Lusk 2002; 2003).

II Purposes of a Hearing-loss Prevention Program

A Hearing loss programs are designed to do the following:

1. Prevent noise-induced hearing loss
2. Reduce worker exposure to harmful noise
3. Identify the progression of hearing loss so preventive measures can be taken
4. Identify temporary hearing loss before it becomes permanent
5. Comply with federal regulations or OSHA-approved state plans (OSHA Noise Standard CFR 1910.95)
   a. OSHA regulations limit work-site noise exposure to 90 dBA time-weighted average (TWA) over an 8-hour work shift. Hearing-loss prevention programs and hearing protection devices (HPDs) are mandatory, as are engineering controls.
   b. Hearing-loss prevention programs (HLPPs) are mandatory in an environment where the daily noise level equals or exceeds 85 dBA over an 8 hour, time-weighted average (TWA); appropriate HPDs are to be provided. Table 16-1 suggests policies regarding HLPPs based on time-weighted averages.

B The rationale for and benefits of a work-site HLPP include:

1. Reduced worker risk for NIHL and other health conditions
2. Better labor-management relations
3. Decreased likelihood of antisocial behaviors resulting from annoyance

TABLE 16-1

Developing a hearing conservation program: suggested policies based on time-weighted average ranges

TWA in dB(A)	Workers included in the HCP	HPD utilization	HPD selection options
84 or below	No	Voluntary	Free choice
85-89	Yes	Optional*	Free choice
90-94	Yes	Required	Free choice
95-99	Yes	Required	Limited choice
100 or above	Yes	Required	Very limited choice

From Royster & Royster, 1990. CRC Press. Reprinted with permission.

* Use of a hearing protective device (HPD) will be required for any worker who shows a significant hearing change, or of all workers if audiometric database analysis results or group hearing trends indicate inadequate protection.

4. Greater job satisfaction, increased productivity, and better quality of life resulting from reducing noise in the workplace
5. Reduced worker fatigue and irritability, improved worker efficiency and job performance
6. Reduced accident rates, illnesses, and lost work time
7. Reduced risk of workers' compensation claims
8. Reduced loss of trained and experienced personnel

III Roles and Responsibilities Related to Hearing-loss Prevention Programs

Hearing-loss prevention programs benefit everyone from management to employees. Prevention, early detection, and reducing noise hazards benefit employees' health and improve workplace morale. In turn, management benefits from improved employee morale, greater job satisfaction, and improved occupational safety (Sutter, 2003)

A An effective hearing loss prevention program requires the following:
1. The support, cooperation, and participation of all levels of management
2. Support of workers, because they are the most knowledgeable about the work environment
3. Cooperation of union leaders, where applicable, and/or the person responsible for work-site safety
4. Review of the OSHA standard (29 CFR 1910.95) or the OSHA-approved state plan, where applicable
5. Review of recommendations for compliance contained in the "NIOSH Practical Guide to Preventing Hearing Loss–96-110, Appendix A – OSHA Standard Compliance Checklist" on website http://www.cdc.gov/niosh/96-110q.html

B Management's roles include:
1. Developing and implementing an HLPP policy, including disciplinary action for noncompliance
2. Identifying program personnel and defining their responsibilities
   a. Provide a qualified physician, an otolaryngologist, or an audiologist to supervise the program.
   b. Identify the program coordinator and other personnel responsible for the program's components.
   c. All participants should be enthusiastic, committed to the HLPP and receive the appropriate training.
3. Providing personnel, space, supplies, and funding for the program
4. Providing all elements of the program to workers free of charge
5. Ensuring that workers exposed to hazardous noise are compliant with the use of hearing protection
6. Making a good-faith effort to eliminate or reduce sources of noise and to reevaluate the noise level when there are changes in exposure
7. Posting appropriate warning signs and ear-protection requirements at entrances to areas with noise levels exceeding 85 dBA
8. Conducting and reviewing annual program evaluations to ensure the quality and effectiveness of the program

C The hearing loss prevention coordinator (who may be an occupational and environmental health nurse) has the following responsibilities:
1. Acquiring certification in hearing conservation
2. Determining the workers who qualify for enrollment in an HCP
3. Taking a brief health and aural history on each worker participating in the program
4. Performing an otoscopic examination and audiometric testing
5. Coordinating the testing schedules and follow-up procedures
6. Keeping accurate, clear, and complete testing and counseling records
7. Selecting, fitting, and monitoring the wearing of appropriate hearing-protection devices
8. Acting as liaison between workers and other members of the team
9. Educating and training workers on how to protect themselves from hearing loss
10. Referring workers to outside sources for further testing or medical treatment when indicated
11. Seeking workers' input for the evaluation of the HLPP
12. Providing regular updates annually to management regarding the HLPP program

D The success of a hearing loss prevention program depends of workers' active participation by doing the following:
1. Provide information relative to current ear conditions, ear diseases and or treatments, and ototraumatic exposure histories in order to promote reliability of the audiogram implementation and interpretation (NIOSH, 1996).
2. Cooperate by following audiometric tester instructions (NIOSH 1996).
3. Inform the audiometric tester if instructions are unclear or if there are personal and/or environmental interferences with the test process (NIOSH, 1996).
4. Comply with the program by wearing appropriate hearing protection.
5. Encourage co-workers to wear hearing protection devices.
6. Report difficulties or safety hazards related to hearing protection use and/or changes in noise levels in the work area.

IV Assessment and Control of Noise Exposure

A If reliable information indicates noise exposure in the work site, noise measurements should be conducted.
1. Noise measurements should be performed by an acoustical engineer, industrial hygienist, occupational audiologist, or a professional proficient in noise-level measurement.
2. Only sound-level meters or noise dosimeters that meet the American National Standards should be used.
3. A sampling strategy that will pick up all continuous, intermittent, and impulse sound levels from 80 to 130 dBA is needed; all sound levels in the total noise measurement should be included.
4. All continuous, intermittent, and impulse noise within an 80-dB(A) to 130-dB(A) range taken during a typical work situation should be included.
5. Workers and/or their representatives should be permitted to observe monitoring.
6. Workers who are exposed to noise at or above an 8-hour TWA of 85 dBA must be notified.

B **Sound-survey results are used to:**
1. Identify areas of the work site where hazardous noise levels exist
2. Identify workers to be included in the HLPP
3. Classify workers' noise exposures to define policies for hearing protection devices and prioritize areas for noise-control efforts
4. Identify safety hazards in terms of interference with speech communication and warning-signal detection
5. Evaluate noise source for noise-control purposes
6. Document noise levels for legal purposes

C **Noise-control measures include engineering controls, administrative controls and personal protective equipment.**
1. *Engineering controls* are the most effective and the most desirable long-term solutions. To determine the type of modification to be used, it is recommended that the noise characteristics be assessed (May, 2000). Common noise control measures may include any of the following:
   a. Elimination of the noise source
   b. Redesign of the process to be quieter
   c. Isolation of the machinery to prevent vibrations and noise from radiating
   d. Building an enclosure around noisy machinery
   e. Using absorptive material on walls and ceilings
   f. Erecting a barrier or noise-reducing curtain around the noisy area
   g. Adding a muffler to noisy tools
   h. Keeping machinery well balanced, oiled, and in good repair
2. *Administrative controls*, including work practices, are implemented when engineering and work-practice controls are not feasible; these include:
   a. Rotating workers to less noisy areas
   b. Performing high-noise tasks when fewer workers are present
3. *Personal protective equipment* is provided when engineering and administrative controls are not feasible; in some cases, it may be used in conjunction with other strategies.
   a. Workers should be provided with appropriate hearing protection devices (e.g. ear plugs, muffs, and helmets).
   b. Workers should have a selection of appropriate styles and types of hearing protection devices; they should be provided at no cost to workers.

V Worker Training and Education

A **Appropriate training and education of workers is essential to a successful program.**
1. Training and education should be conducted initially for new hires and annually for workers who are included in the HLPP; interpreters should be provided when training English as a Second Language (ESL) workers.
2. The characteristics of sound should be described; sound is defined as a complex combination of pure tones found in the environment that result in a vibratory disturbance in the pressure of fluid in the ear and capable of being detected by the organs of hearing.
3. Workers should be told where noise is found.
   a. Cite occupational, recreational, and environmental sources (Table 16-2), including cumulative effects from multiple sources.
   b. Provide examples of different types of noise from actual locations at the work site (where most of the noise exposure occurs).

TABLE 16-2

Some commonly encountered noise levels

Source	dB(A) level	Effect
Jet plane	140	Acoustic trauma: May cause permanent
Gunshot blast (impulse)	140 (pain threshold)	damage to the delicate hair cells of the cochlea
Automobile horn	120	
Rock band	110	Noise-induced hearing loss:
Chain saw	110	Long exposure over 90 dB(A) may eventually
Car racing	110	cause permanent hearing loss
Motorcycle	100	
Subway	90	
Average factory	80-90	
Noisy restaurant	80	Usually will not cause permanent hearing loss
Busy traffic	75	
Conversational speech	65	
Average home	50	
Quiet office	40	
Soft whisper	30	

Sources: Environmental Protection Agency, 1978; Royster & Royster, 1990.

4. The multiple effects of noise (additional to hearing loss) should be described (Lusk 2002; 2003).
    a. Physical problems include effects on the cardiovascular and gastrointestinal systems, headache, stress, and fatigue.
    b. Psychologic problems include annoyance, feeling of isolation among workers, masking of warning shouts and signals, and interference with speech communication.

B **An overview of signs and symptoms of hearing loss should be provided; the fact that awareness of hearing loss usually does not occur until the loss is significant should be emphasized.**
    1. Tinnitus, or ringing in the ear, is a sign of an overtaxed auditory system.
    2. Perception that others are "mumbling" is often a sign of hearing loss.
    3. Occupational hearing loss is usually bilateral; hearing loss in only one ear may be caused by pathologic processes other than occupational exposures or acoustic trauma to that ear.

C **The anatomy and physiology of the outer, middle, and inner ear should be explained; a diagram or model of the parts of the ear is helpful (Figure 16-1).**
    1. The outer ear collects sound waves and funnels them into the ear canal.
    2. In the middle ear, sound impinges on the ear drum and is mechanically transmitted to the bones of the middle ear, known as the malleus, incus, and stapes, and collectively referred to as the ossicular chain. Ossicular movement creates vibrations in the fluid-filled cochlea in the inner ear.
    3. The inner ear transmits sound waves through hair cells in the cochlea that send electrical impulses to the auditory nerve, which transmits the signals to the brain where the sound is interpreted.

D **The different types of hearing loss should be described.**
    1. Hearing loss from acoustic trauma:
        a. Results from a single exposure such as a loud, explosive blast or a blow to the head
        b. May rupture the eardrum and damage the middle and inner ear

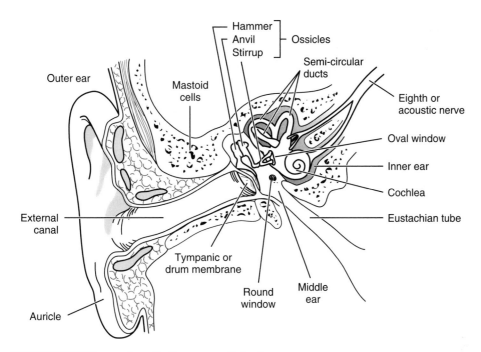

FIGURE 16-1 *Sectional diagram of the human ear*

Courtesy The Sonotone Corporation, Boca Raton, Florida.

2. Sensorineural hearing loss:
   a. Results in changes in the receptive cells; occurs from long-term exposure to noise
   b. Is usually bilateral
   c. Is not usually apparent until hearing loss is severe
   d. Can be caused by trauma, use of certain ototoxic drugs, aging, disease, or heredity
   e. Is usually irreversible, its severity depending on the intensity, frequency, and duration of noise exposure
3. Conductive hearing loss:
   a. Occurs from obstruction of sound through the outer and inner ear
   b. May be caused by wax buildup, presence of a foreign body, ruptured eardrum, infection, otosclerosis, or injury
   c. May be reversed or stabilized by appropriate treatment or surgery

VI Hearing Protection Devices

HPDs should be provided at no cost, or more-expensive devices at minimal cost, for workers to use when engaged in noisy activities outside the workplace. Proper fit is vital for promoting hearing protection.

A **There are a variety of hearing protection devices (HPDs) available to workers.**
1. Ear plugs (aural inserts) are formable or molded, and made of soft material. Many types and styles are available.
   a. Advantages—Small, inexpensive, easy to use, comfortable, can be worn for long periods

    b. Disadvantages—Need to be kept clean; may become contaminated with dirt and grime; may cause allergic reaction in some individuals; may produce wax buildup, are difficult to monitor at a distance

2. Ear muffs (circumaurals) are plastic-foam–filled cuffs that fit snugly against the head and are attached to an adjustable headband.
   a. Advantages—Easy to fit and easy to monitor from a distance
   b. Disadvantages—Expensive, large, and bulky; may be difficult to use with hard hats or respiratory equipment; and may become loose with head movement

3. Canal caps (semiaurals) are ear-plug–like tips connected by a lightweight headband.
   a. Advantages—Suitable for short-duration and off-and-on wearing
   b. Disadvantages—Uncomfortable if worn for long periods; not suitable for areas where the noise level is high

4. Custom-fitted ear plugs are molded to the ear. They may be solid or filtered, to allow speech to enter but reduce harmful noise.
   a. Advantages—Suitable for small or hard-to-fit ear canals; can be filtered for special needs
   b. Disadvantages—The material may shrink; the fit may change if worker gains or loses weight

B HPDs by law must contain a number that reflects the amount of noise that will be reduced by their use.
1. The noise reduction rating (NRR) is determined in laboratories with selected subjects and may not reflect real work situations. OSHA adjusts the NRR by 50% (e.g., 30 dB NRR = 15 dB in the real workplace).
2. The formula that is used in the workplace to obtain the number is to subtract the NRR number from the dB level of noise exposure.
3. OSHA indicates a dB(C) scale is used in NRR and needs to be corrected to dB(A) by subtracting 7 from the NRR [noise level in dB(A) -[NRR -7] = estimated exposure in dB(A)].

C Workers' perceptions and motivations related to the use of HPDs should be evaluated.
1. Barriers to compliance with recommendations should be identified.
2. Strategies to address concerns of workers related to the use of HPDs should be developed.

D The following should be considered when fitting HPDs.
1. Several styles and varying sizes should be offered to the worker.
2. Workers should be evaluated to determine the types of hearing protection best suited to each worker's anatomy and job situation.
3. Workers should be instructed on proper placement, limitations, and care of HPDs.
4. The manufacturers' directions can serve as a guide to proper use.

VII Audiometric Testing

A Audiometric testing is performed to determine baseline hearing and to monitor the effects of noise exposure.
1. The test is implemented under the direction and supervision of an audiologist, otolaryngologist, or qualified physician.

2. Both the test environment and the audiometer must meet criteria set by the American National Standards Institute.
   a. Audiometric testing shall consist of pure-tone, hearing threshold measures at no less than 500, 1000, 2000, 3000, 4000, and 6000 hertz (Hz).
   b. Right and left ears shall be individually tested.
   c. The 8000-Hz threshold should also be tested as an option and as a useful source of information about the etiology of a hearing loss.
3. The test must be performed by a licensed or certified audiologist, otolaryngologist, or physician; or by a technician who is certified by the Council for Accreditation in Occupational Hearing Conservation.
   a. A worker's baseline audiogram is performed at least 14 hours after noise exposure, or at the time of hire for job placement, or when a worker is transferred from a non-noisy to a noisy work site.
   b. The baseline audiogram is used as a reference against which future audiograms are compared.
   c. An annual or periodic audiogram may be performed well into the work shift to provide information on the effectiveness of noise-control measures; it must be taken within one year of the baseline test.
   d. An exit, or termination, audiogram is performed when work-site noise exposure ceases; it is not an OSHA requirement, but it may be important in determining the extent of employer liability for workers' compensation determination.

B **An audiometric evaluation provides information about the extent of hearing loss; the evaluation may include the following:**
1. Calibrating the audiometer at least daily by testing the same individual with stable hearing.
2. Taking a health history and noise-exposure history as follows:
   a. Perform a visual and otoscopic examination of the ears
   b. Explain the purpose of the test
   c. Administer a pure-tone audiometric test
   d. Provide immediate feedback and counseling
3. Recognizing criteria for referral to audiologist, otolaryngologist, or a qualified physician which may include:
   a. An infection in the ear is suspected.
   b. Hearing loss is unilateral.
   c. The worker complains of pain in the ear.
   d. A Standard Threshold Shift (STS) is evident (See VII.C.1. for definition).
   e. The view of the tympanic membrane is obstructed due to cerumen or foreign body (May, 2000).
   f. Hearing loss is rapidly progressing or shows fluctuation (May, 2000).
   g. Other criteria can be determined by a supervising audiologist or physician.

C **Normal hearing, in general, falls within hearing threshold levels between 0 and 25 dB; it may vary slightly from left to right ear and may be age dependent (Figure 16-2).**
1. A *standard threshold shift* (STS), also referred to as *significant threshold shift*, is an average shift in either ear of 10 dB or more at 2000, 3000, and 4000 Hz compared with the baseline audiogram.
   a. An STS may require referral to an audiologist, an otolaryngologist, or a qualified physician.

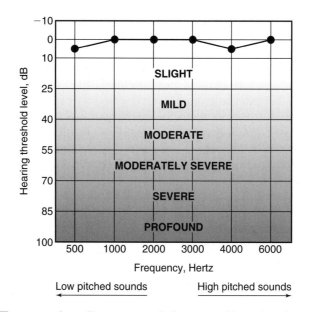

FIGURE 16-2 *Normal audiogram and degrees of hearing loss*

From Royster & Royster, 1990. CRC Press. Reprinted with permission.

    b. Depending upon program supervisor protocol, an exposed worker whose test reveals a possible STS must then be retested within 30 days after the initial test revealing the STS, in order to confirm that a persistent STS has occurred.

    c. If the follow-up audiogram confirms an STS, workers must be notified in writing within 21 days of determination of the STS.

2. A *temporary threshold shift* (TTS) occurs shortly after exposure and improves gradually if the noise has not been too loud or the exposure too long.

    a. The greatest STS recovery occurs in 1 to 24 hours if the worker is removed from exposure.

    b. When a TTS occurs, the adequacy of the HPD should be checked.

3. A *permanent threshold shift* occurs when hearing loss persists after removal from exposure; it is associated with damage to the delicate sensory hair cells in the inner ear. If there is no improvement within one week, the loss is usually permanent.

VIII Monitoring and Evaluating a Hearing-loss Protection Program

A Audiometric test records must include the worker's name, identification number, duties performed at job location, type of hearing protection worn, date of the test, the examiner's name, date of the last audiometer calibration, and the worker's most recent noise exposure assessment.

1. It is advisable to document any worker counseling that was provided.

2. In accordance with 29CFR 1910.20(d), medical monitoring records (audiometric records) shall be retained for at least the duration of the affected employee's employment plus 30 years.

3. Noise exposure monitoring records shall be retained for 30 years.
4. Background-noise measurements of the room where work is performed should be recorded and maintained.
5. Audiometric and noise-exposure records should be accessible upon request to workers, former workers, worker-designated representatives, and others as required by law.
6. If the employer ceases to do business, all records must be transferred to the successor employer and kept in accordance with the law.
7. Documentation that training has occurred is needed; documentation should indicate that interpreters and/or translated documents were used when this is the case.

B **It is essential that the program be evaluated on a regular basis, and that the completeness and quality of the program components be assessed.**
1. Compare annual audiograms with baseline for individuals and groups to determine the success of control measures; identify areas where further controls are needed.
2. Develop a checklist specific to the work environment to ensure that all components of the program are being followed and comply with the appropriate standards.

Ergonomics programs

Work-related musculoskeletal disorders (WMSDs) are among the most costly injuries in terms of the pain and suffering of workers and direct and indirect costs to employers (Box 16-1). Successful prevention of WMSDs requires a multifaceted approach that focuses on prevention and is tailored to the specific needs of the organization. This section describes the elements of comprehensive ergonomics programs and services. Additional information about ergonomics can be found in Chapter 5.

IX Overview of Ergonomics

A **Ergonomics "is the science of designing and arranging the physical environment, equipment and organization of work to most safely and effectively fit the human body of the worker" (AAOHN, n.d.).**

B **The field of ergonomics is concerned with the design of the work site, equipment, and physical environment and the organization of work; it focuses on the interaction of the worker with the job.**

C **Ergonomics is a multidisciplinary science that considers knowledge from four areas.**
1. *Human factors engineering*, also called engineering psychology or cognitive ergonomics, focuses on the perceptual and information-processing requirements and the psychomotor actions of the job.
2. *Anthropometry*, looks at the worker's body size, dimensions, or measurements when designing work space or equipment.
3. *Occupational biomechanics* examines the mechanical properties of the human body and their responses to mechanical stressors.
4. *Work physiology* is concerned with the responses of the body (e.g., respiratory, cardiovascular, and musculoskeletal systems) to the metabolic demands of work.

BOX 16-1

Impact and costs related to work-related musculoskeletal disorders (WMSDs)

- WMSDs account for greater than one third of all occupational injuries and illnesses reported to the Bureau of Labor Statistics each year.
- In 2002, WMSDs accounted for 487,900, or 34% of the injuries and illnesses with days away from work.
- Among major disabling injuries and illnesses, median days away from work in 2002 were highest for carpal tunnel syndrome (30 days).
- Repetitive motion, such as grasping tools, scanning groceries, and typing, resulted in the longest absences from work– a median of 23 days.
- More than 600,000 employees suffer lost-workday WMSDs each year in the United States.

- WMSDs result in an estimated $13 to $20 billion in workers' compensation costs and lost days each year.
- Direct costs associated with WMSDs are estimated between $45 to $54 billion for time and man-power to conduct accident investigations, decreased productivity and quality, job retraining costs, replacement hiring costs, increased absenteeism, decreased worker morale, and litigation costs.
- Not included in these numbers are the musculoskeletal disorders that are not recognized as work related, but are treated under the employee's general medical insurance.
- Pain and suffering to workers and their families are not included either.

Source: Bureau of Labor Statistics, www.bls.gov, NAS, 1999, and IOM 2001.

X Work-Related Musculoskeletal Disorders

A **Injuries or illnesses resulting from poor biomechanics, sometimes referred to as *ergonomic injuries*, are called *work-related musculoskeletal disorders* (WMSDs).**

1. WMSDs typically include soft tissue injuries to the muscles, tendons, ligaments, joints, blood vessels, and nerves.
2. Problems occur in the upper and sometimes lower extremities, cervical spine, and lower back; symptoms of musculoskeletal disorders include pain, swelling, erythema, numbness, and paresthesia.
3. WSMDs exclude injuries from slips, trips, falls, motor vehicle accidents, or being struck by objects.

B **Contributing factors for WMSDs include exposure to hazards related to the following:**

1. Physical factors, such as the physical working conditions
2. Environmental factors, such as hot/cold temperatures, noise, and lighting
3. Work organizational factors, or the "organizational structure of the work environment, such as restrictive, high demand–low control jobs" (Forde, Punnett, & Wegman, 2002)
4. Personal factors and activities outside the workplace

C **WMSDs may result from exposure to the following risk factors:**
1. Awkward postures, such as working with hands above head
2. Forceful exertions, such as high hand force, in gripping an unsupported object or using a pinch grip
3. Highly repetitive motions, such as performing intensive keying
4. Repeated impact, such as using the hand as a hammer
5. Heavy, frequent, and/or awkward lifting
6. Moderate to high hand-arm (segmental) vibration caused by using equipment such as grinders or sanders
7. Whole body vibration, such as occurs when driving heavy equipment
8. Compression at pressure points, or local contact stress, that inhibits nerve function and blood flow
9. Lack of sufficient rest periods or machine-paced work
10. Combinations of any of these conditions

D **Examples of work-related musculoskeletal injuries are muscle strains and tears, ligament sprains, joint and tendon inflammation, pinched nerves, ganglion cysts, and degeneration of spinal discs.**
1. Conditions associated with musculoskeletal injuries include tendinitis, tenosynovitis, epicondylitis, DeQuervain's syndrome, thoracic outlet syndrome, sciatica, trigger finger, synovitis, and rotator cuff syndrome.
2. Nerve entrapment syndromes include carpal tunnel syndrome (median nerve entrapment at the wrist), tarsal tunnel syndrome (tibial nerve entrapment at the ankle), and ulnar nerve entrapment at the elbow or wrist.
3. Another form of peripheral nerve impairment has been termed *hand-arm vibration syndrome*; this is thought to result from vibration such as that experienced with the use of power tools (Galszechy, 1999).

E **Studies suggest that the greater the intensity, duration, and frequency of exposure to physical risk factors, the more likely it is that a worker will sustain a WMSD.**
1. Several studies provide evidence that WMSDs are associated with various work-related conditions.
   a. A NIOSH report concluded that there is "strong evidence of an association between WMSDs and certain work-related physical factors when there are high levels of exposure and especially in combination with exposure to more than one physical factor" (NIOSH, 1997a).
   b. The National Academy of Science (NAS) reported that "scientific evidence shows that musculoskeletal disorders of the lower back and upper extremities can be attributed to particular jobs and working conditions." These conditions include heavy lifting, repetitive and forceful motions, and stressful work environments (Institute of Medicine [IOM], 2001).
   c. The NAS also noted that there is evidence for reducing biomechanical stress on the job, which will then reduce the risk of injuries.
2. Virtually any worker is potentially at risk of exposure to WMSDs.

XI Ergonomic Regulation and Guidelines

A **U.S. workers are protected through the OSHA general duty clause from hazards created by not addressing ergonomic issues in the workplace (Chapter 3).**

B **In 1990, OSHA developed ergonomics program-management guidelines for meat-packing plants.**

C The Americans with Disabilities Act of 1990 and workers' compensation laws also provide a legal framework for ergonomic concerns.

D Some states and some international agencies have developed or are in the process of promulgating regulations requiring workplaces to implement ergonomics programs and services to reduce the incidence of WMSDs.

E In 2002, OSHA developed a four-pronged ergonomics strategy, including a combination of industry-specific and task-specific guidelines, outreach, enforcement, and research.

F Guidelines have been developed for the following high-risk industries: retail grocery, poultry, and nursing homes.

G Shipbuilding industry guidelines are currently being developed, and other industry guidelines will follow.

H Other agencies with ergonomic related regulations or guidelines include the European Union's European Agency for Safety and Health at Work; the International Labour Organization; and the American National Standards Institute.

XII Purposes of Ergonomics Programs and Services

Ergonomics programs and services are designed to:

A Identify potential hazards in the work setting that may require ergonomic interventions

B Provide a framework for the development of strategies to prevent and control work-related hazards

C Reduce workers' exposures to workplace conditions or hazards that can cause or aggravate WMSDs

D Limit the costs related to WMSDs, for both the company and the worker

E Improve productivity and quality of production or service

F Accommodate diverse populations in the workplace

G Help the company comply with health and safety regulations

XIII Ergonomics Programs and Services

A Successful ergonomics programs and services require management leadership and commitment and worker involvement.

   1. The program includes identifying hazards, developing prevention and control strategies, implementing health management techniques, training and educating employees, and conducting a thorough program evaluation.
   2. The approach should "conform with existing programs and business goals, as well as the facilities' culture" (AAOHN, n.d.).

B Management of the organization or company should provide overall leadership and commitment to the ergonomics program; the role of management includes:

   1. Being visibly involved in planning, developing, and implementing the company's ergonomic program.
   2. Demonstrating commitment of time and resources.
   3. Delineating responsibility for the various components of the program.

    a. Assignment of resources

    b. Delegation of authority and responsibility for program components

    c. Assurance of accountability

    d. Implementation of workplace policies that value health and safety as important as productivity and quality

    e. Demonstration of concern for workers' well being

    f. Inclusion of workers in all aspects of the ergonomics program

    g. Training of workers and encouraging their involvement on committees or ergonomics teams to identify hazards and to offer suggestions for abatement, a process called *participatory ergonomics* (Zalk, 2000)

    h. Providing all workers and their union representatives access to the written ergonomic program

  4. The occupational and environmental health nurse may also take a major role in one or all of these functions, either as the organizational manager, or through delegation of some responsibilities.

C **The role of the worker is to:**

  1. Report hazards found in the workplace

  2. Report any symptoms of WMSDs without fear of retribution

  3. Participate in training

  4. Participate on ergonomic teams and joint management/labor safety committees

D *Work-site analysis* **is a health and safety review to identify hazards that cause WMSDs, the risk factors that pose the hazards, and the causes of the risk factors (Chapter 10). See Box 16-2 for a list of common potential risk factors that are considered when planning ergonomic programs and services.**

  1. *Hazards* are those stressors and workplace conditions that pose a potential for harm or development of WMSDs.

  2. *Risk factors* are the elements of the job, or personal attributes, that increase the likelihood that a hazard will cause WMSDs.

  3. The duration of exposure to the risk factor and combinations of risk factors may increase the likelihood of WMSDs.

E *Occupational health surveillance* **"is the process of monitoring the health status of worker populations to gather data on the effects of workplace exposures and using the data to prevent illness or injury" (AAOHN, 1996). Surveillance can be active or passive.**

BOX 16-2

Risk factors associated with work-related musculoskeletal disorders (WMSDs)

- Excessive force
- Repetition
- Awkward, non-neutral postures
- Extreme environmental conditions—hot or cold stress, noise or ineffective lighting
- Vibration—upper extremities or whole body exposures

- Static postures or sustained exertions
- Contact stress
- Psychosocial and work organizational issues, including pace, demand and control provided to the worker

---

NOTE: Risk increases when several hazards are coupled in a single job.

1. *Passive surveillance* is the "collection and analysis of data obtained from existing record sources" that identifies the patterns of injuries and illnesses or potential WMSDs (NIOSH, 1995).
   a. Review of company records provides data to target work areas and work processes for further evaluation, and to prioritize the jobs to investigate for hazards.
   b. Data gathered can be used as baseline information to evaluate efforts of prevention.
   c. Passive surveillance includes multiple data sources.
      1) Workers' compensation records
      2) OSHA 300 log and supplemental records (OSHA Form 301)
      3) Accident/incident reports
      4) Safety meeting minutes or reports
      5) Equipment and tool evaluation records
      6) Costs related to short-term and long-term disability
      7) Group health insurance utilization reports
      8) Absentee and lost workday data, job turnover data
      9) Days away from work or days on job transfer or restriction count
      10) Nurse's daily log
2. *Active surveillance* is the proactive development of methods to collect data to determine trends in WMSDs or identify symptoms that indicate risk for WMSDs.
   a. Symptom surveys, worker questionnaires, and symptom diaries allow workers to track the symptoms they encounter during and after work, relating it to the tasks of their job. Examples include the following:
      1) Discomfort rating scales
      2) Body part maps
   b. These methods depend on worker self-report, which may limit the validity of the information.
   c. The advantage of worker reports is the ability to identify jobs with potential risk factors for WMSDs before full-blown injury or illness occurs.
   d. The data gathered may be useful in evaluating ergonomic interventions.

F *Work-site hazard evaluation* **examines both job demands and human capacities.**
   1. The purposes of a work-site hazard evaluation are to:
      a. Identify hazards that may be risk factors for WMSDs
      b. Identify and correct the causes of the hazards
      c. Examine the interaction of the worker with the job demands
   2. The job demand evaluation examines the components of the work environment, which include:
      a. Tools, machines, and materials
      b. Workstation and the physical environment
      c. Job tasks, including the organization environment in which they are performed
   3. Job hazard analysis encompasses the methods used to analyze job tasks and the performance demands of jobs. A number of analytical tools are available for purchase or use in job analysis.
      a. These methods include direct observation or videotaping of workers and work processes, job function lists, and site surveys.
      b. Tools to assist in the job hazard analysis include videotape, ergonomic checklists, and forms. Chapter 10 presents additional information on hazard analysis.

BOX 16-3

Analytical tools for job hazard analysis

Human Capacities Guidelines
- NIOSH Lifting Equation (http://www.cdc.gov/niosh/94-110.html)
- Liberty Mutual Manual Handling Tables
- ANSI S3.34-1986 (R1997) Hand Arm Vibration Standards (http://webstore.ansi.org/ansidocstore/ find.asp?)
- Physiologic measures, such as heart rate, blood pressure, oxygen consumption, and body temperature are sometimes used to assess the effects of work demands on the body (http://www.cdc.gov/niosh/pdfs/95-119.pdf.)

- Subjective assessments, such as perceived exertion ratings and scales, collect information used to determine human capacity. Normally they are combined with physiologic measures (http://www.cdc.gov/niosh/pdfs/95-119.pdf).

Performance Measure
- Time
- Accuracy
- Frequency
- Amount achieved or accomplished
- Consumption or quantity use

Additional tools may be found via several websites:
http://www.ergoweb.com/
http://www.ergoresources.org/

---

    c. Checklists are used to identify common hazard sources in a timely manner, while ensuring that systematic and standardized procedures are followed.

    d. Videotaping allows time-and-motion analysis to identify risks, such as repetition or awkward and static postures, or to describe regular and irregular activities that are part of the job.

4. Human capacities are an integral part of ergonomics; however, for most job demands, there are not well-defined limits. Some select resources for analytical tools are found in Box 16-3.

    a. Design of workstations can be complemented by use of anthropometric tables and other guidelines.

    b. Multiple guidelines for determining human capacities, coupled with quantifying the human requirements of the job that will minimize the risk of injury, have been researched and published.

    c. When worker's capacities are exceeded by the demands of the job, performance is affected.

G Hazard prevention and control components focus on ways to reduce or eliminate the hazards associated with risk factors for WMSDs. The hierarchy of controls (engineering and administrative controls, personal protective equipment) is the preferred method for controlling and preventing WSMDs.

1. *Engineering controls* aim to remove the hazard or limit its risk in the work process by altering the physical work area, work tools, or work process (Box 16-4).

2. *Administrative controls* are the policies and procedures implemented and supported by management that aim to reduce the worker's exposure to risk

---

BOX 16-4

Considerations for engineering controls

Tool and Equipment Design

Tools and equipment should be:

- Sized to fit the individual user
- Counterweighted to minimize the force necessary to use the tool
- Balanced, so the grip is at the center of gravity
- Designed without sharp edges
- Designed to minimize vibration and minimal rotational forces
- Designed to minimize tension on finger-triggers

Controls and Displays

- Location of controls and displays depends on:
  - Importance, frequency, and sequence of use
  - Anthropometry
- Controls and displays should be visible and accessible
- Controls and displays should be spaced to accommodate personal protective equipment

Workstation and Work Environment Design

Design of workstations should consider:

- Workspace layout
- Work surfaces
- Standing and walking surfaces
- Seating
- Work fixtures
- Materials handling
- Storage
- Lighting
- Noise levels
- Temperature regulation

Work Methods and Process

Work methods and process should consider:

- Work rates
- Sequence of actions
- Job steps

---

factors or hazards; administrative controls also include work-practice controls, the strategies for the manner in which work is performed. Examples include the following:

a. Scheduling strategies to limit time of exposure to specific hazards
   1) Job rotation—Alternating a worker between two or more jobs within a single workday to minimize the exposure to hazards. The jobs or tasks should consist of significantly varied risk factors.
   2) Job enlargement—A form of job rotation that varies the types of risk factors the worker is exposed to in different work tasks.

b. Rest breaks or recovery pauses

c. Training

d. Tools and equipment maintenance schedules

e. Scheduled housekeeping for work areas

f. Providing for worker control over job pace and processes

3. *Personal protective equipment* (PPE) provides a barrier between the worker and the hazard source. Examples of accepted PPE for exposures when ergonomics solutions do not entirely remove the hazard include the following:

a. Vibration attenuation gloves

b. Ear plugs or noise reduction devices

c. Anti-fatigue insoles

d. Knee pads

     e. Temperature control clothing
     f. Eye protection
  4. Wrist supports or splints and back belts are not considered PPE.
     a. Wrist supports or splints are considered immobilization devices; they may be included in medical treatment as part of the health management program.
     b. Multiple studies have concluded that there is no evidence that back belt use reduces the incidence of injury or low back pain.

XIV Training and Education

A **Training and education are integral components of an ergonomics program.**
  1. Ergonomic awareness provides the basic education on ergonomics and WMSDs (Box 16-5).
  2. Job-specific training provides education in the hazards specific to particular job tasks and the methods to avoid the risk factors for WMSDs (See Box 16-5).
  3. Supervisors and managers also need to have training to properly ensure safe work practices and implement ergonomic controls.
  4. Videotaping of hazardous jobs and risk factors can be useful as a training tool (e.g., demonstrating proper and improper work processes and techniques).

B **Training should be conducted:**
  1. In the primary language of the workers
  2. At the appropriate education level of the workers
  3. On paid time
  4. In a method and style appropriate to the workers and workplace

---

BOX 16-5

Contents of ergonomics training

Awareness Training
- Types of WMSDs associated with jobs
- Symptoms of WMSDs
- Recognition and reporting of symptoms
- Hazards
- Risk factors for WMSDs
- Principles of ergonomics (such as neutral postures)
- Workplace analysis methods
- Prevention and control methods
- Workplace policies and procedures for reporting
- Content of the ergonomic program
- Worker's role
- Responsibility for components of program
- Reporting procedures

Job Specific Training
- Job specific hazards
- Tool and equipment maintenance
- Hands-on training for a new job
- New employee safe work practices
- New work processes
- Proper lifting techniques
- Correct body postures and motions
- Use of personal protective equipment (PPE), if any

XV Management of Work-Related Musculoskeletal Disorders (WMSD) as Part of a Comprehensive Ergonomics Program

A *Health care management* **refers to the effective use of available health care resources to ensure early detection, evaluation, and treatment to prevent impairment and disability related to WMSDs.**

    1. The health care management team should include the occupational and environmental health nurse, company physician or other licensed health care provider, physical or occupational therapist, nurse case manager, ergonomist, and the safety/industrial hygiene department.

    2. Health care management for WMSDs encompasses a wide range of activities (Box 16-6).

B **Preplacement physical examinations can be used to identify existing WMSDs, but are not considered useful in screening workers for risk.**

C **Components of health care management may be done within the company or be contracted out to other service providers.**

XVI Documentation and Recordkeeping

A **A written program should be developed that provides the following:**

    1. The basis for documentation of plans

    2. Historical record of activities

    3. Data to use in evaluating the program

B **All training and education records should be maintained and stored.**

    1. Many companies are now using on-line training programs that also track the records and provide notification for updates.

    2. Records should be maintained according to regulations and company policy.

BOX 16-6

Components of health care management

- Health surveillance
- Occupational health history taking
- Early recognition and reporting of symptoms of WMSDs
- Access to evaluation and appropriate conservative treatment, including referral
- Alternative duty or transitional work programs—placing workers into temporary positions to accommodate their functional capacity limitations while recovering from WMSDs
- Job evaluations and periodic workplace walk-throughs
- Education for health care providers on workplace hazards
- Rehabilitation and work hardening—work hardening involves gradually introducing the full workload over time, enabling the worker to build up endurance for the job
- Injury and illness case management
- Recordkeeping and confidentiality

C Documentation of the following data is advised:
1. Risk factors and hazards
2. Worker aggregate and individual symptoms records
3. Injury and illness records
4. Treatment records
5. Hazard prevention and control measures

D Personal health data, such as occupational health histories, treatments, and symptom questionnaires and surveys that contain information that could identify workers should be kept in confidential health files. The information released to other company employees should be aggregate data only.

XVII Program Evaluation

A Ergonomic evaluation can be accomplished by using the quality assessment (i.e., structure, process, outcome) framework developed by Donabedian (1966) (Chapter 9, Section IV).
1. Examples of structural elements to be considered in an ergonomic evaluation:
   a. Evidence of management support and commitment to the program
   b. Adequate human, financial, and training resources to implement and evaluate the program
   c. Policies and procedures supportive of the program
   d. Mechanisms that support worker participation
   e. Support of health and safety identified in the company's mission statement
2. Examples of basics to include in the process evaluation include tracking the actions taken to implement the program and the dates the activities were accomplished:
   a. Establishment of the ergonomic team completed by stated date
   b. Number of workers afforded ergonomic training
   c. Number of requests for ergonomic evaluations of workstations or tools
   d. Number of ergonomic evaluations completed
   e. Number and type of ergonomic solutions implemented
3. Outcome evaluation elements cover the effects achieved or the goal achieved by the ergonomics program or specified components of the program.
   a. Worker outcomes that should be examined include:
      1) Incidence of reported WMSDs
      2) Description of the severity of the WMSDs
      3) Completeness of incident reporting by workers
      4) Worker morale
      5) Worker's quality of life
   b. Organizational outcomes that should be examined include:
      1) Affects of WMSDs on productivity and quality of product or service
      2) Workers' compensation costs related to WMSDs
      3) Number of days on job transfer or restriction or days away from work
      4) Turnover and absenteeism data

B Training and education evaluation must examine both knowledge and skills.

C Videotaping before and after ergonomic interventions provides objective demonstration of ergonomic controls and hazard reduction.

Hazard communication programs and services

The hazard communication standard was promulgated by OSHA in 1983 as a means of reducing risks related to chemical exposure in the American work force. The hazard communication programs and services described in this section provide a guide to assist in compliance with this standard. Some of the suggested elements may not be required but are included as recommendations to ensure successful programs and services. Because no single written program will work for all work sites, programs should be tailored to comply with the law and to protect workers against exposures specific to their work settings.

XVIII Hazardous Chemical Exposure

A It is estimated that over 30 million American workers are exposed to 650,000 hazardous chemicals in more than 3 million worksites (US Department of Labor [USDL], OSHA, n.d.; Washington State Department of Labor and Industries, 2004).

B All known hazardous chemicals or chemical compounds that are not covered under other federal acts are covered under the Occupational Safety and Health Act.

C Standards may vary from one jurisdiction to another; therefore, it is important that occupational and environmental health nurses review the standards applicable to their own jurisdiction.

XIX Purposes of a Hazard Communications Program

Hazard communication programs and services are designed to:

A Ensure that the hazards of all chemicals produced or imported into the workplace are evaluated and that information concerning these hazards is transmitted to employers and workers

B Prevent illness, injury, or death from exposure to hazardous chemicals and substances in the workplace

C Comply with OSHA's Hazard Communication Standard (HCS) 29 CFR 1910.12 and regulations specific to the jurisdiction (Note: OSHA specifically checks for demonstration of compliance through a written program and implementation.)

XX Management Roles and Responsibilities

Management assures of the delivery of effective hazard communication programs and services.

A Management provides workers with a company policy statement that includes the following:
   1. A statement that indicates that the company is committed to protecting the health and safety of its workers
   2. A statement that all workers will be informed of the Hazard Communication Standard requirements

3. A statement indicating that all workers will be informed of known hazardous substances that can cause illness, injury, or death
4. A statement that all workers will be trained at the time of hire, when they move to an area with new hazards, and when a new hazard is introduced into the workplace
5. The identification of individuals (or their job titles) who will be responsible for implementing and managing the hazard communication (HazCom) program
6. A statement that affirms there will be an annual review and update of the company's hazard communication program

B **Management should provide a written program that includes:**
1. A list of hazardous chemicals present in the workplace and the title of the person responsible for ensuring the list is current
2. A description of the policy for proper labeling of chemical containers that includes:
   a. The titles of the persons directly responsible for ensuring container labeling on a day-to-day basis and for the proper labeling of all containers, including those used for the shipping of chemicals
   b. An explanation of the labeling systems used
   c. Procedures to review and update labeling
   d. Identification and explanation of alternatives in container labeling
3. The preparation of material safety data sheets (MSDSs)
4. A description of training content and documentation of worker training about the hazards of chemicals and measures that can be taken to protect workers from dangerous exposures

XXI Description of the Programs and Services

A **The goals and objectives of HazCom programs and services are to:**
1. Identify and assess all chemical substances in the workplace that can pose physical or health hazards to workers
2. Communicate to all workers the presence of potentially hazardous substances in the workplace through training and provision of accessible MSDSs, which must be kept current
3. Train all workers in the safe handling of potentially hazardous substances
4. Properly label all chemical containers with warning notices and the handling and disposal procedures of hazardous substances

B **Communicating hazards requires a common understanding of core terminology.**
1. A *chemical* is any element, chemical compound, or mixture of elements and compounds.
2. A *hazardous chemical* is any chemical that is a health or physical hazard.
   a. *Health hazards* include chemicals that are known carcinogens, toxic or highly toxic agents, agents that damage the reproductive system, irritants, corrosives, sensitizers, hepatotoxins, neurotoxins, agents that act on the hematopoietic system, and agents that damage the lungs, eyes, skin, or mucous membranes.
   b. A *physical hazard* is any chemical for which there is scientifically valid evidence that it is a combustible liquid, compressed gas, or organic peroxide, or that it is explosive, flammable, pyrophoric, unstable (reactive), or water reactive.

XXII Elements of the HazCom Program

A Responsibilities of the occupational and environmental health nurse include:

1. Keeping accurate inventory of all hazardous chemicals and substances used in the workplace
2. Obtaining MSDSs from the manufacturers or suppliers of all chemicals used in the workplace
   a. Maintain MSDS inventory for 30 years
   b. Collaborate with the purchasing department to identify the chemicals that have been purchased or ordered
3. Ensuring that the requirements for training under the state and federal Hazard Communication Standards are met for workers when:
   a. A worker is hired and before starting their specific job
   b. Any hazardous chemical is used in the workplace
   c. Any new physical or health hazard is introduced into the workplace
4. Ensuring that all chemicals are properly labeled and stored
5. Conducting an annual Hazcom program evaluation and developing recommendations for the future
6. Providing management with an annual report relative to program outcomes and recommendations

B Elements of worker training programs are as follows:

1. The program is communicated to all current and new workers at least annually. Accessibility of information is assured via the use of interpreters and translated materials for workers who may not have English as a primary language.
2. The standard is summarized during the training program.
3. The location of the written program must be communicated to workers.
4. The location of the list of hazardous chemical products and the master list and location of MSDSs must be communicated and be "readily accessible" to all workers in their work areas during each work shift. OSHA interprets "readily accessible" to include the use of electronic means such as computers with printers, microfiche machines, the Internet, CD-ROMs, and fax machines, provided there is an adequate backup system in the event of a power failure.
5. The program provides mechanisms for understanding its components; for example, the worker should be able to demonstrate understanding the following:
   a. How to obtain, read and understand the purpose of the MSDSs
   b. The worksite location of and labeling procedures for hazardous chemicals and products
   c. The health and safety hazards of the chemicals used in the workplace
   d. The safe handling and disposal of hazardous chemicals
   e. The signs and symptoms of overexposure such as nausea, vomiting, headache, dizziness, burn, and rash
   f. Emergency procedures for spills and or exposure events
   g. Methods and observations that can be used to detect the presence or release of hazardous chemicals
   h. Controls that are in place to protect workers, such as engineering or administrative controls and personal protective equipment
   i. Where workers can obtain more information about hazardous chemicals

C **All workers are covered by the Hazard Communication Standard; special training procedures are required for contract workers.**

1. All contract workers must be informed of the chemical hazards and the location of the MSDSs.
2. The labeling system of hazardous chemicals used by the company should be explained to contract workers.
3. Contract workers must be provided with appropriate personal protective equipment.
4. Emergency procedures to be used in event of spill and or exposure should be described to contract workers.

D **If workers participate in nonroutine hazardous tasks, training procedures require that the organization:**

1. Provide training for the specific hazardous chemicals to which the workers will be exposed.
2. Provide workers with personal protective equipment appropriate for the specific hazards

XXIII Material Safety Data Sheets (MSDSs)

A **Completion of MSDSs requires the following:**

1. Completion of all items, leaving no blank spaces
2. The generic *and* common names of the chemical
3. A description of the chemical's characteristics (e.g., liquid, vapor, solid, flammable, or explosive)
4. A list of the chemical characteristics that make it hazardous to health, including signs and symptoms of over exposure and any medical conditions that may be aggravated by exposure to the chemical. This list may include the following:
   a. Carcinogens
   b. Corrosives
   c. Highly toxic chemicals
   d. Irritants
5. The primary routes of entry into the body
   a. Absorption
   b. Inhalation
   c. Ingestion
   d. Injection
6. Permissible exposure limits set by OSHA, and threshold limit values (TLVs) set by the American Congress of Governmental Industrial Hygienists (ACGIH)
7. Information on the chemical's listing on a hazardous chemical registry, such as the Annual Report of Carcinogens, if applicable
8. Precautions for safe handling, along with the recommended type of PPE
9. Measures to control exposure to the chemical, such as engineering, work practices, administrative controls, and PPE
10. Emergency and first-aid procedures if a spill and or exposure occurs
11. Date the MSDS was prepared and the name, address, and phone number of the manufacturer or other responsible party

B **The MSDS is required to be printed in English.**

XXIV Trade Secrets

A A *trade secret* is any confidential formula, pattern, process, device, information, or compilation of information that is used in an employer's business and that gives the employer an opportunity to obtain an advantage over competitors who do not know or use it.

B A manufacturer may withhold the identity of a certain chemical when knowledge of that chemical by other manufacturers could give the latter a competitive advantage, except in the following situations:

1. A treating physician or occupational and environmental health nurse determines that a medical emergency exists and the identity of that chemical is necessary for emergency first-aid treatment.

2. In a nonemergency situation, when the name of the chemical is requested in writing by a health professional (e.g., physician, occupational and environmental health nurse, industrial hygienist, toxicologist, or epidemiologist) who is providing occupational and environmental health services to exposed workers for valid reasons described in the OSH Act, a signed confidentiality statement may be required by the manufacturer.

XXV Container Labeling and Warning Requirements

A All chemical containers entering the workplace must be clearly marked with the identity of the chemical, appropriate warnings, and the name of the manufacturer.

B All chemicals transferred to other containers must be marked with the information listed on the original container.

C All unmarked containers must be reported to the program coordinator immediately.

D Generic warning labels are available from the U.S. Department of Transportation for such chemicals as flammable gas, flammable solid, oxidizer, or corrosive.

XXVI Recordkeeping

Although not required by OSHA, keeping records of worker training and education, including the content of the training program and the names and signatures of workers, is important. Well maintained records:

A Document that all workers have been trained in handling and storing products that contain hazardous substances.

B Document that HazCom training has been provided. This is helpful during an audit of workers' compensation claims.

C Assure that there is documentation when interpreters have been used for trainings, and/or translations of documents have been conducted for ESL employees.

XXVII Evaluation

When conducting an evaluation of hazard communication programs and services, the occupational and environmental health nurses and/or others responsible will do the following:

BOX 16-7

Checklist for a hazard communication program

- Obtained a copy of the rule
- Read and understood the requirements
- Assigned responsibility for tasks
- Prepared an inventory of chemicals used in the workplace
- Ensured that containers are properly labeled
- Obtained an MSDS for each chemical

- Prepared a written program
- Made MSDSs available to workers
- Conducted training for workers
- Established procedure to maintain current program
- Established procedures to evaluate completeness and effectiveness of the program

---

Source: U.S. Department of Labor, 1995.
MSDS, Material safety data sheet.

A Observe how chemicals are actually being handled by workers.

B Solicit feedback from workers and management on how the program is working.

C Make a checklist of all elements of the program to ensure that the program is working and complies with appropriate standards (Box 16-7).

NOTE: For further information regarding all facets of program development, implementation, and evaluation see the OSHA Draft Model Training Program for Hazard Communication at: http://www.osha.gov/dsg/hazcom/MTP101703. html.

Drug and alcohol programs and services

It is estimated that substance abuse costs employers billions of dollars each year as a result of increased injuries, fatalities, absenteeism, excessive use of health care benefits, decreased productivity, and theft. To ensure productivity, safety, and solid business practices, many companies are instituting drug free workplace programs; many of these include drug testing.

XXVIII Mandated Drug and Alcohol Programs

A While many employers have voluntarily adopted drug and screening programs, others are required to comply with federal regulations.

1. The Drug-free Workplace Act of 1988 requires employers and employees who are federal grantees, or who are functioning as federal contractors to agree to establishing workplaces that are drug-free as a precondition of receiving Federal agency contracts or grants.

2. The Omnibus Transportation Employee Testing Act of 1991 requires governmental agencies with workers in safety sensitive positions to establish anti-drug programs.

   a. The Omnibus Transportation Employee Testing Act was established by the Department of Transportation's (DOT) Operating Administrations Regulations.

b. In early 1997 the DOT published rules of compliance for all facilities and supplemented the drug testing rules as published in 1988.

c. The DOT reports that since 1991 there has been a decrease in drug and alcohol use in workers who fall under the screening program (McAndrew, 2002).

B **Collectively, the Drug-free Workplace Act of 1988 and the Omnibus Transportation Testing Act of 1991 provide excellent frameworks from which to model drug-free workplace programs (McAndrew, 2002).**

XXIX Establishing a Drug-Free Workplace

A **Drug and alcohol abuse has far-reaching effects in the workplace.**

1. Results of the 2003 National Survey on Drug Use and Health (NSDUH) revealed that 77% of adults aged 18 or older, employed full or part time, were characterized with abuse of, or dependence on, alcohol or drugs (USDL, 2004b).

2. Workers with substance abuse problems are likely to have more absences, worksite accidents and workers' compensation claims (McAndrew, 2002).

3. OSHA's web site for Workplace Substance Abuse (www.osha.gov/SLTC/substanceabuse/) states that between 10% and 20% of America's workers who die on the job test positive for alcohol or other drugs. Industries with the highest rates of drug use are the same as those at a high risk for occupational injuries, such as construction, mining, manufacturing, and wholesale (USDL, OSHA, n.d.2).

4. Alcohol- and drug-related problems have been linked to workplace theft and violence. These factors, along with the enormous health care costs and lost productivity associated with alcohol and drug abuse, result in expenses in the billions of dollars for American corporations (Substance Abuse and Mental Health Service Administration, 1999, USDL, 1998, McAndrew, 2002).

B **Developing an effective drug-free program is challenging.**

1. Key considerations include understanding the current impact of substance abuse on the organization and professional or community partners available to promote success.

2. Prior to the development of drug-free programs and/or drug and alcohol testing programs in the workplace, several steps must be taken (USDL, n.d.2.).

a. Employers must review all laws and regulations applicable to their jurisdiction regarding the regulations and mandatory requirements for drug-free workplace programs, safety sensitive positions, disabilities, rehabilitation, and discrimination.

b. The National Labor Relations Act requires bargaining with unions before changing work rules and policies.

c. Public employers must consider constitutional rights; unreasonable search and seizure is the most common challenge.

C **The 1988 Drug Free Workplace was developed in order to:**

1. Educate small business concerns about the advantages of a drug-free workplace

2. Provide grants and technical assistance in addition to financial incentives to enable small business concerns to create a drug-free workplace

   3. Assist working parents in keeping their children drug free
   4. Encourage small business employers and workers alike to participate in drug-free workplace programs

D **Drug testing is NOT required under the Drug-Free Workplace Act of 1988.**
   1. Understanding the various state and federal regulations that may apply to an organization is a *vital first step before designing a drug-testing program* (USDL, 2004c).
   2. Many employers across the United States are NOT required to test, and many state and local governments have statutes that limit or prohibit workplace testing, unless required by state or federal regulations for certain jobs.
   3. Although not required, many private employers have the right to test for various substances only when drug testing policies and procedures are in accordance with state and federal regulations that may apply to their business or organization (USDL, 2004c, USDL, n.d.3.).
   4. All federal contractors and grantees covered by the Drug-Free Workplace Act of 1988 must provide a drug-free workplace as a precondition of receiving federal agency contracts or grants (USDL, 1998).

E **The Drug Free Workplace Act of 1988 requires that:**
   1. A policy statement specifying the actions that will be taken for those who violate the policy be developed and provided to all covered workers
   2. A drug-free awareness program be established to raise worker awareness of:
      a. The dangers of drug abuse in the workplace
      b. The policy of maintaining a drug-free workplace
      c. Any available drug counseling, rehabilitation, and Employee Assistance Programs (EAP)
      d. The penalties that may be imposed upon employees for drug-abuse violations
   3. Workers be notified under the jurisdiction of federal contract or grant employment that they must:
      a. Abide by the terms of the policy statement
      b. Notify the employer, within five calendar days, if they are convicted of a criminal drug violation in the workplace
   4. The contracting agency be notified within 10 days after receiving notice that a covered employee has been convicted of a criminal drug violation in the workplace
   5. Penalties or satisfactory participation in a drug-abuse assistance or rehabilitation program be imposed on any worker who is convicted of a reportable workplace drug conviction
   6. A good faith effort be made to maintain a drug-free workplace by meeting the requirements of the Act

F **The U. S. Department of Labor (1998) recommends that drug-free workplace programs:**
   1. Balance the rights of workers and the rights of employers
   2. Balance the need to know and rights to privacy
   3. Balance detection and rehabilitation
   4. Balance the respect for workers and the safety of all

G **Key elements of an effective Drug-Free Workplace program are:**
   1. A written policy, including expectations and prohibitions related to drug and alcohol abuse and the consequences of violating the policy

2. Drug and alcohol abuse prevention training for a total of not less than 2 hours for each worker, and additional voluntary drug and alcohol abuse prevention training for workers who are parents
3. Illegal drug testing of workers, with analysis conducted by a drug testing laboratory certified by the Substance Abuse and Mental Health Services Administration (SAMHSA) or approved by the College of American Pathologists for forensic drug testing, and a review of each positive test result by a medical review officer
4. Worker access to an employee assistance program (EAP), including confidential assessment, referral, and short-term problem resolution
5. Continuing alcohol and drug abuse prevention education

XXX Purposes of a Drug and Alcohol Testing Program

A **The purposes of drug and alcohol testing programs are to:**
1. Avoid hiring workers who use illegal drugs
2. Deter workers from abusing drugs and alcohol
3. Identify and refer to treatment those workers who are presently abusing drugs or alcohol

B **Prior to the development and implementation of alcohol and drug screenings, employers should:**
1. Seek thorough legal, medical, and human resources advice (McAndrew, 2002)
2. Bargain with unions before changing work rules and policies
3. During program implementation, protect workers' constitutional rights and prevent unreasonable search and seizure

C **It is important to understand core terms related to drug and alcohol abuse.**
1. A *drug* is any chemical substance that produces physical, mental, emotional, or behavioral changes in the user.
2. *Drug and alcohol abuse* is the use of any drug or alcohol in a medically, socially, or legally unacceptable manner.
3. *Substance abuse* occurs whenever an illegal drug is used, when a prescribed drug is misused, when drugs or alcohol are consumed to the point of physical or mental impairment, or when alcohol is used in an amount or at a time prohibited by an employer's policy.

XXXI Program Components

A **A company policy for a drug-testing program should adhere to applicable state and federal regulations and include the following components:**
1. An explanation regarding why the program is being implemented
2. A description of substance abuse–related behaviors that are prohibited
3. A thorough explanation of the consequences for violations of the policy

B **When developing drug-free policies, employers should:**
1. Involve legal counsel and unions (if applicable) in policy development
2. Include ongoing worker input into policy development
3. Give workers 30 to 60 days' notice before the testing program starts

C **There are several recordkeeping recommendations for drug and alcohol programs.**

1. Records that each worker has been notified of the company policy regarding drug testing should be maintained.
2. Workers should sign a receipt that they received a copy of the policy.
3. Information and training should be provided to workers well before the program begins.
4. Face-to-face training that includes an opportunity for employees to ask questions should be provided.

D **Several administrative issues must be considered when a drug and alcohol program is being developed.**
1. Employers should keep detailed records of their drug and alcohol abuse prevention programs; these will become necessary if and when the program is inspected or audited by federal agencies.
2. Workers' alcohol testing records are confidential; without a signed release they may be released only to the employer and substance abuse professional (and to the DOT, if applicable).
3. Comparison analysis of the costs of drug testing with the costs of accidents, injuries, industrial injury time loss, workers' compensation claims, and productivity before and after initiation of a drug testing program can provide helpful information.

XXXII Methods and Procedures of a Drug and Alcohol Testing Program

A **A successful testing program must contract with reliable, professional laboratories.**
1. Laboratory *certification (and monitoring)* by the Substance Abuse and Mental Health Services Administration (SAMHSA) is required for federally mandated testing. (SAMHSA was formerly the National Institute of Drug Abuse.)
2. The *testing methodology* required by the DOT is a two-stage process, starting with an initial screening test, which, if positive for one or more drugs, is followed by a confirmation test.
   a. The very sensitive initial screening test (immunoassay) looks for the presence or absence of drugs.
   b. The confirmation test is performed for each identified drug with state-of-the-art gas chromatography/mass spectrometry analysis.
3. The *testing program must establish testing protocols*, such as the specific drugs to be tested and the cutoff levels.
   a. The most common drugs tested for (and required by federal testing) are marijuana, cocaine, amphetamines, opiates (including heroin), and phencyclidine.
   b. Other drugs also abused but less commonly tested include barbiturates (including sedatives and tranquilizers), hallucinogens, inhalants, and "designer drugs."
   c. Cutoff (laboratory reporting) levels are established by SAMHSA.

B **The chain-of-custody procedures ensure that the specimen's security, proper identification, and integrity are not compromised.**
1. The procedures track the handling and storage from initial collection to final disposition.
2. A positive test result must be linked back to the individual whose name appears on the specimen bottle label.

3. All personnel who handle the specimen are documented; no unauthorized access to the specimen is possible, and no adulteration or tampering takes place.

C **The Omnibus Transportation Employee Testing Act of 1991 requires that drug testing procedures for most transportation workers include split-specimen procedures.**

1. Each urine specimen is subdivided into two bottles, labeled as *primary* and *split* specimens; both bottles are sent to the laboratory.
2. Only the primary specimen is opened and used for the urinalysis; the split-specimen bottle remains sealed and is stored in the laboratory.
3. If the analysis of the primary specimen confirms the presence of illegal, controlled substances, the worker has 72 hours to request that the split specimen be sent to another SAMHSA-certified laboratory for analysis.

D **To protect worker and employer, a medical review officer (MRO) reviews and interprets all drug test results before they are reported to the employer.**

1. Federal regulations require the MRO to contact the worker in person or by telephone and conduct an interview to determine if there is an alternative medical explanation for the drugs found in the worker's urine specimen.
2. If the worker provides appropriate documentation and the MRO determines that it is legitimate medical use of the prohibited drug, the drug test result is reported to the employer as negative.

E **As a quality assurance measure for the testing laboratory, employers are required by federal regulations to perform blind sample testing. Types of tests include:**

1. *Preemployment,* or *applicant, testing* is conducted to prevent hiring workers with drug or alcohol problems; it is the most popular type of drug testing because it avoids union problems and potential future problems associated with substance-abusing workers.
2. *Post-accident testing* is used to determine if drug or alcohol abuse was a contributing factor in the accident, identify drug and alcohol abusers, and deter drug and alcohol abuse.
3. *Reasonable suspicion testing* is conducted when an employer suspects that a worker is using alcohol or drugs in violation of the company's policy, based on "specific, contemporaneous, and articulable observations concerning the appearance, behavior, speech, or body odor" of the worker (U.S. Department of Transportation, 1994b).
4. *Random testing* is conducted without suspicion that any particular worker is using drugs, and it identifies workers who are abusing drugs or alcohol but have been able to use the predictable testing schedule to escape detection.
   a. Candidates for random testing should be selected using a simple random sampling method so that all workers eligible for testing are equally likely to be tested.
   b. An excellent deterrent and early intervention tool, random testing is recommended for workers in safety- or security-sensitive positions and for workers in companies in which alcohol and drug abuse problems are common.
   c. Federal regulations require random drug testing of at least 50% and random alcohol testing of at least 25% of safety-sensitive workers (the random testing rate is determined annually based upon the random positive rate for each industry).

d. Because alcohol is legal, random alcohol testing must be conducted just before, during, or just after a worker's performance of safety-sensitive duties.

5. *Return-to-duty* and *follow-up testing* are conducted when a worker who has tested positive for drugs and been removed from the workplace returns to work or to performing safety-sensitive duties.

   a. federal regulations require that follow-up tests must be unannounced and that a minimum of six tests must be conducted in the first 12 months after a worker returns to duty; follow-up testing and monitoring may continue for up to 5 years.

   b. The frequency of the follow-up tests should depend on the characteristics of the abused drug and the worker's abuse-related behavior.

F **Federal regulations require that breath testing for alcohol be done with evidential breath-testing devices approved by the National Highway Traffic Safety Administration.**

G **Some federal regulations require certain categories of safety-sensitive workers to report *any* medical use of controlled substances.**

H **Federal regulations pertaining to alcohol-related conduct mandate that a worker's performance of safety-sensitive functions is prohibited under the following circumstances:**

1. If an alcohol breath test indicates an alcohol concentration of 0.04 or greater
2. While using alcohol
3. Within 4 hours after using alcohol
4. When worker uses alcohol within 8 hours after an accident or until tested
5. When worker refuses to submit to an alcohol test

XXXIII Employee Assistance Programs

EAPs provide a support system and counseling services for workers and for management. Chapter 14 provides additional information about EAPs.

A **EAPs may consist of formal programs, a listing of available resources, or participation in consortia (groups or associations of employers) that provide testing and other related services.**

B **EAPs must be viewed as a confidential source of help.**

C **Workers must understand that EAPs will not shield them from disciplinary action if behavior continues.**

XXXIV Training and Education

A **Supervisors are responsible for the following activities:**

1. Observe and document unsatisfactory job performance
2. Confront workers about unsatisfactory job performance according to company procedures
3. Recognize and manage drug crisis situations
4. Understand the policy and their role in its implementation
5. Understand the effects of substance abuse
6. Feel comfortable with evaluating work performance and understand performance evaluation procedures

7. Know how to refer to individuals qualified to diagnose and offer assistance for drug and alcohol problems

B **Comprehensive employee education programs and services should:**
   1. Provide information about the dangers and effects of alcohol and drug abuse
   2. Describe the impact of substance abuse on safety, productivity, and the company's bottom line
   3. Describe program components, the EAP, and testing procedures and protocols
   4. Describe the signs and symptoms of drug and alcohol abuse
   5. Describe regulatory requirements and the employer's policy and procedures
   6. Explain how and where workers can get help for drug and alcohol problems

XXXV Consequences of Drug and Alcohol Abuse and Return to Duty

A **The consequences of drug and alcohol misuse must be defined before the worker begins the drug and alcohol testing program.**

B **Workers who abuse drugs or alcohol must be immediately removed from safety-sensitive functions. Return to duty requires the following:**
   1. Evaluation by a substance-abuse professional
   2. Compliance with any treatment recommendations
   3. A return-to-duty drug or alcohol test (with the result of the alcohol test less than 0.02)
   4. The worker to be subject to unannounced follow-up drug or alcohol tests

International travel health and safety program

International travel health knowledge and expertise is critical for the occupational and environmental health nurse who provides travel counseling, administers immunizations, or is responsible for the coordination and administration of the organization's international health and safety program (Butcher, 2004). The travel health and safety program described in this section provides guidelines that can be used by the occupational and environmental health nurse to reduce the risk to the personal health and safety of the traveler.

XXXVI International Business and the International Work Force

A **According to a study by the Society for Human Resource Management (2004), 134 American companies operating globally generated 31% of their revenues outside of the United States; 39% of the respondents believe that their expatriate population will increase in 2004.**
   1. Expatriates, their families, and business travelers are at risk of exposure to infectious disease, foodborne illnesses, injuries, and threats to personal safety and security.
   2. Long-term assignees may suffer from emotional and mental health conditions associated with isolation, culture shock, and family conflict (Rosselot, 2004).

3. As the world economy becomes increasingly global, management will look toward the occupational and environmental health nurse to partner with them in understanding the health and safety risks facing international assignees, their families, and business travelers.

B **International travel health and safety programs are designed to:**
   1. Prepare workers for travel and international assignment
   2. Provide consultation and recommendations
   3. Ensure physical and emotional fitness for travel and work assignment
   4. Prevent illness and injury
   5. Provide appropriate vaccinations
   6. Ensure, to the greatest extent possible, the personal safety of the traveler

XXXVII Roles and Responsibilities Related to International Travel Programs

Employers and occupational and environmental health nurses work together to develop and implement effective travel health and safety programs.

A **Employers are primarily responsible for:**
   1. Developing travel policies and procedures, including emergency evacuation or escape protocols
   2. Allocating sufficient resources for the program
   3. Providing appropriate travel agency services and travelers' assistance program vendors
   4. Providing health and safety information appropriate to the traveler's destination
   5. Requesting security information from destination hotels or other accommodations (dead bolts and view holes on doors, fire safety, 24-hour security, safety-deposit boxes, etc.)
   6. Providing the medications, supplies, vaccinations, and counseling necessary for the traveler's health and safety
   7. Assessing and evaluating available health care services in locations where workers will be living or visiting and identifying resources for health or safety emergencies
   8. Educating workers of the international travel health program prior to implementation and regularly communicate changes or updates as travel health and safety issues develop

B **Occupational and environmental health nurse's primary responsibilities include the following:**
   1. Obtain the traveling worker's health history
      a. Determine past or present significant physical or mental health conditions, injuries, or surgeries
      b. Identify health conditions and risks factors that could compromise travel plans, such as cardiovascular, pulmonary, endocrine, musculoskeletal, neuropsychiatric, or mental health issues
      c. List any scars or permanent identifying marks on the worker's body in case identity of the traveler needs to be confirmed
      d. Review any health problems encountered related to previous travel
      e. List all current medications (prescription and nonprescription)

    f. Review current health, vision, and dental status and provide appropriate interventions or referrals

    g. List all allergies (medications, food, plants, insects, vaccines, etc.)

2. Determine and provide appropriate immunizations
   a. Review worker's immunization status
   b. Determine which vaccines are required or recommended for the traveler's destination
   c. Administer appropriate vaccines or provide resources to obtain those vaccines
   d. Report adverse vaccine reactions to the local health authorities
3. Conduct a physical exam based on health and safety risk, duration of travel or assignment, and destination (Butcher, 2004)
4. Perform laboratory and other diagnostic tests as appropriate; these may include:
   a. Complete blood count, chemistry panel, urinalysis, blood type
   b. Human immunodeficiency virus (HIV) (as required by country)
   c. Tuberculin skin test (PPD—purified protein derivative)
   d. Chest x-ray (as required by country)
   e. Electrocardiogram (ECG) as appropriate for age and risk
   f. Health surveillance screening appropriate for job assignment (e.g., pulmonary function testing, audiogram)
5. Review special health and safety considerations for the traveler, such as pregnancy or recent surgery
6. Provide counseling for occupational, environmental, and psychologic health and safety risks, including recommended country specific counseling.
7. Refer the worker for treatment of travel-related problems and follow up on referral recommendations

C The traveling worker also has responsibilities; these include the following:
1. Maintain a current passport and obtain visa and other necessary documents
2. Ensure that adequate time is available for administration of vaccines before departure, usually 4 to 6 weeks
3. Prepare a travel itinerary with contact information and leave a copy with family and office staff
4. Confirm travel arrangements (tickets, hotel accommodations, car rental, etc.)
5. Review and follow all safety procedures recommended in the travel policy and procedure manual
6. Prepare an emergency contact list
7. Consider obtaining and carrying personal medical record
8. Obtain a sufficient amount of maintenance prescriptions from primary care provider and carry written prescriptions
9. Obtain and wear emergency medical identification to alert emergency personnel of chronic medical conditions, severe allergies, or other health conditions

XXXVIII Health and Safety Education for Travel

A The safety of the traveler is affected by multiple factors in international workplaces. Safety issues should be addressed as follows:
1. Because business travelers usually travel alone, discuss personal safety, such as avoiding drawing attention to oneself as a "business traveler;"advise traveling in casual attire and being alert to surrounding activities.

2. Provide current information on the political and social climate of the traveler's destination, such as risk of terrorism, kidnapping, theft, and crime
3. Encourage the use of travelers' checks or bank cards instead of carrying large sums of currency
4. Discuss methods to reduce risk of theft of important documents and personal property
5. Review the traveler's itinerary
   a. Length of stay at each destination
   b. Type of work to be performed (office versus field work)
   c. Specific hazards associated with the work to be done
   d. Type of accommodations (e.g. housing, utilities, and services available)

B **Business travel frequently results in stress for the traveler.**
1. Business travel differs from tourism; the following factors may add to the stress of business travelers:
   a. Sleep disturbances
   b. Isolation
   c. Cultural differences
   d. Job performance requirements
   e. Tight schedules
   f. Sudden departures
   g. Separation from family and home
   h. Fear of the potential for kidnapping and terrorism
2. If a worker is traveling internationally for a short-term assignment, it may be appropriate to:
   a. Discuss living accommodations and schedules
   b. Help the traveler understand the culture of the destination country and advise on culturally appropriate dress and behaviors
   c. Provide the traveler with resources for health care or emergency situations
   d. Provide information on safe driving in destination country
3. Workers who have long-term international assignments may need assistance dealing with loneliness, job demands, living in hotels, and traveling alone. In order to prepare the worker for this assignment, it may be helpful to:
   a. Offer training and country-specific cultural programs
   b. Provide a copy of the appropriate evacuation procedure and be clear about instructions
   c. Identify resources for health or psychologic concerns for the traveler (e.g., an employee assistance counselor, if available, or insurance for health care)
   d. If the traveler's family will also be living abroad, provide information on housing accommodations, the lifestyle and culture of the destination country, and schooling options for dependents.

C **Health threats can be very different in the international work environment.**
1. In many countries, illnesses such as "traveler's diarrhea" can be caused by food or water contaminated with bacteria, viruses, or parasites; the following high-risk foods should be avoided:
   a. Undercooked meat, poultry, or seafood, which may contain harmful organisms
   b. Raw fruits or vegetables, which may contain harmful bacteria if not thoroughly washed with a chlorine solution

    c. Tap water, including ice made from tap water, which may be unchlorinated and contaminated with fecal material

    d. Unpasteurized dairy products, which may contain organisms such as the salmonella bacteria

2. Prevention of illness may be further enhanced by the following recommendations:

    a. Give hepatitis A vaccine for high endemic areas

    b. Drink bottled water; purify water through boiling for at least 10 minutes, or use water-purification tablets as recommended

    c. Follow the basic principles for safe handling of foods

    d. Follow the basic principles of good hygienic practice

3. Management of traveler's illnesses may include the following:

    a. Oral rehydrating fluids (electrolyte solutions) for diarrhea

    b. Prophylactic antibiotics to prevent certain bacteria-caused illnesses

    c. Good hygienic practices to avoid reinfection (e.g., proper disposal of contaminated items, thorough hand washing)

4. Assemble an appropriate medical emergency kit (Box 16-8)

BOX 16-8

Traveler's medical kit recommendations

- **Essential Items**

  An adequate supply of medications for health conditions specific to the traveler

  Additional prescriptions (with generic name) as determined by physician

  Copies of medical and eyeglasses

  Disposable thermometers (Fever Scan) prescriptions

- **Nonprescription Items**

  Analgesic (aspirin, acetaminophen, ibuprofen)

  Antibiotic skin ointment (Bacitracin, Betadine, Mycitracin)

  Antiseptic (providone iodine)

  Anticonstipation (many brands of laxatives are available)

  Antidiarrheal (lopermide [Immodium AD], bismuth subsalicylate [Pepto Bismol])

  Anti-motion sickness (meclizine [Bonine], dimenhydrinate [Dramamine])

  Antihistamines (diphenhydramine [Benadryl])

  Adhesive bandages (Band-Aids, Curad)

  Antacids (Tums, Rolaids, Maalox)

  Oral rehydrating salts (available at sporting goods stores)

  Water purification tablets

- **Prescription Items**

  Altitude sickness prophylactics (acetazolamide [Diamox])

  Antibiotics (oral doxycycline, ciprofloxacin, or erythromycin)

  Antimalarials (mefloquine, choloquine, or doxycycline)

  Sleeping medications (Halcion, Restoril)

- **Additional Medical Supplies**

  Disposable syringes and needles

  Latex gloves

  Skin closures (Steri-Strips)

  Suture removal kit

XXXIX Control of Prevalent Communicable Diseases

A Although vaccines have significantly controlled many communicable diseases in America and other developed countries, these diseases may still be endemic in developing countries.

1. It is imperative that the occupational and environmental health nurse assess immunization status and, if necessary, administer required and recommended vaccines.

2. Health maintenance recommended immunization information and schedules can be found at the Centers for Disease Control and Prevention's (CDC) National Immunization Program web site: http://www.cdc.gov/nip/default.htm

   a. Recommendations based on age and risk factors include immunization for tetanus and diphtheria; hepatitis A and B; influenza; pneumovac; measles, mumps and rubella (MMR), and polio.

   b. Other country-specific recommended or required vaccinations for travel may include yellow fever, typhoid, cholera, rabies, meningococcal meningitis, and Japanese encephalitis. Refer to the CDC's Yellow Book or Travel Health web site for requirements (http://www.cdc.gov/travel/).

B Malaria is one example of a preventable disease that can affect an international worker.

1. Malaria is a febrile illness caused by four different species of the protozoan parasite Plasmodium: *Plasmodium falciparum, P. vivax, P. ovale* and *P. malariae* (World Health Organization, 2004).

   a. Malaria caused by *P. falciparum* results in severe disease and increased mortality risk.

   b. *Plasmodium* is transmitted via infected saliva following the bite of the female *Anopheles* mosquito.

2. Signs and symptoms of malaria include:

   a. Fever, which is the "most indicative" sign of malaria infection (Butcher, 2004)

   b. Other signs and symptoms, which include chills, headache, nausea, vomiting, myalgia and diarrhea

3. Risk of malaria is directly related to mosquito exposure.

   a. Because malaria is spread by mosquitoes, the risk is greatest in areas where mosquito activity is high.

   b. The highest rate of mosquito activity occurs in Africa, where mosquitoes carry the malaria parasite.

   c. Risk of exposure is highest between dusk and dawn when mosquito activity is the highest.

   d. The risk increases during rainy and hot seasons.

4. Prevention of malaria involves avoiding mosquito exposure.

   a. Stay indoors during increased mosquito activity

   b. If outdoors, wear long-sleeved clothing, long pants and hat

   c. Use repellents containing DEET (acronym for the chemical N, N-diethyl-3-methylbenzamide)

   d. Sleep under mosquito bed netting treated with a permethrin insecticide (USDHHS, 2003)

   e. Sleep in screened or air-conditioned rooms if possible

5. Control is achieved through antimalarial medications.

   a. Antimalarial medications (chemoprophylaxis) include mefloquine, doxycycline, chloroquine, and atovaquone/proguanil (USDHHS, 2003).

   b. There is currently no vaccine against malaria.

6. Delay of appropriate treatment can result in serious illness or death.
   a. Travelers who have not taken prophylactic medications, are in an area resistant to the medications they were treated with, or cannot access urgent medical care, can be given a self-treatment course of atovaquone/proguanil at the onset of flu-like symptoms and/or fever.
   b. If atovaquone/proguanil was given as prophylaxis, another self-treatment medication should be given (USDHHS, 2003).
   c. Self-treatment is only a temporary measure, and prompt health evaluation is imperative.

C **Other country-specific diseases of concern include dengue fever, monkeypox, Lassa fever, plaque, and tuberculosis (Butcher, 2004). Recommendations for prevention and traveler education can be found at the CDC Travel Health web site (http://www.cdc.gov/travel/).**

D **Individuals traveling abroad may be at risk for contracting sexually transmitted diseases (STDs) if they engage in sex while abroad; thus the health care provider must include education specific to STDs.**
   1. Individuals assigned to long-term assignments abroad are more likely to engage in casual sex than are short-term travelers.
   2. Discuss the risk of engaging in casual sex abroad.
   3. Encourage the use of condoms and other safe sex practices.
   4. Warn about the effects of alcohol and drugs, which may contribute to careless sexual behavior.
   5. Discuss cultural attitudes concerning prostitution in the traveler's destination country.

NOTE: Table 16-3 provides information regarding other selected physiologic health hazards.

XL Post-Travel Evaluation for Long-Term Travelers

This type of evaluation is usually not necessary for short-term travelers; however, it should be performed when indicated.

A **Provide immediate evaluation for signs or symptoms of illness.**

B **Post-travel assessment is traveler specific and may include the following:**
   1. History and physical examination, including laboratory and other diagnostic tests such as:
      a. Complete blood count, chemistry panel, and urinalysis
      b. Stool for ova and parasites if returning from high-risk area
      c. Tuberculosis skin test (PPD)
      d. Chest x-ray (as required by country)
      e. Health surveillance screening appropriate for job exposures (e.g., pulmonary function testing, audiogram)
   2. Post-travel debriefing includes:
      a. A discussion of problems encountered during travel/stay
      b. Recommendations for future travelers
      c. Referral to a primary health care provider for routine health maintenance screening as appropriate
      d. Referral for routine vision and dental screening as appropriate

TABLE 16-3

Selected physiologic health hazards

Jet lag: Jet lag is the disruption of the traveler's sleep–wake cycle. It usually occurs when traveling over two or more time zones

Risk factors	Prevention
Insomnia	Adjust sleep schedule
Fatigue	Drink extra fluids (preferably water)
Poor concentration	Reduce coffee and alcohol consumption
Irritability	Exposure to light may help in resetting circadian rhythm
Headache	
Myalgia	

Altitude sickness: Altitude sickness is a cluster of symptoms caused by lack of oxygen. The symptoms may include headache, shortness of breath, lightheadedness, fatigue, insomnia, loss of appetite, and nausea. It can be life threatening.

Risk factors	Prevention	Treatment
Ascent over 6000 feet	High carbohydrate diet	Descent and rest
Rapid ascent without acclimation	Extra fluid intake	Aspirin or acetaminophen
Obesity	Reduce strenuous activity	
Strenuous activity at high altitudes	Slow, gradual descent	Diamox
Use of sleeping pills or sedatives	Acetazolamide (250 mg every 8 hours for 3-5 days before ascent)	
Previous history of altitude sickness		

C Obtain worker's feedback to assist in the evaluation of the international health and safety program.

1. Use this information to analyze the program's effectiveness and efficiency
   a. Analyze the cost/benefit ratio of the program's elements
   b. Evaluate the *overall* effectiveness and cost of program
2. Make revisions as appropriate based on this information

REFERENCES

American Association of Occupational Health Nurses. (n.d.). *Ergoresources* Retrieved November 14, 2004, from http://www.ergoresources.org/

American Association of Occupational Health Nurses. (1996R, reviewed 6/03 and 8/04). *Position statement: occupational health surveillance.* Retrieved November 14, 2004, from http://www.aaohn.org/practice/positions/upload/position_surveillance-2.PDF.

Butcher, C. A. (2004). International health program: preventing health problems associated with living abroad. *AAOHN Journal, 52*(2), 77-85.

Centers for Disease Control and Prevention. (2003). *Health information for international travel 2003-2004.* Retrieved October 2004, from http://www.cdc.gov/travel/

Donabedian, A. (1966). Evaluating the quality of medical care. *Milbank Fund Quarterly, 44*(3), 166-206.

Forde, M. S., Punnett, L., & Wegman, D. H. (2002). Pathomechanisms of work-related musculoskeletal disorders: conceptual issues. *Ergonomics, 45*(9), 619-630.

Galszechy, T. (1999). The effects of vibration on hands and arms: Clinical brief. *AAOHN Journal, 47*(3), 117-119.

Institute of Medicine (IOM). (2001). *Musculoskeletal disorders and the workplace: low back and upper extremities.* National Academies of Sciences (NAS), National Academies Press. Washington DC Retrieved November 14, 2004, from http://www.nap.edu/books/0309072840/html/

Lipscomb, D. M. (2003). The impact of NIHL upon quality of life. Council for Accreditation in Hearing Conservation Newsletter *Update, 15*(2), 7, 10.

McAndrew, K. G. (2002). Drug and alcohol screening in the workplace. Advisory. *AAOHN Journal, 50*(1), 8.

National Academies of Sciences (NAS), Commission on Behavioral and Social Sciences and Education. (1999). *Work-related musculoskeletal disorders: report, workshop, summary and workshop papers.* National Academies Press. Retrieved November 14, 2004, from http://books.nap.edu/catalog/ 6431.html.

National Institute for Occupational Safety and Health (NIOSH). (1995). *Cumulative trauma disorders in the workplace: Bibliography.* Retrieved November 14, 2004, from http:// www.cdc.gov/niosh/pdfs/95-119.pdf.

National Institute for Occupational Safety and Health (NIOSH). (1997a). *Musculoskeletal disorders and workplace factors: a critical review of epidemiologic evidence for work-related musculoskeletal disorder of the neck, upper extremity, and low back.* Retrieved November 14, 2004, from http:// www.cdc.gov/niosh/ ergoscil. html.

Rosselot, G. (2004). Travel health nursing: Expanding horizons for occupational health nurses. *AAOHN Journal, 52*(1), 28-41.

Royster, J. D., & Royster, L. H. (1990). *Hearing conservation programs: Practical guidelines for success.* Chelsea, MI: Lewis Publishers.

Substance Abuse and Mental Health Services Administration (SAMHSA). (n.d.). *Worker drug use and worksite policies and programs: Results from the '94 & '97 National Household Survey on Drug Abuse.* Retrieved November 17, 2004, from http:// www.oas.samhsa.gov/ NHSDA/A-11/toc.htm-TopOfPage

Substance Abuse and Mental Health Services Administration (SAMSHSA). (1999*). Fact Sheet: Workplace substance abuse related violence and security issues.* Retrieved February 25, 2005, from www.workplace.samhsa.gov/ SubstanceAbuse/ WPViolence/Violence InWP.pdf

Suter, A. H. (2003*). Hearing conservation manual* (4th ed.). Milwaukee, WI: Council for Accreditation in Occupational Hearing Conservation.

U.S. Department of Labor. (n.d.1). *OSHA Protocol for developing industry and task specific ergonomic guidelines.* Retrieved November 14, 2004, from: http://www.osha.gov/ SLTC/ ergonomics/guidelines_protocol.html

U.S. Department of Labor. (n.d.2). *Drug Free Workplace Advisor.* Retrieved November 17, 2004, from http://www.dol.gov/asp/programs/drugs/workingpartners/ dfwpadvisor.asp

U.S. Department of Labor. (n.d.3). *Working partners for an alcohol and drug free workplace.* Retrieved November 17, 2004, from http://www.dol.gov/dol/ workingpartners.htm

U S. Department of Labor. (1998). *Working partners advisor.* Retrieved November 11, 2004, from www.dol.gov/ asp/programs/drugs/workingpartners/dfwadvisor.asp

U.S. Department of Labor. (2004b). Survey: 2003 National Survey on drug use and health (NSDUH) reveals the vast majority of drug and alcohol abusers work. *Drug Programs. What's New?* Retrieved November 11, 2004, from http:// www.dol.gov/asp/programs/drugs/said/WhatsNewa9ae.html?ID=1667

U.S. Department of Labor. (2004c). *Frequently Asked Questions. Drug Testing.* Retrieved February 26, 2005, from http://www.dol.gov/elaws/asp/drugfree/drugs/ screen92.asp

U.S. Department of Labor. Occupational Safety and Health Administration. (2004c). *Guidelines for retail grocery stores–ergonomics for the prevention of musculoskeletal disorders* (OSHA Publication 3192). Retrieved November 14, 2004, from http://www.osha.gov/ ergonomics/guidelines/retailgrocery/retailgrocery.html.

U.S. Department of Transportation. (1994b, February). Alcohol and drug rules. 49 CFR 382 et. al., 49 CFR Part 40, *Federal Register*.

Washington State Department of Labor and Industries, Industrial Safety and Health Division. (1993). *Understanding "Right to Know."* P413-000 (3/93). Olympia, WA: Washington State Department of Labor and Industries, Industrial Safety and Health Division.

World Health Organization. (2004). *International travel and health*. Retrieved October 2004, from http:// www.who. int/ith/

Zalk, D. M. (2000). Grassroots ergonomics: initiating an ergonomics program utilizing participatory techniques. *Annals of Occupational Hygiene, 45*(4), 283-289.

OTHER RESOURCES

California Department of Industrial Relations. (2003). *Ergonomics in action: a guide to best practices for the food processing industry*. Retrieved November 14, 2004, from http://www.dir.ca.gov/ dosh/dosh_publications/ Erg_Food_ Processing.pdf

California Department of Industrial Relations. (1999). *Easy ergonomics*. Retrieved November 14, 2004, from http://www.dir.ca.gov/dosh/dosh_pu blications/ EasErg2.pdf.

GMAC Global Relocation Services, National Foreign Trade Council, Society for Human Resource Management Global Forum. (2004) *Global relocation trends: 2003/2004 survey report*. Retrieved October 2004 from http://www. nftc.org/default/ hr/GRTS 2003-4.pdf.

National Institute for Occupational Safety and Health (NIOSH). (2004). *Noise and hearing loss prevention: porkplace solutions*. Retrieved September 21, 2004, from http:// www.cdc.gov/niosh/ topics/ noise/workplacesolutions/ hearingch.

National Institute for Occupational Safety and Health (NIOSH). (1997b). *Elements of ergonomics programs: a primer based on workplace evaluations of musculoskeletal disorders*. Retrieved November 14, 2004, from http://www.cdc.gov/niosh/ ephome2.html.

National Institute for Occupational Safety and Health (NIOSH). (1997c). *Worker protection: Private sector ergonomics programs yield positive results* (Letter Report, 08/27/97, GAO/HEHS-97-163 [Online]). Retrieved November 14, 2004, from http://www.cdc.gov/niosh/ gaergo.html.

Ostendorf, J. S., Rogers, B., & Bertsche, P. K. (2000). Ergonomics: CTD management evaluation tool. *AAOHN Journal 48*(1), 17-24.

Rogers, B. (2003). *Occupational and environmental health nursing: concepts and practice* (2nd ed). Philadelphia: Saunders.

Rose, S. (Ed.). (2001). *International travel health guide* (12th ed.). Hampton, MA: Travel Medicine Inc. Retrieved October 15, 2004, from https://www. travmed. com/index. html.

U.S. Department of Labor. (1991). *Ergonomics program management guidelines for meatpacking plants*. Retrieved November 14, 2004, from http://www.osha-slc.gov/ Publications/osha3123. pdf.

U.S. Department of Labor. (2004a). *OSH Act, section5, 1970, amended January 1, 2004*. Retrieved November 14, 2004, from http://www.osha.gov/pls/osha web/owadisp.show_document?p_table =OSHACT&p_id=2743.

U.S. Department of Labor (2004d). Can I drug test? *Frequently Asked Questions, Workplace Health and Safety, Drug-Free Workplac*e Retrieved November 11, 2004, from www.dol.gov/dolfaq/go-dol faqafc1.html?faqid=405&faqsub=Drug %2DFree+Workplace&faqtop=Workpla ce+Safety+%26+Health&topicid=2

U.S. Department of Labor, Occupational and Safety Health Administration (2003). *Draft model training program for hazard communication*. Retrieved October 11, 2004, from http:// www. osha. gov/dsg/hazcom/MTP101703. html

U.S. Department of Labor. Occupational Safety and Health Administration (2004a). *Guidelines for Poultry Processing: Ergonomics for the Prevention of Musculoskeletal Disorders* (OSHA 3213-09N). Retrieved November 14, 2004, from http:// www.osha.gov/ ergonoics/guidelines/poultryprocess-ing/ poultryprocessing.html.

U.S. Department of Labor. Occupational Safety and Health Administration (2004b). *Guidelines for Nursing Homes: Ergonomics for the Prevention of Musculoskeletal Disorder*. Retrieved November 14, 2004, from http://www. osha.gov/ ergonomics/guidelines/ nursinghome/index.html.

U.S. Department of Labor, Occupational and Safety Health Administration

(2005). *Health and Safety Topics: Workplace Substance Abuse*. Retrieved, February 22, 2005, from http:/ /www.osha.gov/SLTC/substanceabuse/

Wassell, J. T., Gardner, L. I., Landsittel, D. P., Johnston, J. J., Johnston, J. M., (2000). A prospective study of back belts for prevention of back pain and injury. *Journal of the American Medical Association*, 284 (21), 2727-2732.

SECTION THREE

Advancing Professionalism in Occupational and Environmental Health Nursing

∼

CHAPTER

17

Research

BONNIE ROGERS

Through research, occupational and environmental health nurses can improve the health and safety of the workplace, and, ultimately, the quality of workers' lives. Research is essential to support and expand the knowledge base for occupational and environmental health nursing practice. This chapter focuses on basic elements in the research process, research priorities, funding sources, evaluation criteria, communication of research findings, and the use of research findings, which are critical to advancing this specialty practice.

I Professional Mandates for Research

A According to the AAOHN's Standards of Occupational and Environmental Health Nursing (Standard X, Research): The occupational and environmental health nurse uses research findings in practice and contributes to the scientific base in occupational and environmental health nursing to improve practice and advance the profession (AAOHN, 2004).

1. AAOHN supports occupational and environmental health nursing research by encouraging participation and providing resources (through the AAOHN Foundation) to conduct research, and by publishing research in the *AAOHN Journal*.

2. The occupational and environmental health nurse engages in research through activities such as identifying researchable problems; designing and conducting research; disseminating research findings; writing research grant proposals; and collaborating with other disciplines on research studies.

B The American Nurses Association (ANA) Standards of Clinical Nursing Practice (Standard VII, Research) says, "The nurse uses research findings in practice" (ANA, 1998).

1. The nurse uses research data to develop the plan of care and interventions.

2. The nurse participates in research activities as appropriate to the individual's education and position.

II Research Roles of Occupational and Environmental Health Nurses by Education Level

A Associate Degree/Diploma: The occupational and environmental health nurse identifies clinical problems for research, such as identifying that there is a cluster of workers with similar health complaints coming to the occupational health unit from a certain department, assists in the development of the research and data collection activities, and uses research as a basis for clinical practice.

B Baccalaureate Degree: The occupational and environmental health nurse evaluates research for applicability to practice; works with skilled researchers to develop research projects; uses research to refine and extend the practice, for example, using a specific intervention such as a support group for diet control that has been reported in the research literature; and discusses research findings with colleagues.

C Master's Degree: The occupational and environmental health nurse provides expertise related to the research problem, care delivery, and the research process; analyzes the practice problems within the context of the scientific process; collaborates with other disciplines in scientific investigations such as by helping to design the research study; supports the conduct of research; disseminates research findings; encourages the integration of research into practice; and contributes to an environment supportive of nursing research.

D Doctoral Degree: The occupational and environmental health nurse develops and conducts independent and collaborative investigations with other scientists; develops methodologies such as survey tools or research protocols for scientific inquiry into phenomena relevant to the practice of occupational and environmental health and safety; uses analytical methods and integrates findings to explain and extend scientific knowledge to nursing practice; develops and tests interventions to improve worker health and safety; acquires research grant support; disseminates findings; and provides leadership for integrating research findings into practices.

III Purposes of Research

Purposes of research in occupational and environmental health are to (Polit & Hungler, 2004; Rogers 2003):

A Help identify and solve problems relevant to nursing practice.

B Improve the effectiveness of nursing care through scientific inquiry using a systematic process.

C Advance the body of knowledge in the occupational and environmental health nursing discipline.

IV Ethics in Research

A To protect all study participants' rights, the investigator must provide participants with the following:
  1. Description of study purpose
  2. Discussion of risks and benefits; informal consent
  3. Assurance of confidentiality (and of anonymity, where appropriate)
  4. Specification of a contact person

B *Consent* to participate in the research must be obtained from each study participant.
  1. Consent usually covers an explanation of the study, procedures used, risks, invasion of privacy, and methods used to protect the identity of the participants (i.e., anonymity or confidentiality).

a. *Anonymity:* Protection of participants in a study such that even the researcher cannot link the participants with the information collected.

b. *Confidentiality:* Protection of participants in a study such that their identities will not be linked to the information they provide and that individually identifiable information collected will not be divulged.

c. *Risks and benefits:* A description of any risk involved related to the research such as potential harm from a needlestick during blood collection or invasion of privacy.

2. Consent is usually obtained with a written statement from participants, or it may be described by the researcher in a cover letter notifying participants to voluntarily return survey forms; in these cases, return of the survey implies consent.

3. Special circumstances may be related to informed consent, such as literacy or non–English-speaking workers. The researcher must ensure that study participants have a full understanding of research procedures, which may include reading the consent statements or interpreting information for the participant.

C Research is usually approved by an ethics committee commonly referred to as an institutional review board (IRB). This committee oversees the ethical treatment of study participants and assesses the study's impact on them. It is the IRB's responsibility to:

1. Evaluate and determine if any research-related risks are reasonable in relation to anticipated benefits of the research.

2. Determine if adequate procedures and safeguards are in place to ensure privacy and confidentiality, including informed consent procedures, particularly for vulnerable populations.

3. Approve or disapprove the research or ask that modifications be made.

V   Research Development

This section outlines the scientific process for the conduct of research and the logical steps needed to develop a research proposal. Box 17-1 lists the steps in the research process.

BOX 17-1

Steps in the research process

- Formulate the problem
- Review the literature
- Develop a theoretical framework
- Formulate hypothesis/question(s)
- Identify research variables
- Operationalize variables
- Select research design
- Specify population
- Conduct pilot studies
- Select sample
- Collect data
- Organize data for analysis
- Analyze data
- Interpret results
- Communicate findings

NOTE: There may be some variation in the conduct of pilot studies.

A **Identification of the problem**
1. The problem that is identified should consist of a situation that needs a solution and that will contribute to improving practice.
2. The problem is relevant to contemporary nursing practice and is stated clearly and precisely.
3. Research of the problem will contribute to the body of nursing knowledge.
4. Research of the problem will explain, describe, and predict behaviors, and will test strategies or interventions to modify or improve outcomes.

B **Significance of the study**
1. The research problem needs to address the "so what?" question.
2. The importance of the problem should be explained by describing its critical characteristics, pointing out gaps in the literature, and presenting possible solutions.

C **Literature review**
1. The literature is discussed to help the researcher critically evaluate existing research and provide a context or frame of reference for the study.
2. Literature sources may include previous studies relevant to clinical or substantive articles, conceptual or theoretical understanding, and methodologic readings.
3. Material for review and inclusion should be current but also capture long-standing issues and classical articles.
4. When conducting a literature search, the researcher can use several resources, such as print indexes and electronic databases (Box 17-2), or consult with a reference librarian. In any search, key words, text words, or subject headings can be used to identify articles that may be valuable.
5. When critiquing a research study, the following should be considered:
   a. Clarity, logic, and understandability of the study
   b. Currency of the study and its applicability to practice
   c. Strength of the questions and hypotheses and that they are addressed in the analysis
   d. Theoretical framework, if used
   e. Appropriate design, sample, and interpretation of findings
   f. Protection of participants' rights
   g. Limitations
6. Literature should be analyzed and synthesized.

BOX 17-2

Common electronic databases used in occupational and environmental health

- **CINAHL:** Cumulative index to nursing and allied health literature
- **MEDLINE:** Medical literature on-line
- **TOXNET:** Toxicology database
- **EMBASE:** Exerpta Medica

- **NIOSH TIC:** NIOSH database
- **TOXLINE:** Toxicology
- **HSDB:** Hazardous substance database
- **RTECS:** Registry of toxic effects of chemical substances

NOTE: Search home pages of federal and state agencies (e.g., OSHA, EPA, NIOSH) for links to other sources of databases.

D Problem statement/formulation
1. The problem statement introduces the topic, explains the importance of the problem, and states what the research intends to study.
2. The problem statements may be grounded within a theoretical framework (links and explains the relationships among different theories) or conceptual framework (building blocks of theories). However, not all research studies may be sufficiently developed to have these frameworks (e.g., descriptive studies).
3. There are three types of questions (Brink & Wood, 1988):
   a. Type I research question: Expression of a single concept with the stem beginning with "what." Little or no knowledge about the topic exists. Example: What are occupational and environmental health nurses' attitudes about providing health promotion activities at work?
   b. Type II research question: Examines relationships between two or more concepts or variables. Example: What is the relationship between stress and injury?
   c. Type III research question: Builds on type I and II questions and examines a causal relationship using an experimental design. Asks why. Example: Why does an increase in stress result in increased musculoskeletal disorders?

E Formulation of hypothesis, if appropriate
1. Hypotheses require a theoretic basis and are used to test an idea.
2. A hypothesis suggests a relationship among two or more variables and is used when the researchers can predict an outcome. Example: Stress reduction programs are likely to reduce musculoskeletal disorders.

F Definition of terms
1. *Conceptual definitions* explain interrelationships among concepts (e.g., self-esteem and eating disorders).
2. *Operational definitions* guide the implementation of the study (e.g., an occupational and environmental health nurse can be defined as a registered nurse who provides for and delivers health and safety services to employees, employee populations, and community groups).

G Methodology
1. Designs: Many types of designs can be used to answer research questions. Designs fall into two major categories (Polit & Hungler, 2004).
   a. *Experimental designs* are used to test research hypotheses and infer causal relationships.
      1) A true experiment requires random assignment of participants, a control group, and manipulation of a treatment or intervention (independent variable) for the experimental group. Example: Randomly assign participants to two groups; administer treatment to one group; and measure the outcome or effect in both groups.
      2) *Quasi-experimental designs* include manipulation of the treatment or intervention; however, this design lacks either a control group or random assignment of participants.
      3) *Preexperimental designs* manipulate the variable or treatment in only one group (i.e., no comparison group or randomization), and measure the effect.
   b. *Nonexperimental designs* are used when the research does not support an experiment (e.g., survey). Two broad categories are included:

1) *Descriptive studies* are designed to observe and describe the phenomenon under investigation and are not concerned with relational variables.
2) *Ex post facto* (sometimes called *correlational*) research examines relationships between variables (that have already occurred) and *implies* a correlation (e.g., smoking and lung cancer).

2. Variables
   a. Dependent variable: This is the study variable under investigation (i.e., the outcome variable).
   b. Independent variable: This is the variable that is presumed to have an effect or influence on the dependent variable. In an experimental design, it is the treatment or intervention.
   c. Example: Is absenteeism higher among workers who work straight or rotating shifts?
      1) Dependent variable: absenteeism
      2) Independent variable: shift work

3. Research instruments/measurements
   a. Instrumentation
      1) Existing instruments or tools are often available for the researcher to use. The researcher should search the literature carefully for available instruments that can be used or modified to answer the research questions.
      2) If no instruments or tools are available, the researcher may need to develop and pilot test a new tool.
   b. Reliability and validity of the instrument
      1) The *reliability* of an instrument is its degree of consistency in measuring responses of the attribute under study. Types of reliability measurements include the following:
         a) *Stability,* which refers to the extent to which the same results are obtained on repeated administrations of the instrument (also referred to as *test-retest*).
         b) *Internal consistency,* wherein all of items included measure a certain attribute, not some other tangential attribute.
         c) *Equivalence,* wherein the instrument produces the same (or equivalent) results when administered by two different observers or raters.
      2) *Validity* refers to the degree to which an instrument measures what it is supposed to measure. Examples include the following:
         a) Content validity, which is concerned with the sampling adequacy of the content area being measured.
         b) Criterion-related validity, which focuses on the relationship or correlations between the instrument and some outside criterion (e.g., an instrument to measure self-performance would be validated by manager ratings).

4. Population and sample
   a. The target population includes all persons who fit the characteristics the researcher wants to study and to whom the results can be generalized. Not all members of a population can be included in a study, so a sample may be used.
   b. The sample size needs to be adequate within the context of the design and problem under investigation.

1) Use the largest sample possible to provide for more representation of the population under study as smaller samples are less accurate estimates of the population. However, if there is reason to believe the population may be relatively homogeneous, a smaller sample may be adequate.

2) Effect size is important to consider. This is a statistical expression of the relation between two variables or the magnitude of difference between groups. If there is reason to believe the relationship between two variables is weak, a larger sample will be needed.

3) The sample size must be large enough to satisfy the statistical tests being used.

c. Depending on participant availability, time, and resources, different types of samples may be used.

1) Probability sampling: All elements or subjects have an equal chance of being included. Types of samples include random, stratified random, systematic random, and clusters.

2) Nonprobability sampling: Participant selection is not based on chance (e.g., the participants are volunteers). Types of samples include convenience, quota, purposive, and snowball.

3) Probability sampling is more representative of the population; the results of studies that rely on probability sampling are less subject to bias and can be generalized more easily.

5. Data collection: This is the phase of the study wherein the researcher gathers the data specific to the purpose and questions. Several methods can be used depending on what types of data are needed.

a. *Interview:* A generally structured approach with specific or open-ended questions that can be asked face to face or via the telephone

b. *Questionnaire:* A written response to survey items, using a structured format *that typically uses a scale* (e.g., strongly agree to strongly disagree or a yes/no response) or open-ended questions

c. *Observation:* Systematic observation of participants and recording of data for later analysis

d. *Physiologic:* Methods for measuring biophysiologic data, such as blood and urine samples, electrocardiograms, etc.

e. *Record review:* Gathering data from charts related to specific indices or criteria under investigation

f. *Focus group:* A group interview with participants assembled to answer questions on a given topic

6. *Data analysis:* During this phase, the researcher examines the data using statistical approaches, analyzes relationships between the data and the research questions, and forms conclusions and recommendations.

a. *Quantitative data* provide descriptive statistics and comparative analysis about phenomena measured at the nominal, ordinal, interval, or ratio levels. The higher the level of measurement, the more powerful the results.

1) *Nominal level* measurement (lowest level) is simply the assignment of numbers to classify data into mutually exclusive categories (e.g., 1 = male, 2 = female).

2) *Ordinal level* measurement involves the sorting of elements on the basis of their relative standing to each other, yielding a ranking (e.g., 1 = completely independent to 5 = completely dependent).

    3) *Interval level* measurement yields equivalent distance between numerical values on scales (e.g., temperature scale).

    4) *Ratio level* measurement (highest level) permits numerical calculations or operations and has an absolute zero.

  b. *Qualitative data* provide descriptions about phenomena and help generate hypotheses.

  c. *Descriptive analysis* discusses what was found in the study. Common descriptions include the following:

    1) Frequency distributions (i.e., counts of the number of times a value was obtained) presented in tables or graphs that report the overall summary of group characteristics

    2) Summary of a group's characteristics when describing ages, educational levels, etc. (i.e., mean [average], range [highest score minus the lowest score in a given distribution]), and the standard deviation degree to which scores deviate from each other])

  d. *Inferential analysis* begins to specify relationships between variables.

7. Interpretation of findings

  a. Clearly state the answers to research questions, which hypotheses were supported or not supported, and formulate conclusions and recommendations.

  b. Discuss findings within the context of the practice discipline and suggest future research.

  c. State to whom the findings are generalized, paying attention to how the sample was selected.

NOTE: For purposes of developing research proposals, the researcher should explain the data analysis plans in detail, based on the scientific design of the study.

VI Research Dissemination

A **It is essential to disseminate research findings to build knowledge, improve practice, and share results with colleagues (Overman, 2002).**

B **Most original research is published in peer-reviewed journals, such as the *AAOHN Journal*.**

  1. Articles generally provide an abstract, background information, methodology, findings, and discussion sections.

  2. Although providing scientific information is critical, research reports should also be reader friendly and applied to practice.

C **Research is also disseminated through presentations at scientific meetings and may be discussed in work settings where the research work was conducted.**

VII Research Utilization

A **Practice application: Implementation of research into nursing practice is guided by its significance, the degree to which results can be generalized to populations, and the feasibility of implementation, including an analysis of cost-benefit issues.**

B **Evaluation: Several factors should be considered before implementing findings into practice, including critical review of the literature, sample**

representativeness, adequate study design, ethicality, reliability and validity of measurements, consistency with other studies, and cost-effectiveness.

VIII Research Priorities

A Based on guidance from the membership about important research topics to advance the profession and improve the practice, updated occupational and environmental health nursing research priorities have been published (Box 17-3) (Rogers et al., 2000).

B The National Institute for Occupational Safety and Health has published National Occupational Research Priorities, grouped into three categories (NIOSH, 1996). Note: These may be soon updated.

1. Disease and injury
   a. Allergic and irritant dermatitis
   b. Asthma and chronic obstructive pulmonary disease
   c. Fertility and pregnancy abnormalities
   d. Hearing loss
   e. Infectious diseases
   f. Low-back disorders
   g. Musculoskeletal disorders of the upper extremities
   h. Traumatic injuries
2. Work environment and work force
   a. Emerging technologies
   b. Indoor environment
   c. Mixed exposures
   d. Organization of work
   e. Special populations at risk

BOX 17-3

Research priorities in occupational and environmental health nursing

1. Effectiveness of primary health care delivery at the work site
2. Effectiveness of health promotion nursing intervention strategies
3. Methods for handling complex ethical issues related to occupational and environmental health
4. Strategies that minimize work-related health outcomes (e.g., respiratory disease)
5. Health effects resulting from chemical exposures in the workplace
6. Occupational hazards of health care workers (e.g., latex allergy, blood-borne pathogens)
7. Factors that influence workers' rehabilitation and return to work
8. Effectiveness of ergonomic strategies to reduce worker injury and illness
9. Effectiveness of case-management approaches in occupational illness and injury
10. Evaluation of critical pathways to effectively improve worker health and safety and enhance maximum recovery and safe return to work
11. Effects of shift work on worker health and safety
12. Strategies for increasing compliance with or motivating workers to use personal protective equipment.

---

3. Research tools and approaches
   a. Cancer research methods
   b. Control technology and personal protective equipment
   c. Exposure assessment methods
   d. Health services research
   e. Intervention effectiveness research
   f. Risk assessment methods
   g. Social and economic consequences of workplace illness and injury
   h. Surveillance research methods

IX Evaluating Research

The following elements should be considered when critically evaluating research reports (Giuffree, 1998; Rogers, 1995; Rogers, 2003).

A **Title: Indicates clearly to the reader the intent and topic of the investigation.**

B **Abstract**
   1. Provides a clear but concise statement of purpose
   2. Summarizes the data analysis
   3. Describes important findings

C **Problem statement and purpose**
   1. Provides an introduction to the study topic, including the importance and need for the study.
   2. Identifies variables, basic design, population studied, and data collection methods.

D **Theoretic foundation**
   1. The selected framework is relevant to the research and is understandable.
   2. There is a clear link between the problem and the framework.

E **Literature review**
   1. The literature specific to the problem was reviewed primarily from primary (original) sources in scientific, peer-reviewed journals.
   2. Recent and past empirical studies are progressively presented and provide the context and scope of the problem.
   3. The research reviewed is critically analyzed, gaps are identified, and synopsis with implications for the rationale for the study is provided.
   4. The review is clear, concise, and understandable.

F **Methodology**
   1. Research questions are clearly stated and hypotheses show a relationship between variables.
   2. Variables are conceptually and operationally stated and are amenable to measurement.
   3. The research design is clearly indicated, providing the overall statement for the conduct of the research.
      a. Experimental
         1) Participants are randomly assigned, the control group is identified and adequate, and the intervention is clear and measurable.
         2) Threats to validity of the design are controlled.
      b. Nonexperimental

1) The best design method to address the research questions is selected and variables are controlled for in the design.
2) Comparison groups, if used, are equivalent and representative.

4. Participants and sample
   a. The target population is defined and participants are ascertained.
   b. The sample should be representative of the population and the sample size adequate for the statistical analysis and scientific rigor.

5. Instrumentation
   a. Instruments or tools used should be clearly described and should ask questions pertinent to the research questions or hypotheses.
   b. Validity and reliability data are provided.
   c. Newly developed instruments or tools should be adequately tested and described.

6. Data collection procedures
   a. Methods used to collect the data (e.g., reviews, questionnaires, physiologic measurements) are clearly described.
   b. Data collection procedures are internally consistent.
   c. The setting for data collection is described.
   d. Participants rights are protected.

7. Data analysis
   a. Demographics of the sample are provided and described.
   b. A description of statistical procedures used for data analysis, including levels of measurement appropriate to the questions, is provided.
   c. Research questions or hypotheses are addressed with appropriate descriptive and inferential statistics.
   d. Results are reported and interpreted correctly.
   e. Tables and graphs are used to clarify results and are reported in a way that allows the reader to evaluate the results.

8. Interpretation and conclusions
   a. Findings that address the research questions are discussed along with their statistical significance and what that means.
   b. Findings are discussed within the context of existing knowledge and gaps are identified.
   c. Application of the findings to nursing practice and a discussion of practical strategies are given.
   d. Methodologic problems and limitations are discussed.
   e. The degree to which the findings can be generalized is addressed.
   f. Suggestions for further research are made.

X Funding Research

Good research is not feasible if it cannot find funding.

A **There are many sources of support for the conduct of research. Table 17-1 lists selected sources of funding.**
   1. Professional societies (e.g., AAOHN, ANA)
   2. Government agencies (e.g., NIOSH, DOE, OSHA)
   3. Foundations (e.g., Macy Foundation, Robert Wood Johnson)
   4. Voluntary agencies (e.g., American Cancer Society, American Heart Association
   5. Corporations

TABLE 17-1

Selected organizations for research funding for health related projects

Organization	Application deadline
Agency for Healthcare Research and Quality (AHRQ) Rockville, MD Phone: 301-427-1364 http://www.ahcpr.gov	February 1, June 1, October 1; January 15, May 15, September 15, for small grants
American Association of Occupational Health Nurses Foundation Atlanta, GA Phone: 770-455-7757 http://www.aaohn.org	December 1
American Cancer Society New York, NY Phone: 1-800-227-2345 http://www.cancer.org	April 1, October 15
American Federation on Aging Research New York, NY Phone: 212-703-9977 http://www.afar.org	December 15
American Lung Association New York, NY Phone: 212-315-8700 http://www.lungusa.org	October 1 November 1
American Nurses' Foundation Silver Spring, MD Phone: 301-628-5000 http://www.ana.org	June 1
March of Dimes Foundation White Plains, NY Phone: 914-428-7100 http://www.modimes.org/	Varies
Metropolitan Life Foundation New York, NY Phone: 212-578-7049 http://www.Metlife.com	None
Ruth Mott Fund Flint, MI Phone:810-233-0170 http://www.activistcash.com/ foundation.cfm/did/465	March, July, November
National Institute for Nursing Research Bethesda, MD Phone: 301-496-0207 http://www.nih.gov/ninr	February 1, June 1, October 1
National Institute for Occupational Safety and Health Atlanta, GA Phone: 1-800-356-4674 http://www.cdc.gov/niosh/	February 1, June 1, October 1
National Institutes of Health (Cancer; Eye; Heart, Lung & Blood; Allergy/Infectious Diseases; Arthritis/Musculoskeletal/Skin; Child Health; Diabetes/Digestive/Kidney; Environmental Health; General Medical; Drug Abuse; Mental Health; Alcohol; Neuro/Communicative Disorders) Bethesda, MD Phone: 301-496-4000 http://www.nih.gov Inquire for contact for individual institute	February 1, June 1, October 1
National Science Foundation Arlington, VA Phone: 703-292-5111 http://www.nsf.gov	None
PPG Industries Foundation Pittsburgh, PA Phone: 412-434-3131 http://www.ppg.com	September

TABLE 17-1

Selected organizations for research funding for health related projects—cont'd

Prudential Foundation	None
Newark, NJ	
Phone: 973-802-4791 http://www.prudential.com	
Robert Wood Johnson Foundation	None
Princeton, NJ	
Phone: 888-631-9989 http://www.rwjf.org	
Sigma Theta Tau International	March 1
Indianapolis, IN	
Phone: 317-634-8171 http://www.nursingsociety.org	

B The AAOHN Foundation, established in 1998, has several research awards available to fund competitive applicants for researchable topics. (See AAOHN website for information.)

C The researcher should consider the research topic as it relates to the mission of the funding source before applying (Rogers, 1996; 2003).

REFERENCES

American Association of Occupational Health Nurses (AAOHN). (2004). *Standards of occupational and environmental health nursing*. Atlanta: AAOHN.

American Nurses Association. (1998). *Standards of clinical nursing practice* (2nd ed). Washington, DC: ANA.

Brink, P. J., & Wood, M. J. (1988). *Basic steps in planning nursing research*. Boston: Jones and Bartlett.

Giuffre, M. (1998). Critiquing a research article. *Journal of Perianesthesia Nursing, 13*, 104-108.

National Institute for Occupational Safety and Health (NIOSH). (1996). *National occupational research agenda*. Cincinnati, OH: USDHHS, CDC, NIOSH.

Polit, D., & Hungler, B. (2004). *Nursing research: principles and methods*. Philadelphia: Lippincott.

Rogers, B. (1995). Critically evaluating research studies. *AAOHN Journal, 43*, 54-55.

Rogers, B. (1996). Researchability and feasibility issues in conducting research. *AAOHN Journal, 44*, 58-59.

Rogers, B., Agnew, J., & Pompeii, L. (2000). Research priorities in occupational health nursing. *AAOHN Journal, 48*, 9-16.

Rogers, B. (2003) *Occupation and environmental health nursing: concepts and practice*. St. Louis: Saunders.

18

Professional Issues: Advancing the Specialty

Eleanor McCarthy Chamberlin and Elizabeth Lawhorn

Professional development is the process by which the occupational and environmental health nurse maintains professional competency and contributes to the professional growth of self and others. The purpose of this chapter is to provide an overview of issues and activities that are related to professionalism in occupational and environmental health nursing.

I   Professional Associations

A **The American Association of Occupational Health Nurses (AAOHN) is the professional association of nurses engaged in the practice of occupational and environmental health nursing.**

1. The major roles and responsibilities of AAOHN are as follows:
    a. Defines the scope of practice and sets standards for occupational and environmental health nursing practice (AAOHN, 2004a) (Appendix VII)
    b. Develops standards of professional conduct for the occupational and environmental health nurse as described in the AAOHN Code of Ethics (AAOHN, 2003a) (Appendix VIII)
    c. Promotes the health and safety of work and community environments
    d. Promotes and provides continuous learning opportunities for occupational and environmental health nurses and professionals
    e. Advances the profession by encouraging and facilitating research
    f. Advocates for occupational and environmental health nursing in business, government, and other professional areas
    g. Responds to issues critical to the practice of occupational and environmental health nursing; responses are reported in the following publications:
       1) Governmental affairs action alerts
       2) Position statements and advisories, such as "Confidentiality of Employee Health Information" and "Occupational Health Surveillance"
       3) Competencies and performance criteria for occupational and environmental health nurses
2. The *AAOHN Journal* is the official journal of AAOHN. It provides information related to occupational and environmental health nursing practice, advisories, continuing education modules, and research literature.

B **AAOHN is guided by its vision and mission statements (www.aaohn.org).**
1. AAOHN's vision is that "work and community environments will be healthy and safe."
2. AAOHN's mission is to ensure that occupational and environmental health nurses "are the authority on health, safety, productivity, and disability management for worker populations."
3. AAOHN achieves its mission through the following activities:
   a. Advancing the profession by offering a number of cutting-edge professional and leadership development, networking, and career opportunities
   b. Protecting the profession by advocating for legislation, regulations, and public policy that positively impact occupational and environmental health nursing
   c. Guiding the profession by providing a number of tools to address the distinct role these nurses play in business. These tools include a code of ethics, standards of practice, competencies, self-assessment, a peer-reviewed journal, monthly newsletters, weekly e-news, and a current and up-to-date web site.
   d. Promoting the profession through a marketing and public relations campaign that emphasizes the value of occupational and environmental health nurses to employers, employees, government, and other important groups

C **AAOHN Opportunities for Growth**
1. AAOHN's website (www.aaohn.org) provides an array of resources for occupational and environmental health nurses such as:
   a. Networking, which can be accomplished through two valuable resources for members, the discussion forum for members only and the member directory
   b. Self-assessment tool and foundation blocks
   c. CE modules, advisories, practice Q&A's
   d. Mentor partnership programs
   e. Public policy, which includes updates in the ProHealth Alert section; it provides an interactive tool for elective officials and contact information
   f. Career resources, which include employment job listings online
   g. Advocacy tools for worksite health and safety issues
   h. 24/7 access to AAOHN's website
2. AAOHN's monthly member-focused newsletter and weekly e-news provides:
   a. Updates on AAOHN events, products, and services
   b. Briefs on governmental issues concerning the profession
   c. Information on practice issues
   d. Resources for career building

II Professional Credentialing in Nursing

Obtaining and maintaining high-quality nursing care for the public good is the basis of any process used in credentialing nurses, nursing education, and nursing services (ANA, 1979); credentialing is a complex process intended to define levels of practice and associated knowledge, skills, abilities, and competencies.

A **Credentialing is an umbrella term that includes processes that assure clients, consumers, and the public that a practitioner has the qualifications and competencies necessary to practice nursing according to pre-established standards.**

1. The credentialing process may require registration, certification, licensure, and accreditation.
    a. Credentialing programs "aid the profession by encouraging and recognizing professional and institutional achievement" (Rabenstein & Lewis, 1998).
    b. Credentialing mechanisms affecting occupational and environmental health nurses "include licensure and certification of individuals and accreditation of educational and health care organizations" (Olson, Verrall & Lundvall, 1997).
2. *Certification* is "the formal recognition of the specialized knowledge, skills, and experience demonstrated by the achievement of standards identified by a nursing specialty to promote optimal health outcomes" (American Board of Nursing Specialties [ABNS], 2005).
3. According to the American Nurses' Credentialing Center [ANCC], 2005a:
    a. Certification validates nurses' specialty knowledge.
    b. Certification provides an opportunity for the certified nurse to demonstrate his or her professional competence and to meet nationally recognized standards in a nursing specialty.
    c. Certification "is a testimonial of [the certificant's] dedication to nursing, bringing greater accountability to the profession."

B **Major credentialing processes**

1. *Accreditation* is broadly defined as "a voluntary, self-regulatory process by which governmental, non-governmental, and voluntary associations or other statutory bodies grant formal recognition to programs or institution that meet stated quality criteria" (ABNS, 2005b).
    a. The American Board of Nursing Specialties, established in 1991, serves as the accrediting board for specialty nursing certification programs (Box 18-1 provides an overview of the value of ABNS certification to nursing certification organizations.)
    b. The National Organization for Competency Assurance (NOCA), established in 1977, sets quality standards for credentialing organizations; the National Commission for Certifying Agencies (NCCA) is the accreditation body of NOCA (http://www.noca.org/ncca/ncca.htm).
2. An *academic degree* is awarded to an individual upon completion of pre-established requirements in a field of study.
    a. An academic degree forms the basis for nursing practice and is a fundamental pre-requisite to entry into practice through licensure.
    b. Additional degrees in nursing signify advanced or more focused education in a specialty or subspecialty.
3. *Licensure* is the process by which an agency of government grants permission to engage in a given profession or occupation.
    a. Granting a license signifies that the bearer of the license has attained the minimal degree of competency in a particular field.
    b. This process is intended to ensure that the public health, safety, and welfare will be reasonably well protected (Joel, 2003).
    c. Licensure also authorizes the use of a particular title or designation.

BOX 18-1

The value of American Board of Nursing specialties accreditation

Organizations with accredited examination programs (such as the American Board for Occupational Health Nurses) have indicated that ABNS accreditation:

- Gives more prestige and legitimacy to the credential and the specialty
- Reflects the certification program's attainment of the highest quality standards of the industry
- Presents the certification program in a positive manner, particularly in comparison to other nursing certification programs that are not ABNS-accredited
- Allows ABNS to satisfy employer and regulatory requirements
- Promotes the recruitment and retention of certificants
- Offers an opportunity to gain valuable feedback on the rigor

and value of the examination and certification renewal policies and procedures

- Is useful when responding to a candidate's concerns or questions about certification and examination policies and procedures
- Is the only accreditation offered specifically for specialty nursing certification programs
- Reinforces the ability to maintain excellence by continuing to meet the standards
- Provides structure and guidelines for the certification process
- Provides specialty practice with credibility as a *nursing* specialty
- Makes examinations legally defensible by ensuring that they are of the highest quality from a validity and reliability standpoint.

Source: ABNS, 2005b.

---

4. *Certification* is a voluntary process that involves the formal recognition of specialized knowledge, skills, and experience demonstrated by achievement of standards identified by a nursing specialty to promote optimal health outcomes. Certification validates nursing specialty knowledge (ABNS, 2005b).

C The American Board for Occupational Health Nurses (ABOHN) is an independent, autonomous, nursing-specialty certification board.
   1. ABOHN is the sole certifying body for occupational and environmental health nursing in the United States. The ABOHN certification program is accredited by both the American Board of Nursing Specialties (ABNS) and the National Certification Credentialing Agency (NCCA) of the National Organization for Competency Assurance (NOCA).
   2. ABOHN's role in occupational and environmental health nursing includes:
       a. Setting criteria and standards for certification
       b. Establishing sound policies and procedures for achieving and maintaining certification
       c. Using the definitions and standards of occupational and environmental health nursing practice established by AAOHN
       d. Providing a peer review certification that attests that certified occupational and environmental health nurses have met standards for knowledge, experience, and education in the specialty

    e. Basing the content of examinations on independent research that validates current practice in occupational and environmental health nursing

D **Two core and two subspecialties certifications are currently available in occupational and environmental health nursing.**

1. Core certification includes:
   a. *Certified Occupational Health Nurse* (COHN): The COHN credential is available to registered nurses whose role is more focused on direct care and provision of services. The COHN credential does not require a bachelor's degree. COHN roles include clinician, coordinator, advisor, and case manager.
   b. *Certified Occupational Health Nurse-Specialist (COHN-S):* The COHN-S credential is available to registered nurses with a bachelor's degree or higher and whose practice is more focused on program management and administration. COHN-S roles include: educator, manager, clinician, consultant, and case manager.

2. Requirements for certification in occupational and environmental health nursing as a COHN or COHN-S include:
   a. Licensure as a registered nurse in the state(s) of practice
   b. Current practice in occupational and environmental health nursing
   c. Experience in an occupational and environmental health nursing role
   d. Continuing education in topics related to occupational and environmental health nursing
   e. Successful completion of a scientifically valid national examination

3. Core certification as a COHN or a COHN-S is required as a prerequisite prior to becoming eligible to apply for subspecialty certification; the subspecialties currently available through ABOHN include:
   a. Case Manager (COHN/CM or COHN-S/CM): Case management is defined by AAOHN as a distinct role for occupational and environmental health nurses who specialize in the coordination of client's health services from the onset of injury or illness to a safe return to work or an optimal alternative (AAOHN, 2004b).
   b. Safety Manager: (COHN/SM or COHN-S/SM): To be eligible for the ABOHN Safety Manager credential, the practice of the COHN or COHN-S includes at least 25% safety functions. This certification validates the knowledge, skills, and abilities of many occupational and environmental health nurses who function in an expanded role that includes responsibility for safety functions and programs (ABOHN, 2004).

4. In addition to COHN or a COHN-S core credential, requirements for achieving a subspecialty credential include:
   a. Additional contact hours in area of specialty (case management or safety management)
   b. Focused practice time and/or other experience in the area of specialty
   c. Successful completion of a scientifically valid national examination

III Competency in Occupational and Environmental Health Nursing

The code of ethics, standards of practice, core curriculum, and competencies provide the basis for the scope of practice, knowledge, skill, and the legal and ethical framework in occupational and environmental health nursing.

A *AAOHN Code of Ethics and Interpretive Statements* (AAOHN, 2003a)—Provides a guiding ethical framework for decision making and evaluation of nursing actions as occupational and environmental health nurses fulfill their professional responsibilities to society and the profession (Appendix VIII).

B *Standards of Occupational and Environmental Health Nursing* (AAOHN, 2004a)—Delineates concepts and principles to support the knowledge base for occupational and environmental health nursing (Appendix VII).

C *Competencies in Occupational and Environmental Health Nursing* (AAOHN, 2003b)—Provides guidelines that address the continuum of practice experience and are applicable to every occupational and environmental health nurse in every practice role; performance criteria were developed for each competency (see Appendix VI).
   1. The AAOHN defines competency as an outcome-oriented statement of mastery of a particular skill or ability.
   2. The full text describing these competencies can be obtained from AAOHN at http://www.aaohn.org/practice/competencies.cfm
   3. Based on these competencies, a self-assessment tool was developed to assist occupational and environmental health nurses identify their professional strengths (knowledge, skills, and abilities), identify and prioritize their learning needs, and organize a self-directed plan to meet these needs.

IV Strategies for Advancing the Discipline and Practice

The AAOHN Standards of Occupational and Environmental Health Nursing (2004a), Standard VIII: Professional Development, states: "The occupational and environmental health nurse assumes accountability for professional development to enhance professional growth and maintain competency." Occupational and environmental health nursing is advanced through education, research, continuing education, practice, and other professional activities.

A Academic education in safety and health
   1. Occupational Safety and Health Education and Research Centers (ERCs), funded by the National Institute for Occupational Safety and Health, are the primary vehicles for training and educating occupational health and safety professionals, including occupational and environmental health nurses, industrial hygienists, occupational physicians, and occupational safety professionals (For a list of ERCs, see http://www.aaohn.org/member_services/career/upload/ERC-List-2.doc).
   2. These ERCs provide academic, research, continuing education, and outreach programs.
   3. Other schools of nursing offer academic degrees and coursework related to occupational health and safety.

B Research (see Chapter 17)
   1. The occupational and environmental health nurse participates in research activities at levels appropriate to the individual's education and experience, which may include problem identification, critical analysis of reported research, research project participation, acting as a resource person, and collaborating with colleagues.

2. The occupational and environmental health nurse develops grant proposals commensurate with education and experience.
3. The occupational and environmental health nurse uses research findings in the development of policies, procedures, and guidelines.

C Continuing education
  1. The occupational and environmental health nurse assumes accountability for professional development to enhance professional growth and maintain competency.
     a. Exercising responsibility in the profession requires learning, applying, and assessing knowledge pertaining to occupational and environmental sciences, technology, information systems, and research; this is a required commitment throughout the occupational and environmental health nurse's professional career.
     b. As nurses in occupational and environmental health assume increased responsibility, there is an obligation to take steps to maintain and increase competency. It is generally accepted that professionals are well prepared and qualified for the functions they perform.
  2. The occupational and environmental health nurse determines continuing education needs, initiates independent learning opportunities, seeks additional academic/continuing education, and evaluates learning for effectiveness.
  3. Organizational resources are allocated for professional growth activities.
  4. The occupational and environmental health nurse acts as a role model and student mentor.
  5. The occupational and environmental health nurse facilitates learning of colleagues through discussion, demonstration, and quality improvement techniques.
  6. The occupational and environmental health nurse incorporates new knowledge into practice, based on scientific research.
  7. The occupational and environmental health nurse meets continuing education requirements for certification, licensure, etc.

D Practice
  1. Occupational health nursing practice is characterized by professionalism and professional commitment.
     a. *Professionalism* describes the conduct or qualities that characterize a practitioner in a particular field or occupation.
     b. *Professional commitment* is carried out in accordance with occupational health nursing standards, scope of nursing practice, and an ethical code.
     c. The occupational and environmental health nurse maintains a professional image and exhibits a high level of respect and dignity for the profession.
  2. All nurses are accountable to the client and society for actions taken in nursing practice.
  3. The occupational and environmental health nurse demonstrates practice accountability by validating desired outcomes.
  4. The occupational and environmental health nurse facilitates the leadership role by recognizing the value of and using professional resources.
  5. The occupational and environmental health nurse is guided by standards of practice, which are criteria-based and measurable and ensure accountability to the profession (AAOHN, 2004a).

6. The occupational and environmental health nurse practices within an ethical framework to make ethical judgments for decision making in practice (AAOHN, 2004c).

E **Growth of the profession**

1. Key elements to advancing occupational and environmental health nursing practice include:
   a. Creating and communicating a vision statement
   b. Creating and communicating a mission statement
   c. Developing and communicating the outcomes for the organization
2. The implementation of these elements is carried out by the AAOHN Board of Directors and the members of the association.
   a. The AAOHN Board of Directors is responsible for creating/developing and communicating these changing elements.
   b. The current level of success in advancing occupational and environmental health nursing practice will be possible only with the continuing and complete participation of each member.
3. The occupational and environmental health nurse supports the growth of the profession through the following activities:
   a. Membership in professional associations
   b. Serving on association committees and boards
   c. Assuming leadership positions in elected capacity
   d. Coordinating and expanding services into the occupational health/managed care area to meet the challenges of the current health care environment.
4. The occupational and environmental health nurse acts as a role model in the following ways:
   a. Applies concepts of autonomy, influence, fairness, and risk taking to the professional role
   b. Supports education to increase knowledge and expertise
   c. Supports research as the foundation for professional practice
   d. Precepts students regarding the professional role and knowledge enhancement
5. See Box 18-2 for examples of achieving professional development

V Role Expansion

The role of the occupational and environmental health nurse will continue to expand. In collaboration with other professionals, the occupational and environmental health nurse will assume new responsibilities.

A *Case management* **responsibilities and opportunities will require conducting job analyses and functional-capacity job assessments and working with community agencies to provide the most appropriate and cost-effective services for employees and family members with complex illnesses and injuries.**

B *Environmental health* **responsibilities and opportunities will include analyzing aggregate data related to incidence/prevalence, epidemiologic trends and patterns, and work practices related to injury/illness events (Rogers, 2002).**

C *Management* **responsibilities and opportunities will include conducting cost-benefit analyses of available internal and external health care services,**

BOX 18-2

Examples of professional development

Scenario 1

Mary is a 43-year-old occupational and environmental health nurse who is committed to continuing education. She also believes that becoming certified in occupational health nursing is essential to advancing her career. Mary understands the importance of saving her company money while protecting the health and safety of workers. Although she has been successful in effecting significant cost savings and reducing injury rates, her accomplishments were not reflected in her salary until she became certified. Mary wished to contribute more effectively to occupational and environmental health nursing practice. After practicing for several years, she successfully ran for a position on the AAOHN Board of Directors. Through her experience on the board, Mary was empowered to further improve employee health and safety by effecting legislation through her participation in governmental and professional affairs activities. Mary continues as an AAOHN Board member as an advocate, promoting AAOHN and respect for occupational and environmental health nurses and the profession, through collaboration and mentoring.

Scenario 2

Debbie believes she developed skills and professionalism early in her career, in great part through participation in her local chapter of AAOHN. The focus of her efforts was the improvement of worker health and safety at the local, state, and national levels of the organization. At the local level she served as vice president; and her focus was education and professional development. At the state level she held several offices, including president, vice president, and governmental affairs chair. Early in her career as an occupational and environmental health nurse, Debbie spent time as a nurse manager in a major chemical company, designing, developing, and implementing occupational health programs. Debbie demonstrated her expertise and leadership skills while interacting with and gaining the respect of varied other disciplines for herself and her profession. Over the past 17 years Debbie has been involved both personally and professionally in occupational and environmental health nursing and continues to be an inspiration and mentor to her colleagues.

---

participating in the selection and design of benefits and benefit programs, and providing expertise in program design, implementation, and management and outcome measurement.

D *Primary care* responsibilities/opportunities will be in consumer education related to health promotion, disease prevention, self-care, and appropriate access to a reformed health care system; nurse-managed primary care delivery at the work site for employees and their families; and provision of international health care services to traveling employees (O'Brien, 1995; Rogers, 2002).

E *Consulting* opportunities will provide expertise in occupational and environmental health to colleagues, government, and the private sector for the purpose of improving workers' health.

F *Presenter/speaker* responsibilities and opportunities will be increasingly available and will serve as an excellent forum not only for professional development within our specialty, but also for enhancing collaborative efforts with other colleagues, organizations, agencies, and disciplines.

G *Entrepreneurial* responsibilities/opportunities will allow individuals the ability to promote and manage business with leadership and managerial goals while providing expertise, which is essential as a nurse entrepreneur.

VI Partnerships in Occupational and Environmental Health

A Collaboration: The occupational and environmental health nurse collaborates with a multidisciplinary team in assessing, diagnosing, planning, implementing, and evaluating care of workers.
1. Collaboration often occurs with physicians, industrial hygienists, toxicologists, safety professionals, and ergonomists to identify, monitor, and control workplace hazards and promote a healthy workplace.
2. Collaboration among professionals and others is essential to providing appropriate interventions and treatments of high quality.
3. Collaboration with employers and employees is essential to establish and maintain a healthy and safe working environment.
4. Collaboration with external agencies supports safe and healthful work and community environments.
   a. Governmental agencies and programs (e.g., Occupational Safety and Health Administration, National Institute for Occupational Safety and Health, Environmental Protection Agency, Agency for Toxic Substance and Disease Registry)
   b. Voluntary agencies (e.g., American Heart Association, American Cancer Society, American Diabetes Association)
   c. Nursing organizations (e.g., American Nurses' Association)
   d. Other specialty organizations (e.g., National Safety Council) and professional associations (e.g., American Industrial Hygiene Association)

B Advocacy: The occupational and environmental health nurse has a responsibility to be an advocate for occupational and environmental health nursing practice and the work force and community populations served.
1. The following activities help the nurse fulfill this responsibility within occupational and environmental health nursing.
   a. Active involvement in professional associations at all levels
   b. Participation on AAOHN committees and task forces charged with developing practice guidelines, vision, mission, for the organization, etc.
   c. Assuming a leadership role and serving as a mentor and role model for the professional development of peers, colleagues, and others
2. The following activities help the nurse fulfill this responsibility outside occupational and environmental health nursing.
   a. Increasing awareness of the scope of occupational and environmental health practice among other organizations, associations, agencies, specialty practices, and health care professionals

b. Getting involved and encouraging and empowering peers to participate in discussions with their state and federal legislators
   1) State legislators need to be knowledgeable and informed about issues that are relevant to occupational and environmental health.
   2) Occupational and environmental health nurses should be alert to new legislation, and to changes and challenges to existing legislation that affect the health and safety of workers and worker populations.

REFERENCES

American Association of Occupational Health Nurses. (2003a). *AAOHN code of ethics and interpretative statements*. Atlanta, GA: AAOHN.

American Association of Occupational Health Nurses. (2003b). Competencies in occupational and environmental health nursing. *AAOHN Journal, 51*(7), 290-302.

American Association of Occupational Health Nurses. (2004a). *Standards of occupational and environmental health nursing*. Atlanta, GA: AAOHN.

American Association of Occupational Health Nurses. (2004b). The occupational health nurse as case manager. [Position Statement]. Atlanta, GA: AAOHN.

American Board for Occupational Health Nurses, Inc. (ABOHN). (2004c). *Announcement: New Certification Opportunity*. Retrieved on April 7, 2005 from http://www.abohn.org/

American Board of Nursing Specialties (ABNS) (2005a) ABNS: Providing Excellence in Nursing Certification: Home page. Retrieved on April 6, 2005 from http://www.nursingcertification.org/index.html.

American Board of Nursing Specialities ABNS) (2005b). ABNS: Providing Excel-lence in Nursing. Frequently Asked Questions. http://www.nursingcertification.org/faq.htm-2.

American Nurses Association. (1979). *The study of credentialing in nursing: A new approach. American Journal of Nursing,* 79(4), 674-683.

American Nurses Credentialing Center (2005). *ANCC Certification-Opening a world of opportunities*. Retrieved on April 7, 2005 from http://www.nursingworld.org/ancc/cert.html

Joel, L. A., (2003). *Dimensions of professional nursing*, 9th ed. McGraw-Hill Inc., New York, NY.

O'Brien, S. (1995). Occupational health nursing roles: Future challenges and opportunities. *AAOHN Journal, 43*(3), 148-152.

Olson, D. K., Verrall, B., & Lundvall, A. M. (1997). Credentialing: Concerns and issues affecting occupational health nursing. *AAOHN Journal, 45*(5), 231-238.

Rabenstein, K. I., & Lewis, C. K. (1998). Certification: positioning nurses for the 21st century. *Imprint, 45*(1), 33, 47.

Rogers, B. (2002). *Occupational health nursing: Concepts and practice*. Philadelphia: Saunders.

APPENDIX

I

Occupational and Environmental Health and Safety Resources

Professional Associations

American Association of Occupational Health Nurses, Inc. (AAOHN), Suite 100, 2920 Brandywine Road, Atlanta, GA 30341, phone (770) 455-7757, fax (770) 455-7271.

American College of Occupational and Environmental Medicine (ACOEM), 1114 N. Arlington Heights Road, Arlington Heights, IL 60004, phone (847) 818-1800, fax (847) 818-9266.

American Conference of Governmental Industrial Hygienists, Inc. (ACGIH), 1330 Kemper Meadow Dr., Suite 600, Cincinnati, OH 45240, phone (513) 742-2020, fax (513) 742-3355.

American Industrial Hygiene Association (AIHA), 2700 Prosperity Avenue, Suite 250, Fairfax, VA 22031, phone (703) 849-8888, fax (703) 207-3561.

American Public Health Association (APHA), 800 I Street NW, Washington, DC 2000-3710, phone (202) 777-APHA, fax (202) 777-2534.

American Society for Safety Engineers (ASSE), 1800 East Oakton, Des Plaines, IL 60018-2187, phone (847) 699-2929, fax (847) 768-3434.

Human Factors and Ergonomics Society, P.O. Box 1369, Santa Monica, CA 90406, phone (310) 394-1811, fax (310) 394-2410.

National Safety Council (NSC), 1121 Spring Lake Drive, Itasca, IL 60143-3201, phone (630) 285-1121, fax (630) 285-1315.

Certifying Organization

American Board for Occupational Health Nurses, Inc. (ABOHN), 201 East Ogden Road, Suite 114, Hinsdale, IL 60521-3652, phone (630) 789-5799; (888) 842-2646, fax (630) 789-8901.

Publications

Journals

AAOHN Journal, the official journal of the American Association of Occupational Health Nurses, published monthly by SLACK, Inc., 6900 Grove Road, Thorofare, NJ 08086-9447.

American Industrial Hygiene Association Journal, the official journal of the American Hygiene Association, published monthly by the American Industrial Hygiene Association, 2700 Prosperity Avenue, Suite 250, Fairfax, VA 22031.

American Journal of Occupational Medicine, published monthly by Wiley Interscience, Box 1057, Mount Sinai School of Medicine, One Gustave Levy Place, New York, NY 10029-6574.

Applied Occupational and Environmental Hygiene, an international journal published monthly by Applied Industrial Hygiene, Inc., a wholly owned subsidary of ACGIH (American Conference of Governmental Industrial Hygienists, Inc.), 1330 Kemper Meadow Dr., Cincinnati, OH 45240.

Journal of Occupational and Environmental Medicine, the official journal of the American College of Occupational and Environmental Medicine, published monthly by Lippincott Williams & Wilkins, 530 Walnut Street, Philadelphia, PA 19106.

Journal of Occupational Health Psychology, published quarterly by the Educational Publishing Foundation, 750 First Street NE, Washington, DC 20002-4242.

Safety and Health, published monthly by the National Safety Council, 1121 Spring Lake Drive, Itasca, IL 60143.

Books

DiBenedetto, D. V., Harris, J. S., & McCunney, R. S. (1998). *OEM Occupational health and safety manual, Version 2.1*. Beverly, MA: OEM Press.

Fleming, L. E., Herzstein, J. A., & Bunn, W. B. (1997). *Issues in international occupational and environmental medicine*. Beverly, MA: OEM Press.

Harris, J. S., Belk, H. D., & Wood, L. W. (1992). *Managing employee health care costs: Assuring quality and value*. Boston: OEM Press.

Levy, B. S. & Wegman, D. H. (2000). *Occupational Health: Recognizing and preventing work-related disease and injury* (4th ed.). Philadelphia: Lippincott Williams & Wilkins.

Menzel. N. N. (1998). *Workers' comp management from A to Z: A "how to" guide with forms* (2nd ed.). Beverly, MA: OEM Press.

Moser, R. (1999). *Effective management of occupational and environmental health and safety programs* (2nd ed.). Beverly Farms, MA: OEM Press.

Rogers, B. (2003). *Occupational and environmental health nursing: Concepts and practice* (2nd ed.). Philadelphia: WB Saunders (NOTE: At this writing, a second edition is in process.)

Sources of Internet/Computer Information

AAOHN Home Page, http://www.aaohn.org provides information on association products and services and links to practice resources, including topic discussion forums.

CIN: Computers, Informatics, Nursing, Lippincott Company Publishing, 12107 Insurance Way, Suite 114, Hagerstown, MD 21740. Can be accessed through http://www.nursingcenter.com.

The Nurse Executive Guide to Directing and Managing Information Systems, The Center for Health Care Information Management (CHIM), 900 Victors Way, Suite 124, Ann Arbor, MI 48108.

OSHA ComputerLed Information System (OCIS), U.S. Government Printing Office, Washington, DC 20402-9325, phone (202) 783-3238. Contains agency documents, technical information, and training materials on CD-ROM.

THE ONLINE JOURNAL OF NURSING INFORMATICS (OJNI) is a source of peer-reviewed, original, high-quality scientific papers, review articles, and practice-based articles related to nursing informatics. American Nurses Association http://nursingworld.org

Sources of Technical Information

CHEMTREC: 24-hour hotline to provide information about chemicals. To obtain information call (800) 262-8200 or (703) 741-5523 or go to http://www.chemtrec.org/

TOXNET: Comprehensive database that provides toxicity data on chemicals, available though Melars Management Section, National Library of Medicine, Building 38, Room 4N421, 8600 Rockville Pike, Bethesda, MD 20894, phone (800) 638-8480.

Poison Control Centers: These centers are located in every state. Each has a 24-hour hotline to provide emergency information and referrals. Information about centers can be found on the inside covers of local phone directories.

National Pesticide Telecommunications Network: A cooperative effort of Oregon State University and the U.S. Environmental Protection Agency that provides objective, science-based information about a wide variety of pesticide-related subjects. To obtain information call (800) 858-7378.

Government Resources

Agency for Toxic Substances and Disease Registry (ATSDR), ATSDR, 1600 Clifton Road, NE, Atlanta, GA 30033.

Clearinghouse on Health Indexes, U.S. Department of Health and Human Services, Centers for Disease Control and Prevention, National Center for Health Statistics, Division of Data, Hyattsville, MD 20782, phone (301) 458-4636.

Environmental Protection Agency (EPA), Public Information Center, PM-211B, 401 M Street SW, Washington, DC 20460.

National Institute of Environmental Health Sciences (NIEHS), National Institutes of Health, Public Health Service, U.S. Department of Health and Human Services, P.O. Box 12233, Research Triangle Park, NC 27709.

National Institute of Nursing Research, National Institutes of Health, Public Health Service, U.S. Department of Health and Human Services, Building 45, Room AN-12, 45 Center Drive MSC 6300, Bethesda, MD 20892-6300.

National Institute for Occupational Safety and Health (NIOSH) *Headquarters,* 200 Independence Ave. SW, Washington, DC 20201, phone (800) 35-NIOSH or (800) 356-4674.

Occupational Safety and Health Administration (OSHA), U.S. Department of Labor, 200 Constitution Avenue NW, Washington, DC 20210. Films and printed material available through regional OSHA offices, or through OSHA Publications Office, 200 Constitution Avenue NW, Washington, DC 20210, phone (202) 219-4667, fax (202) 219-9266.

Office of Occupational Health Nursing, Occupational Safety and Health Administration, Directorate of Technical Support, Room 4618, 200 Constitution Avenue NW, Washington, DC 20210, phone (202) 693-2120.

International Agencies, Organizations, and References

International Labour Office Occupational Safety and Health Branch (ILO-SHB), Bureau International de Travail-Service de la securité et de l'hygiène du travail (BIT-Sec-Hyg), and Information Safety and Health Information Center, 4 route des Morillons, CH-1211 Geneva 22 (Switzerland).

International Labour Office (ILO). (1997). *Encyclopedia of occupational health and safety* (4th ed.). Geneva, Switzerland: International Labour Organization.

International Occupational Safety and Health Information Centre, Centre international & information de securité et d'hygiène du travail (CIS). IL0, 4 route des Morillons, CH-121 Geneva 22 (Switzerland).

International Organization for Standardization (ISO), Organization internationale de normalization. 1 rue de Varembe, CH-1211 Geneva 20 (Switzerland).

Pan American Health Organization and Regional Office for the Americas of the World Health Organization (PAHO), 525 Twenty-third Street NW, Washington, DC 20037.

Regional Office for Europe of the World Health Organization (WHO-EURO-Environmental Health Service), Scherfigvej 8, DK-2100 Copenhagen (Denmark).

World Health Organization (1995). *Global strategies on occupational health for all: The way to health at work.* Geneva: World Health Organization.

World Health Organization-Office of Occupational Health (WHO-OCH). Organization Mondiale de la Sante–Office de la médicine du travail (OMS-OCH). 20 rue Appia, CH-1211 Geneva 27 (Switzerland).

International Travel Safety and Health Program Resources

American Society of Tropical Medicine and Hygiene, 60 Revere Drive, Suite 500, Northbrook, IL 60062, phone (708) 480-9592, fax (708) 480-9282.

Centers for Disease Control and Prevention, Atlanta, GA 30333

- CDC Hot Line (recorded messages 24 hours a day), phone (404) 332-4559
- http://www.cdc.gov/travel.html

Heymann, D.L. (Ed.). (2004). *Control of communicable diseases manual* (18th ed.). Washington, DC: American Public Health Association.

International Society of Travel Medicine, P.O. Box 871089, Stone Mountain, GA 30087-0028, phone (770) 736-7060, fax (770) 736-6732, e-mail: bcbistmaol.com.

International Travel Safety and Health Program (TRAVAX). Travel Health Information Services, phone (608) 831-2331, fax (414) 774-4060.

Jong, E.C. & McMullen, R. (Eds.) (2003). *The travel and tropical medicine manual.* Philadelphia: WB Saunders.

Medical College of Wisconsin International Travel Clinic, Milwaukee, WI, phone (414) 805-3666. http://www.intmed.mcw.edu/travel.html.

Occupational Health and Safety Tools

General Information Resources

Foundation Blocks: A Guide to Occupational & Environmental Health Nursing: A series of subject-specific modules designed to provide valuable information, templates, and tools for the practicing occupational and environmental health nurse.

Success Tools: Strategies for Thriving and Surviving in Business: Includes three modules to help occupational health professionals succeed in the business environment.

Sources for Inspection Checklists

Kornberg, J.P. (1992). *The workplace walk-through*. Boca Raton, FL: Lewis Publishers.

Sources for Accident Investigation

U.S. Department of Labor, Bureau of Labor Statistics, *Evaluating Your Firm's Injury and Illness Record,* Reports 813 and 814, available from regional OSHA offices.

Information on Process Safety Reviews

Ignatowski, A. J. & Rosenthal, I. (2001). The Chemical Accident Risk Assessment Thesaurus: A Tool for Analyzing and Comparing Diverse Risk Assessment Processes and Definitions. *Risk Analysis, 21* (3), 513-532.

OSHA 3133 *Process Safety Management-Guidelines for Compliance,* OSHA Publications Office, 200 Constitution Avenue NW, Washington, DC, phone (202) 219-4667.

Ergonomic Tools and References

ANSI S3.34-1986 (R1997) Hand Arm Vibration Standards American National Standard Guide for the Measurement and Evaluation of Human Exposure to Vibration Transmitted to the Hand. ANSI S3.34-1986 (R1997). Available for purchase at the ANSI Web site at http://web.ansi.org/default.htm.

Department of Energy ErgoEASER–Ergonomics Education, Awareness, System Evaluation and Recording (ErgoEASER) software package. U.S. Department of Energy, Office of Environment, Safety, and Health (1995). Can be downloaded from the Department of Energy Web site at http://tis.eh.doc.gov/others/ergoeaser/download.htm.

Moore, J.S. & Garg, A. (1995). The Strain Index: A proposed method to analyze jobs for risk of distal upper extremity disorders. *American Industrial Hygiene Association Journal, 56,* 443-458.

- http://www.satx.disa.mil/hscoemo/tools/strain.htm.
- NOTE: See additional resources in Appendix IV: Web Sites.

Guidelines for Respirator PPE Health Clearance

American National Standards Institute (ANSI) 88.6, *Respirator Use Physical Qualifications for Personnel,* ANSI, 11 West 42nd Street, New York, NY 10036.

Resources for Direct Care Activities

The Agency for Healthcare Research and Quality, in association with the American Association of Health Plans (AAHP) and the American Medical Association (AMA), established a *National Guidelines Clearinghouse*™ (NGC), a public resource for evidence-based clinical practice guidelines http://www.guideline.gov

Centers for Disease Control and Prevention

- Guidelines for occupational infectious disease (ftp://ftp.cdc.gov/pub/Publications/mmwr/rr/rr4618.pdf) or the post exposure prophylaxis

- Recommendations for health care workers exposed to HIV
- (ftp://ftp.cdc.gov/pub/Publications/mmwr/RR/RR4707.pdf).

- Publications and resources
- (http://www.cdc.gov/nip/publications/ACIP-list.htm) The Adult Immunization Acton Plan can be found at http://www.cdc.gov/od/nvpo/adult.htm.

- Delivery of a vaccine program http://www.cdc.gov/epo/mmwr/preview/mmwrhtml/rr4901a1.htm.

First aid: OSHA Directive CPL 2-2.53–Guidelines for First Aid Programs can be accessed at http://www.osha-slc.gov.

Guidelines for Preventing Workplace Violence for Health Care and Social Service Workers (USDL, OSHA, 1998) can be used to design engineering and administrative controls and for post-incident response and evaluation. Available on-line at http://www.osha.gov/

The *Guide to Clinical Preventive Services* (3rd ed.) provides research-based screening recommendations for the clinician (U.S. Preventive Services Task Force, 2004).

Healthy People 2010, objectives on immunizations in Chapter 14: Immunizations (http://www.health.gov/healthypeople).

Preplacement resources: Federal OSHA standards (http://www.osha.gov), the Americans with Disabilities Act (http://www.usdoj.gov/crt/ada/adahom1.htm), and other mandated programs; for example, the Department of Transportation (http://www.dot.gov) preplacement programs.

Prevention Dissemination and Implementation: Put Prevention into Practice is a program of the Office of Disease Prevention and Health Promotion (http://www.ahrq.gov/clinic/ppipix.htm); includes health education materials, *The Clinician's Handbook of Preventive Services,* and other resources.

Workplace Violence: AAOHN provides multiple resources on their website related to this important issue; these include a position statement, a workplace violence fact sheet, a policy platform statement, and a description of their alliance with OSHA focusing on workplace violence.

APPENDIX

II

Glossary

Accident: An undesired event causing harm to people, property, or the environment, possibly causing additional losses by interrupting the conduct of business.

Accident investigation: A fact-finding procedure to identify the pertinent factors that allow accidents to occur, with the aim of preventing similar future accidents.

Administrative controls: Supervisory and management practices that promote safe work behaviors to eliminate or limit exposure to hazards.

Air-purifying respirator: A type of personal protective equipment (PPE) that uses filters or adsorbents to remove toxic materials from inhaled air.

Area sample: A sample most commonly collected when doing environmental monitoring to detect where contaminants are most likely to be generated, creating a "map" of levels present.

Assigned protection factor: The minimum anticipated protection provided by a properly functioning respirator or class of respirators to a given percentage of properly fitted and trained users.

Atmosphere-supply respirator: A type of PPE that uses bottled or compressed air via an airline or a tank worn by the worker to protect against inhalation of toxic or oxygen-deficient atmospheres.

Atmospheric monitoring: The testing of air over time to detect the presence and measure the concentration of airborne contaminants to which a worker is being exposed.

Benchmarking: using a point of reference as a means to measure and compare performance, services, and products.

Budgeting: The process by which programs and activities are quantified into monetary terms for the purpose of planning and managing resources for a given time period.

Case management: A process of coordinating an individual client's total health care services to achieve optimal, quality care delivered in a cost-effective manner (AAOHN, 2004a).

Common law: The legal precedents that have been established as a result of decisions handed down in past cases within a given jurisdiction.

Confidentiality: The implicit promise that information divulged to another will be respected and not released or repeated.

Confined space: An area not designed for human occupancy, with limited entry and egress and often with inadequate ventilation, thus presenting a potential hazard to a worker inside it.

Consensus standard: A standard accepted among professionals and professional organizations and regarded as a guideline, representative of general opinion; it is, however, not legally enforceable unless quoted in a regulation of a legislative body.

Containment: The practice of enclosing a hazardous unit or container inside another container in event of a leak or release of a contaminant or toxin.

Contingent workers: A category of workers also known as floaters, regular part-time, formal intermittents, limited duration hires, informal intermittents, casuals, contract labor services, independent contractors, leased workers, or temporary help services workers.

Dilution ventilation: The circulation of fresh air into the work site to dilute to an acceptable exposure level a contaminant that is emitted into work-site air.

Direct-reading instrument: An instrument that provides immediate data on the contents of the surrounding atmosphere.

Documentation: The written communication of information that is the basis of the legal occupational health record.

Engineering controls: Devices or methods that stop hazards at their source or in the pathway of transmission before they can reach the worker; engineering controls do not depend on the worker to control their effectiveness.

Environmental health: Promoting health and quality of life by preventing or controlling those diseases or deaths that result from interactions between people and their environment (Centers for Disease Control and Prevention [CDC], 2005).

Epidemiology: The study of the distribution and determinants of health-related states or events in specified populations, and the application of this study to the control of health problems. (From *epi*, meaning *upon*; *demos*, meaning *people*; and *logos*, which means *science*.)

Ergonomics: The study of the interaction between humans and their work, ergonomics is concerned with the design of the work site, equipment, physical environment, and organization of work in order to fit them to the worker.

Exposure monitoring: Often done by or with the aid of an industrial hygienist, it is the quantitative assessment of work-site exposures to hazards that are recognized, suspected, or reasonably predictable, based on other preliminary hazard identification methods.

Federal Reserve discount rate: The rate at which the Federal Reserve Bank lends funds to its member banks.

Focused inspections: Periodic inspections of a workplace that target specific processes, equipment, or work areas; investigate an accident; evaluate a reported health or safety hazard; or investigate complaints about such things as a strange odor or loud noise.

Grab sample: An air sample collected over a short period, which may range from a few seconds to less than 2 minutes.

Gross national product (GNP): The total final value of domestic goods and services produced in a national economy over a particular period, usually one year.

Hazard analysis: Procedures used to assess workplace contaminants and associated worker exposures relating to probability of occurrence, severity of consequences, and vulnerability of workers using planned strategies and foresight to ensure the most productive and thorough evaluation of contaminants in the workplace are performed (OSHA, 2003).

Hazardous energy control: A device or method that prevents contact between the worker and the sources of hazardous energy.

Hazardous energy source: Sources, such as electrical energy, chemical reactivity, thermal extremes, mechanical energy, and physical energy, that may be harmful to work with.

Hazards: Work-site conditions that present the potential for harm or damage to people, property, or the environment. Hazards are classified as physical, chemical, biological, psychological, or mechanical.

Health promotion: A process that supports positive lifestyle changes through corporate policies, individual efforts to lower risk of disease and injury, and the creation of an environment that provides a sense of balance among work, family, personal, health, and social concerns.

Incidence rate: An epidemiologic term that describes the occurrence of new disease or injury per unit of time among persons at risk

Incident historical review: The compilation and analysis of accidents and near misses that have occurred over a selected period of time.

Industrial hygiene: The anticipation, recognition, evaluation, and control of environmental factors or stresses arising in or from the workplace, which can cause injury, sickness, impaired health and well-being, or significant discomfort among workers or among citizens.

Informatics nurse: A nurse who "is involved in activities that focus on the methods and technologies of information handling in nursing. Informatics nursing practice includes the development, support, and evaluation of applications, tools, processes, and structures that help nurses to manage data in direct care of patients/clients" (American Nurses Association, 2005).

Informed consent: A decision made with a complete understanding of a treatment or action, including risks, benefits, and alternative treatments; informed consent must be obtained without coercion or deception.

Integrated disability management: A comprehensive approach to integrating all disability benefits, programs, and services to help control the employer's disability costs and to return the employee to work as soon as possible and maximize the employee's functional capacity.

Integrated, or **long-term, sample:** A sample that consists of a known volume of air drawn through an appropriate medium for a sampling period of less than 1 hour to a full 8 hours, reflecting the length of time of a worker's overall exposure.

Information management systems: A means to collect, access, and apply large amounts of information from many sources to effectively manage all aspects of the occupational health unit.

Isolation: Interposition of a barrier between a hazard and those who might be affected by that hazard.

Job hazard analysis: The process of carefully studying and recording each step of a job to identify safety and health job hazards and to determine the best way to perform the job to reduce or eliminate those hazards. Also known as *job safety analysis.*

Local exhaust: Removal of contaminated air from the point of origin, away from the worker's breathing zone, through a scrubber or cleaning system to the outside atmosphere.

Machine safeguarding: Eliminating hazards of pinch-, nip-, or shear-points at which it is possible to be caught between the moving parts of a machine or between the materials and the moving parts of a machine.

Malpractice: A type of negligence that involves professional misconduct or unreasonable lack of skill.

Managed care: Any form of health plan that initiates selective contracting between providers, employers, and insurers to channel employees/patients to a specified set of cost-effective providers (a provider network); these providers have procedures in place to ensure that only medically necessary and appropriate use of health care services occurs.

Multiple chemical sensitivity: A condition that has been described as a chemically-induced immune system dysfunction, a low-grade yeast infection, a psychologic response to low-level chemical exposures, antioxidant vitamin deficiencies, and various other causes.

Negligence: The failure to perform one's duties according to acceptable standards.

Net national product: The gross national product less capital consumption allowance (allocated costs for depreciation of capital equipment).

Noise exposure assessment: Measurements of sound-pressure levels, expressed in terms of decibels (dB).

Occupational and environmental health nursing: The specialty practice that "provides for and delivers health and safety programs and services to workers, worker populations and community groups. The practice focuses on promotion and restoration of health, prevention of illness and injury and protection from work related and environmental hazards" (http://www.aaohn.org/press_room/fact_sheets/profession.cfm).

Occupational health surveillance: The "process of monitoring the health status of worker populations to gather data on the effects of workplace exposures and using data to prevent injury and illness" (AAOHN, 2004b).

Occupational illness: Any abnormal condition or disorder, other than one resulting from an occupational injury, caused by exposure to environmental factors associated with employment.

Occupational injury: Any injury, such as a cut, fracture, sprain, or amputation, that results from a single incident in the work environment.

Permissible exposure limits: Standards promulgated by the Occupational Safety and Health Administration that refer to 8-hour, time-weighted averages of airborne exposure to a hazard over 5 working days per week.

Personal protective equipment: Devices, such as respirators, gloves, or special clothing and shoes, that are worn by workers to protect against hazards in the workplace.

Prevalence rate: An epidemiologic term that describes the proportion of the population that has a particular condition at a given time or during a given period.

Primary care: The provision of integrated, accessible health care services by clinicians who are accountable for addressing a large majority of personal health care needs, developing a sustained partnership with patients, and practicing in the context of family and community (Donaldson, Yordy, & Vanselow, 1994).

Primary prevention: Health promotion and health protection measures that prevent the occurrence of disease.

Privatization: A system in which government services are sold or transferred to private businesses and corporations.

Process safety review: A careful evaluation of what could go wrong and what safeguards must be implemented to prevent hazardous chemical releases, explosions, or other process accidents.

Quantity reduction: Reducing the amount of hazardous substances on hand by storing only those amounts that will actually be needed and consumed in a reasonable time, rather than storing large amounts of material over long periods of time. Reducing the amount stored reduces the potential hazard in the event of a leak, spill, or release.

Risk: The possibility of injury or illness occurring.

Screening: Testing people who are as yet asymptomatic for the purpose of classifying them with respect to their likelihood of having a particular disease.

Secondary prevention: Early detection and treatment of disease so that its progression is slowed or its complications limited; *screening* is a secondary prevention measure.

Self-contained breathing apparatus: Respirable air carried in a tank on the back of the user.

Sentinel health event—occupational: A preventable disease, disability, or untimely death that is occupationally related and whose occurrence may: (1) provide the impetus for epidemiologic or industrial hygiene studies; or (2) serve as a warning signal that materials substitution, engineering control, personal protection, or health care may be required.

Site survey/walk-through: A worksite inspection not related to any particular incident, area, or piece of equipment.

Standard industrial classification (SIC): Reference to a four-digit number used by the Bureau of Labor Statistics to classify industries according to type.

Standards of care: Actions that the average, reasonable, and prudent health care provider would perform in similar circumstances; also known as "reasonable and customary care."

Standards of nursing practice: Standards developed by professional nursing associations to guide practice and provide practitioners with a framework for evaluating practice.

Tertiary prevention: The prevention of disability; includes rehabilitative efforts.

Threshold limit values: Guidelines for rating exposure to hazardous substances that are developed by the American Conference of Governmental Industrial Hygienists; they are published annually by that organization and generally refer to 8 hours of time-weighted average exposure in a 5-day week.

Toxic Substances Control Act: A law that requires documentation of worker allegations of previously unrecognized adverse health effects from new chemicals, mixtures, or processes.

Toxicology: The study of adverse effects of chemicals on biologic systems.

Work-conditioning, or work-hardening, program: A "highly structured, goal-oriented, individualized treatment program designed to maximize the person's ability to return to work" (Commission on Accreditation of Rehabilitation Facilities, 1991).

Workers' compensation: A publicly funded insurance system that provides for lost wages, medical costs, and rehabilitation for persons who experience an occupational injury or illness.

Workplace violence: Harassment, threats, and actual physical assaults in the workplace.

REFERENCES

American Association of Occupational Health Nurses (2004a). *Advisory: Case management*. Atlanta, GA: AAOHN Publications.

American Association of Occupational Health Nurses (2004b). *AAOHN position statement: Occupational health surveillance*. Atlanta, GA: AAOHN Publications.

American Nurses Association (2005). *Informatics nurse certification*. American Nurses Certification Center. Retrieved February 13, 2005 from http://nursingworld.org/ancc/certification/cert/certs/informatics.html.

Centers for Disease Control and Prevention (CDC) (2005). Environmental health page. Definition retrieved March 11, 2005 from http://www.cdc.gov/node.do/id/0900f3ec8000e044.

Commission on Accreditation of Rehabilitation Facilities (1991). *Standards manual for organizations serving people with disabilities*. Tucson, AZ: Commission on Accreditation of Rehabilitation Facilities.

Donaldson, M., Yordy, K., & Vanselow, N. (Eds.). (1994). *Defining primary care: An interim report*. Washington, DC: National Academy Press.

Institute of Medicine (1995). *Nursing, health and the environment: Strengthening the relationship to improve the public's health*. Washington, DC: National Academy Press.

APPENDIX

III

Acronyms

AACN: American Association of Colleges of Nursing

AAIN: American Association of Industrial Nurses (AAOHN's name until 1977)

AAOHN: American Association of Occupational Health Nurses, Inc.

ABOHN: American Board for Occupational Health Nurses, Inc.

ACGIH: American Conference of Governmental Industrial Hygienists

ACOEM: American College of Occupational and Environmental Medicine

ADA: Americans with Disabilities Act

AED: Automatic external defibrillator

AFL: American Federation of Labor

AIHA: American Industrial Hygiene Association

ANA: American Nurses Association

ANSI: American National Standards Institute

APHA: American Public Health Association

ASSE: American Society of Safety Engineers

ATSDR: Agency for Toxic Substances and Disease Registry

BLS: Bureau of Labor Statistics (USDL)

BPR: Business process reengineering

CAOHC: Council for Accreditation in Occupational Hearing Conservation

CARF: Commission on Accreditation of Rehabilitation Facilities

CCM: Certified Case Manager

CDC: Centers for Disease Control and Prevention

CDL: Commercial driver's license

CFR: Code of Federal Regulations

CIO: Council of Industrial Organizations

CISD: critical incident stress debriefing

CLIA: Clinical Laboratory Improvement Amendments

CO: Carbon monoxide

COBRA: Consolidated Omnibus Budget Reconciliation Act

COHC: Certified Occupational Hearing Conservationist

COHN: Certified Occupational Health Nurse

COHN/CM: Certified Occupational Health Nurse/Case Manager

COHN-S: Certified Occupational Health Nurse-Specialist

COHN-S/CM: Certified Occupational Health Nurse-Specialist/Case Manager

COHN/SM: Occupational Health Nurse/Safety Manager

COHN-S/SM: Occupational Health Nurse-Specialist/Safety Manager

CPI: Consumer Price Index

CPR: Cardiopulmonary resuscitation

CPWR: Center to Protect Workers' Rights

CQI: Continuous quality improvement

CTD: Cumulative trauma disorder

dB: Decibel

dBA: A sound-pressure measurement derived by using an A-weighted scale that combines frequency with intensity

D-C: Demand-control

DFW: Drug-Free Workplace Act

DI: Disposable income

DOE: Department of Energy

DOT: Department of Transportation

EAP: Employee assistance program

EBD: Evidential breathing device

EBRI: Employee Benefit Research Institute

EBT: Evidential breath testing

EEOC: Equal Employment Opportunity Commission

EPA: Environmental Protection Agency

ERC: Education and Research Center (funded by NIOSH)

ERISA: Employment Retirement Income Security Act

FAA: Federal Aviation Administration

FDA: Food and Drug Administration

FFDCA: Federal Food, Drug and Cosmetic Act

FHWA: Federal Highway Administration

FIFRA: Federal Insecticide, Fungicide, and Rodenticide Act

FLSA: Fair Labor Standards Act

FMCSA: Federal Motor Carrier Safety Administration

FMEA: Failure mode and effect analysis

FMLA: Family and Medical Leave Act

FRA: Federal Railroad Administration

FTA: Federal Transit Administration

FTE: Full-time equivalent

GAO: Government Accounting Office

GATT: General Agreement for Trade and Tariffs

GIS: Geographic information system

GNP: Gross national product

HazCom: Hazard communication

HazMat: Hazardous materials

HAZOP: Hazard and operability

HCFA: Health Care Financing Administration

HCP: Hearing conservation program

HCS: Hazard Communication Standard (29 CFR 1910, 1915, 1917, 1918, 1926, 1928)

HCW: Health care worker

HEDIS: Health Plan Employer Data Information Set

HEPA: High efficiency particle air

HIPAA: Health Insurance Portability and Accountability Act

HLPP: Hearing-loss prevention program

HMO: Health maintenance organization

HPD: Hearing protection device

Hz: Hertz

ICOH: International Commission on Occupational Health

ILO: International Labour Organization

IMS: Information management system

INS: Informatics nurse specialist

IPA: Independent practice association

ISO: International Organization for Standardization

JCAHO: Joint Commission for Accreditation of Health Care Organizations

JSA: Job safety analysis

LC_{50}: Lethal concentration, 50%

LD_{50}: Lethal dose, 50%

MCS: Multiple chemical sensitivity

MRI: Magnetic resonance imaging

MRO: Medical review officer

MSDS: Material safety data sheet

NAFTA: North American Free Trade Act

NAS: National Academy of Science

NCEH: National Center for Environmental Health

NCQA: National Committee for Quality Assurance

NGO: Nongovernmental organization

NHTSA: National Highway Traffic Safety Administration

NIDA: National Institute of Drug Abuse

NIEHS: National Institute of Environmental Health Sciences

NIHL: Noise-induced hearing loss

NINR: National Institute for Nursing Research

NIOSH: National Institute for Occupational Safety and Health

NRC: National Research Council

NRR: Noise reduction rating

NSC: National Safety Council

OHNAC: Occupational Health Nurse in Agricultural Communities

OSH Act: Occupational Safety and Health Act (1970)

OSHA: Occupational Safety and Health Administration

OSHRC: Occupational Safety and Health Review Commission

OTC: Over-the-counter

PCP: Primary care provider

P-E: Person-environment

PEL: Permissible exposure limits (OSHA exposure limits)

POS: Point-of-service

PPE: Personal protective equipment

PPI: Producer Price Index

ppm: Parts per million

PPO: Preferred provider organization

PT: Physical therapy

RCRA: Resource Conservation and Recovery Act

REL: Recommended exposure level

RFC: Residual functional capacity

RSD: Reflex sympathetic dystrophy

RSPA: Research and Special Programs Administration

RTW: Return-to-work

SAMHSA: Substance Abuse and Mental Health Services Administration

SARA: Superfund Amendments and Reauthorization Act (1986)

SHE-O: Sentinel health event–occupational

SIC: Standard industrial classification

SSDI: Social Security Disability Insurance

STD: Sexually transmitted disease

STEL: Short-term exposure levels

STS: Standard threshold shift (also referred to as significant threshold shift)

TCM: Telephonic case management

TLD: Thermal luminescent dosimeter

TLV: Threshold limit value (ACGIH-recommended exposure limit)

TPA: Third-party administrator

TQM: Total quality management

TSCA: Toxic Substances Control Act

TTS: Temporary threshold shift

TWA: Time-weighted average

USDOC: United States Department of Census

USDA: United States Department of Agriculture

USDHHS: United States Department of Health and Human Services

USDL: United States Department of Labor

USDL, BLS: United States Department of Labor, Bureau of Labor Statistics

USPHS: United States Public Health Services

UV: Ultraviolet

VPP: Voluntary Protection Program (OSHA)

WB: Women's Bureau (USDL)

WBS: Work breakdown structure

WHO: World Health Organization

WMSD: Work-related musculoskeletal disorder

APPENDIX

IV

Websites

Agency for Toxic Substance and Disease Registry: http://www.atsdr.cdc.gov

Airline safety information: http://www.airsafe.com

American Association of Occupational Health Nurses: http://www.aaohn.org

American Board of Independent Medical Examiners: http://www.abime.org

American Board for Occupational Health Nurses: http://www.abohn.org

American College of Occupational and Environmental Medicine: http://www.acoem.org

American Conference of Governmental Industrial Hygienists: http://www. acgih.org

American Industrial Hygiene Association: http://www.aiha.org

American National Standards Institute: http://www.ansi.org

American Public Health Association: http://www.apha.org

American Society of Safety Engineers: http://www.asse.org

Association of Occupational and Environmental Clinics: http://www.aoec.org

Association of Occupational Health Professionals: http://www.podi.com/aohp

Bureau of Labor Statistics: http://www.bls.gov

Case Management Society of America: http://www.cmsa.org

CCH Annual Unscheduled Absence Survey: http://www.cch.com/hr

CCOHS Health & Safety Internet Directory: http://www.ccohs.ca/resources/occupati.html

Centers for Disease Control and Prevention: http://www.cdc.gov

Centers for Medicare & Medicaid Management: http://www.cms.gov

Children's Environmental Health Network: http://www.cehn.org

CHEMTREC: http://www.cwc-chemical.com

Council for Accreditation on Occupational Hearing loss: http://www.caohc.org

CTD News. Workplace solutions for repetitive stress injuries online: http://www.ctdnews.com

Disability Fact Book: http://www.jhaweb.com

ErgoWeb—the Place for Ergonomics: http://www.ergoweb.com

ErgoResources: http://www.ergoresources.org/

Enviro-Net: http://www.enviro-net.com

Human Factors and Ergonomics Society: http://hfes.org/HFES.html

Institute for Health & Productivity: http://www.ihpm.org

Institute of Medicine (IOM): http://www.iom.edu

Integrated Benefits Institute: http://www.ibiweb.org

Mercer/March Employer's Time Off & Disability Programs: http://www.mercerHR.com

National Archives and Records Administration: Federal Register: http://www.gpoaccess.gov/fr/index.html

National Association of County and City Health Officials: http://www.naccho.org

National Center for Health Statistics: http://www.cdc.gov/nchs/fastats/osh.htm

National Environmental Education and Training Foundation: http://www.neetf.org

National Institute for Occupational Safety and Health: http://www.cdc.gov/niosh

National Institute of Environmental Health Sciences: http://www.niehs.nih.gov

National Library of Medicine: http://www.nlm.nih.gov

National Safety Council: http://www.nsc.org

National Pesticide Telecommunications Network: http://ace.orst.edu/info/nptn

Occupational Safety and Health Administration: http://www.osha.gov

Occupational Health Clinics: http://www.aoec.org

Office of Homeland Security: http://www.dhs.gov

Society of Occupational and Environmental Health: http://www.soeh.org

Travel Health Information: http://www.cdc.gov/travel/

Travel Tips, Health and Safety: http://www.prevmed.com

U.S. Department of Labor: http://www.dol.gov

U.S. Department of Health and Human Services: http://www.hhs.gov

U.S. Department of Transportation: http://www.dot.gov

U.S. Department of Travel Warning and Consular Information: http://www.travel.state.gov

U.S. Environmental Protection Agency: http://www.epa.gov

Watson Wyatt Annual Staying@Work Survey: http://www.watsonwyatt.com

APPENDIX

V

Occupational Safety and Health Administration Act of 1970

To assure so far as possible every working man and woman in the Nation safe and healthful working conditions and to preserve our human resources.

1. By encouraging employers and employees in their efforts to reduce the number of occupational safety and health hazards at their places of employment, and to stimulate employers and employees to institute new and to perfect existing programs for providing safe and healthful working conditions;

2. By providing that employers and employees have separate but dependent responsibilities and rights with respect to achieving safe and healthful working conditions;

3. By authorizing the Secretary of Labor to set mandatory occupational safety and health standards applicable to businesses affecting interstate commerce, and by creating an Occupational Safety and Health Review Commission for carrying out adjudicatory functions under the Act;

4. By building upon advances already made through employer and employee initiative for providing safe and healthful working conditions;

5. By providing for research in the field of occupational safety and health, including the psychological factors involved, and by developing innovative methods, techniques, and approaches for dealing with occupational safety and health problems;

6. By exploring ways to discover latent diseases, establishing causal connections between diseases and work in environmental conditions, and conducting other research relating to health problems, in recognition of the fact that occupational health standards present problems often different from those involved in occupational safety;

7. By providing medical criteria which will assure insofar as practicable that no employee will suffer diminished health, functional capacity, or life expectancy as a result of his work experience;

8. By providing for training programs to increase the number and competence of personnel engaged in the field of occupational safety and health;

9. By providing for the development and promulgation of occupational safety and health standards;

10. By providing an effective enforcement program which shall include a prohibition against giving advance notice of any inspection and sanctions for any individual violating this prohibition;

11. By encouraging the States to assume the fullest responsibility for the administration and enforcement of their occupational safety and health laws by

providing grants to the States to assist in identifying their needs and respon-sibilities in the area of occupational safety and health, to develop plans in accordance with the provisions of this Act, to improve the administration and enforcement of State occupational safety and health laws, and to conduct experimental and demonstration projects in connection therewith;

12. By providing for appropriate reporting procedures with respect to occupa-tional safety and health procedures which will help achieve the objectives of this Act and accurately describe the nature of the occupational safety and health problem;

13. By encouraging joint labor-management effort to reduce injuries and disease arising out of employment.

Competencies in Occupational and Environmental Health Nursing*

AAOHN has identified nine categories of competencies for occupational and environmental health nurses.

- Clinical and Primary Care

- Case Management

- Work Force, Workplace and Environmental Issues

- Regulatory/Legislative

- Management

- Health Promotion and Disease Prevention

- Occupational and Environmental Health and Safety Education and Training

- Research

- Professionalism

Three levels of performance criteria have been developed for each competency:

- *Competent*: The occupational and environmental health nurse's role is one of mastery and an ability to cope with specific situations.

- *Proficient*: The nurse perceives the client situation as a whole based on previous experience, focusing on relevant aspects of a situation.

- *Expert*: The nurse has extensive experience and a broad knowledge base and is able to grasp a situation quickly and initiate appropriate action.

*The complete text of AAOHN's Competencies in Occupational and Environmental Health Nursing, including the performance criteria, can be obtained from AAOHN.

APPENDIX

VII

Standards of Occupational and Environmental Health Nursing*

Standard I: Assessment

The occupational and environmental health nurse systematically assesses the health status of the client(s).

Standard II: Diagnosis

The occupational and environmental health nurse analyzes assessment data to formulate diagnoses.

Standard III: Outcome Identification

The occupational and environmental health nurse identifies outcomes specific to the client.

Standard IV: Planning

The occupational and environmental health nurse develops a goal-directed plan that is comprehensive and formulates interventions to attain expected outcomes.

Standard V: Implementation

The occupational and environmental health nurse implements interventions to attain desired outcomes identified in the plan.

Standard VI: Evaluation

The occupational and environmental health nurse systematically and continuously evaluates responses to interventions and progress toward the achievement of desired outcomes.

Standard VII: Resource Management

The occupational and environmental health nurse secures and manages the resources that support occupational health and safety programs and services.

Standard VIII: Professional Development

The occupational and environmental health nurse assumes accountability for professional development to enhance professional growth and maintain competency.

*The complete text of AAOHN's Standards of Occupational and Environmental Health Nursing can be obtained from AAOHN (www.aaohn.org).

Standard IX: Collaboration

The occupational and environmental health nurse collaborates with clients for the promotion, prevention, and restoration of health within the context of a safe and healthy environment.

Standard X: Research

The occupational and environmental health nurse uses research findings in practice and contributes to the scientific base in occupational and environmental health nursing to improve practice and advance the profession.

Standard XI: Ethics

The occupational and environmental health nurse uses an ethical framework as a guide for decision making in practice.

APPENDIX

VIII

American Association of Occupational Health Nurses' Code of Ethics*

Occupational and environmental health nurses:

- Provide healthcare in the work environment with regard for human dignity and client rights, unrestricted by consideration of social economic status, personal attributes, or the nature of the health status.

- Promote interdisciplinary collaboration with other professionals and community agencies in order to meet the health needs of the client.

- Strive to safeguard employees' rights to privacy by protecting confidential information and releasing information only upon written consent of the employee or as required or permitted by law.

- Through the provision of care, strive to provide quality care and to safeguard clients from unethical and illegal actions.

- Licensed to provide health care services, accept obligations to society as professionals and responsible members of the community.

- Maintain individual competence in health nursing practice, based on scientific knowledge, and recognize and accept responsibility for individual judgements and action, while complying with appropriate laws and regulation (local, state, and federal) that impact the delivery of occupational and environmental health services.

- Participate, as appropriate in activities such as research that contribute to the ongoing development of the profession's body of knowledge while protecting the rights of subjects.

*The complete text of AAOHN's Code of Ethics, including the preamble and interpretive statements, can be obtained from AAOHN.

APPENDIX

IX

Legislation Related to Occupational Health and Safety

1936 Walsh-Healy Act

1938 Federal Food, Drug and Cosmetic Act (FFDCA)

1947 Federal Insecticide, Fungicide, and Rodenticide Act (FIFRA)

1948 Federal Water Pollution Control Act (later called the Clean Water Act)

1955 Clean Air Act

1965 Shoreline Erosion Protection Act

1966 Solid Waste Disposal Act

1969 Federal Coal Mine and Safety Act

1969 National Environmental Policy Act (NEPA)

1970 Consumer Product Safety Act (CPSC)

1970 Clean Air Act (amended 1977)

1970 Federal Railroad Safety Act (amended 1974, 1975, 1976) (DOT)

1970 Hazardous Materials Transportation Control Act (amended 1975, 1976) (DOT)

1970 Occupational Safety and Health Act (OSH Act)

1970 Pollution Prevention Packaging Act

1970 Resource Recovery Act

1971 Lead-Based Paint Poisoning Prevention Act

1971 Coastal Zone Management Act

1972 Marine Protection, Research, and Sanctuaries Act

1972 Ocean Dumping Act

1972 Noise Control Act

1972 Federal Water Pollution Act (amended and renamed Clean Water Act in 1977)

1972 Federal Insecticide, Fungicide, and Rodenticide Act

1973 Rehabilitation Act (EEOC)

1973   Endangered Species Act

1974   Safe Drinking Water Act (amended 1977)

1974   Shoreline Erosion Control Demonstration Act

1974   Employee Retirement Income Security Act

1975   Hazardous Materials Transportation Act

1976   Resource Conservation and Recovery Act (RCRA)

1976   Toxic Substances Control Act (TSCA)

1977   Surface Mining Control and Reclamation Act

1978   Lead Standard

1978   Cotton Dust Standard

1978   Uranium Mill-Tailings Radiation Control Act

1980   Asbestos School Hazard Emergency Response Act

1980   Carcinogens Standard

1980   Comprehensive Environmental Response, Compensation, and Liability Act (CERCLA or Superfund)

1982   Nuclear Waste Policy Act

1983   Noise Standard

1984   Asbestos School Hazard Abatement Act

1986   Asbestos Hazard Emergency Response Act

1986   Superfund Amendments and Reauthorization Act (SARA)

1986   Emergency Planning and Community Right-to-Know Act (EPCRA)

1986   Consolidated Omnibus Budget Reconciliation Act (COBRA)

1987   Clean Water Act Reauthorization

1988   Indoor Radon Abatement Act

1988   Lead Contamination Control Act

1988   Medical Waste Tracking Act

1988   Ocean Dumping Ban Act

1988   Shore Protection Act

1990   National Environmental Education Act

1990   Clean Air Act Amendment

1990   Oil Prevention Act (OPA)

1990   Pollution Prevention Act (PPA)

1990   Americans with Disabilities Act

1991   Omnibus Transportation Employee Testing Act

1993   Family Medical Leave Act

1994   North American Free Trade Act (NAFTA)

1996   Food Quality Protection Act (FQPA)

1996   Health Insurance Portability and Accountability Act, 1996

1999   Chemical Safety Information, Site Security and Fuels Regulatory Act

2002   Homeland Security Act

INDEX

A

Absenteeism, 110
Accidents, 429
Accreditation, 535, 536b
Acronyms, 557-561
Active surveillance, 488
Addiction behaviors, 424
Adjusted (standardized) rates, 126
Administrative controls
  for hazards associated with WMSDs, 489-490
  for noise exposure, 477
  for occupational exposures, 143
  prevention and control approaches focusing on, 279-285
Adult education
  central principles of, 433
  effective presentations, 437, 441-448
  motivating adults to learn, 436-437
  philosophies of, 434-436
  self-directed learning, 433-434
  teaching methods and techniques, 437, 438t-440t
Adult health risk profile, 318-321
Adult preventive care flow sheet, 314-317
Advanced practice nursing, 295
Advocacy
  for children in workforce, 46-47
  for community populations served, 542-543
  environmental, 160-161
  for the practice, 542
Age of workers, 42-44
Aging, as endogenous factor, 133-134
Agricultural workers, 53-56
Airborne contaminants, 143
Alcohol use
  CAGE questionnaire, 425b
  drug and alcohol programs, 499-506
All-Hazard Disaster Management Plan, 373
Alternative workers, 48-50

American Association of Occupational Health Nurses (AAOHN), 533-534
  behavioral objectives, 435b
  position on ethics, 95
  professional mandates for research, 519
American Board for Occupational Health Nurses, 536-537
American Board of Nursing Specialties, 536b
Americans with Disabilities Act (ADA), 49, 77-79, 486
Analytic studies in epidemiology, 127
Antagonism between toxins, 132
Arsenic, 134-135
Asbestos, 137
Asphyxiants, 130, 140-141
Assembly work, 145
Assessment
  environmental health, 155-158
  as first step in case management process, 340-342
  of noise exposure, 269, 476-477
  of occupational health and safety programs, 237-239
  of occupational injury and illness, 23-24
  qualitative and observational, of work site, 141
  vulnerability assessment, 374-375
Assumption-of-risk defense, 13
Asthma, 159, 173
Atmospheric monitoring, 269-270
Attributable risk, 125
Audiometric testing, 480-482
Audiovisuals, 442-443
Authorization letter, 89
Automatic systems, 275-276

B

Back injury, 144
Balance of trade, 102-103
Behavior change theories, 416-420
Behavioral sciences, 149-150
Behavioral theories, 188-189
Benchmarking, 206-207
Benefits
  cash, 331-332
  definition of, 331
  of disaster planning and preparedness in workplace, 370-371

Benefits—cont'd
  health care, 36
  indemnity, 332
  for nonoccupational illness and injury, 357-359
  workers' compensation, 94-95, 111
Benzene, 138
Beryllium, 135-136
Best practices in record keeping, 87-88
Bias in epidemiologic studies, 127-128
Biologic hazards
  challenges to prevention of, 18
  in health care industry, 60, 61t
Biologic weapons, 391-393
Biosafety cabinet, 292
Biosafety levels for infectious agents, 291t
Biotransformation, 133
Bisphenol A exposure, 160
Black lung, 138
Body mass index, 426, 427t
Brainstorming, 437
Brownfields, 176
Budgeting
  methods for, 192
  steps in process of, 192-193
Buildings, high-rise, 388
Business Continuity Plan, 371-372
Business plan, 251-252
Business Process Reengineering, 189
Business travel, health and safety education for, 508-510
Businesses
  day-to-day communication, 202-203
  employers' trends affecting, 110
  health and safety program implementation, barriers to, 242
  megatrends, 108-109
  regulatory constraints on, 109-110
  risk of attack, 39
  21st century issues, 109
  and technology explosion, 109
  and workers' compensation, 111

C

Cadmium, 136
CAGE questionnaire, 425b
Campaigning approaches, 161

Page numbers in *italic* indicate figures; those followed by t indicate tables, and by b, boxes.

Cancellation/discontinuation of program, 252
Cancer awareness, 429
Capital expenditure budgets, 192
Capitalism, 101
Carbamates, 140
Carbon disulfide, 138
Carbon monoxide, 141, 175
Carcinogens, 130
Case advocacy, 160
Case management
　disability. *See* Disability case management
　onsite, 360-361
　outcome and cost savings, 248
　in program evaluation, 245-246
　telephonic, 361-362
　tertiary prevention related to, 323
Case manager role, 28, 540
Case study, as teaching method, 437, 439t
Case-control study, 127
Cash benefits, 331-332
Centers for Disease Control (CDC), 167-168
Centers for Medicare and Medicaid Services (CMS), 83
Certification, 536-537
Certified Occupational Health Nurse, 537
Certified Occupational Health Nurse-Specialist, 537
Cervical spine injury, 144
Chain-of-custody procedures, 503-504
Chaos theory, 187, 189
Characteristic-specific rates, 125
Charts used in presentations, 446b
Chemical hazards
　forms and effects of, 17-18
　and hazard communication program, 494
　to health care workers, 60-61
Chemical inventories, 262-263
Chemicals
　asphyxiants, 140-141
　exposure to, 153-154
　multiple chemical sensitivity, 273
　toxicity criteria for, 130
　transformation of, 133
　as weapons, 394-396
Children
　and environmental health, 158-160
　in workforce, 44-48
Chromium, 136
Class action suits, 161
Class advocacy, 160
Clean Air Act, 165

Client-centered information management systems, 216-217
Clinical decision making, 307-309
Clinical Laboratory Improvement Amendments (CLIA), 82-83
Clinician role, 28
Coaching, as staff development activity, 198-199
Coal dust exposure, 138
Cognitive conflict, 194
Cohort study, 127
Cold environmental conditions, 145
Collaboration
　with external agencies, 542
　multidisciplinary, 3-4
Collaborative approaches, 161
Common law, 71
Communicable diseases, 511-512
Communication. *See also* Hazard communication program
　about environmental risks, 164-165
　delivery of a presentation, 446-448
　as immediate cause of incidents, 262b
　as major disaster response need, 383
　skills in, 200-205
　strategies, as emergency procedures, 400-401
　systems, in office management programs, 229-230
Communism, 101
Community
　advocacy for community populations served, 542-543
　environmental risks in, 175-179
　health services for, 24-25
　international, occupational health and safety programs in, 15-17
Competency
　general environmental health, 179-180
　in occupational and environmental health nursing, 25, 337, 537-538
Competitiveness, national and global, 105-106
Comprehensive containment approaches
　administrative elements, 290, 292
　engineering elements, 290
Comprehensive Environmental Response, Compensation, and Liability Act, 165
Compression disorders, 144

Computer-enhanced education, 437
Concurrent document review, 248
Confidence interval, 126
Confidentiality
　considered in health and safety programs, 251
　as ethical responsibility, 96-97
　in research, 521
　of worker health information, 231-232
Conflict resolution, 201-202
Conflict-related hazards, 389-390
Conflicts of interest, 97-99
Confounding in epidemiologic studies, 128-129
Consistency of the association, 124
Construction workers, 56-58
Consultant role, 28, 542
Consultation services by OSHA, 76
Consumer price index (CPI), 101
Consumer Product Safety Commission, 168
Contaminants
　airborne, 143
　drinking water, 177
　indoor air, 173
　industrial, 169-170
Contest strategies, 161
Contingency Plan, 372
Contingency theory, 189
Contingent workers, 48-50
Continuing education, 539
Continuous monitors, 271
Continuous quality improvement, 204-205, 328
Contributory negligence, 13
Control strategies for occupational exposures, 143
Corporate director, 28
Correlational research, 524
Corrosives, 130
Cost evaluations for health and safety programs, 249-250
Counseling services, 29
Countermeasures in injury epidemiology, 147-148
Covered entity, 92
Credentialing in nursing, 534-537
Critical thinking, 193
Cross-sectional study, 127
Crude rates, 125
Customer service, 209
Cutaneous route of exposure, 131-132

D
Data analysis
　and data collection, 525-526, 529
　as step in case management process, 342-343

Data sources in epidemiology, 124-125
Decision making
  clinical, 307-309
  in management process, 193-194
Deductible, 332
Delayed recovery, indicators of, 340b
Demand-control model, 463
Demographic and social trends
  implications for occupational and environmental health nurse, 41
  supportive and explanatory data on, 35-37
Demonstration, as teaching method, 437, 439t
Department of Agriculture (USDA), 166
Department of Defense (DOD), 167
Department of Energy (DOE), 167
Department of Health and Human Services (DHHS), 167-168
Department of Transportation (DOT), 79-82, 166
Descriptive studies, 524
  in epidemiology, 127
Developing countries, 15-17
Diagnosis
  formulation of, 342
  of illness, early, 322-323
Diet and health promotion, 426
Direct care
  clinical decision making in, 307-309
  evaluating outcomes, 323, 328
  health history, 300-302
  knowledge needs for, 298-300
  levels of prevention applied to, 310-313, 322-323
  physical examination, 302-306
  practice guidelines, 309-310
  primary emphasis of, 298
  professional practice concepts, 295-296
  range of services, 296-298
  resources for, 549-550
Disability case management
  assessment step, 340-342
  data analysis and formulation of diagnoses, 342
  delivery models, 360-362
  evaluation step, 343-345
  federal acts affecting, 360
  historical perspective, 333-337
  implementation step, 343
  important terms in, 331-333
  integrated disability management programs, 359-360
  planning step, 342-343

Disability case management—cont'd
  practice settings and providers, 337
  return to work, 345-359
  team roles and responsibilities, 338-340
Disability classifications, 95
Disability management, 323
  integrated, 114
Disabled workers, 51-53
Disaster planning and preparedness, 369-377
  appendices to include in written plan, 405-406
  emergency preparedness/ disaster management plan, 397-405
  hazard-specific considerations
    conflict-related, 389-390
    natural, 386-387
    technologic, 387-389
    for terrorism, 390-397
Disaster response
  command post, 381
  communications, 383
  defensive or offensive, 378
  emergency operations center, 381
  evacuation of facility, 383-384
  first response, 378
  Incident Command System, 379-380
  including environmental protection considerations, 384
  magnitude-appropriate activities, 378-379
  National Incident Management System, 379
  news media and, 382
  notification stage, 377-378
  reduction of legal liability and, 381-382
  resources, 382-383
Disasters
  Disaster Life Cycle model, 367
  emergencies, 366-367
  events, 365-366
  Jennings Disaster Nursing Management Model, 367-369
  recovery from, 385-386
  timeline model for, 367
Discussions, as teaching method, 437, 438t
Disposable income, 101
Distance education, 437
Documentation
  important characteristics of, 83-84
  pertaining to ergonomics program, 492-493
  of progress toward standards of performance, 204

Documentation—cont'd
  purposes of, 83
  regular evaluation of, 247
Dose of agent, 130-131
Dose-response relationship, 124, 132
Dosimetry, personal, 270
Drinking water, safe and reliable, 177
Drug and alcohol programs
  drug testing program, 502-505
  employee assistance programs, 505
  establishing drug-free workplace, 500-502
  mandated, 499-500
  and return to duty, 506
  training and education, 505-506
Drug-Free Workplace Act of 1988, 499-501
Dusts, respirable, 137-138

E
Ear anatomy, 479
Earning capacity, 332
Earthquakes, 387
Ecologic stress model, 464-465
Ecologic study, 127
Economic impacts
  on individual, 104-105
  of occupational injury and illness, 22
  of stress, 462
Economic indicators, 102
Economics
  balance of trade, 102-103
  key terms in, 101-102
  of United States, 103
Education
  academic, in safety and health, 538
  adult, 433-448
  for children in workforce, 47
  continuing, 539
  distance, 437
  in drug and alcohol programs, 505-506
  in ergonomics program, 491
  health and safety, for travel, 508-510
  incorporation of environmental health concepts, 180-181
  level of, research roles by, 519-520
  specialized, 29
  of workers, in hearing loss prevention, 477-479
Educator role, 28
Effects of toxins, 132
Effort-reward imbalance model, 463
Electronic databases, 522b

Elimination or substitution, as control strategy, 274
E-mail, 229, 230b
Emergencies, 366-367
Emergency Action Plan, 371
Emergency Management Plan, 372-373
Emergency operations center, 381
Emergency preparedness, 283
Emergency preparedness/disaster management plan
  annual review and update of, 404-405
  emergency procedures as part of, 400-403
  purposes of, 397-398
  recovery procedures, 403-404
  requiring input from multiple sources, 398-400
  site specificity of, 398
Emergency response
  operations, 284
  planning, 246-247
  team drills, 404
Emergency Response Plan, 372
Emotional intelligence, 185-186
Employee Assistance Programs (EAPs), 505
  external and internal models, 432
  objectives of, 431-432
  role of occupational and environmental health nurse in, 432-433
Employers
  legal defenses for, 13
  responsibilities related to international travel programs, 507
  role in case management process, 339
  trends affecting business, 110
Empowerment, 189
End goals, 190-191
Endogenous factors, 133-134
Engineering controls
  for hazards associated with WMSDs, 489
  for noise exposure, 477
  for occupational exposures, 143
  prevention and control approaches focusing on, 274-279
Entrepreneurial role, 542
Environmental advocacy, 160-161
Environmental assessment at work site, 238
Environmental health
  accessing information and the Right to Know, 169-172
  assessment, 155-158
  chemical, radiologic, and biological risks, 154-155

Environmental health—cont'd
  children and, 158-160
  environmental justice and advocacy, 160-161
  federal agencies, 165-168
  and industrial pollutants, 179
  magnitude of health issues, 153-154
  nurses' roles in, 179-181, 540
  public health infrastructure, 168-169
Environmental health risks
  assessment, 161
  communication, 164-165
  in the community, 175-179
  in the home, 172-174
  management, 161-162
  in schools, 174-175
Environmental justice, 160
Environmental management systems, 285
Environmental Protection Agency (EPA), 165-166
Environmental protection considerations in disaster response, 384
Environments
  community, environmental risks in, 175-179
  home, health risks in, 172-174
  school, environmental risks in, 174-175
  work, 4, 59-61
Epidemic events, 272
Epidemiology
  bias and confounding in studies of, 127-129
  data sources, 124-125
  environmental, 156-157
  inferential statistics, 126
  injury epidemiology, 147-149
  measures of association, 124
  rates, comparisons and types of, 125-126
  screening, 129
  study designs, 126-127
  terms and principles, 123-124
Equipment
  availability of, 239-240
  emergency, 405
  location of, 276
  personal protective, 143, 285-290, 477, 490-491
  respiratory, 288
Ergonomic analysis, 264
Ergonomics
  evaluating risk factors, 145-146
  high-risk jobs, 145
  improvements, 146
  as multidisciplinary science, 483
  terms and principles, 143-144
  work-related musculoskeletal disorders, 144-145, 484-485, 492

Ergonomics programs
  documentation and record keeping, 492-493
  ergonomic regulation and guidelines, 485-486
  evaluation of, 493
  hazard evaluation at workplace, 488-489
  hazard prevention and control, 489-491
  leadership in, 486-487
  management of WMSDs as part of, 492
  occupational health surveillance, 487-488
  purposes of, 486
  training and education, 491
  work site analysis, 487
Ethical issues
  concerning research, 520-521
  definitions and principles of ethics, 96
  ethical conflicts, 96-99
  professional position on ethics, 95
  regarding direct care, 297
  in telephonic case management, 362
Ethylene oxide, 139
Evacuation of facility, 383-384, 401
Evaluation
  audiometric, 481
  in case management process, 343-345
  of ergonomic program, 493
  of ergonomic risk factors, 145-146
  of hazard communication program, 498-499
  of health and safety program, 242-248
  of health promotion programs, 423-424
  of hearing loss protection program, 482-483
  post-travel, for long-term travelers, 512-513
  of psychosocial health interventions, 468
  of research, 528-529
  of work site hazards, 488-489
Evolution
  of occupational and environmental health nursing, 24-25
  of occupational and environmental health nursing practice, 121-123
  of occupational health and safety, 7, 9, 12-13
Ex post facto research, 524
Exclusive remedy, 332
Excretion of toxins, 133

Executive summary of business plan, 251
Exogenous factors, 134
Experimental designs to test research hypotheses, 523
Experimental study designs, 126
Explosive devices, 396-397
Exposure data, 125
Exposure monitoring
   assessment of noise exposure, 269, 476-477
   atmospheric monitoring, 269-270
   continuous monitors, 271
   ionizing and nonionizing radiation monitoring, 270
   sampling, 268-269
   temperature monitoring, 270-271
Exposure records, 86, 88-90, 142
Exposures
   acute and chronic, 131
   to asphyxiants, 140-141
   to chemicals, 153-154, 494
   major routes of
      cutaneous, 131-132
      ingestion, 132
      inhalation, 131
   to metals, 134-137
   occupational
      control strategies for, 143
      health history, 301-302, 303-307
   to pesticides, 140
   potential environmental, 155-156
   to radiation, 393-394
   to respirable dusts, 137-138
   to solvents, 138-140
Extranets, 227
Eye and face protective equipment, 286

F
Facilitating the work of others, 194-200
Fagerstrom test for nicotine dependence, 425
Family and Medical Leave Act (FMLA) of 1993, 79
Farms, supersized, 178
Fate of toxins, 133
Federal Insecticide, Fungicide, and Rodenticide Act, 165
Federal law, 71
Federal Motor Carrier Safety Administration (FMCSA), 79-81
Federal Reserve discount rate, 101
Federal Response Plan, 372
Federalism, increased, 109-110
Feedback, discussed in Task Cycle® Phase 4, 200-205
Fellow servant rule, 13

Female workers
   implications for occupational and environmental health nurses, 41
   supportive and explanatory data on, 40
Fertilizers, 178
Financial budgets, 192
Financial projection in business plan, 252
Fire prevention, 387-388
Firewall, 228
First aid, 87b
Focused inspections, 257-258
Food and Drug Administration (FDA), 166-167
Food pyramid, 426, 428
Food Quality Protection Act, 166
Foot protection, 286-287
Forearm/elbow injury, 144
Formaldehyde, 139
Fractures, risk factor analysis for, 147t
Functional capacity evaluation, 332
Funding of research, 529-531

G
Gatekeeper, 332
Gender, as endogenous factor, 133
General Agreement for Trade and Tariffs (GATT), 107
General contractors, 56
Genetic differences, as endogenous factor, 133
Global marketplace, 107
Global warming, 177
Globalization of trade, 17
Goals
   of business plan, 251-252
   development, for health and safety program, 240-241
   discussed in Task Cycle® Phase 1, 190-191
   national health, 15
   of occupational health and safety, 3-4
   of strategic planning, 186
   Theory of Goal Setting, 419
Government agencies
   and legislation, 8-9b
   and regulatory agencies, 30
Government sources, 547-548
Gross domestic product, 102
Gross national product, 102
Growth opportunities through AAOHN, 534

H
Half-life of toxins, 133
Hand protection, 286
Harassment, as psychosocial hazard, 457
Harm Reduction Model, 416

Hazard communication program
   chemical exposures, 494
   container labeling and warning requirements, 498
   elements of worker training programs, 496
   evaluation of, 498-499
   goals and objectives of, 495
   management roles and responsibilities, 494-495
   MSDSs, 497
   purposes of, 494
   record keeping, 498
   responsibilities of occupational and environmental health nurse, 496
   terminology of, 495
   trade secrets, 498
   training procedures for contract workers, 497
Hazardous energy control, 276-278
Hazardous materials, 388, 403. See also Material safety data sheets (MSDSs)
Hazards
   to agricultural workers, 55t
   assessment of, 23
   biologic, 18, 60, 61t
   chemical, 17-18, 60-61
   construction materials, 57t
   disaster-potential, 365t
   environmental, affecting children, 158-160
   ergonomic: high-risk jobs, 145
   evaluation and analysis, 264-273
   exposure monitoring, 268-271
   identification of, 256-264, 374
   industry standards, 265-267
   mechanical, 18-19
   natural, 386-387
   physical, 17, 62b
   psychologic and emotional, 61
   psychosocial, 19, 453-460
   risk analysis for, 267-268
   technologic, 387-389
   worker populations analysis, 271-273
   workplace, 122, 255-256
      evaluation of, 488-489
Head protection, 287
Health
   determinants of, 122
   goals of, national, 15
   related threats, in international work environment, 509-510
Health Action Process Approach, 420
Health and Productivity Management, 114
Health and safety education for travel, 508-510
Health Belief Model, 413, 415

Health care. *See also* Direct care
  benefits, 36
  24-hour model of, 114
  reform, 113
  services, changes in payment
    for, 334-335
  timely, as goal of RTW
    program, 346, 356
  workers, 58-63
Health care management, for
  WMSDs, 492
Health clinics, onsite, 110
Health history
  comprehensive, 300-301
  limitations of, 302
  for occupational and
    environmental exposure,
    301-302, *303-307*
  problem-specific, 301
Health Insurance Portability and
  Accountability Act of 1996
  (HIPAA), 90-93
Health maintenance organization
  (HMO), 113
Health outcomes
  evaluation of, 323, 328
  resulting from programs and
    services, 247-248
Health promotion
  behavior change theories and
    models, 416-420
  direct care and, 298
  Employee Assistance
    Programs, 431-433
  focuses of, 410
  health models, 413, 415-416
  historical overview, 409
  levels of prevention, 420
  lifestyle and, 424-431
  national objectives of, 413
  program framework, 420-424
  program levels, 412
  and risk reduction, 150
Health Promotion Model, 415
Health Promotion Planning
  Model, 415
Health Resources and Services
  Administration, 168
Health risk appraisal, 422b
Health services
  modern approaches to, 149
  public and community, 24-25
Health services coordinator role,
  28
Health-illness continuum, 465
Healthy People 2010, 15, 16b, 413,
  414t
Hearing loss, noise-induced,
  473-474
  in farm workers, 54
Hearing loss prevention program
  assessment and control of
    noise exposure, 476-477
  audiometric testing, 480-482

Hearing loss prevention
    program—cont'd
  hearing protection devices,
    479-480
  monitoring and evaluation of,
    482-483
  purposes of, 474-475
  roles and responsibilities
    related to, 475-476
  worker training and education,
    477-479
Hearing protection, 286
  devices, 479-480
Heavy and civil engineering
    construction contractors,
    56
n-Hexane, 139
High complexity testing, 83
High-rise buildings, 388
Hippocrates, 4
Historical perspective
  on case management, 333-337
  on health promotion, 409
  on management theories,
    187-189
  on occupational and
    environmental health
    nursing, 24-25, 26b-27b
  on work and occupational
    health, 4-7
History
  health, 300-302, *303-307*
  as part of business plan, 251
Home environments, health risks
    in, 172-174
Homeland Security advisory sys-
    tem recommendations, *39*
Host factors, endogenous and
    exogenous, 133-134
Hours worked, 35
Housekeeping practices, 281
Human relations, 188
Hurricanes, 386-387
Hydrogen cyanide, 141
Hygiene, industrial, 141-143
Hypothesis formulation, 523
Hysteria, epidemic (mass), 272

I
Illness
  early diagnosis and treatment
    of, 322-323
  immediate reporting of, 346
  nonoccupational, benefits for,
    357-359
  prevention of. *See* Prevention
    of occupational injury and
    illness
  reported as Privacy Cases,
    85-86
  work-related, 19-22
Image, of occupational and envi-
    ronmental health nurse,
    209

Immigration impacts on
    workforce, 31-32
Immunizations, 310
Implementation
  of disaster plan, 377
  of health and safety program,
    241-242
  of health promotion program,
    423
  of occupational and
    environmental health
    information system,
    223-224
  of plan for case management,
    343
Incendiary devices, 394
Incidence rate, 123
Incident analysis, 260-261
Incident Command System,
    379-380
Incident historical review,
    261-262
Indemnity benefits, 94-95, 332
Indemnity plan, 332
Independent medical
    examination, 332
Industrial hygiene
  airborne contaminants, 143
  hazard recognition, 141-142
  occupational exposures,
    control strategies for, 143
  sampling methods, 142-143
Industrial hygienists, 4
Industrial nursing, 24
Industrial pollutants, 179
Industrial revolution, 6
Industrial settings for practice, 30
Industry standards in hazard
    identification, 265-267
Infectious agents, recommended
    biosafety levels for, 291t
Inferential statistics in epidemio-
    logy, 126
Information
  on environmental risks,
    accessing, 169-172
  finding on Internet, 225-227
  health: protected, 91-93
  methods for gathering, 248-249
  on occupational injury and
    illness, sources for, 22
  technical, sources for, 547
Information management
  client-centered systems,
    216-217
  implications for occupational
    and environmental health
    nursing, 230-232
  Internet, 224-227
  intranets, 227
  office management programs,
    229-230
  security, 227-229
  selecting systems of, 217-224

Informed consent, 72-73
Infrastructure, public health, 168-169
Ingestion route of exposure, 132
Inhalation route of exposure, 131
Injury
  due to awkward positions, 144-145
  early diagnosis and treatment of, 322-323
  epidemiology of, 147-149
  lost-time, 346
  nonoccupational, benefits for, 357-359
  prevention of. *See* Prevention of occupational injury and illness
  reported as Privacy Cases, 85-86
  WMSDs, 144-145, 484-485, 492
  work-related, 19-22
Inspections
  focused, 257-258
  pre- and post-inspection activities, 256-257
Institute of Medicine, recommendations of, 180-181
Institutional review board, 521
Instructors, motivational, 436
Insurers and third-party administrators, 30, 339
Integrated disability management, 114
Integrated pest management, 174b
Intelligence, emotional, 185-186
Interest rates, 102
International (expatriate) workers, 63-64
International organizations, 16-17, 548
International travel health and safety program
  control of prevalent communicable diseases, 511-512
  health and safety education for travel, 508-510
  international business and workforce, 506-507
  post-travel evaluation for long-term travelers, 512-513
  resources, 548
  roles and responsibilities related to, 507-508
Internet
  finding information on, 225-226
  guidelines for assessing health information on, 226-227
  protocols, 224-225
  terms, 225
  utility of, 226
Interpersonal relationships and work, 452-453

Intervention studies, 126
Intervention wheel, in public health, *120*, 121-122
Interviews
  evaluating ergonomic risk factors, 145
  as method of gathering information, 248-249
  structured, 196
Intranets, 227
Inventories, chemical, 262-263
Ionizing radiation monitoring, 270
Irritants, 130

J
Jennings Disaster Nursing Management Model, 367-369
Jet lag, 513t
Job analysis, 332
Job hazard analysis, 259-260, 488-489
Job safety analysis form, *260*
Job stress, prevention of, 466b
Justice, environmental, 160

K
Kyoto Agreement, 162b

L
Labeling of containers, 498
Labor unions, 9, 12
  role in case management process, 340
  workers in, 50-51
Laboratory testing, 82-83
  in drug and alcohol testing program, 503
Labor-force statistics, 102
Lead exposure, 136, 175
  in children, 159
  in home, 172-173
Leadership
  associated responsibilities, 183-184
  business and industry approaches, 183
  delineated in business plan, 252
  in ergonomics program and services, 486-487
  organizational, levels of, 184
  requiring vision and relationship, 184-186
Learning contracts, 437, 438t
Lectures, 437, 438t
Legal defenses for employers, 13
Legal issues
  access to employee medical and exposure records, 88-90
  ADA legislation, 77-79
  Clinical Laboratory Improvement Amendments (CLIA), 82-83

Legal issues—cont'd
  considered in health and safety programs, 251
  documentation, 83-84
  Family and Medical Leave Act (FMLA) of 1993, 79
  HIPAA, 90-93
  OSH Act (Public Law 91-596), 73-77
  record keeping, 84-88
  regarding direct care, 297-298
  relevant legal concepts, 72-73
  responsibilities of occupational and environmental health nurse, 73
  sources of law, 71-72
  U.S. Department of Transportation, 79-82
  workers' compensation, 93-95
Lethal dose (LD_{50}), 132
Licensure, 535
Lifestyle, 134
  and health promotion, 424-431
Likert scale, 188
Linear change, 186-187
Listening, 201
Literature review
  in research development, 522
  in research evaluation, 528
Litigation, strategies for avoiding, 341b
Lockout/tagout, *279*
Logistical steps in preparing for presentations, 443, 446
Low back pain, RTW for, 349-355

M
Machinery
  farm, 54
  machine guard, *277-278*
Macroeconomics, 102
Malaria, 511-512
Malpractice, 73
Managed care, 113-115, 332, 336
Management process, 189-208
  Task Cycle® Phases 1 through 6, 190-208
Management roles and responsibilities in hazard communication program, 494-495
Management styles, 197-198
Management support, considered in health and safety programs, 251
Management theories, historical perspective on, 187-189
Manager/administrator role, 28, 540-541
Manganese exposure, 137, 159
Manual materials handling, 145
Marketing strategy, described in business plan, 252

Marketplace
  domestic and international,
    105-106
  global, 107
Mass hysteria, 272
Mass shootings, 390
Material safety data sheets
    (MSDSs), 141-142,
    262-263, 497
Materials and services manage-
    ment, 283-285
Maximum medical improvement,
    332-333
Measures of association, in
    epidemiology, 124
Mechanical hazards, 18-19
  mechanical stress, 144, 146
Mechanical integrity programs,
    278-279
Media tools for presentations,
    444t-445t
Medical controls, 283
Medical examination
  and ADA, 78-79
  independent, 332
Medical kit for travelers, 510b
Medical records, 86, 88-90
Medical review officer, 504
Medical surveillance, 313, 322
Megatrends, 108-109
Mentoring, 198
  as teaching method, 437, 439t
Mercury, 137, 159, 178
Metals, exposure to, 134-137
Methylene chloride, 139
Microeconomics, 102
Middle Ages, 4-5
Migrant workers, 53
Minority workers
  implications for occupational
    and environmental health
    nurses, 42
  supportive and explanatory
    data, 41-42
Mission of occupational health
    and safety, 3-4
Mistreatment, as psychosocial
    hazard, 457
Mitigation, 375-376, 388
Model of Health Promotion
    Behavior, 416
Moderate complexity testing, 83
Monitoring
  of exposure, 268-271
  of hearing loss protection
    program, 482-483
  of management process,
    205-207
Motivation
  of adults, to learn, 436-437
  as key to mentoring, training,
    and coaching, 200
  as management theory focus,
    188

Multiple chemical sensitivity, 273
Musculoskeletal disorders,
    work-related (WMSDs),
    144-145, 484-485, 492
Mutagens, 130
Mutual Aid Plan, 372

N
National Environmental
    Education Act, 166
National health goals, 15
National Incident Management
    System, 379
National Institute for
    Occupational Health and
    Safety (NIOSH), 168
  Agricultural Initiative, 54
National Institute of
    Environmental Health
    Sciences (NIEHS), 168
Near-miss incident, 260
Needlestick injury, 60
Negligence
  contributory, 13
  nursing, 72
Negotiation, 201-202
Net national product, 102
Networking, 200
Neurotoxins, 153-154
News media, disaster coverage
    by, 382
Nicotine dependence,
    Fagerstrom test for, 425
Nightingale, Florence, 119
Nitrous dioxide, 175
Noise exposure assessment, 269,
    476-477
Noise-induced hearing loss,
    473-474
  in farm workers, 54
Nominal group technique, 437
Nonexperimental designs,
    523-524
Nonionizing radiation monitor-
    ing, 270
North American Free Trade Act
    (NAFTA), 107
Nuclear Regulatory Commission
    (NRC), 167
Nuclear weapons, 393
Nurse practitioner, 28
Nursing
  advanced practice, 295
  disaster, 366
  industrial, 24
  negligence, 72
  occupational and environmen-
    tal health. See
    Occupational and environ-
    mental health nursing
  professional credentialing in,
    534-537
  representation in OSHA policy
    making, 77

Nursing informatics
  applications of, 216
  definition of, 215-216
Nursing science
  in context of public health,
    119-121
  evolution of occupational and
    environmental health
    nursing practice, 121-123
Nutrition, 134

O
Obesity, 134
Observational assessment of
    work site, 141
Occupational and environmental
    health nurse
  case managers, 334
  focus of, 3
  future opportunities and chal-
    lenges, 31-32
  general environmental health
    competency for, 179-180
  and HIPAA, 92-93
  image of, 209
  implications of
    age of workers, 43-44
    agricultural workers, 55-56
    alternative workers, 50
    business trends, 112-113
    children in workforce, 46-48
    construction workers, 58
    demographic changes, 37-38
    disabled workers, 52-53
    economics, 108
    females in workforce, 40-41
    health care workers, 61, 63
    international (expatriate)
      workers, 64
    minorities in workforce,
      41-42
    technologic trends, 38
    workers in labor unions, 51
  legal responsibilities of, 73
  and managed care, 116
  practice settings for, 30-31
  roles and responsibilities of,
    27-29
    in case management, 338
    in EAPs, 432-433
    regarding international
      travel programs, 507-508
  specialized education, 29
  tools available to, 216-217
Occupational and environmental
    health nursing
  competency in, 25, 337, 537-538
  history and evolution of,
    24-25, 26-27b
  implications of information
    management, 230-232
  model for, 5
  practice of. See Practice
  principles important to, 96

Occupational and environmental
    health nursing—cont'd
relevance of epidemiology, 124
research priorities in, 527b
Occupational health
    direct care in, knowledge
        needs for, 298-300
    historical perspective on, 4-7
    information management in,
        215-232
    surveillance, 487-488
Occupational health and safety
    evolution of, 7, 9, 12-13
    mission and goals of, 3-4
    tools, 549
Occupational health and safety
        programs
    assessment, 237-239
    costs, 249-250
    drug and alcohol programs,
        499-506
    ergonomics programs, 483-493
    evaluation of, 242-249
    hazard communication
        programs, 494-499
    hearing loss prevention
        programs, 473-483
    implementation, 241-242
    in international community,
        15-17
    international travel programs,
        506-513
    issues related to, 251-252
    planning, 239-241
Occupational physicians, 4
Occupational Safety and Health
        Act of 1970, 14
    Public Law 91-596, 73-77
Occupational Safety and Health
        Administration (OSHA),
        14, 167
    policy making, nursing
        representation in, 77
    regulations requiring emer-
        gency plans, 370t
    requirements for record
        keeping, 85-86
    standards requiring medical
        surveillance, 75b
    states and territories with, 74b
Occupational Safety and Health
        Review Commission
        (OSHRC), 77
Occupational setting
    health promotion programs in,
        429-431
    managing psychosocial factors
        in, 451-468
Occupational stress
    definitions and facts about, 460
    ecologic approach to, 464-465
    job conditions leading to,
        460-461
    models of, 462-463

Odds ratio, 125
Office management programs,
    229-230
Office work, ergonomic hazards
    of, 145
Omnibus Transportation
    Employee Testing Act of
    1991, 81-82, 499-500, 504
Online recruiting, 195-196
Onsite case management,
    360-361
Operating budgets, 192
Organization of work, 451-452
Organizations
    culture and climate of,
        185, 452
    effects of stress on, 462
    for research funding for
        health-related projects,
        530t-531t
Organized labor, 7, 9-12
Organochlorines, 140
Organophosphates, 140
Outcome elements in program
    evaluation, 247-248
Outcomes evaluation
    in case management process,
        344-345
    direct care and, 323, 328
Outcomes management, 206
Outreach for children in work-
    force, 47
OVINDICATES mnemonic, 309
Ozone, 175-176

P
Particulate matter, 175
Partnerships in occupational and
    environmental health,
    542-543
Passive surveillance, 488
Perchlorate exposure, 160
Performance goals, 190
Performance management
    process, 203-205
Performance reinforcement,
    207-208
Permanent disabilities, total and
    partial, 95
Permanent threshold shift, 482
Permissible exposure limits, 143
Persistent bioaccumulative toxics
    (PBTs), 176
Personal protective equipment,
    143
    characteristics of, 285
    for hazards associated with
        WMSDs, 490-491
    for noise control, 477
    regulations related to,
        285-286
    types of, 286-290
Person-environment fit model,
    462-463

Pesticides
    exposure to, 140
    in food production, 178
    home use, 173
    as PBTs, 176
Pharmacology, compared with
    toxicology, 157t
Pharmacotherapy, for
        hazardous material
        exposure, 396t
Philosophies of adult education,
    434-436
Physical activity, 426, 429
Physical examination
    methods for conducting,
        305-306
    preplacement, 310-311
    purposes of, 302-303
    techniques for, 304-305
Physical hazards, 17
    in health care settings, 62b
Physicians
    occupational, 4
    role in case management
        process, 338-339
Planning
    in case management process,
        342-343
    disaster, 369-377
    discussed in Task Cycle® Phase
        2, 191-194
    emergency response, 246-247
    health and safety program,
        239-241
    in health promotion program,
        420-423
    strategic, 186-187
Plausibility of the association,
    124
Point-of-service plan (POS), 114
Policies and procedures
    for health and safety program,
        242
    in management process,
        205-206
    regarding computerized infor-
        mation security, 227-229
Political economy, 102
Pollution Prevention Act, 166
Polycholorinated biphenyls
    (PCBs), 159
Population-based health outcome
    data, 124-125
Post-travel evaluation for long-
    term travelers, 512-513
Potentiation, 132
Power
    in inferential statistics, 126
    managerial, sources of, 208b
Power outages, 388
Practice
    advancement of, 539-540
    basic legal concepts relevant
        to, 72-73

Practice—cont'd
clinical, guidelines for, 309-310
professional and regulatory
parameters of, 295-296
research role in, 29-30
roles and responsibilities in,
27-29
scientific foundations of
epidemiology, 123-129
ergonomics, 143-146
industrial hygiene, 141-143
injury epidemiology,
147-149
nursing science, 119-123
social and behavioral sciences, 149-150
toxicology, 130-141
settings for, 30-31
case management services,
337
standards of, 25
Precautionary Principle, 163b
PRECEDE model, 415
Preferred provider organization
(PPO), 114
Preindustrial age, 5
Presentations
delivery of, 446-448
effective, 437
elements and types of, 441
logistical considerations, 443,
446
preparation of, 441-442
use of audiovisuals, 442-443
Presenteeism, 110
Presenter/speaker role, 542
Prevalence, in epidemiology, 123
Prevention and control measures
for workplace violence,
456b
Prevention of occupational injury
and illness, 23-24
administrative controls focus,
279-285
comprehensive containment
focus, 290, 292
engineering controls focus,
274-279
hazard evaluation and analysis, 264-273
personal protective equipment
focus, 285-290
recognition and identification,
255-264
Preventive maintenance, 278-279
Primary barriers, engineering
elements including, 290
Primary care, 295, 541
Primary prevention
and direct care, 310-311
and health protection programs, 420
Prime rate, 102
Privacy Rule of HIPAA, 91-92

Problem identification, 522
Problem solving, discussed in
Task Cycle® Phase 2,
191-194
Problem statement/formulation,
523
Process elements, in program
evaluation, 245-247
Process safety review, 263-264
Producer Price Index (PPI), 102
Professional associations,
533-534, 545
Professional development,
541b
Project management, 191-192
Protected health information,
91-93
Protection Motivation Theory,
420
Psychosocial factors
characteristics of workers, 453
interpersonal relationships and
work, 452-453
interventions promoting psychosocial health, 468
in occupational setting, managing, 465-468
occupational stress, 460-461
ecologic approach to,
464-465
models of, 462-463
organization of work, 451-452
stress effects on workers and
on organizations, 461-462
Psychosocial hazards
internationally recognized
problem of, 19
mistreatment and harassment,
457
shift work, 458-459
stresses, 459-460
unemployment and underem-
ployment, 457-458
workplace violence, 453-457
Public health
infrastructure, 168-169
nursing science in context of,
119-121
Public pressure, 12-13
Publications, 545-546
p-value, 126

Q
Qualitative assessment of work
site, 141
Quality assurance
in drug and alcohol testing
program, 504-505
evaluative elements in, 243t
Quality control in managed care,
114-115
Quality outcomes, defining and
evaluating, 115
Quality reviews, 249

Questionnaires
CAGE, 425b
on employee perception, 263
evaluating ergonomic risk
factors, 145

R
Radiation
exposure to, 393-394
monitoring for, 270
Random drug testing, 504-505
Randomized clinical trials, 126
Rate ratio, 125
REACH policy, 170-172
Reasonable accommodation, 78
Recommended exposure levels,
143
Record keeping
best practices in, 87-88
for emergency preparedness
plan, 402
for ergonomics program,
492-493
for hazard communication
program, 498
OSHA requirements for,
85-86
regular evaluation of, 247
and worker medical records,
86
Records review, 258-259
Recovery Plans, 372
Recruitment strategies, 195b
Reference checks, 196-197
Rehabilitation, 333
Rehabilitation specialists, 339
Reinforcement of performance,
discussed in Task Cycle®
Phase 6, 207-208
Relationship, as requirement of
leadership, 185-186
Relative risk, 125
Reliability of research instrument, 524
Repetitive motion disorders,
21, 144
Reports
mandatory, in disaster
recovery, 385-386
oral, 441
Research
on children in workforce, 47-48
dissemination of, 526
epidemiologic, 123
ethics in, 520-521
evaluation of, 528-529
funding of, 529-531
involvement in, 538-539
multidisciplinary, 180-181
priorities, 527-528
professional mandates for, 519
purposes of, 520
in social sciences, 149
utilization of, 526-527

Research development
   identification of problem, 522
   literature review, 522
   methodology, 523-526
   problem statement/formula-
      tion, 523
   steps in research process, 521b
Researcher role, 28
   by education level, 519-520
Reserves, 333
Residual functional capacity, 333
Resource Conservation and
   Recovery Act, 165
Resources
   available to meet program and
      service needs, 239-240
   as major disaster response
      need, 382-383
   occupational and environmen-
      tal health and safety,
      545-550
Respirable dusts, exposure to,
   137-138
Respirators, *289*
Respiratory protection, 287-290
Response preparedness step in
   disaster planning, 376-377
Retrospective chart audit, 248
Return to work (RTW), 333, 336,
   345-359
Return-to-duty drug or alcohol
   test, 506
Review grid for occupational
   health system, *221-223*
Right to Know, concerning
   environmental risks,
   169-172
Rights under FMLA, 79
Risk analysis
   in disaster management plan,
      375
   in hazard identification, 267-268
Risk assessment, environmental
   health, 161
Risk communication, environmental health, 164-165
Risk factor analysis, for injury
   occurrence, 147t
Risk factors
   ergonomic, evaluating, 145-146
   for WMSDs, 485
Risk management, 29
   definition of, 333
   environmental health, 161-162
   plan, 372
Risk score formula, 268b
Risks
   chemical, biological, and radio-
      logic, 154-155
   environmental health, 172-179
   perceptions of, factors
      affecting, 164t
   reduction of, and health
      promotion, 150

Roles and responsibilities
   expansion of, 540-542
   of management, in hazard
      communication program,
      494-495
   of occupational and environ-
      mental health nurse, 27-29
   in case management, 338
   in EAPs, 432-433
   related to
      hearing loss prevention
         programs, 475-476
      international travel
         programs, 507-508

S
Safe Drinking Water Act, 165
Safe driving tips, 429b
Safety committees, 280
Safety engineers, 4
Safety officers, 29
Safety promotion, 282-283
Safety training, 280-281, 290
Sample size, 524-525
Sampling
   conducted for all exposure
      types, 268-269
   methods, in industrial hygiene,
      142
   surface, 271
Scheduling
   proper, 281
   for shift work, 458b
School environments, environ-
   mental risks in, 174-175
Screening
   in epidemiology, 129
   as secondary prevention
      measure, 311-313
Search engines, 225-226
Secondary barriers, engineering
   elements including, 290
Secondary prevention
   and direct care, 311-313,
      322-323
   and health protection pro-
      grams, 420
Security of computerized health
   information, 227-229, 231
Self-care actions, *411-412*
Self-directed learning, 433-434
Sensitivity of screening test, 129
Sensitizers, 130
Sentinel health event, 273
Serious health condition, 80b-81b
Sexual harassment, 457
Shift work, 458-459
Shoulder injury, 144
Silica exposure, 138
Simulation, as teaching method,
   437, 440t
Site survey, 256-257
Site-management systems, 217
Skin disorders, 21-22

Skin protection, 286
SLIDE rule for corrections to
   documentation, 84
Slips and falls, 148t
SOAP formula for documenta-
   tion, 84t
Social activism, 12-13
Social Learning Theory, 417-419
Social sciences, 149-150
Socialism, 102
Software, malicious, 228
Solvents, exposure to, 138-140,
   160
Specialty trade contractors, 56
Specificity of screening test, 129
Spill Prevention, Control and
   Countermeasures Plan, 372
Stages of change model, 418t
Standard threshold shift, 481-482
Standards of care, judging, 115
Standards of performance, 204
State law, 71-72
Statistical significance, tests of,
   126
Statute of limitation, 73
Statutes, 71
   regarding indemnity benefits,
      94-95
Storage of hazardous materials,
   276
Strategic planning, 186-187
Strength of the association, 124
Stress
   critical incident, 403
   effects on
      organizations, 462
      workers, 461-462
   epidemic, 272
   as exogenous factor, 134
   health promotion and, 424-426
   as leading problem, 36-37
   mechanical, 144, 146
   in modern workplace, 459-460
   occupational, 460-461
   psychologic, in health care
      workers, 62b
   travel-related, 509
   workplace designs reducing,
      275b
Stroke, RTW for, 358
Structural elements, in program
   evaluation, 242-245
Structured interviews, 196
Styles of management, 197-198
Substance abuse
   clinical evaluation for, 323
   definition of, 502
   toluene, 139
Superfund sites, 176
Surface sampling, 271
Surveillance
   occupational health, 487-488
   as secondary prevention
      measure, 313, 322

Surveys on employee perception, 263
Synergistic effects, 132
Systems model, 463
Systems theory, 189

T
Target population, 524
Task Cycle®
  Phase 1: Making goals clear and important, 190-191
  Phase 2: Planning and problem solving, 191-194
  Phase 3: Facilitating the work of others, 194-200
  Phase 4: Obtaining and providing feedback, 200-205
  Phase 5: Monitoring and adjusting the process, 205-207
  Phase 6: Reinforcing performance, 207-208
Tax cuts, 103
Teaching
  effective, 434
  methods and techniques of, 437, 438t-440t
Team building, 199-200
Technical information sources, 547
Technologic trends, 38
  businesses and, 109
Telephonic case management, 361-362
Temperature monitoring, 270-271
Temporality of the association, 124
Temporary disabilities, total and partial, 95
Temporary threshold shift, 482
Temporary workers, 49-50
Tendinitis, 324b-327b
Teratogens, 130
Terrorism
  biologic agents, 391-393
  chemical weapons, 394-396
  definition of, 390
  incendiary device, 394
  nuclear and radiologic, 393-394
  weapons of mass destruction, 391
Tertiary prevention
  and direct care, 323
  and health protection programs, 420
Testing
  audiometric, 480-482
  drug and alcohol, programs for, 502-505
  high complexity, 83
  waived, 82
Theory of Goal Setting, 419

Theory of Planned Behavior, 419
Theory of Reasoned Action, 419
Theory of Social Behavior, 420
Third-party administrator, 333
  role in case management process, 339
300 Log (OSHA), 85-86
Threshold limit value guidelines, 143
Thriving economy, 104-105
Timeline
  of disaster recovery, 385
  model, for disasters, 367
Time-weighted average ranges, 474t
Titles of HIPAA law, 90-91
Tobacco smoke, environmental, 159, 173
Toluene, 139
Tornadoes, 402
Torso protection, 287
Tort, 72
Total absence management, 335
Total Health Management, 114
Total Quality Management, 189
Toxic Substances Control Act, 165
Toxic waste dumps, 158
Toxicology
  dose-response relationship, 132
  endogenous and exogenous host factors, 133-134
  environmental, 157-158
  exposures and their effects
    asphyxiants, 140-141
    metals, 134-137
    pesticides, 140
    respirable dusts, 137-138
    solvents, 138-140
  fate of toxins in body, 133
  major exposure routes, 131-132
  nature of effects, 132
  terms and principles, 130-131
Toxins
  effects of, 132
  fate in body, 133
  potential toxic effects by system, 135t
Trade globalization, 17
Trade secrets, 498
Trade status of United States, 106-107
Training
  in drug and alcohol programs, 505-506
  in ergonomics program, 491
  as immediate cause of incidents, 262b
  for older workers, 43b
  safety, 280-281, 290
  as staff development activity, 198
  of workers, in hearing loss prevention, 477-479

Transactional Theory, 419
Transformation of toxins, 133
Transitional work, 333, 347b-348b, 356-357
Transtheoretical Theory, 417
Travel, international, 506-513
Trichloroethylene, 139-140

U
Underemployment, 457-458
Underreporting of work-related incidents, 20
Unemployment
  among disabled workers, 51-52
  low, 104-105
  as psychosocial hazard, 457-458
United States
  changes in national economy, 105
  economic state of, 103
  international trade status of, 106-107
  national and global competitiveness of, 105-106
Universalism, 187
Utilization review
  and case management firms, 30-31
  definition of, 333

V
Validity of research instrument, 524
Variables in research development, 524
Vendor-contracted programs, 241-242
Ventilation, 276
Verbal theories, 416
Vibration-induced injury, 145-146
Videotaping, in risk evaluation, 146
Violence in workplace, 37, 273, 389-390, 453-457
Virtual offices, 36
Viruses, computer, 228
Vision, as requirement of leadership, 184-185
Voluntary Protection Program of OSHA, 76-77
Vulnerability assessment, 374-375

W
Wage loss, 333
Waived testing, 82
Walk-through, 256-257
Warning labels, 498
Warning signs, 281-282
Web sites, 562-564
Wipe sampling, 271
Work
  injury and illness related to, 19-22
  interpersonal relationships and, 452-453

Work—cont'd
 meaning of, 453
 modified/transitional, 323
 and occupational health,
   historical perspective, 4-7
 organization of, 451-452
 of others, facilitating, 194-200
 performance, measuring, 462
 permits, 281
 skilled, demand for, 38
 transitional, 333, 347b-348b,
   356-357
Work environment, 4
 of health care industry, 59-61
 international travel, 509-510
 and stress, 460-461
Work practices, controlling,
   279-280
Work restriction management,
   219-220
Work site analysis, 487
Worker populations
 age of, 42-44
 analysis of, 271-273
 demographic and social
   trends, 35-38
 female, 40-41
 minority, 41-42
 technologic trends and, 38
Workers
 age of, 42-44
 agricultural, 53-56
 assessment related to, 237
 changes affecting, 31

Workers—cont'd
 characteristics of, 453
 children, 44-48
 construction, 56-58
 contingent and other
   alternative, 48-50
 disabled, 51-53
 female, 40-41
 in health care, 58-63
 international (expatriate), 63-64
 in labor unions, 50-51
 medical and exposure records,
   86
 minority, 41-42
 motivation of, 189
 occupational injuries, 20-21
 in postindustrial era, 6-7
 role in case management
   process, 338
 safety-sensitive, 81-82
 stress effects on, 461-462
 training
   in hazard communication
     program, 496-497
   in hearing loss prevention,
     477-479
 traveling, responsibilities of, 508
Workers' compensation
 benefits, 94-95, 111
 compensable injuries and illnesses under, 94
 design of system of, 93
 history of, 13-14
 managed, 114

Workforce
 children in, 44-48
 females in, 40-41
 health care industry, 58-63
 immigration impacts on,
   31-32
 international, 506-507
 minorities in, 41-42
Workplace
 assessment, 238-239
 changes affecting, 31
 disaster planning and preparedness, 370-371
 drug-free, 500-502
 engineering designs, 274-275
 ethical dilemmas in, 97-99
 hazards, 122
 health promotion program,
   410, *421*
 impacts of occupational hazards on, 17-19
 international, 63-64
 sampling, 142
 social activism and, 12-13
 stress in, 459-460
 violence in, 37, 273, 389-390,
   453-457
Work-related musculoskeletal
   disorders (WMSDs),
   144-145, 484-485, 492
Wrist/hand injury, 145
Writing, business, 202-203
Written emergency plan,
   405-406